CLINICAL VETERINARY ONCOLOGY

CLINICAL VETERINARY ONCOLOGY

Edited by

Stephen J. Withrow, DVM

Diplomate, American College of Veterinary Surgery
Diplomate, American College of Veterinary Internal Medicine
  (Oncology)
Professor of Surgery/Oncology
Chief, Clinical Oncology
Comparative Oncology Unit
Veterinary Clinical Sciences
College of Veterinary Medicine and Biomedical Sciences
Colorado State University
Fort Collins, Colorado

E. Gregory MacEwen, VMD

Diplomate, American College of Veterinary
  Internal Medicine (Oncology/Medicine)
Professor of Medicine/Oncology
Department of Medical Sciences
Associate Dean for Clinical Affairs
School of Veterinary Medicine
Affiliate Professor, Department of Veterinary Science
College of Agriculture and Life Sciences
Associate Member, Wisconsin Clinical Cancer Center
Department of Human Oncology
School of Medicine
University of Wisconsin–Madison
Madison, Wisconsin

With 24 contributors

J.B. Lippincott Company
Philadelphia
Grand Rapids, New York, St. Louis, San Francisco
London, Sydney, Tokyo

Acquisitions Editor: Susan Gay
Sponsoring Editor: Kathy Crown
Manuscript Editor: Terry Shutz
Project Editor: Linda J. Stewart
Indexer: Helene Taylor Associates
Design/Production Coordinator: Caren Erlichman
Production Manager: Carol A. Florence
Compositor: Monotype Composition Company
Printer/Binder: Halliday Lithograph

6 5 4 3 2 1

Library of Congress Cataloging in Publication Data

Clinical veterinary oncology.

  Includes bibliographies and index.
  1. Veterinary oncology.   I. Withrow, Stephen J.
II. MacEwen, E. Gregory.
SF910.T8C58   1989   636.089'6994   88-27210
ISBN 0-397-59784-4

The editors, authors and publisher have exerted
every effort to ensure that drug selection and
dosage set forth in this text are in accord with
current recommendations and practice at the time
of publication. However, in view of ongoing
research, changes in government regulations, and
the constant flow of information relating to drug
therapy and drug reactions, the reader is urged to
check the package insert for each drug for any
change in indications and dosage and for added
warnings and precautions. This is particularly
important when the recommended agent is a new
or infrequently employed drug.

Dr. Robert S. Brodey
1927–1979

A leader in veterinary oncology. We will always remember him for his tireless effort to advance the field of oncology, teach principles of surgery and, most important, to preserve nature.

We dedicate this book to this fine man.

CONTRIBUTORS

Mark W. Dewhirst, DVM, PhD
Associate Professor, Division of Radiation
  Oncology
Duke University Medical Center
Durham, North Carolina

Richard R. Dubielzig, DVM
Diplomate, ACVP
Associate Professor of Pathology
Department of Pathobiological Sciences
School of Veterinary Medicine
University of Wisconsin–Madison
Madison, Wisconsin

William D. Hardy, Jr., VMD
Memorial Sloan Kettering Cancer Center
New York, New York

Suzanne Hetts, MS, PhD
Director, CHANGES: Support for People and
  Pets
Colorado State University Veterinary Teaching
  Hospital
College of Veterinary Medicine and
  Biomedical Sciences
Colorado State University
Fort Collins, Colorado

Mary Kay Klein, DVM, MS
Resident, Comparative Oncology Unit
Department of Veterinary Clinical Sciences
College of Veterinary Medicine and
  Biomedical Sciences
Colorado State University
Fort Collins, Colorado

Ilene D. Kurzman, MS, EdD
Assistant Scientist
Department of Medical Sciences
School of Veterinary Medicine

University of Wisconsin–Madison
Madison, Wisconsin

Laurel S. Lagoni, MS
Assistant Director, CHANGES: Support for
  People and Pets
Colorado State University Veterinary Teaching
  Hospital
College of Veterinary Medicine and
  Biomedical Sciences
Colorado State University
Fort Collins, Colorado

Susan Margaret LaRue, DVM, MS
Diplomate, ACVS
National Cancer Institute Fellow in Radiation
  Biology
Department of Radiation and Radiation
  Biology
College of Veterinary Medicine and
  Biomedical Sciences
Colorado State University
Fort Collins, Colorado

Richard A. LeCouteur, BVSc, PhD
Diplomate, ACVIM (Neurology)
Associate Professor, Department of Clinical
  Sciences
College of Veterinary Medicine and
  Biomedical Sciences
Colorado State University
Fort Collins, Colorado

E. Gregory MacEwen, VMD
Diplomate, ACVIM (Oncology/Medicine)
Professor of Medicine/Oncology
Department of Medical Sciences
Associate Dean for Clinical Affairs
School of Veterinary Medicine
Affiliate Professor

Department of Veterinary Sciences
College of Agriculture and Life Sciences
Associate Member, Wisconsin Clinical Cancer
    Center, Department of Human Oncology
School of Medicine
University of Wisconsin–Madison
Madison, Wisconsin

Peter S. MacWilliams, DVM, PhD
Diplomate, ACVP
Clinical Associate Professor, Department of
    Pathobiological Sciences
Clinical Pathologist, Veterinary Medical
    Teaching Hospital
School of Veterinary Medicine
University of Wisconsin–Madison
Madison, Wisconsin

Dennis W. Macy, DVM, MS
Diplomate, ACVIM (Medicine/Oncology)
Associate Professor of Medicine/Oncology
Department of Veterinary Clinical Sciences
College of Veterinary Medicine and
    Biomedical Sciences
Colorado State University
Fort Collins, Colorado

Gregory K. Ogilvie, DVM
Diplomate, ACVIM (Medicine)
Assistant Professor of Medicine/Oncology
Comparative Oncology Unit
Department of Veterinary Clinical Sciences
College of Veterinary Medicine and
    Biomedical Sciences
Colorado State University
Fort Collins, Colorado

Rodney L. Page, DVM, MS
Diplomate, ACVIM (Medicine)
Assistant Professor of Medicine/Oncology
Department of Companion Animal and Special
    Species
School of Veterinary Medicine
North Carolina State University
Raleigh, North Carolina

Nancy C. Postorino, DVM
Resident, Comparative Oncology Unit
Department of Veterinary Clinical Sciences
College of Veterinary Medicine and
    Biomedical Sciences

Colorado State University
Fort Collins, Colorado

Robert C. Rosenthal, DVM, MS, PhD
Diplomate, ACVIM (Medicine/Oncology)
Assistant Professor, Medicine/Oncology
Department of Medical Sciences
School of Veterinary Medicine
Affiliate Member, Department of Veterinary
    Sciences
College of Agriculture and Life Sciences
Associate Member, Wisconsin Clinical Cancer
    Center
University of Wisconsin–Madison
Madison, Wisconsin

Rodney C. Straw, BVSc
Diplomate, ACVS
Assistant Professor, Surgery/Oncology
Comparative Oncology Unit
Department of Veterinary Clinical Sciences
College of Veterinary Medicine and
    Biomedical Sciences
Colorado State University
Fort Collins, Colorado

Steven J. Susaneck, DVM, MS
Diplomate, ACVIM (Medicine)
Staff Oncologist
Animal Emergency Clinic
Houston, Texas

James F. Swanson, DVM, MS
Diplomate, ACVO
Staff Ophthalmologist
Campbell Road Animal Clinic
Houston, Texas

Richard E. Thoma, DVM
Director, Town and Country Animal Clinic
Cheektowaga, New York

Donald E. Thrall, DVM, PhD
Diplomate, ACVR
Professor of Radiology
Department of Anatomy, Physiological
    Sciences and Radiology
School of Veterinary Medicine
North Carolina State University
Raleigh, North Carolina

Steven L. Wheeler, DVM, MS
Diplomate, ACVIM (Medicine)
Assistant Professor, Department of Veterinary
   Clinical Sciences
College of Veterinary Medicine and
   Biomedical Sciences
Colorado State University
Fort Collins, Colorado

Stephen J. Withrow, DVM
Diplomate, ACVS
Diplomate, ACVIM (Oncology)
Professor of Surgery/Oncology
Chief, Clinical Oncology

Comparative Oncology Unit
Department of Veterinary Clinical Sciences
College of Veterinary Medicine and
   Biomedical Sciences
Colorado State University
Fort Collins, Colorado

Karen M. Young, VMD, PhD
Assistant Professor of Clinical Pathology
Department of Pathobiologic Sciences
School of Veterinary Medicine
University of Wisconsin–Madison
Madison, Wisconsin

PREFACE

The field of clinical veterinary oncology has grown remarkably in the last 10 years, as evidenced by increased coverage in journals, a proliferation of textbooks, and expansion of training programs in the field, as well as by the establishment and growth of the Veterinary Cancer Society and sanction of the discipline by board certification under the American College of Veterinary Internal Medicine in 1988.

Historically, clinical veterinary oncology was characterized by strong opinions based on weak data. Unusual case reports and small anecdotal case series predominated the literature, as did pathologic descriptions with an emphasis on morphology and metastatic distribution. In recent years, more attention to controlled and randomized therapeutic trials that are stratified for histologic grade, clinical stage, and other prognostic variables has enhanced the understanding of this complex disease. It is clear that cancer is no more "one disease" than is kidney disease or heart failure. A given histological type of cancer is likely to have different natural behavior and response to treatment depending on anatomic location and species differences. Because tumors may be biologically or therapeutically heterogeneous, careful analysis of all variables is required in management of the patient with cancer and interpretation of end results.

In *Clinical Veterinary Oncology* we have tried to assemble a text that is clinically relevant for the general veterinary practitioner and veterinary medical student and a helpful reference for the veterinary oncologist. In an attempt to be concise and clinically relevant, it is possible that some areas in the vast volume of literature have not been cited. The essentials of etiology, epidemiology, and biologic behavior have been provided for each tumor type, but the emphasis is on treatment. We have tried to keep the text as practical as possible. A crucial advance in clinical oncology has been the increased awareness that the best treatment for a cancer patient is a multidisciplinary approach utilizing a combination of surgery, radiation therapy, chemotherapy, and other modalities. We have tried to emphasize this approach whenever possible.

The text is divided into three major areas. The first section covers the biology and diagnoses of cancer (Chapters 1–7), the second section deals with principles of cancer therapy (Chapters 8–15), and the final section concentrates on management of specific cancers (Chapters 16–32). Our contributors were chosen because of their expertise in a specific area, and all chapters were reviewed by a surgical oncologist (SJW) and a medical oncologist (EGM) to give the book balance and a diverse perspective. We thank the contributing authors for their expert thoughts and ideas, and the staff of J.B. Lippincott, especially Linda J. Stewart our Project Editor, for their patience and dedication to this project. In particular, we acknowledge the expert typing and advice of Mrs. Helen Mawhiney at Colorado State University. Finally, and most importantly, we thank our families for their unselfish support during the long hours dedicated to making this book a reality.

Rapid changes in our fundamental biologic understanding of cancer and the advent of more aggressive therapeutic approaches to its management are a healthy sign for the discipline of clinical veterinary oncology. In the course of this progress it is conceivable that some historically accepted data in this text will be outdated soon. That new information will force a revision of this book.

It is our desire to provide the reader with the most current information and a better understanding of cancer biology, diagnostic approaches, therapeutic interventions, and prognostic variables. Cancer is not *always* curable, but in most cases the patient can be helped to an improved quality and quantity of life.

Stephen J. Withrow, DVM
E. Gregory MacEwen, VMD

CONTENTS

CHAPTER 1
Why Worry About Cancer in Pet
Animals?
Stephen J. Withrow 1

CHAPTER 2
Cancer Overview: Epidemiology,
Etiology, and Prevention
E. Gregory MacEwen 3

CHAPTER 3
Cancer Pathology
Richard R. Dubielzig 16

CHAPTER 4
Mechanisms of Invasion and Metastasis
Robert C. Rosenthal. 23

CHAPTER 5
Paraneoplastic Syndromes
Gregory K. Ogilvie. 29

CHAPTER 6
Cytologic Techniques in Cancer
Diagnosis
Peter S. MacWilliams 41

CHAPTER 7
Biopsy Principles
Stephen J. Withrow 53

CHAPTER 8
Surgical Oncology
Stephen J. Withrow 58

CHAPTER 9
Chemotherapy
Robert C. Rosenthal. 63

CHAPTER 10
Radiation Therapy
Donald E. Thrall and Mark W.
Dewhirst 79

CHAPTER 11
Immunology and Biologic Therapy of
Cancer
E. Gregory MacEwen 92

CHAPTER 12
Cryosurgery
Stephen J. Withrow 106

CHAPTER 13
Hyperthermia
Mark W. Dewhirst, R. L. Page, and
Donald E. Thrall 113

CHAPTER 14
Photodynamic Therapy
Richard E. Thoma 124

CHAPTER 15
New Developments in Cancer Therapy
Ilene D. Kurzman and E. Gregory
MacEwen. 128

CHAPTER 16
Tumors of the Skin and Subcutaneous
Tissues
Steven J. Susaneck and Stephen J.
Withrow. 139

CHAPTER 17
Mast Cell Tumors
Dennis W. Macy and E. Gregory
MacEwen. 156

CHAPTER 18
Soft Tissue Sarcomas
E. Gregory MacEwen and Stephen J.
Withrow. 167

CHAPTER 19
Tumors of the Gastrointestinal System
The Oral Cavity
Stephen J. Withrow 177

xiii

Salivary Glands
Stephen J. Withrow 190
Esophageal Cancer
Stephen J. Withrow 190
Exocrine Pancreas
Stephen J. Withrow 192
Gastric Cancer
Stephen J. Withrow 193
Hepatic Tumors
Nancy C. Postorino 196
Tumors of the Intestinal Tract
Rodney C. Straw. 200
Perianal Tumors
Stephen J. Withrow 209

CHAPTER 20
Tumors of the Respiratory System
Stephen J. Withrow 215

CHAPTER 21
Tumors of the Skeletal System
Susan Margaret LaRue and Stephen J.
Withrow 234

CHAPTER 22
Tumors of the Endocrine System
Stephen L. Wheeler. 253

CHAPTER 23
**Tumors of the Female Reproductive
System**
Mary Kay Klein. .283

CHAPTER 24
Tumors of the Mammary Gland
E. Gregory MacEwen and Stephen J.
Withrow 292

CHAPTER 25
Tumors of the Male Reproductive Tract
Nancy C. Postorino and Stephen J.
Withrow 305

CHAPTER 26
Tumors of the Urinary System
Stephen J. Withrow 312

CHAPTER 27
Tumors of the Nervous System
Richard A. LeCouteur 325

CHAPTER 28
Ocular Tumors
James F. Swanson and Richard R.
Dubielzig 351

CHAPTER 29
Hematopoietic Tumors
29a. Feline Retroviruses
William D. Hardy and E. Gregory
MacEwen. 362
**29b. Canine Lymphoma and Lymphoid
Leukemias**
E. Gregory MacEwen and Karen M.
Young 380
**29c. Canine Myeloproliferative
Disorders**
Karen M. Young and E. Gregory
MacEwen. 394
29d. Plasma Cell Neoplasms
E. Gregory MacEwen 402

CHAPTER 30
Miscellaneous Tumors
30a. Hemangiosarcoma
E. Gregory MacEwen 412
30b. Thymoma
Stephen J. Withrow 418
**30c. Canine Transmissible Venereal
Tumors**
E. Gregory MacEwen 421
30d. Mesothelioma
Richard R. Dubielzig and E. Gregory
MacEwen. 425

CHAPTER 31
**Designing Clinical Cancer Trials: Basic
Considerations**
E. Gregory MacEwen 429

CHAPTER 32
**The Veterinarian's Role in Pet Loss:
Grief Education, Support, and
Facilitation**
Laurel S. Lagoni, Suzanne Hetts,
and Stephen J. Withrow 436

APPENDIX A
**Guidelines for Handling Cytotoxic
Agents**
E. Gregory MacEwen 446

APPENDIX B
  WHO Staging Forms 448

INDEX 490

CLINICAL VETERINARY
ONCOLOGY

1

WHY WORRY ABOUT CANCER IN PET ANIMALS?

Stephen J. Withrow

One reason veterinarians need to be concerned about cancer in pet animals is because its prevalence is increasing.[1] *Prevalence* denotes the number of diagnosed cases per year without reference to *incidence*—the ratio of prevalence to population at risk. The increased prevalence of cancer is at least in part related to the increased life expectancy of pet animals. Since cancer is generally a disease of the older animal, the price pets pay for living longer is an increased likelihood of developing cancer. The greater life-span is a result of better nutrition, increased use of vaccinations (preventing many previously fatal contagious diseases), better preventive and therapeutic medical practices, better leash laws, and possibly a deeper devotion to pet animals within the last 10 to 20 years.

Cancer is a major cause of pet animal death.[2] This is a difficult statement to document, but it is supported by a study that determined the cause of death in a series of over 2000 autopsies. In that study, 45% of dogs that lived to 10 years or older died of cancer.[3] Regardless of age, 23% of dogs presented for autopsy died of cancer.

Breakthroughs in treatment of human cancer have received a great deal of exposure through newspapers, magazines, radio and television. Although progress in cancer treatment is slow, pet owners are aware of what can be done. With the increased and optimistic media coverage, pet owners are becoming more knowledgeable and demanding in seeking care for the animal with cancer. Veterinarians need to be prepared for their demands.

More open acknowledgment of the human-animal bond has elevated the importance of pet animals in many owners' eyes. Some owners consider their pet more important than any human being.[4] Proper care of these animals will be of increasing importance to many owners.

Cancer is a common and serious disease for human beings. Many pet owners have had or will have a personal experience with cancer in themselves, a family member, or a close friend. Keeping this in mind, the veterinarian should approach the owner of the pet with cancer in a positive, compassionate, and knowledgeable manner. Frequently the veterinary profession has taken a negative approach (sometimes characterized as "test and slaughter") to cancer. This attitude is not only a detriment to the pet; it may also arouse the owner's unfounded fears that cancer in humans is not treatable. We owe it to our pet animal patients and their owners to be well informed on current treatment methods for cancer.

Pet animals with spontaneously developing cancer provide an excellent opportunity to study many aspects of the disease from etiology to treatment. Provided that studies are done in a humane fashion, they may unlock clues to improving the outlook for this disease in animals and people.[5,6] Some of the aspects of pet animal cancer that make pets attractive comparative models are:

1. Pet dogs and cats are outbred animals (like humans) as opposed to some strains of rats, mice, and other animals used in laboratory experiments. The animal rights movement, by making investigations of new treatment methods more difficult to perform on normal laboratory animals, is also enhancing the appeal of studies of cancer in pets.

2. The cancers seen in practice develop spontaneously, whereas in experiments, they are induced by carcinogens or transplanted. Spontaneous cancers may behave in a significantly different fashion than induced or transplanted cancers.

3. Pets share the same environment as their owners and may serve as sentinels for changes in the patterns of cancer development seen in humans.

4. Pets have a higher incidence of some cancers (*e.g.*, osteosarcoma, non-Hodgkin's lymphoma, among others) than humans. Including pets in cancer studies will allow more cases of those forms of the disease to be studied.

5. Most animal cancers progress at a more rapid rate than the same cancers in humans. They can therefore be studied more rapidly and the results extrapolated to humans.

6. Because fewer established "gold standard" treatments exist in veterinary medicine, it is easier and morally acceptable to attempt new forms of therapy rather than wait until all known treatments have failed, as is common in the human condition. This lat-

itude in clinical trials must not be abused. We have an obligation to provide known effective treatment while at the same time planning well-designed prospective clinical trials of newer treatment methods.

7. Pet animal cancers are more akin to human cancers than are rodent tumors in terms of size and cell kinetics. Dogs and cats also share with humans certain characteristics of physiology and metabolism for most organ systems and drugs. This allows better comparison of treatment modalities such as surgery, radiation, and chemotherapy between animals and man to be made.

Owners who seek treatment for their pet animals with cancer are a devoted and compassionate subset of the population. Working with them can be a very satisfying aspect of a sometimes frustrating specialty. They are almost always satisfied with an honest and aggressive attempt to cure or palliate the disease of their pet.

Clinical and comparative oncology is a rapidly growing field of study. More training programs are being developed each year. Eventually they will funnel a wider distribution of experienced veterinarians into practice, research, and teaching. Through study and treatment of cancer in pet animals, the veterinarian can hope to improve the outlook for all victims of cancer.

REFERENCES

1. Dorn CR: Epidemiology of canine and feline tumors. Comp Cont Educ 12:307–312, 1976

2. Animal health survey. In Companion Animal News, p. 12. Englewood, CO, Morris Animal Foundation, August 1986

3. Bronson RT: Variation in age at death of dogs of different sexes and breeds. Am J Vet Res 43:2057–2059, 1982

4. Quakenbush J: Pet loss and human emotion. Vet Cancer Soc Forum, Purdue University, 1985

5. Richardson RC: Spontaneous canine and feline neoplasms as models for cancer in man. Kal Kan Forum 2:89–94, 1983

6. Gillette EL: Spontaneous canine neoplasms as models for therapeutic agents. In Fidler IJ, White RJ (eds): Design of Models for Testing Cancer Therapeutic Agents, pp. 185–192 New York, Van Nostrand Reinhold Co, 1982

2

CANCER OVERVIEW: EPIDEMIOLOGY, ETIOLOGY, AND PREVENTION

E. Gregory MacEwen

Cancer is one of the leading causes of death in dogs and cats today. As a result of improved veterinary care, pet animals are living much longer and are thus more susceptible to diseases of old age such as tumors. Compared to man, dogs develop tumors twice as frequently, but cats only half as frequently. In a survey of animal neoplasms in Alameda County, California, in 1968, the estimated annual rates for tumors of all sites were 381.2 per 100,000 dogs at risk and 155.8 per 100,000 cats at risk.[1] The location and incidence of various tumors depend on a number of variables, predominantly age, breed, sex, and geographic location. Figures 2-1 and 2-2 present the epidemiologic features of cancer by major sites in dogs and cats.

ETIOLOGY OF CANCER

Cancer is a collective category of many different diseases affecting different organs and tissues of the body. At the cellular level, cancer is characterized by uncontrolled cell growth. Cancer cells appear to have undergone a process of transformation from the normal phenotype to a malignant phenotype capable of autonomous growth. Several theories attempt to explain malignant transformation of normal cells:

1. Mutation(s) can alter the genetic makeup of the somatic cell.
2. Aberrant differentiation of normal cells results in alterations in cellular differentiation and disruption of cellular regulatory mechanisms.
3. Normal cellular genes (called proto-oncogenes) acquire the ability to induce neoplastic transformation.

It has been suggested that retroviruses, point mutations, deletions, and DNA rearrangements may activate proto-oncogenes to become transforming genes. It is conceivable that cellular oncogenes can be damaged by carcinogens (most of them are mutagens) causing inappropriate expression of these genes that results in uncontrolled growth leading to cancer. Carcinogens can be chemicals, radiation, or viral agents that

3

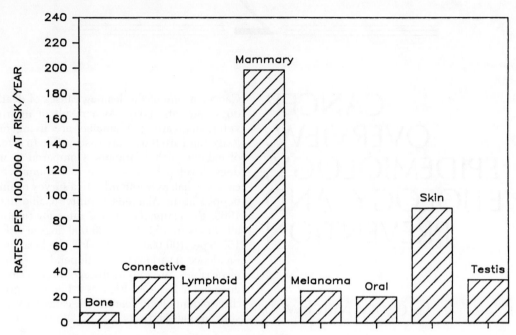

Figure 2-1. Incidence of canine tumors by site of origin.

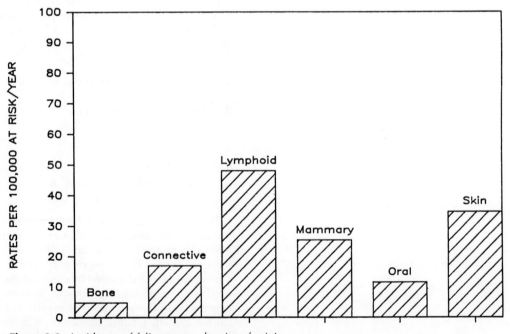

Figure 2-2. Incidence of feline tumors by site of origin.

induce mutations affecting cellular oncogenes either by changing properties of gene products or altering their expression at inappropriate times or to inappropriate cells during normal growth and development of organisms.

As our understanding of the causes of cancer unfolds, it is becoming apparent that a *minority* of cancers are genetically fated to appear, while *most* cancers are caused by environmental factors. For example, in humans, it is expected that one out of four people now alive will contract cancer. Some epidemiologists have suggested that as many as 80% to 90% of human cancers may be related to the environment and life-style[2] and that about 40% of cancers in men and 60% in women in the United States could be attributed to dietary factors.[3]

Most of the information regarding etiology of cancer is derived from epidemiologic studies in humans or experimental studies using rodents. In this chapter much of the information regarding etiology will be based on human and rodent studies. When it is known, information regarding dogs and cats will be presented.

The most generally accepted concept of carcinogenesis is that it is a prolonged process that starts when a cell is exposed to some mutagen *(initiator)* that can interact with DNA, usually affecting only one or two nucleotide base pairs.[4] On the other hand, viruses are carcinogenic because they lead to integration of a protovirus into host chromosomes. Most chemical initiators are unstable and do not last long in the environment. Thus, a more usual carcinogenic sequence is exposure to a stable but toxic chemical (*e.g.*, aflatoxin B1) that has to be detoxified in an organ such as the liver and, in the process, is turned into a highly active derivative that interacts with DNA. In short, most carcinogenic initiators are created within the body as the result of metabolic activation. Most cells possess effective methods for repairing DNA. They are, therefore, able to undo most of the damage caused by initiating carcinogens, if there is sufficient time before they have to duplicate their DNA. It follows that initiators are sometimes made more effective if they interact with the DNA during cell division.

The second stage (promotion) of carcinogenesis is brought about by agents or substances called *promoters*.[5] These will affect cell differentiation, provoke cell proliferation, and induce the initiated cell to express the transformed phenotype. The third stage of carcinogenesis is termed the *progression phase* and is the time when the initiated cell becomes a tumor. This process is influenced by hormones, immune response, nutrition, and vascularization of transformed cells.

GENETIC FACTORS

In the dog certain breeds have a higher incidence of cancer than others. These include the boxer, Airedale terrier, German shepherd, Scottish terrier and golden retriever.[6] The reason for this is unknown but three factors must be considered: (1) In the process of intensive breeding and selection, oncogenes may have inadvertently been selected along with the desired morphologic traits. (2) Once selected the oncogenes may have been transmitted to the offspring, and (3) members of these breeds may have a genetically determined deficient immune surveillance system. Genes governing the amount of pigment present in an animal's skin are important to the development of certain cancers. For example, heavily pigmented breeds such as the cocker spaniel and Scottish terrier have a higher incidence of malignant melanoma.[6] Lightly pigmented cats tend to develop more squamous cell carcinoma (on the pinnae and dorsal facial areas) than darkly pigmented cats.[6] Giant breed dogs, such as the Great Dane, Irish wolfhound, and St. Bernard, among others, have a higher incidence of osteosarcoma, although body weight may contribute as much as genetics to the development of bone neoplasms.[6]

HORMONES

Hormones apparently induce neoplasia both directly and in concert with known carcinogenic agents. Estrogen has been shown to bind covalently to DNA, and diethylstilbestrol can induce mutation and neoplastic transformation in tissue culture.[7] Most studies have shown that hormones probably act to enhance the replication and progression of a few cells already potentially neoplastic as a result of other initiating events.

Intact female dogs develop mammary tumors seven times more frequently than dogs spayed at 2 years or less.[1] Estrogen exposure (or a combination of hormones) early in life (first few years) may initiate tumor development, and the tumor may not manifest itself for many years.[8] Another hormone-related tumor is the perianal gland adenoma, which has a very low incidence in females and castrated males.[9] Prostatic cancer is also thought to be hormonally induced; it occurs much less frequently in castrated dogs.

CONGENITAL FACTORS

Ocular dermoids in dogs are the best example of congenital tumors, which tend to be very rare. These growths are probably related to an abnormality in embryogenesis rather than to hereditary factors.

TRAUMA

Trauma is thought to play a role in the etiology of osteosarcoma in giant breed dogs. It may be that repeated microtrauma to the metaphyses, via weight-bearing stresses, may initiate the development of osteosarcomas. This is supported by the fact that 60% of bone tumors developing in dogs occur in the front leg, which bears more weight than the rear leg. Osteosarcoma of the leg is more common than osteosarcoma of the arm in man. Osteosarcomas have also been associated with delayed healing of fractures and with metallic fixation devices.[10,11] Squamous cell carcinomas have developed at the site of chronic infection and previous burns.[12] Intra-ocular sarcomas in cats seem to be associated with traumatic injuries to the lens.[13]

RADIATION

There are two major types of radiation that are thought to play a role in the etiology of cancer: ultraviolet (UV) radiation and ionizing radiation.[14]

UV Light. The cumulative dosage or exposure to UV radiation is a function of the amount of ozone in the stratosphere, atmospheric conditions (cloudiness, presence of aerosol, and so forth), latitude, and exposure duration. Of these, the thickness of the stratospheric ozone layer is the major determinant.[15] Lack of pigmentation has been associated with squamous cell carcinomas on the pinnae and dorsal facial area of cats, the ocular region in cattle, and the nasal region in collies and Shetland sheepdogs. It has also been associated with squamous cell carcinoma in the flank of Dalmatians. These tumors tend to occur most commonly in areas of the country with a lot of sunlight or high elevation.

Ionizing Radiation. Ionizing radiation is characterized by localized release of energy sufficient to break strong chemical bonds. The subcategories of ionizing radiation are electromagnetic radiation, such as x-ray and gamma rays, and particulate radiation, including electrons, protons, neutrons, alpha particles, and heavy ions.

The oncogenic effect of ionizing radiation depends on the dose delivered, the type of radiation used, and the mode of delivery. The biologic effects that x-rays and gamma rays induce are thought to be caused by the production of free radicals. One electron is removed from O_2 to form the free radical O_2^-, which may be the agent that ultimately affects DNA.[16] Particle radiation, with its high linear energy transfer (LET), can interact directly with critical targets within the cell. In particular, it causes specific break points in the chromosome and activation of cellular oncogenes.

Some studies show that humans can have a higher incidence of chronic leukemias, thyroid tumors, and breast cancer from exposure to radiation, and a higher incidence of lung cancer from exposure to radioactive ores (a condition primarily affecting miners).[16a] In the home, radon (^{222}Rn), which emits from the ground, is associated with increased lung cancer risk.[14] In humans, there is a 1% incidence of second primary cancers after therapeutic radiation. In dogs, radiation-induced tumors have been reported to occur from 30 to 78 months after radiation therapy.[17,18] These occurrences are very rare and should not preclude the use of radiotherapy.

Strontium-90 has been shown to cause bone cancer in dogs and some lymphoproliferative tumors in some experimental studies. High doses of radium, plutonium, and radiothorium have also been shown to produce osteosarcomas in dogs.[19]

PARASITES

Spirocerca lupi has been associated with the development of esophageal fibrosarcomas (in 34% of cases studied) and osteogenic sarcomas (in 66% of cases studied). The parasite is found in the esophageal tumor. Because of epizootiological and dietary factors, *S. lupi* is found mainly in hounds, but it has been reported in the fox, wolf, jackel, lynx, jaguar, snow leopard, and domestic cat. It is usually associated with ingestion of infected chicken parts.[20]

The eggs of *S. lupi* are passed in the feces of the infected host and hatch only after they have been ingested by a coprophagous beetle (dung beetle). The larvae become encystic in the beetle and if the beetle is eaten (typically by a chicken, which, thus infected, is in turn eaten by the recipient host), the larvae may then penetrate the stomach wall of the host, migrate the wall, and reach the gastroepiploic arteries, the celiac arteries, and then the aorta. Once they reach the thoracic cavity, they pass out of the aorta and eventually migrate to the esophagus. The adult worms may induce tumors in the esophagus, stomach, or aorta. These tumors tend to metastasize in 54% of cases and hypertrophic pulmonary osteoarthropathy (HPO) is a common sequel in two-thirds of the cases. It is thought that the parasite may secrete a chemical carcinogen.

TRANSPLANTATION

The only known transplantable tumor is the transmissible venereal tumor (TVT). The tumor is transmitted by the transplantation of whole cells to another host. Dogs appear to be the only hosts.[21,22] TVT is usually transmitted from an infected host to the recipient by means of coitus, licking, or trauma. Dogs infected with TVT can also transmit the tumor to other parts of their own bodies by licking. TVT has been experimentally transplanted in foxes. It tends to be more common in southern regions (southern USA, Caribbean Islands, Africa, for example). The greater the number of stray dogs in an area, the higher the incidence of TVT. There is no evidence that TVT is caused by a virus. TVT cells contain 56 chromosomes (normal canine cells have 78 chromosomes); this finding has remained constant after many years.

CHEMICAL CARCINOGENS

Chemical carcinogens may be active in their primary form (direct acting), or they may need to be modified in the body before becoming active (procarcinogen). The annual production of synthetic organic chemicals in the United States has doubled approximately every 8 years since 1940. At present the Environmental Pro-

tection Agency (EPA) lists 44,000 chemicals used commercially. Of the 7000 chemicals tested, 1500 have been found to be carcinogenic. There are two ways to test a chemical for carcinogenic activity. One method involves the use of laboratory rodents, and the other tests for mutagenic activity in bacteria (Ames Test).

The following substances (partial listing) have been associated with carcinogenesis:[24,25]

1. *Hydrazines.* Dialkylhydrazines have been shown to induce colon tumors in laboratory animals.
2. *Bracken fern.* Indirect evidence for carcinogenicity is derived from observations that milk from cows fed high levels of bracken fern contained compounds shown to be carcinogenic in rats. Carcinomas of the intestines, urinary bladder, and kidneys were observed in rats fed high levels of fresh or powdered milk from cows that had consumed 1 g of bracken fern per kilogram of body weight daily for approximately 2 years.
3. *Cycasin.* This substance, found in certain plants, has been used as a source of starch for people and livestock in tropical and subtropical regions for many years. High rates of liver cancer have been thought to be associated with the ingestion of cycasin in cycacl nuts.
4. *Pyrrolizidine alkaloids.* Derived from nonedible plants that may contaminate foodstuffs and food grains, these have been shown to produce liver cancers in rodents.
5. *Asbestos.* Asbestos is reported to be a cause of mesothelioma in man and is a suspected cause in dogs. Mesotheliomas in dogs have been shown to occur when owners worked with asbestos, either as an occupation or a hobby.
6. *Food additives.* Nearly 3000 substances (direct additives) are intentionally added to foods. In addition, several thousand chemicals (indirect additives and contaminants) find their way into food through chemical treatment of crops, during food processing, or from packaging materials.

    Nitrate and nitrite, used as preservatives in many foods, can be converted to *N*-nitroso compounds. Most *N*-nitroso compounds are carcinogenic in many species of laboratory animals. Epidemiologic studies suggest that these compounds are carcinogenic in man.

Acrylonitrite, a food packaging material, contaminates foods and is a confirmed carcinogen in rodents.

Polyvinylchloride (PVC) is an indirect food additive due to contamination from packaging material. Tumor incidence has been shown to increase with exposure to vinyl chloride, and occupational exposure in man has been associated with cancer of the liver, brain, respiratory tract, and lymphatic system.

7. *Environmental contaminants.* These include:

Pesticides. Common organochloride pesticides (for example, toxaphene and chlordane) are carcinogenic in some rodent species. Other compounds such as Kepone (chlordesone), hexachlorobenzine, and perhaps heptachlor (with chlordane) and lindane, present carcinogenic risk to humans and animals.

Polycyclic aromatic hydrocarbons (PAHs). PAHs are contaminants from smoking and broiling foods and have been found to be carcinogenic in laboratory animals. Occupational exposure of humans to PAHs is associated with an increased incidence of skin and lung cancer.

Polychlorobiphenyls (PCBs). PCBs are persistent in the environment. They occur in fish, meat, and dairy products and are carcinogenic in rodents, producing tumors of the liver.

Air pollutants. Various substances contaminate our environment from combustion of petroleum products. Evidence that air pollutants cause cancer in animals comes from autopsy data suggesting that canine lung cancer and tonsillar tumors occur more frequently in dogs from urban than from rural environments.

8. Chemotherapy agents. Cyclophosphamide has been reported to cause bladder cancer in dogs.[26]

NUTRITION

Studies of the association between diet and cancer have focused on cancers of the gastrointestinal tract, the breast, the prostate, and to a lesser extent, the respiratory tract and urinary bladder. Most of the evidence presented is based on human or experimental rodent studies.

1. *Total dietary intake.* There is indirect evidence that total caloric intake is associated with an increase in cancer incidence. Much of the risk is in association with obesity. In laboratory animals, the incidence of tumors is lower and the life-span is much longer for animals on a restricted diet.[27,28]

2. *Lipids.* Epidemiological studies have shown an association between dietary fat and the occurrence of cancer of the breast, prostate, and large bowel. Similar studies have been done in laboratory animals to show the same correlation of fat intake to tumor incidence.[29] When fat intake is low, polyunsaturated fats appear to be more effective than saturated fats in enhancing tumorigenesis, especially in mammary tumors.[30]

3. *Carbohydrates.* There is some suggestive evidence that high intake of refined sugar or starch may increase the incidence of breast cancer, but laboratory studies using animal models have failed to prove this.[31,32] However, excessive carbohydrate consumption contributes to caloric excess, which in turn has been implicated as a modifier of carcinogenesis.

4. *Fiber.* Some studies have shown that high fiber diets are associated with a lower risk of colon cancer in man.[33,34] Fiber may help to dilute or inactivate fecal mutagens by increasing stool bulk.[35]

5. *Vitamins and minerals.*
   a. Vitamin A. Studies have shown a lower incidence of cancer (lung, larynx, and bladder) with increased A and carotenoid intake.[36] Laboratory studies have shown an increased susceptibility to chemical carcinogens in vitamin A-deficient animals.[37]
   b. Vitamin C. Little evidence exists in human studies to show a protective effect of increased vitamin C intake (except for some evidence of reduced stomach and esophageal cancers), but in laboratory studies vitamin C can inhibit the formation of carcinogenic N-nitroso compounds both *in vitro* and *in vivo.*[36,37]
   c. Vitamin E. Vitamin E also inhibits the formation of N-nitroso amines *in vitro*

and *in vivo.*[38] Little evidence exists to show antitumor activity.

d. Selenium. Many studies have shown selenium to have anticarcinogenic activity and to protect against a wide variety of tumors.[39–41]

e. Iron. Laboratory studies have shown that iron deficiency can be associated with an increased susceptibility to chemically induced tumors. In one study, iron deficiency increased the onset of chemically induced liver tumors.[42]

f. Zinc. A zinc deficiency increases the incidence of and shortens the lag time for the induction of tumors in rats given carcinogens.[43]

g. Calcium. Calcium salts lower the toxicity of bile acids and slow the rate of intestinal cell duplication; they may lower the incidence of colon cancer.[44]

6. *Inhibitors of carcinogenesis.* Certain foods, such as carotene-rich vegetables and cruciferous vegetables (cabbage, broccoli, cauliflower, and brussels sprouts), are associated with reductions in tumors in rodents.

IMMUNOLOGY

A high incidence of cancer is associated with immunodeficient conditions. Individuals with congenital immunodeficiencies have a 2% to 4% incidence of cancer. Non-Hodgkin's lymphomas account for over half of these malignancies.[45] There is also a high incidence of non-Hodgkin's lymphoma (about 25 to 60 times greater than expected) in transplantation patients on high doses of immunosuppressive therapy. Squamous cell carcinoma also occurs 10 to 20 times more often than expected in transplantation patients.[45] (see Chapter 11).

ONCOGENIC VIRUSES

Oncogenic viruses can be divided into two groups: (1) DNA and (2) RNA. The DNA viruses can be further divided into (a) the enveloped double-stranded DNA herpesviruses and (b) the naked double-stranded DNA papova- and adenoviruses. All oncogenic viruses either contain DNA or, in the case of RNA viruses, contain an enzyme called *RNA-dependent DNA polymerase* or *reverse transcriptase*, which can make DNA from viral RNA (Tables 2-1 and 2-2).[47,48]

Upon infection, viral RNA is converted to double-stranded DNA and stably integrated into the host genome. The viral genome or the proviral genome (in retroviruses) contains vegetative genes related to the replication of the virus and one or more transforming genes or oncogenes whose protein products trigger cellular proliferation. In DNA viruses, transforming genes appear to be intrinsic viral genes; in retroviruses, by contrast, the oncogene is derived from the cellular genome. In both, it is the continuous expression, the transforming gene, that is responsible for tumorigenesis.[49–53]

Following integration of viral DNA, the transforming gene or oncogene is transcribed, probably from some viral promoter, and the oncogenic protein is found in each transformed cell. How the oncogene protein causes cell proliferation is unknown. Two hypotheses have been proposed: (1) The transforming protein acts directly on cellular DNA to modulate gene expression or cellular DNA replication and thereby stimulates cell proliferation; and (2) the transforming protein affects a structured element of the cell (*e.g.,* the cytoplasmic membrane) related to cellular growth control. Further information regarding viral integration and cellular transformation may be obtained from the literature.[47,49,50,54]

RISK FACTORS AND PREVENTION FOR SPECIFIC TUMOR TYPES

Most of the evidence for the prevention of cancer comes from studies in humans and rodents. This summary represents current evidence regarding the risk factors and preventive approaches for some of the common tumors.[37, 55–65]

UPPER ALIMENTARY TRACT CANCER

Risk Factors. In North America and other Western countries, smoking and alcohol consumption are associated with cancers of the mouth and the esophagus. Certain nitrosamines, found at appreciable levels in tobacco and chewing tobacco, are thought to be associated with cancers of the oral cavity. The nutritional intake of green or yellow vegetables and fruits containing vitamins C and A may protect against the development of oral and esophageal cancers. Oral cancers are common in cats and dogs, but no

Table 2-1.   DNA Viruses Associated with Cancer

VIRUS GROUP (OR FAMILY)	VIRUS MEMBER	ABBREV.	NATURAL HOST	ASSOCIATION WITH ONCOGENICITY
Papovaviruses	Polymavirus	Py	Mouse	Wide variety of tumors (particularly sarcomas in hamsters, mice, and rats)
	Simian virus 40	SV 40	Monkey	Lymphocytic leukemia, ependymomas, lymphosarcoma, reticulum cell sarcoma, and osteogenic sarcoma in hamsters; tumors in mice and rats
	Papillomaviruses Human	HPV 5	Human	Squamous cell carcinoma in humans
		HPV 6	Human	Squamous cell carcinoma in humans
		HPV ?	Human	Laryngeal papilloma in humans
	Shope		Rabbit	Squamous cell carcinoma in domestic rabbits
	Bovine	BPV	Cow	Esophageal papilloma in cow
	Mastomys		*Mastomys natalensis*	Invasive acanthomas in mastomys
Herpes B virus	Hepatitis B virus	HBV	Human	Primary hepatocellular carcinoma in humans
Adenoviruses	Human types		Human	Undifferentiated sarcomas and neoplastic lymphomas in hamster, mouse, rat, and mastomys
	Simian		Monkey	Sarcomas in hamster, rat, and mouse
	Bovine type 3		Cow	Sarcomas in hamster
	Avian	CELO	Chicken	Sarcomas in hamster
Herpes viruses	Herpes simplex (types 1 & 2)	HSV HSV 1 HSV 2	Human	Uterine cervical and vulvar carcinomas in humans; adenocarcinoma and fibrosarcoma in hamsters
	Cytomegalovirus	CMV	Human	Prostatic carcinoma, uterine cervical carcinoma in humans
	Epstein–Barr virus	EBV	Human	Burkitt's lymphoma, nasopharyngeal carcinoma, and Hodgkin's disease in humans
	Marek's disease virus	MDV	Chickens	Neurolymphomatosis in chickens
	Herpesvirus ateles	HVA	Spider monkeys	Lymphoma in marmosets, owl monkeys, and rabbits
	Herpesvirus saimiri	HVS	Squirrel monkeys	Lymphoma in marmosets, owl monkeys, and rabbits
	Herpesvirus sylvilagus		Rabbit	Lymphoma in rabbits
	Guinea pig herpesvirus	GPHV	Guinea pig	Lymphocytic leukemia in guinea pigs
Poxviruses	Yaba monkey tumor virus		Monkey	Benign skin tumors of monkeys and other primates
	Rabbit fibroma virus		Rabbit	Fibromas in cottontail and domestic rabbits
	Myxomavirus		Rabbit	Fibromas in South American forest rabbit and lethal disease in domestic European rabbits

Table 2-2.   RNA Viruses Associated with Cancer

VIRUS GROUP (OR FAMILY)	VIRUS MEMBER	ABBREV.	NATURAL HOST	ASSOCIATION WITH ONCOGENICITY
Avian, quail retroviruses	Sarcoma (Rous)	RSV	Chicken	Sarcoma in chicken, turkey, duck, hamster, monkey
	Leukemia	ALV	Chicken	Leukemia in chicken, turkey
Murine retroviruses	Sarcoma	MSV	Mouse	Sarcoma in mouse, rat, hamster, cat
	Leukemia	MuLV	Mouse	Leukemia, lymphoma in mouse, rat, hamster
	Murine mammary tumor (Bittner)	MMTV	Mouse	Adenocarcinoma in mouse
Feline retroviruses	Sarcoma	FeSV	Cat	Sarcoma in cat, dog, rabbit, monkey
	Leukemia	FeLV	Cat	Leukemia and lymphoma in cat
Primate retroviruses	Simian sarcoma	SiSV	Woolly monkey	Fibrosarcoma in marmoset
	Gibbon ape leukemia	GALV	Gibbon ape	Lymphosarcoma in ape
	Mason-Pfizer	MPMV	Monkey	Mammary carcinoma in monkey
Human retroviruses	T-cell leukemia	HTLV	Human	Cutaneous adult T-cell leukemia/lymphoma

specific risk factors have been identified except for dark pigmentation for melanoma and largeness of breed for oral fibrosarcoma. Some studies report that males have a higher incidence of melanomas and fibrosarcoma than females.

Preventive Approaches. In man, reduced intake of alcohol and tobacco should be associated with a reduction in oral and esophageal cancer. Proper dietary intake of vitamins C and A, as well as sufficient trace elements such as zinc, magnesium, and iron, may help prevent oral and esophageal cancer. In animals, no known preventives have been identified.

STOMACH CANCER

Risk Factors. An increased incidence of gastric cancer has been associated with high consumption of dried and salted fish, pickled vegetables, and smoked fish, along with low fresh vegetable and fruit intake. Studies in animal models have shown that salt can act as a cocarcinogen, enhancing the effect of stomach carcinogens. In man a lower risk has been associated with high consumption of yellow and green vegetables and fruits, suggesting that vitamin A or beta carotene may be protective. Stomach cancer is very rare in dogs and even rarer in cats. No specific etiological factors have been identified in animals.

Preventive Approaches. In humans, decreasing the use of salted, pickled, or smoked foods should reduce the risk of gastric cancer. Increased intake of vegetables and fresh fruit may be of value.

LARGE BOWEL CANCER

Risk Factors. High fat diets, low fiber diets, and low calcium intake tend to be the predominant factors associated with colon cancer. The specific carcinogens causing large bowel cancer are not known, but several leads have emerged. Colon bacteria have been shown to produce certain fecal mutagens by the desaturation of bile acids. Mutagens are also produced on charcoal-broiled fish and meats, and also on fried meat and fried fish. Some of the carcinogens have been classified as *heterocyclic amines*, which have been shown to induce neoplasms in the mammary gland, intestines, pancreas, bladder, and liver in rodents.

Preventive Approaches. A reduction in dietary fat or an increase in dietary fiber will reduce the probability of developing large bowel cancer. Certain vegetables, such as brussels sprouts and cauliflower, contain indol derivatives that can act as enzyme inducers and, under certain conditions, seem to inhibit the carcinogenic process. Dietary intake of calcium salts can lower the toxicity of bile acids and slow the rate of intestinal cell duplication and thus may inhibit potential tumor development.

PANCREATIC CANCER

Risk Factors. In humans, consumption of alcohol, tobacco smoking, and coffee drinking have been implicated, but not yet proven responsible, in the development of pancreatic cancer. Intake of dietary fat has also been correlated with pancreatic cancer. In experimental studies, feeding animals diets high in unsaturated fat after exposure to a carcinogen produced an increase of pancreatic carcinomas in hamsters and rats. In dogs and cats no particular risk factors have been identified.

Preventive Approaches. Since tobacco use and high fat diets may be risk factors, it is possible that reduction in these substances may have a preventive effect.

MAMMARY CANCER

Risk Factors. Dogs develop more mammary tumors than any species except mice. Canine mammary tumors are found four times more commonly in unspayed bitches than in spayed bitches.[1] Ovariohysterectomy before the first estrus cycle has resulted in a sevenfold decrease in the risk of developing mammary tumors. The cat also has a high incidence of mammary tumors, but the role of hormones in their development is less clear. The annual incidence of mammary tumors in intact female cats is 32 per 100,000, but the incidence among neutered female cats is 20 per 100,000. Thus, intact cats have a much greater risk of developing mammary tumors than do neutered female cats, though the difference between intact and neutered animals isn't as great as it is in the dog.

In rodent models and in studies in human beings, dietary fat appears to be a risk factor for developing breast cancer. When female rats are exposed to carcinogens such as 7,12-dimethyl-benz(a)anthracene (DMBA) and N-nitrosomethylurea (nmu) those fed diets with 20% fat developed mammary gland cancer significantly more frequently than those fed diets containing 0.5% to 5% fat. Dietary fat may elicit its tumor-enhancing effects by altering host endocrine metabolism, thus stimulating mammary epithe-lium. Polyunsaturated fats seem to be more effective promoters of mammary tumor development than are saturated fats. Caloric restriction can inhibit the effect of a high fat diet.

Preventive Approaches. In humans, reductions of the level of dietary fat from 40% to 20% or 25% of calories, consumed, especially if accompanied by a reduced overall caloric intake, might help prevent the development and recurrence of mammary cancer. In humans, it has been suggested that menhaden oil (from fish oils) may inhibit the development of breast cancer.

The most significant way of preventing breast cancer in both dogs and cats is early ovariohysterectomy. The procedure should be performed prior to the first estrus. Obesity has been associated with breast cancer development in women and should be prevented in dogs and cats.

PROSTATE CANCER

Risk Factors. In general, populations that have a high risk of breast, colon, and endometrial cancer also have a high risk of prostate cancer. An association with diet has been documented for breast and colon cancer, and dietary fat may also play a role in the etiology of prostate cancer. Some studies have shown that vegetarians have a lower incidence of prostate cancer, presumably owing to a lower intake of fat. No specific etiological factors have been identified in the development of prostatic cancer in dogs, but significantly, prostatic adenocarcinoma is rare in castrated dogs.

Preventive Approaches. As for other nutritionally linked cancers, a 50% reduction in total fat intake may serve to lower the risk of prostatic cancer for humans. Other nutritionally important approaches may involve using micronutrients such as zinc or selenium. Castration may help to prevent prostatic tumors in dogs.

SKIN TUMORS

Risk Factors. In humans and in experimental animals, protracted or frequent exposure to high doses of UV radiation can be associated with the development of carcinomas of the skin. Experimental evidence suggests that UV radiation initiates mutagenic effects in many cells, but that they do not develop into cancer. There is now a renewed interest in the role of immune surveillance in the apparent suppression of initiated cells. It is suggested that UV radiation affects Langerhans' cells, which are antigen-presenting cells in the epidermis and are important sentinels of the immune system. These effects result in the development of suppressor T-lymphocytes, which interfere with the rejection of the tumors.

People are protected from the sequelae of UV radiation-induced damage by two distinct types of mechanisms. First, pigment, hair, and skin thickness all reduce the absorbed dose. Second, human cells repair UV radiation-induced DNA damage with great speed.

UV radiation has been associated with solar dermatitis and squamous cell carcinoma in white cats and with nasal squamous cell carcinoma in collies and Shetland sheepdogs living in sunny climates.

Preventive Approaches. Skin tumors can be prevented by keeping susceptible cats and dogs out of sunlight during the peak daylight hours, or by applying sunscreening lotions to susceptible areas. Tatooing the areas exposed to sunlight is another effective tumor inhibitor.

CONCLUSIONS

Because we live in an environment saturated with many diverse chemicals, in the air, the water supply, and the food supply, it is important that we know and understand the mechanisms by which chemicals and various agents can induce neoplastic transformation. Identification of offensive chemical agents and their specific mechanisms of tumor induction will require many years of extensive research. Rarely is the etiology so simple that blame can be placed entirely on one agent. The long latent period from initiation and promotion to clinical detection of cancer, coupled with the multiplicity of causative agents, makes rapid detection of specific etiologic agents a most difficult task. It will be virtually impossible to test for potential carcinogenic activity all of the many compounds being produced that we, as well as animals, are exposed to. As veterinarians it is our responsibility to try to minimize exposure of our patients and ourselves. Furthermore, it is our responsibility to remain as open minded and as cur-

rently informed as we can be regarding the proven and potential adverse effects of various chemical compounds. The prevention of cancer will depend on a number of factors, such as an understanding of the mechanism of cellular transformation, the identification of specific carcinogens, educational programs to minimize exposure, and where necessary, regulatory legislation to control the manufacture and dissemination of known carcinogens.

REFERENCES

1. Dorn CR: Survey of animal neoplasms in Alameda and Contra Costa Counties, California. II. Cancer morbidity in dogs and cats from Alameda County. J Natl Cancer Inst 40:307–318, 1968

2. Higginson J, Muir CS: Environmental carcinogenesis: Misconceptions and limitations to cancer control. J Natl Cancer Inst 63:1291–1298, 1979

3. Wynder EL, Gori GB: Contribution of the environment to cancer incidence: An epidemiologic exercise. J Natl Cancer Inst 58:825–832, 1977

4. Pitot HC: Principles of cancer biology: Chemical carcinogenesis. In DeVita VT, Hellman S, Rosenberg SA (eds): Cancer: Principles and Practice of Oncology, 2nd ed, pp 79–100. Philadelphia, JB Lippincott, 1985

5. Boutwell RK: The function and mechanism of promoters of carcinogenesis. Crit Rev Toxicol 2:419–443, 1974

6. Priester WA, McKay FW: The Occurrence of Tumors in Domestic Animals, p. 152. Natl Cancer Inst Monogr No. 54, Washington DC, US Govt Printing Office, 1980

7. Jaggi W, Lutz WK, Schlatter C: Covalent binding of ethinylestradiol and estrone to rat liver DNA in vivo. Chem Biol Interact 23:13–18, 1978

8. Lemon HM: Experimental basis for multiple primary carcinogenesis by sex hormones. Cancer 40:1825–1832, 1977

9. Nielson SW, Aftosmis J: Canine perianal gland tumors. J Am Vet Med Assoc 144:127–135, 1964

10. Sinibaldi KR, Rosen H, DeAngelis M: Tumors associated with metallic implants in animals. Clin Orthop 118:257–266, 1976

11. Knecht CD, Priester WA: Osteosarcoma in dogs: a study of previous trauma, fracture and fracture fixation. J Am Anim Hosp Assoc 14:82–84, 1978

12. Theilan GH, Madewell BR: Tumors of the skin and subcutaneous tissue. In Theilan GH, Madewell BR (eds), Veterinary Cancer Medicine, 2nd ed. Philadelphia, Lea & Febiger, 1987

13. Dubielzig RR, Everitt J, Shadduck JA, et al: Clinical and morphological features of post traumatic ocular sarcomas in cats. Vet Pathol (in press)

14. Upton AC: Physical carcinogenesis: Radiation-history and sources. In: Becker FF (ed), Cancer: A Comprehensive Treatise, Vol 1, pp. 387–403. New York, Plenum Press, 1978

15. Committee on Impacts of Stratospheric Change, National Research Council. Halocarbons: Environmental effects of chloroflouromethane release. Washington, DC, National Academy of Sciences Press, 1976

16. Biaglow JE: The effects of ionizing radiation of mammalian cells. J Chem Educ 58:144–156, 1981

16a. Kohn HI, Fry RJM: Radiation carcinogenesis. N Engl J Med 310:504–511, 1984

17. Thrall DE, Goldschmidt MH, Evans SM, et al: Bone sarcoma following orthovoltage radiotherapy in two dogs. Vet Rad 24:169–173, 1983

18. Thrall DE, Goldschmidt MH, Biery DN: Malignant tumor formation at the site of previously irradiated acanthomatous epulides in four dogs. J Am Vet Med Assoc 178:127–132, 1981

19. Theilen GH, Madewell BR: Tumors of the skeleton. In Theilen GH, Madewell BR (eds), Veterinary Cancer Medicine, 2nd ed, p. 471. Philadelphia, Lea & Febiger, 1987

20. Bailey WS: Parasites and cancer: Sarcomas in dogs associated with *Spirocerca lupi*. Ann NY Acad Sci 108:890–923, 1963

21. Epstein RB, Bennett BT. Histocompatibility typing and course of canine venereal tumors transplanted into unmodified random dogs. Cancer Res 34:788–793, 1974

22. Yang TJ, Jones JB: Canine transmissible veneral sarcoma: Transplantation studies in neonatal and adult dogs. J Natl Cancer Inst 51:1915–1918, 1973

23. Cohen D: The biological behavior of the transmissible venereal tumor in immunosuppressed dogs. Eur J Cancer 9:253–258, 1973

24. Palmer S, Mathews RA: The role of nonnutritive dietary constituents in carcinogenesis. Surg Clin North Am 66:891–915, 1986

25. Chemicals, Industrial Processes and Industries Associated with Cancer in Humans. IARC Monogr Eval Carcinog Risk Chem Hum (Suppl) 4, 1982

26. Weller RE, Wolf AM, Oyejide A: Transitional cell carcinoma of the bladder associated with cyclophosphamide therapy in a dog. J Am Anim Hosp Assoc 15:733–736, 1979

27. Sarkar NH, Fernandes G, Telang NT, et al: Low-calorie diet prevents the development of mammary tumors in C3H mice and reduces circulating prolactin level, murine mammary tumor virus expression, and proliferation of mammary alveolar cells. Proc Natl Acad Sci USA 79:7758–7762, 1982

28. Tucker MJ: The effect of long-term food restriction to tumors in rodents. Int J Cancer 23:803–815, 1979

29. Tannenbaum A: The genesis and growth of tumors. III. Effects of a high fat diet. Cancer Res 2:468–475, 1942

30. Walsh CW, Aylsworth CF: Enhancement of murine mammary tumorigenesis by feeding high levels of dietary fats. A hormonal mechanism. J Natl Cancer Inst 70:215–221, 1980

31. Hems G: The contribution of diet and childbearing to breast-cancer rates. Br J Cancer 37:974–982, 1978

32. National Academy of Sciences: Diet, Nutrition, and Cancer, pp. 7-1 to 7-7. Washington, DC, National Academy Press, 1982

33. Modan B, Barrell V, Lubin F, et al: Low fiber intake as an etiologic factor in cancer of the colon. J Natl Cancer Inst 55:15–18, 1978

34. Dales LG, Friedman GD, Ury HR, et al: A case-control study of relationship of diet and other traits to colorectal cancer in American Blacks. Am J Epidemiol 109:132–144, 1979

35. Watanabe K, Reddy BS, Weisburger LH, et al: Effects of alfalfa, pectin and wheat bran on azoxymethane or methylnitrosourea-induced colon carcinogenesis in F344 rats. J Natl Cancer Inst 63:141–145, 1979

36. Mettlin C: Dietary factors for cancer specific sites. Surg Clin North Am 66:917–929, 1986

37. Williams GM, Weisburger JH. Food and cancer: Cause and effect? Surg Clin North Am 66:873–889, 1986

38. Mirvioh SS. The etiology of gastric cancer. J Natl Cancer Inst 71:631–647, 1983

39. Birt DF, Lawson TA, Julius AD: Inhibition by dietary selenium of colon cancer induced in the rat by bis (2-oxopropyl) nitrosamine. Cancer Res 42:4455–4459, 1982

40. Ip C: Prophylaxis of mammary neoplasia by selenium supplementation in the initiation and promotion of chemical carcinogenesis. Cancer Res 41:4386–4390, 1981

41. Jacobs MM: Selenium inhibition of 1,2-dime-thylhydrazine-induced colon carcinogenesis. Cancer Res 43:1646–1649, 1983

42. Vitale JJ, Broitman SA, Vavrousek–JaKuba E, et al: The effects of iron deficiency and the quality and quantity of fat on chemically induced cancer. Adv Exp Med Biol 91:229–242, 1978

43. Fong LYY, Sivak A, Newberne PM: Zinc deficiency and methylbenzylnitrosamine-induced esophageal cancer in rats. J Natl Cancer Inst 6:145–150, 1978

44. Lipkin M, Newmark H: Effect of added dietary calcium in colonic epithelial-cell proliferation in subjects at high risk for familial colonic cancer. N Engl J Med 313:1381–1384, 1985

45. Kersey JH, Spector BD, Good RA: Immunodeficiency and cancer. Adv Cancer Res 18:211–230, 1973

46. Hoover T, Fraumeni JF Jr: Risk of cancer in renal-transplant recipients. Lancet 2:55–57, 1973

47. Bishop JM: The molecular biology of RNA tumor viruses: A physician's guide. N Engl J Med 303:675–682, 1980

48. Madewell BR, Theilen GH. Etiology of cancer in animals. In Theilen GH, Madewell BR (eds), Veterinary Cancer Medicine, 2nd ed, p. 13. Philadelphia, Lea & Febiger, 1987

49. Slamon DJ, et al: Expression of cellular oncogenes in human malignancies. Science 224:256–259, 1984

50. Bishop JM: Cellular oncogenes and retroviruses. Ann Rev Biochem 52:301, 1983

51. Tooze J (ed): DNA Tumor Viruses. Cold Spring Harbor, NY, Cold Spring Harbor Laboratory, 1980

52. Tevethia SS, Flyer DC, Tjian R: Biology of simian virus 40 (SV40) transplantation antigen (TrAg). Virology 107:13–23, 1980

53. Bishop JM: Enemies within: The genesis of retrovirus oncogenes. Cell 23:5–6, 1981

54. Bishop JM. Viral oncogenes: Curiosity or paradigm? Research Frontiers in Aging and Cancer, pp. 155–159. Natl Cancer Inst Monogr No. 60, Washington, DC, US Govt Printing Office, 1980

55. Theilan GH, Madewell BR, Gardner MB: Hematopoietic neoplasms, sarcomas and related conditions, Parts I and II. In Theilan GH, Madewell BR (eds), Veterinary Cancer Medicine, 2nd ed, pp. 345–381. Philadelphia, Lea & Febiger, 1987

56. Correa P, Cuello C, Fajardo LF, et al: Diet and gastric cancer: Nutritional survey in a high-risk area. J Natl Cancer Inst 70:673–678, 1983

57. Gold EB, Gordis L, Diener MD, et al: Diet and other risk factors for cancer of the pancreas. Cancer 55:460–467, 1985

58. Hill MJ: Environment and genetic factors in gastrointestinal cancer. In Sherlock P, Morson BC, Barbara L, et al (eds): Precancerous Lesions of the Gastrointestinal Tract. New York, Raven Press, 1983

59. Dhom G: Epidemiologic aspects of latent and clinically manifest carcinoma of the prostate. J Cancer Res Clin Oncol 106:210–218, 1983

60. Doll R, Peto R: The causes of cancer: Qualitative estimates of avoidable risks of cancer in the United States today. J Natl Cancer Inst 66:1191–1308, 1981

61. Reddy BS, Cohen L, McCoy GD, et al: Nutrition and its relationship to cancer. Adv Cancer Res 32:237–245, 1980

62. Miller AB: Nutrition and the epidemiology of breast cancer. In Reddy BS and Cohen LA (eds): Diet, Nutrition and Cancer: A Critical Evaluation, Vol 1, Macronutrients and Cancer, pp. 67–76. Boca Raton, FL, CRC Press, 1986

63. Schottenfeld D, Fraumeni JF Jr (eds): Cancer Epidemiology and Prevention. Philadelphia, WB Saunders, 1982

64. Willett WC, MacMahon B: Diet and cancer—an overview, Part I. N Engl J Med 310:633–638, 1984

65. Greenwald P: Prevention of cancer. In DeVita VT, Hellman S, Rosenberg SA (eds): Cancer: Principles and Practice of Oncology, 2nd ed, p. 197. Philadelphia, JB Lippincott, 1985

3

CANCER PATHOLOGY

Richard R. Dubielzig

NEOPLASIA

A neoplasm is a tissue mass characterized by persistent, excessive, and disorganized cell growth that is unresponsive to normal control mechanisms. A neoplasm can be benign or malignant (see Table 3-1). Benign and malignant tumors can originate from virtually any cell in the body; they therefore give rise to a broad spectrum of clinical problems. Benign tumors may cause significant (clinical) problems by compression of local tissue, cosmetic disfigurement, or the production of biologically active chemical factors. Malignant tumors can destroy tissue by invasion or distant metastasis. Oncologists and pathologists must work together as a team in order to understand neoplastic disease and attempt to treat animals that develop it.

THE DISCIPLINE OF PATHOLOGY

Pathology is, in its broadest sense, the study of disease. A more usual understanding of the discipline of pathology focuses on the study of morbid anatomy, which is the study of structural alterations associated with disease. Structural abnormalities often suggest specific pathogenic mechanisms that can help in the understanding of the causes of disease. For the purposes of this chapter, morbid anatomy is used more specifically as a diagnostic tool. A trained pathologist well versed in the art of recognizing structural alternations is a diagnostician. Surgical pathology is the specialized niche within the broad discipline of pathology which deals with the application of morbid anatomy strictly for diagnostic purposes.

SURGICAL PATHOLOGY

The surgical pathologist should be a member of the clinical team. The surgical pathologist's responsibility is to suggest, as accurately as possible, a diagnosis based upon interpretation of the morphological changes associated with disease states. Usually, but not exclusively, this

Table 3-1.   Features of Benign and Malignant Neoplasia

	BENIGN	MALIGNANT
Differentiation	Cells well differentiated	Anaplastic cells
	Tissue organization suggests tissue of origin	Tissue lacking organization
Boundaries of lesion	Sharply delineated, often encapsulated	Locally infiltrated
Nature of growth	Expansive causing compression of surrounding tissues	Infiltration causing destruction of surrounding tissues
Mitosis	Rare	Common
Rate of growth	Slow	Rapid
Metastases	Absent	Often but not always
Clinical results	Danger due to compression of local tissues, hormone production, or cosmetic disfigurement	Additional danger due to tissue destruction, tumor necrosis, metastatic disease

means interpretation of the histopathological changes in biopsy material from diseased patients. Veterinary pathologists have been providing a diagnostic service for quite some time. With the recent advances in specialized clinical fields within veterinary medicine, the science of veterinary surgical pathology has the opportunity to make great strides.

Veterinary surgical pathologists and veterinary clinical oncologists working together can benefit patient care and achieve scientific advancement of their closely related fields.

CLASSIFICATION SYSTEMS (NOMENCLATURE) IN VETERINARY ONCOLOGY

The task of accurately naming and categorizing disease processes should fall under the jurisdiction of the discipline of pathology. Unfortunately, pathologists have been slow and unenthusiastic in responding to this task. In order for veterinarians from diverse specialties and institutions to converse accurately, a systematic disease nomenclature is required. Nowhere is the necessity for accurate and concise nomenclature more important than in dealing with neoplasia. Within surgical pathology there has been a historical emphasis on accurate classification and subclassification of neoplasms. Periodically organizations such as the World Health Organization attempt to standardize nomenclature.[1,2] These efforts have been extremely help-

ful in achieving standardized nomenclature within human surgical pathology.

Widely divergent nomenclature and classification systems are used at different institutions and by different specialty groups within the field of veterinary medicine. Communication between clinicians and pathologists from different institutions and different fields can be fraught with complications because of unfamiliarity with classification criteria and nomenclature use.

A major challenge that needs to be addressed by the veterinary oncology community is to formulate a standardized nomenclature dealing with animal neoplasia. A successful classification system must satisfy several criteria. First, the system must be useful to a wide range of specialists with an interest in cancer, including morphologists, radiologists, clinical oncologists, and microbiologists. Second, the system must be flexible enough to allow new and sophisticated techniques to contribute an ever-expanding list of physical characteristics to various categories of neoplasms. Although the information needed to accurately categorize neoplasia must be extracted from diverse fields of expertise, it should be the responsibility of the pathologists to accurately maintain and put forward standardized nomenclature because morphological criteria are the accepted method for clinical diagnosis. Thirdly, when new evidence is presented suggesting that tumors once thought of as distinct entities are in fact different stages of a similar disease process, then the nomenclature needs to be modified. Conversely, if tumors previously thought to be identical are found to have differing biological behaviors or expected responses to therapeutic modalities, then the nomenclature should reflect these differences.

From a practical point of view, tumor nomenclature is in many instances generic. Table 3-2 summarizes the generic naming of common animal tumors once the cell of origin is known and a distinction between benign and malignant status is made. It must be realized that a generic tumor such as fibrosarcoma in a dog may well have different implications than fibrosarcoma in a horse. Furthermore, fibrosarcoma of the oral cavity in a dog may be expected to behave differently from fibrosarcoma of the abdominal cavity. As long as the information is available to subcategorize these tumors on the basis of criteria suggesting differing identities, the nomenclature remains easy. Canine oral fibrosarcoma is still an adequate name to distinguish the growth from canine abdominal fibrosarcoma. The problem arises when morphological or biological parameters suggest uniqueness within a subcategory of neoplasia. Tumors displaying such uniqueness should receive unique names. Incorporation of human nomenclature into veterinary oncology is acceptable only if the human and animal diseases are similar by morphologic, biologic, and therapeutic criteria.

PROBLEMS AFFECTING MORPHOLOGICAL INTERPRETATION

PROCUREMENT OF TISSUE (THE BIOPSY)

In order to optimize the chances of accurate morphological diagnosis a large amount of tissue, including both tumor and tumor margins, needs to be examined. Careful thought must then be given in determining the most appropriate biopsy procedure. An understanding of the tumors most likely to occur in the affected tissues and knowledge of the difficulties and importance of accurate diagnosis are essential in order to properly manage the patient. Consultation with the surgical pathologist prior to biopsy in order to choose the most appropriate technique may be warranted in selected cases.

TISSUE FIXATION

Tissue fixation may involve several techniques by which tissue degradation (autolysis) is halted and morphological preservation is enhanced. Autolysis is the enzymatic degradation of cellular and tissue structures. Chilling of the tissue slows the process of autolysis. Chemical fixatives can be used to inactivate enzymes associated with tissue breakdown and protect structural molecules. Many new applications of microwave heat have great potential as fixation methods.[3]

Chemical fixatives are the most common means of tissue preservation in surgical pathology. Ten percent buffered neutral formaldehyde fixative satisfies many of the essential criteria for an all purpose fixative.

For adequate fixation 10-unit volumes of formalin are needed for each unit volume of tissue to be fixed. Formalin has excellent penetrating capabilities; however, fixation is always more rapid with smaller amounts of tissue. A good rule to follow when possible with regard to tissue fixation is to remove a small segment of tissue from an area likely to be solid tumor tissue for rapid fixation and fix the remaining tissue anatomically undisturbed. When choosing tissues to be examined by histopathology, it is often important to include definable anatomical landmarks and also margins between normal and abnormal tissue. The excised margins should be sampled to assess invasion into surrounding tissue.

Once fixation has occurred (it takes approximately 24 hours), the volume of formaldehyde compared to tissue is no longer crucial. The tissue must be kept moist. Formaldehyde-soaked cotton is convenient for mailing samples.

A common error in frigid climates is to place the fixed biopsy in an outdoor mailbox. Freezing can cause artifacts in fixed tissues, making histopathology useless.

Occasionally special fixation properties are sought that can be best accomplished by chemical fixatives other than formaldehyde. The advantages and disadvantages of several fixatives are discussed below.

Quick Freezing. Fixation by quick freezing using liquid nitrogen has the advantage of being rapid and leaving the chemical nature of both enzyme and structural proteins unaltered, thus enhancing immunohistochemistry. The disadvantages of freeze fixation are:

1. Liquid nitrogen is inconvenient to work with.

Table 3-2.   Examples of Generic Classification of Animal Tumors

TISSUE OF ORIGIN	BENIGN	MALIGNANT
I. Simple (composed of one single neoplastic cell type)		
A. Tumors of mesenchymal origin		SARCOMAS
1. Connective tissue and derivatives		
Fibrous tissue	Fibroma	Fibrosarcoma
Myxomatous tissue	Myxoma	Myxosarcoma
Fatty tissue	Lipoma	Liposarcoma
Cartilage	Chondroma	Chondrosarcoma
Bone	Osteoma	Osteosarcoma
2. Vascular endothelium—lymph vessels	Hemangioma Lymphangioma	Hemangiosarcoma Lymphangiosarcoma
3. Blood cells and related cells		
Hematopoietic cells		Myeloproliferative disease
Lymphoid tissue		Malignant lymphomas Plasmacytoma (multiple myeloma)
Mast cells	Mastocytoma	Mast cell sarcoma
4. Muscle		
Smooth muscle	Leiomyoma	Leiomyosarcoma
Striated muscle	Rhabdomyoma	Rhabdomyosarcoma
B. Tumors of epithelial origin		CARCINOMAS
1. Stratified squamous	Squamous cell	Squamous cell or epidermoid carcinoma
2. Skin adnexal glands		
Sweat glands	Sweat gland adenoma	Sweat gland carcinoma
Sebaceous glands	Sebaceous gland adenoma	Sebaceous gland carcinoma
3. Epithelium lining		
Glands or ducts—well-differentiated group	Adenoma Papilloma Papillary adenoma	Adenocarcinoma Papillary carcinoma Papillary adenocarcinoma
	Cystadenoma	Cystadenocarcinoma
Poorly differentiated group		Medullary carcioma Undifferentiated carcinoma
C. Tumors of neural tube or neural crest origin		
1. CNS—astrocyte	Astrocytoma Oligodendrioglioma	Malignant astrocytoma Malignant oligodontria
2. Peripheral nerve—Schwann cell	Schwannoma	(Variable nomenclature)
3. Melanocytic	Melanoma	Malignant melanoma
II. Mixed (more than one neoplastic cell type, usually derived from one germ layer)—Canine mammary gland	Canine mixed mammary tumor	Malignant mixed mammary tumor Mesenchymal ?
III. Compound (more than one neoplastic cell type derived from more than one germ layer)—Gonads	Teratoma dermoid cyst	One or more elements become malignant, e.g., squamous cell carcinoma arising in a teratoma (teratocarcinoma)

2. Tissue must be maintained frozen, thus making storage difficult.
3. Tissue must be cut on a cryostat.

Bouin's Solution. Bouin's solution is used to impart rigidity. Tissues that are naturally soft, delicate, or semiliquid even after formalin fixation can be maintained in better anatomical configuration with Bouin's fixation. Some examples of tissues commonly fixed in Bouin's are retina, bone marrow, and intestinal mucosa. The disadvantages of Bouin's fixative are that it is relatively expensive; it leaves a bright yellow stain; and the tissues must be washed and placed in 70% alcohol after fixation.

Glutaraldehyde. Glutaraldehyde is used for fixation of tissue for electron microscopy. It gives the best fixation of any of the aldehyde fixatives in terms of preservation of morphological detail. Because glutaraldehyde is extremely poor in penetrating tissue, only small tissue fragments can be successfully fixed in it. And because it is toxic and caustic, it must be used extremely carefully.

PROBLEMS IN INTERPRETATION

The object of histopathological examination of biopsy material is to provide an accurate and timely diagnosis and prognosis. The successful accomplishment of this goal depends upon several factors.

1. Correct clinical evaluation of the patient, including the choice of the most appropriate biopsy technique.
2. Tissue fixation and delivery to the histopathology laboratory.
3. Delivery of an accurate, concise, and complete description of the pertinent clinical facts with the biopsy tissue.
4. Skillful and speedy processing of the tissue by the histopathology laboratory.
5. Thorough examination of the tissue by a veterinary pathologist adequately experienced in veterinary surgical pathology.
6. A clearly worded histopathology report that addresses the pertinent clinical questions (diagnosis, prognosis, and special considerations).

Successful interpretation of pathological material obviously depends upon the experience and qualifications of the pathologist. Extensive experience in interpretation of biopsy material in domestic animals is essential if the morphological findings are to be accurate and meaningful. Medical (rather than veterinary) pathologists are occasionally asked to make pathological interpretations on animal tissues. Animal tumors differ importantly from human tumors in regard to the significance of morphological features. Practitioners relying on medical pathologists to diagnose animal tumors may receive inaccurate interpretations. Many veterinary schools, state diagnostic laboratories, and private veterinary pathology laboratories provide excellent histopathology services, often including telephone consultations. Practitioners interested in clinical oncology are encouraged to choose one of these and learn to work closely with the pathologist.

SURGICAL PATHOLOGISTS AND TUMOR STAGING

Important to a complete staging protocol is the pathologist's interpretation of morphological features of the tumor that may predict its biologic behavior. This is accomplished by several means.

The size of the initial tumor is recorded, and the presence or absence of local infiltrative disease, vascular invasion, lymph node metastasis, and distant metastatic disease are assessed and recorded. The presence or absence of lymph node metastasis may be determined histologically at the time of biopsy or excision by examination of the draining lymph node.

Morphological criteria related to prognosis need to be developed for each tumor type. Information such as tumor size, clinical stage, location, and so forth should be correlated to pathologic features. Prospective studies of a large series of cases are the best method to address these issues. Relatively few animal cancers have been examined with this goal in mind.

The standard features thought to be significant in characterizing malignancy are the features of cellular and tissue differentiation (Table 3-1). Growth patterns causing tissue disorganization, variable cellular morphology, increased nuclear to cytoplasmic ratio, abnormal irregular nuclear patterns, numbers of mitotic figures, and the presence or absence of abnormal mitoses are cellular features thought to be significant in predicting malignancy. In practice, however, many tumors exhibit different features in different locations or may exhibit features of morphological malignancy and yet remain biologically benign.

RESEARCH DIRECTIONS IN VETERINARY ONCOLOGY AND PATHOLOGY

The veterinary scientific community has a unique perspective on oncological research. By using manipulative animal models the basic processes of oncogenesis can be studied in an attempt to elucidate the underlying mechanisms of oncogenesis and cancer expression. New technologies useful in diagnosis, morphological classification, and treatment of spontaneous animal cancers mandate updated approaches to understanding the biological behavior of spontaneous animal cancer. Studies concentrating purely on morphology of cancers are unlikely to solve the basic questions regarding the natural history of animal cancers. For this reason it is essential that the pathologist collaborate with clinical oncologists, epidemiologists, radiologists, and cell biologists. Many recent technological advances are of particular interest to morphologists studying spontaneous cancer. Morphological classification of tumors is undergoing a major change with the advent of immunohistochemical staining techniques.[4] The binding of monoclonal antibodies to different cellular components makes it possible to study cellular differentiation on the basis of cytochemical phenomena rather than purely morphological phenomena.

The technologies of immune identification are rapidly becoming more accessible at the ultrastructural level and are making it possible to directly match immunocytochemical phenomena with ultrastructural morphology. This will have an effect not only on tumor classification but also on understanding the events leading to cellular differentiation and oncogenesis at the cellular and subcellular level.

Genetic probes will allow researchers to identify specific genetic sequences in the genome of host cells and will provide a powerful tool useful in identifying particular genetic abnormalities responsible for animal cancers.[5] Genetic sequences associated with oncogenic viruses can be identified in material from spontaneous cancers. It is very likely that these techniques will aid greatly in the classification of spontaneous neoplasms caused by oncogenic viruses or specific genetic redistribution abnormalities.

Electron probe microanalysis is a technique whereby microscopic foreign deposits can be identified chemically by computer analysis of the energy released following electron bombardment. The chemical composition of tissue abnormalities, including the quantitative and qualitative analysis of foreign materials, can be determined with a great deal of accuracy. These techniques are likely to prove valuable in studies combined with epidemiological surveys where exposure to foreign particulates is thought to be a possible contributing factor in oncogenesis; respiratory neoplasms and mesothelioma are among the tumors that should be studied with these techniques.

In conclusion, the study of spontaneous animal cancers has come a long way in that the basic categorization and biology of many different types of cancers affecting virtually every tissue of the body in different species of animals are known and recognized. Surgical pathology as a specialized entity within veterinary pathology is in its infancy; the advancement and nurturing of this science in cooperation with clinical oncology and other specialties with both clinical and basic research implications is sure to further our understanding of animal cancers. Many of the studies that have already been accomplished in human oncology need to be duplicated in veterinary oncology, but care must always be used to ascertain that these studies are done by people with a comprehensive knowledge of animal diseases and animal cancers.

REFERENCES

1. Beveridge WIB, Sobin LH: International histological classification of tumors of domestic animals, Part 1. Bull WHO 50:1, 1974
2. Beveridge WIB, Sobin LM: International histological classification of tumors of domestic animals, Part 2. Bull WHO 53:137, 1976
3. Leong, Duncis: A method of rapid fixation of large biopsy specimens using microwave irradiation. Pathology 18:222–232, 1987
4. Baumal R, Kahn HJ, Bailey D, Phillips MJ, Hanna W: The value of immunohistochemistry in increasing diagnostic precision of undifferentiated tumors by the surgical pathologist. Histochem 16:1061–1078, 1984
5. Grady WW, Chang L, Lewia KJ: In situ viral DNA hybridization in diagnostic surgical pathology. Hum Pathol 18:535–543, 1987

GLOSSARY

Neoplasia: "New growth," a neoplasia is a tissue characterized by persistent excessive and disorganized cell growth unresponsive to normal control mechanisms.

Tumor: The classical definition of a tumor is any localized tissue mass. However, the term is commonly used synonymously with neoplasia.

Benign: A neoplasm is classified as benign when its behavioral characteristics are relatively innocuous (see Table 3-1).

Malignant: Neoplasms are classified as malignant when their behavioral characteristics lead to rapid serious clinical complications as a result of aggressive proliferation (see Table 3-1). Neoplasms exhibiting vascular or lymphatic spread are considered malignant.

Mitotic index: The mitotic index is the number of dividing cells per 1000 cells examined. Mitotic index is usually estimated as the number of mitotic cells per high power (40 ×) field.

Rosettes: Cells clustered in such a way as to form a circle are called rosettes. Formation of rosettes suggests epithelial or tubular differentiation. Some rosettes have specific diagnostic significance.

Pseudorosettes: Cells clustered around blood vessels often appear to form a tubular structure by virtue of the circular arrangement. Pseudorosettes do not indicate tubular differentiation but may have diagnostic significance.

Scirrhous, sclerotic, or desmoplastic: These terms are usually used interchangeably and suggest an exaggerated fibrous tissue component usually coexisting with a malignant epithelial neoplasm. The fibrous proliferation in a desmoplastic reaction is not part of the neoplasm but rather an exaggerated body response.

Pleomorphic: Pleomorphic cells have dramatic variation in appearance within the tissue.

Palisading: Cells that line up with their long accesses parallel and their nuclei forming a row are said to be palisading. This can be an indication or epithelial differentiation, or it can suggest a particular pattern or diagnosis among mesenchymal tumors.

Hyperplasia: An increase in size of a tissue or organ caused by an abnormal but not neoplastic increase in the number of cells is called hyperplasia. Hyperplasia can be diffuse or nodular. Nodular hyperplasia is distinguished from neoplasia by demonstrating that the change is a physiological reparative response or by showing that the tissue organization is the same as that of normal tissue.

Hypertrophy: An increase in the size of a tissue or organ caused by an increase in the size of individual cells with no increase in cell numbers is called hypertrophy.

Dysplasia: Abnormal tissue development in dysplasia. The word has very broad usage in pathology, but the use most appropriate to oncology is cellular dysplasia. Cellular dysplasia is characterized by variation in the size and shape of the cell or nucleus. Abnormalities in tissue organization are also seen. It should be emphasized that cellular dysplasia is not a neoplastic change.

Anaplasia: The structural features of a cell that suggest malignancy are anaplasia. These include lack of differentiation, increased nuclear size, irregular nuclear folding, unusual clumping of chromatin, large or numerous nucleoli, and lack of cellular orientation within the tissue.

Metaplasia: The abnormal transformation of differentiated tissue of one type into differentiated tissue of another type is metaplasia.

4

MECHANISMS OF INVASION AND METASTASIS

Robert C. Rosenthal

Metastasis is the transfer of cancer cells from a primary site to distant organs. The ability to invade and metastasize is the only characteristic unique to malignant neoplasms. Metastatic disease, not the primary tumor, is responsible for most therapeutic failures and patient deaths in clinical oncology.[1] The inability of localized forms of therapy (surgery, radiation) to eradicate a malignancy presents conceptual challenges in the therapy of residual or micrometastatic disease. Often the biologic behavior of the disease is known well enough to allow a prognosis to be made with some assurance. As primary and supportive therapies improve, however, increased life-spans may reveal as yet unrecognized patterns of metastasis in canine and feline patients.

The Veterinary Medical Data Program of the National Cancer Institute reports an overall rate of metastasis (excluding leukemia/lymphoma and not specifying at what point in the course of the disease the diagnosis was made) of 21.5% for canine malignancies and 22.7% for feline malignancies.[2] Because this report includes only those cases seen in selected veterinary schools at a time when veterinary oncology was just beginning to develop, the true figures may well be higher than those reported. It is, of course, impossible to know how many instances of metastatic disease could have been effectively managed with appropriate therapy. Nonetheless, it is clear that the problem of dealing with metastatic disease is an important one. Ultimately, its resolution will depend on an understanding of the metastatic process, and such an understanding will be of great benefit to the clinician in offering meaningful advice to the owner of a cancer patient.

PATHOGENESIS

Metastasis is a complex, multistep process. The successful establishment of a metastatic lesion follows vascularization of the primary tumor, invasion of local tissues, release of cells from the primary site, their dissemination to distant sites, arrest in the microcirculation of organs, extravasation, and infiltration and proliferation at the new location.[3] Only a very small number of tumor cells are able to survive and complete the process.

Once the primary tumor has become well vascularized, invasion of host tissues and penetration of blood vessels and/or lymphatics are important subsequent steps. Tumor angiogenesis factor from the neoplasm stimulates host endothelial cells to grow into the tumor. The newly formed vessels have loose junctions between endothelial cells and lack a fully developed basement membrane, tumor cells thus have easy access to the systemic circulation.[4] Poorly vascularized tumors are less likely to metastasize than are those with an abundant blood supply. Both tumor cell motility and tumor-elaborated enzymes may play a part in these processes, but exact mechanisms are not entirely clear. Invasion of local tissues by tumor cells seems to depend on tumor cell dedifferentiation and the dissociation of cells along an invasion front. Tumor cells have the capacity to move into local areas of interstitial edema and proliferate further while gaining an advantage over normal cells in the competition for oxygen and other nutrients.[5] Several enzymes, including hydrolases, collagenases, and plasminogen activator, have also been implicated in the process. In addition, some malignant cells from highly metastatic neoplasms are known to have high levels of collagenase IV, an enzyme specific for the major structural protein of basement membranes found between parenchymal cells and connective tissue.[6]

Much attention has been given to the question of hematogenous spread in sarcomas as opposed to lymphatic spread in carcinomas, but in fact, the interstitial, lymphatic, and venous compartments offer an interconnected system for disseminating cells. A tumor cell that initially enters the interstitial space may pass through both the lymphatic and vascular systems before it again gains access to the interstitium, where it re-establishes as a proliferating metastasis.[1,7] Within the elastin fibers of arteries and arterioles, protease inhibitors can block the enzyme-dependent invasive process; however, tumor cells generally are able to invade thin-walled capillaries and lymphatics. Once inside a vessel, tumor cells may be carried to another site or may initiate some growth and later release emboli.

Fewer than 0.01% of cells gaining access to the circulatory system survive to form metastases.[3] The remainder fall victim to circulatory turbulence and various immunologic hazards. The longer a tumor cell circulates, the less likely it is to establish a metastatic focus. When tumor cells eventually come to rest, they take advantage of the normal endothelial cell shedding that exposes capillary basement membranes. A continuation of the process by means similar to the early invasive events of the primary tumor then occurs.[5]

REGIONAL LYMPH NODES AND IMMUNE RESPONSE

The response and role of regional lymph nodes are important considerations in the spread of a malignancy. Normal lymph nodes can be an effective temporary barrier to tumor spread.[8] In a cancer patient, a clinically palpable lymph node draining the area of a primary neoplasm might be a result of either hyperplasia of the node or active growth of tumor cells. Fine-needle aspiration can be a helpful technique in distinguishing the two phenomena, but its success is highly dependent on the proficiency of both the clinician obtaining the specimen and the cytologist evaluating the slide.[9] A definitive determination of whether the node is neoplastic may require incisional or excisional biopsy and histopathologic evaluation. A hyperplastic response may indicate a beneficial reactivity to a neoplastic process. Inactive, lymphocyte-depleted lymph nodes, on the other hand, might be associated with a poor prognosis. Functionally, the immunologic response of the regional lymph node is important early in the metastatic process when tumor cells may stimulate cytotoxic T-cells. Later, however, tumor progression seems to promote suppressor T-cell activity in the regional node and allow tumor growth and nodal metastasis.[10] By the time the node is grossly involved with the tumor cells, the regional lymph node is no more important than any other source of lymphocytes (distant nodes, peripheral blood) in providing an immunologic defense.[11]

The effect of the immune system's response varies from tumor to tumor, and no broad generalizations are possible. Suppression of cell-mediated immunity can increase, decrease, or have no effect on the incidence of metastasis. Currently, the clinical importance of humoral immunity against tumor antigens is also unknown. Either an increase or a decrease in numbers of metastases is theoretically possible and depends on the relative effects on helper and suppressor T-lymphocyte subpopulations and their subsequent actions.[1] At this time, there is no consensus regarding the removal of enlarged regional lymph nodes; however, in most cases, an enlarged node draining a region with a malignancy is probably no longer an effective immunologic barrier if the node enlargement is due to the presence of cancer cells. Clinical studies in a number of human tumors have shown that removal of regional lymph nodes, whether they are involved with tumor or not, does not improve cure rates compared with observation of the nodes without surgical intervention.[12] The prospective therapeutic and diagnostic benefit of nodal excision needs to be studied further in specific tumor systems of clinical importance in veterinary medicine.

DIAGNOSIS

The presence or absence of metastases may have important prognostic and therapeutic implications; often this becomes the deciding factor in an owner's decision to initiate treatment or not. A confirmed histopathologic diagnosis of the primary tumor is vital because this information helps guide the search for metastatic disease. Occasionally, the metastatic focus will be diagnosed first and will suggest an undetected primary site. Malignancies that present in such a manner are characterized by obscurity of the primary tumor and its infidelity to expected biologic behavior.[13] In some cases, further, more complex diagnostic techniques (computerized tomography, electron microscopy, special stains) might be needed to help detect an unknown primary tumor. More commonly, metastases are suggested by the known biologic behavior of the primary tumor.[13] Repeated physical examinations, coupled with radiographic, cytologic, and other diagnostic means, further support the diagnosis. Although fewer reliable tumor markers are known for canine and feline tumors than for tumors in humans, certain paraneoplastic manifestations may signal the presence or growth of an unsuspected metastasis after a primary

tumor is removed. Hypoglycemia, hypercalcemia, and hyperestrogenism are three examples of conditions with well-recognized clinical effects that may occur in conjunction with a metastasis.[14]

The most commonly used technique to diagnose metastatic disease is the thoracic radiograph, an undeniably valuable procedure for distinguishing a wide variety of neoplastic diseases. Well-positioned, good quality, lateral and ventrodorsal thoracic radiographs are sufficient for diagnosis in most cases. It is also helpful to have two readers interpret the films independently. If the presence of a lesion is questionable, an additional lateral view from the opposite side is strongly advised.[15] Both greater air contrast and a larger lesion-to-film magnification factor on the "up" side contribute to improved visualization. A lesion usually must be at least 2 to 3 mm in diameter in a small patient such as a cat and 5 to 10 mm in diameter in larger canine patients in order to be visualized radiographically. It is not yet clear whether nuclear imaging is able to detect pulmonary metastases before conventional radiography can. Abdominal radiographs are sometimes helpful in detecting sublumbar lymphadenopathy of possible metastatic origin. Bone films can also be useful in assessing the spread of primary bone tumors.[16] Nuclear imaging of bony lesions with ^{99m}Tc may reveal functional changes before radiographs can show morphologic changes, but the true role of nuclear imaging in this setting is not yet clear in veterinary oncology.[16a–c] Recently, lymphoscintigraphy has been suggested as another useful nuclear imaging procedure for the diagnosis of nodal metastasis of canine neoplasia.[17–19]

As mentioned above, cytologic samples taken by fine-needle aspiration can be of great benefit in the diagnosis of metastatic disease. This technique and the criteria for evaluation have been well described in the veterinary literature[20–22a] (see chapter 6).

FACTORS AFFECTING "CURE"

For veterinary oncologists, the goal of curing established metastatic disease remains, for the most part, elusive. "Cure" implies that the patient has been rid of the last remaining cancer cell that might be potentially lethal. Less stringently, it suggests that therapy has destroyed a sufficient fraction of the viable tumor cell population so that the surviving cells can never reestablish the clinically recognizable disease. Chemotherapeutic destruction is influenced by drug cell kill, population growth kinetics, and tumor heterogeneity. Killing cancer cells is a tremendous task. A detectable metastasis has probably undergone 20 or more doublings and often contains as many as several million to billions of cells; even undetected micrometastases can be composed of significant numbers of cells. Theoretically, metastases undergo Gompertzian growth—that is, a prolonged doubling time and a decreased growth fraction as a function of time. The pattern suggests that early chemotherapeutic intervention should be able to attack a higher proportion of actively cycling cells.[23] It is difficult, however, to determine with certainty the most effective schedule for even one drug, let alone many drugs or combined modalities. Conceptually, these problems are compounded as the heterogeneous nature of neoplasia is considered.[1,24]

The concept of tumor heterogeneity is now widely accepted.[1,24,25] Malignant neoplasms are composed of subpopulations of cells with unique metastatic potentials, different drug sensitivities, and various other diverse behavioral characteristics. Indeed, some neoplasms may demonstrate different characteristics during the course of the disease. For example, not all tumor cells show uniform progression. The potential diversity of response by different subpopulations of a primary neoplasm (as well as its scattered metastases) suggests that the chemotherapist will face many frustrations in combating disseminated neoplastic disease.[1] Responsiveness of a primary lesion does not guarantee responsiveness of a metastatic lesion; the latter may have a different pattern of drug resistance. Indeed, metastases themselves may metastasize and thus add to the complexity of the problem.[26] Clearly, there are many unanswered questions.

THERAPY FOR METASTATIC DISEASE

Each cancer treatment modality (including those usually considered local therapy) has proponents who feel their therapy can contribute to the successful management of metastatic disease. Although surgery for gross metastatic disease may be feasible from a theoretic point of view,

it would seem that chemotherapy or immunotherapy hold the most promise for dealing with established, although perhaps undetectable, metastases that might contain up to a million cancer cells (micrometastases).[23a] This promise is, however, largely unrealized at this point and very difficult to evaluate. Both chemotherapy and immunotherapy could theoretically kill "the last cancer cell" and provide a cure, but in fact, combinations, schedules, and responses vary greatly. In every case, sound chemotherapeutic guidelines must be kept in mind when treating both metastatic disease and a primary tumor.[27] One should be wary of broad generalizations regarding the best therapy; each tumor type, indeed, each tumor patient, must be considered as a singular challenge.

The use of activated macrophages to kill established metastases has shown promise. Macrophages, which have been recognized to kill tumor cells, can be activated by lymphokines (MAF) or bacterial cell-wall products (muramyl peptides, MDP and MTP). Liposomes can be used to deliver MDP to the reticuloendothelial system and activate tumoricidal macrophages.[28] Again, perhaps only small tumors will be treatable by this method, and the best use of this modification of a biologic response remains to be defined. This approach is being investigated as one means of combating micrometastatic canine osteosarcoma.[29,29a] Other biological response interventions have also been investigated but await practical application.[30,31]

A different approach to the problem is the use of selective antimetastatic drugs. Because metastasis is a multistep process, the successful establishment of a metastasis depends on the successful completion of each step in the process. Selective antimetastatic agents interfere with the process of dissemination in the host by mechanisms not involved with the inhibition of tumor cell replication. These diverse mechanisms may lead to increased adhesiveness of tumor cells, improved endothelialization in tumor blood vessels, anticoagulation, decreased procoagulant activity of tumor cells, and decreased platelet aggregation.[32,33] A number of agents have these capabilities, but they are effective only in preventing metastasis formation and do not affect established metastasis. Because some metastatic spread is likely to have occurred by the time of diagnosis, the clinical application of selective antimetastatic agents is unclear.

They should, however, have a broad spectrum of efficacy and limited systemic toxicity, and they may be used as an adjunct to chemotherapy or immunotherapy.

REFERENCES

1. Fidler KJ, Hart JR: Principles of cancer biology: Biology of cancer metastases. In DeVita VT, Hellman S, Rosenberg SA (eds): Cancer: Principles and Practice of Oncology, pp. 80–92. Philadelphia, JB Lippincott 1982

2. Preister WA, McKay FW (eds): The Occurrence of Tumors in Domestic Animals. Natl Cancer Inst Monogr No. 54, 1980

3. Poste G, Fidler IJ: The pathogenesis of cancer metastasis. Nature 283(1):139–146, 1980

4. Folkman J: Tumor invasion and metastasis. In Holland JF, Frei E (eds): Cancer Medicine, pp. 167–177. Philadelphia, Lea & Febiger, 1982

5. Gabbert H: Mechanisms of tumor invasion: Evidence from in vivo observations. Cancer Metastasis Rev 4:293–309, 1985

6. Liotta LA, Garbisa S, Tryggvason K: Biochemical mechanisms involved in tumor cell penetration of the basement membrane. In Liotta LA, Hart IR (eds): Tumor Invasion and Metastasis, pp. 319–333. The Hague, Martinis Nijhoff, 1982

7. Scanlon EF: The process of metastasis. Cancer 55:1163–1166, 1985

8. Fisher B, Saffer E, Fisher ER: Studies concerning the regional lymph node in cancer: IV-tumor inhibition by regional lymph node cells. Cancer 33(3):631–636, 1974

9. Chu EW, Marten SE: Fine needle aspiration cytology of metastases. In Liotta LA, Hart IR (eds): Tumor Invasion and Metastasis, pp. 495–510. The Hague, Martinis Nijhoff, 1982

10. Tachibana T, Yoshida K: Role of the regional lymph node in cancer metastasis. Cancer Metastasis Rev 5:55–66, 1986

11. Fidler IJ, McWilliams RW: Role of the regional lymph node in neoplasia: Cellular mediated reactivity in vitro by autologous regional or distant lymph nodes or peripheral blood lymphocytes of dogs with spontaneous neoplasm. Immunol Commun 7(4):325–335, 1975

12. Cady B: Lymph node metastases—Indicators, but not governors of survival. Arch Surg 119:1067–1072, 1984

13. Nissenblatt MJ: The CUP syndrome (carcinoma unknown primary). Cancer Treat Rev 8:211–224, 1981

14. Weller RE: Paraneoplastic disorders in companion animals. Comp Cont Ed Pract Vet 4(5):423–428, 1982

15. Lang J, Wortman JA, Glickman LT, et al: Sensitivity of radiographic detection of lung metastases in the dog. Vet Rad 27(3):74–78, 1986

16. LaRue SM, Withrow SJ, Wrigley RH: Radiographic bone surveys in the evaluation of primary bone tumors in dogs. J Am Vet Med Assoc 188(5):514–516, 1986

16a. Hurd C, Cantorell HD, Hahn KA: Nuclear scintigraphy as a prognostic tool for canine osteosarcoma. Proc Vet Cancer Soc 7:1, 1988

16b. Berg J, Lamb C, O'Callaghan MW: Bone scintigraphy in the initial evaluation of 70 dogs with primary bone tumors. Proc Vet Cancer Soc 7:1, 1988

16c. Ogilvie GK, Allhands RV, Reynolds HA, et al: Clinical utilization of radionuclide imaging to identify malignant mammary tumor bone metastases in the dog. Proc Vet Cancer Soc 7:33, 1987

17. Norris AM, Harauz G, Gunes NE, et al: Lymphoscintigraphy in canine mammary neoplasia. Am J Vet Res 42(2):195–199, 1982

18. Metcalf MR, Rosenthal RC, Setterr LC, et al: Canine ventral body wall lymphoscintigraphy: A comparison of ^{99m}Tc-antimony sulfide colloid and ^{99m}Tc-dextran as lymphoscintigraphic agents. Vet Rad 27(5):155–160, 1986

19. Rodgers KS, Barton CL, Hightower D: Canine lymphoscintigraphy using technetium-99m labled dextran. Proc Vet Cancer Soc 6:6, 1986

20. Perman V, Alasker RD, Riis RC: Cytology of the Dog and Cat. South Bend, IN, American Animal Hospital Association, 1979

21. Rebar AH: Handbook of Veterinary Cytology. St. Louis, Ralston Purina, 1978

22. Roszel JF: Cytologic procedures. J Am Anim Hosp Assoc 17(6):903–910, 1981

22a. McMillan MC, Kleine LJ, Carpenter JL: Fluoroscopically guided percutaneous fine-needle aspiration biopsy of thoracic lesions in dogs and cats. Vet Rad 29(3):194–197, 1988

23. Schabel EM: Concepts for systemic treatment of micrometastasis. Cancer 35(1):15–24, 1975

23a. Withrow SJ, Straw RC, Richter SC, et al: Pulmonary metastasectomy for canine osteosarcoma. Proc Vet Cancer Soc 8:2, 1988

24. Spreafico F, Mantovan A, Giavazzi R, et al: Metastatic potential of metastases, tumor cell heterogeneity and therapeutic implications. Recent Results Cancer Res 80:1–8, 1982

25. Fidler IJ: Tumor heterogeneity and the biology

of cancer invasion and metastasis. Cancer Res 38(10):2651–2660, 1978

26. Hoover HC, Ketcham AS: Metastasis of metastases. Am J Surg 130:405–411, 1975

27. Rosenthal RC: Chemotherapy. In Slatter DH (ed), Textbook of Small Animal Surgery, pp. 2405–2417. Philadelphia, WB Saunders, 1985

28. Fidler IJ: Destruction of heterogeneous metastasis by tumoricidal macrophages. Proceedings of the 36th Annual Symposium on Fundamental Cancer Research: Cancer Invasion and Metastasis, pp. 53–55. Houston, MD Anderson Hospital and Tumor Institute, 1983

29. Smith BW, MacEwen EG, Manley P, et al: Liposome-encapsulated muramyl tripeptide as treatment of metastatic disease in canine ostersarcoma: Preliminary findings. Proc Vet Cancer Soc 6:5, 1986

29a. MacEwen EG, Kurzman ID, Rosenthal RC, et al: Therapy of osteosarcoma in dogs with intravenous injection of liposome-encapsulated muramyl tripeptide. J Natl Cancer Inst (in press)

30. Nomi S, Pellis NR, Kahan BD: Antigen-specific therapy of experimental metastases. Cancer 55:1296–1302, 1983

31. Helicappell R, Schirrmacher V, von Hoegen P, et al: Prevention of metastatic spread by postoperative immunotherapy with virally modified autologous tumor cells. I. Parameters for optimal therapuetic effects. Intl J Cancer 37:569–577, 1986

32. Giraldi T, Sava G: Selective antimetastic drugs (review). Anticancer Res 1(1):163–174, 1981

33. Bastida E: The metastatic cascade: Potential approaches for the inhibition of metastasis. Sem Thromb Hemostat 14(1):66–72, 1988

5

PARANEOPLASTIC SYNDROMES

Gregory K. Ogilvie

The symptoms produced by cancer are commonly viewed as manifestations of direct or metastatic involvement of a part of an animal's body. Tumors can also produce important nonmetastatic alterations of the metabolism and function of virtually all body parts. These systemic effects of cancer are known as paraneoplastic syndromes; they are often entirely unrelated to the normal physiologic activities of the mature tissue in which the tumor originated. Paraneoplastic syndromes are usually caused by the production and release into the circulation of unusual amounts or varieties of micromolecules. The best characterized paraneoplastic syndromes are those produced by a polypeptide hormone secreted by the tumor and distributed by the circulation to distant sites. There are many nonendocrine organ-associated paraneoplastic syndromes for which there is no known etiologic substance or macromolecule. Indeed, in veterinary medicine, the cause of the vast majority of paraneoplastic syndromes is not known. Although not rare, paraneoplastic syndromes develop in a minority of veterinary cancer patients. These syndromes will be recognized in a greater percentage of cancer-bearing animals as awareness of the syndromes expands. A partial list of paraneoplastic syndromes and associated malignant conditions seen in animals is listed in Table 5-1.

The importance of paraneoplastic syndromes is often underestimated. Clinically, they can cause greater morbidity than the malignant tumor. They may be the first sign of a malignancy and may be so severe that appropriate therapy for the underlying cancer is not initiated.

This chapter will review some of the most common paraneoplastic syndromes in veterinary medicine. For the interested reader, several excellent reviews are available.[1-3]

CANCER CACHEXIA

A profound state of malnutrition and wasting is a frequent and important systemic effect of cancer. The weight loss observed in cancer patients in spite of adequate nutritional intake

Table 5-1. Paraneoplastic Syndromes and Associated Tumors

CANCER CACHEXIA	HEMATOLOGIC-HEMOSTATIC ABNORMALITIES
Multiple tumors	*Anemia*
ECTOPIC HORMONE PRODUCTION	Multiple tumors
Hypercalcemia producing factors	*Disseminated intravascular coagulation*
Lymphoma	Hemangiosarcoma
Mammary adenocarcinoma	Thyroid carcinoma
Multiple myeloma	Inflammatory carcinoma
Epidermoid carcinoma	Multiple other tumors
Anal sac apocrine gland adenocarcinoma	*Leukocytosis*
Parathyroid tumors	Lymphoma
Gastric carcinoma	Multiple other tumors
Thyroid carcinoma	*Thrombocytopenia*
Nasal carcinoma	Lymphoma
Thymoma	Mammary adenocarcinoma
Hypoglycemia producing factors	Nasal adenocarcinoma
Hepatocellular carcinoma	Mast cell tumor
Oral melanoma	Hemangiosarcoma
Hemangiosarcoma	Fibrosarcoma
Salivary gland adenocarcinoma	*Hyperproteinemia*
Hepatoma	Multiple myeloma
Plasmacytoid tumor	Lymphoma
Lymphoma	RENAL MANIFESTATIONS
Leiomyosarcoma	*Nephrotic syndrome*
Erythropoietin	Multiple myeloma
Primary or metastatic renal tumors	*Renal disease due to hypercalcemia, amyloid, paraproteins*
Lymphoma	Multiple tumors
Hepatic tumor	FEVER
ACTH	Multiple tumors
Primary lung tumor	NEUROLOGIC ABNORMALITIES
HYPERTROPHIC OSTEOPATHY	Lymphoma
Primary lung tumor	Myelomonocytic neoplasia
Rhabdomyosarcoma (bladder)	Thymoma
Lung metastases	Beta cell tumor
Esophageal sarcomas	Primary lung tumor

is termed cancer cachexia. Unfortunately, cancer cachexia has an estimated incidence of 45% to 87% in hospitalized human patients.[4,5] Since the annual incidence rate of cancer is higher in dogs than in people,[6] cancer cachexia has the potential of being an even more significant problem in dogs.[7]

Human patients affected with cancer cachexia have a decreased quality of life, decreased response to treatment, and a shortened survival time when compared to people with similar neoplastic disease who do not have cachexia.[4,8,9] The tremendous prognostic significance of cancer cachexia is illustrated by the finding that survival of people affected with some cancers is more accurately predicted on the degree of cachexia present than on whether the person receives treatment.[10,11]

Although the underlying mechanisms of cancer cachexia are complex, alterations in carbohydrate, lipid, and protein metabolism are most important in the pathogenesis of this disorder. The profound alterations observed in carbohydrate metabolism result in a net energy gain by the tumor and a net energy loss by the host. Glucose is the preferred substrate for energy production by tumor cells. Instead of completely oxidizing to yield 36 moles of adenosine triphosphate (ATP) per mole of glucose and forming carbon dioxide and water as it does in most normal cells, glucose in cancer cells enters glycolysis and is incompletely metabolized; it yields only two moles of high energy phosphate bonds in the form of ATP and forms lactate as an end product.[4,10,12] This inefficient metabolism requires large quantities of glucose to meet energy needs and deprives host cells of the glucose they need.[10] In order to meet such large glucose requirements, the lactate produced by the tumor is converted back to glucose by host hepatocytes. The host incurs an additional energy expenditure of 12 molecules of ATP for every glucose molecule produced from lactate.[10] The end result is a shift in carbohydrate metabolism by the host from energy-producing oxidative pathways to energy-requiring gluconeogenic pathways with a net energy gain by the tumor and a net energy loss by the host.[4,10,13] In cancer-bearing animals glucose intolerance is seen before cachexia is noted.[13]

In cancer cachexia, protein degradation exceeds protein synthesis, and the result is a negative nitrogen balance.[4,14,15] Since all protein is functional, net protein loss in cancer cachexia results in compromised host bodily functions including cell-mediated and humoral immunity, gastrointestinal function, and wound healing. An increase in breakdown of host proteins is required to supply amino acids for protein synthesis by tumors and to supply amino acid substrates for accelerated gluconeogenesis in the host liver.[4,14,15] Since fatty acids cannot serve as gluconeogenic precursors, besides lactate, amino acids are the primary substrate for gluconeogenesis in cancer cachexia.

The majority of weight loss in cancer cachexia is due to depletion of body fat. Patients with cancer have increased fat lysis, which correlates with increased levels of free fatty acids and plasma lipoproteins.[16,17] Tumor cells have difficulty using lipids as a fuel source, while the host tissues can continue to oxidize lipids for energy.[17]

Cancer cachexia is most commonly recognized clinically as weight loss in spite of adequate nutritional intake, an increase in infections due to an impaired immune system, and decreased wound healing. The treatment for this important paraneoplastic syndrome includes such supportive care as dietary therapy. With dietary manipulation, cancer cachexia may be abated and in some cases reversed.[5,14] Detrimental effects, such as increased rate of tumor growth or rate of metastasis, have not been demonstrated in human patients receiving dietary therapy for cancer cachexia. Diets that contain 30% to 50% of nonprotein calories as fat instead of carbohydrate decrease glucose intolerance, fat loss,

and tumor growth and increase host weight, nitrogen, and energy balance.[4,5,16,17]

Although research identifying the optimum diet for cancer-bearing dogs and cats has not been done, some general principles apply. The first is that the patient should receive nutritional elements orally or by other means through the gastrointestinal tract whenever possible. Whenever oral feeding is not possible, nasogastric, gastrostomy and enterostomy tube feeding should be used.[18] Because diets that provide calories as fat combined with adequate amino acids to achieve nitrogen balance have been shown to promote the greatest host improvement with the least evidence of tumor stimulation, the following diet has been recommended for the cancer-bearing dog and cat:[19]

RECIPE FOR ORAL NUTRITIONAL SUPPORT OF DOGS OR CATS WITH CANCER

1 lb ground beef, cooked but not drained
¼ lb liver
½ cup cooked rice
1 teaspoon vegetable oil
2 teaspoons bone meal
Yield: 1.5 lb

RECIPE FOR TUBE FEEDING FOR NUTRITIONAL SUPPORT OF DOGS OR CATS WITH CANCER

¼ cup vegetable oil
½ lb above recipe
2½ cups of electrolyte solution

Cancer-bearing dogs and cats should be fed nutritionally adequate diets of 1.5 to 3 times the calories of their basal energy requirement (BER = 30 [wt in kg] + 70). Delivery of food should be achieved gradually over 24 to 72 hours.

ECTOPIC HORMONE PRODUCTION

HYPERCALCEMIA

Cancer is the most common cause of hypercalcemia in the dog and cat. Tumors that have been reported to be associated with hypercalcemia in dogs and cats are lymphoma, apocrine gland adenocarcinoma of the anal sac, multiple myeloma, thyroid carcinoma, mammary adenocarcinoma, tumors infiltrating bone, and neoplasia of the parathyroid gland.[20] Lymphoma is the most common cause of tumor-associated hypercalcemia (pseudohyperparathyroidism); a large percentage of dogs with hypercalcemia secondary to lymphoma will have the mediastinal form of the disease. The incidence of hypercalcemia in veterinary patients is not known; however, up to 30% of human cancer patients develop this paraneoplastic syndrome during the course of their disease.[21]

Several mechanisms are associated with the development of hypercalcemia in human and animal cancer patients, including lytic bone metastases, true hyperparathyroidism occurring simultaneously with the malignant disease, ectopic tumor-produced parathormone (PTH), tumor-produced prostaglandins (PGE_1, PGE_2), and tumor-produced osteoclast-activating factor (OAF).[2,3,20,22] Despite the identification of the etiopathogenesis of hypercalcemia in select cases, the cause of the electrolyte abnormality in the majority of animals is not known. Other differentials that must be considered when an animal is presented for true hypercalcemia ($Ca^{++} > 12$ mg/dl) include laboratory error, error in interpretation (e.g., young growing dogs), hyperproteinemia due to dehydration, acute renal failure, vitamin D and calcium toxicosis, granulomatous disorders, non-neoplastic disorders of bone, hypoadrenocorticism, and chronic disuse osteoporosis.[23]

It is important to interpret calcium in relation to serum albumin and the blood pH. A correction formula that takes the albumin into account is as follows:

$$\text{adjusted calcium (mg/dl)} = [\text{calcium (mg/dl)} - \text{albumin (g/dl)}] + 3.5$$

Acidosis results in an increase in the free, ionized fraction of calcium and can magnify the observed clinical signs associated with hypercalcemia.

The predominant clinical manifestations of hypercalcemia due to malignant disease usually result from alterations in renal function.[23] The first thing noted is an inability to concentrate urine. There is a decreased sensitivity to pH of the distal convoluted tubules and collecting ducts. The vasoconstrictive properties of calcium decrease renal blood flow and glomerular filtration rate (GFR). The epithelium undergoes degenerative changes, necrosis, and calcification. The progressive renal disease is noted clinically as polyuria, polydipsia, vomiting, hyposthenuria, and dehydration. Calcium can also affect the gastrointestinal, cardiovascular and neurologic systems directly; it causes anorexia, vomiting, constipation, bradycardia, hypertension, skeletal muscle weakness, depression, stupor, coma, and seizures.

The diagnosis of the cause of hypercalcemia due to malignant disease may be difficult. Frequent associated laboratory findings include azotemia, normo- or hypophosphatemia, hypercalciuria, hyperphosphaturia, hypernaturia, and decreased GFR as noted during a creatinine clearance study. Table 5-2 reviews the laboratory findings for the more common causes of hypercalcemia.

The identification and specific treatment of the underlying cause of hypercalcemia should be the primary objective in each case. Premature and inappropriate administration of symptomatic therapy may interfere with the identification of the source of the electrolyte abnormality. The treatment of hypercalcemia that results from neoplastic diseases involves the appropriate use of surgery, chemotherapy, radiation therapy, and biological response modifiers.

It is often necessary to use symptomatic therapy while searching for the underlying cause or administering specific therapy. The overall goals of symptomatic therapy include increasing renal

Table 5-2.   Hypercalcemia: Differential Diagnoses

DISEASE	SERUM Ca^{++}	SERUM PO$_4$	BONE LESION	TISSUE MINERAL- IZATION
Primary hyperparathyroidism (parathyroid tumors)	High	Low	+ + + +	+ + +
Vitamin D intoxication	High	High	+/−	+ + + +
Bone metastases (mammary, prostatic tumors, etc.)	High	Normal– elevated	+ + + +	+ +
Pseudohyperparathyroidism (lymphoma, nasal tumors, etc.)	High	Low	+/−	+ + +

excretion of calcium, inhibiting bone reabsorption, promoting calcium deposition in soft tissues, and promoting external loss of calcium.[23] The severity of the hypercalcemia and the resulting clinical signs will dictate the choice of treatment agents and their dosages. The administration of 0.9% NaCl (45–80 ml/kg every 24 hrs) intravenously is effective in expanding the extracellular fluid volume, increasing GFR, decreasing renal tubular calcium reabsorption, and enhancing calcium and sodium excretion. The thiazide diuretic furosemide (1–4 mg/kg BID IV or PO) is often administered concurrently to well-hydrated hypercalcemic patients; the drug inhibits calcium resorption at the level of the ascending loop of Henle. Prednisone (0.5–1 mg/kg BID PO) is very effective in treating hypercalcemia because it inhibits OAF, prostaglandins, vitamin D, and the absorption of calcium across the intestinal tract. The glucocorticoid is also cytotoxic to some tumors, notably lymphoma, the most common malignant cause of hypercalcemia. Therefore, caution is indicated when administering prednisone; the drug may obscure the extent of the tumor and thus delay a diagnosis of lymphoma and appropriate therapy. Other treatments that may be considered in unusual cases include calcitonin, mithramycin, prostaglandin synthetase inhibitors, and oral phosphate.[23] My limited experience with calcitonin (4–8 international units/kg SQ, given once) suggests that the drug causes a dramatic, rapid reduction in calcium levels, which may remain low for days. Mithramycin is also very effective (25 μ/kg IV, once or twice weekly).

HYPOGLYCEMIA

Insulinoma is one of the most common causes of hypoglycemia (blood glucose < 70 mg/dl) in the dog. In addition, non-islet cell tumors that are sources of ectopic hormone production have also been shown to cause hypoglycemia in man and dogs.[24-27] The majority of non-islet cell tumors associated with the paraneoplastic syndrome of hypoglycemia in the dog are hepatocellular carcinomas; other reported tumors include a hepatoma, plasmacytoid tumor, lymphoma, leiomyosarcoma, oral melanoma, hemangiosarcoma, and a salivary gland adenocarcinoma.[25-28] In contrast to insulinomas, which produce excessive quantities of insulin, extra-

pancreatic tumors in the dog have been associated with hypoglycemia, which produces low to low-normal insulin levels.[25] Possible mechanisms of hypoglycemia in cases of extrapancreatic tumors include secretion of an insulinlike substance, accelerated use of glucose by the tumor, and failure of gluconeogenesis or glycogenolysis by the liver. The most common differential diagnoses of hypoglycemia include hyperinsulinism, hepatic dysfunction, adrenocortical insufficiency, hypopituitarism, extrapancreatic tumors, starvation, sepsis, and laboratory error.

Clinical signs associated with hypoglycemia in companion animals are generally seen when the blood glucose falls below 45 mg/dl. Neurologic signs predominate because carbohydrate reserve is limited in neural tissue and brain function depends on an adequate quantity of glucose. The neurologic signs include weakness, disorientation, and seizures that may progress to convulsions, coma, and death. Hypoglycemia is a potent stimulus for the release of catecholamines, growth hormone, glucocorticoids, and glucagon. These substances tend to compensate for hypoglycemia by promoting glucogenolysis. It is not possible to identify the cause of hypoglycemia in many extrapancreatic tumors. Insulin-producing tumors may be diagnosed by identifying elevated insulin levels in association with low blood glucose concentrations. Periodic sampling during a 72-hour fast may be necessary to identify times when the blood glucose is dramatically reduced and the insulin level elevated. Although controversial, the amended insulin-glucose ratio has been advocated as a method to help diagnose insulin-producing tumors in domestic animals.[29]

$$\frac{\text{serum insulin } (\mu U/ml \times 100)}{\text{serum glucose } (mg/dl) - 30} =$$
amended insulin-glucose ratio

Values above 30 are suggestive of a diagnosis of an insulinoma or other insulin-producing tumor.

Surgical extirpation is the treatment of choice for tumors that produce hypoglycemia. In the case of insulinomas, a partial pancreatectomy may be indicated; iatrogenic pancreatitis and diabetes mellitus are recognized complications. Medical management is often necessary before, during, and after definitive therapy, especially in cases of insulinomas where the metastatic rate is high. Prednisone (0.5–2 mg/kg divided BID PO) is often effective in elevating blood glucose levels by inducing hepatic gluconeogenesis and decreasing peripheral utilization of glucose.[30] Diazoxide (10–40 mg/kg divided BID PO) is effective in elevating blood glucose levels by directly inhibiting pancreatic insulin secretion and glucose uptake by tissues, enhancing epinephrine-induced glycogenolysis, and increasing the rate of mobilization of free fatty acids.[30,31] Diazoxide's hyperglycemic effects can be potentiated by concurrently administering hydrochlorothiazide (2–4 mg/kg daily PO). Propranolol (0.2–1.0 mg/kg. PO TID), a β-adrenergic-blocking agent, may also be effective in increasing blood glucose levels by blocking insulin release through the blockage of β-adrenergic receptors at the level of the pancreatic beta cell, inhibition of insulin release by membrane stabilization, and alteration of peripheral insulin receptor affinity.[32] Combined surgical and medical management of pancreatic tumors has been associated with remission times of a year or more.

ERYTHROPOIETIN

The glycoprotein hormone, erythropoietin, is normally produced by the kidney in dogs and cats and by the carotid bodies of cats. Excessive erythropoietin levels result in increased red cell production by increasing the differentiation of early stages of red blood cells. Tumors that have infrequently been shown to induce a pathologic increase in the red blood cell mass by direct or indirect means include renal cell tumors, lymphoma, and hepatic tumors.[33] A renal tumor mass may cause local kidney hypoxia and induce excess erythropoietin production leading to a secondary inappropriate erythrocytosis. Tumors of the kidney may produce erythropoietin directly.[33] Other causes of polycythemia include dehydration, pulmonary and cardiac disorders, venoarterial shunts, Cushing's disease, the chronic administration of adrenocortical steroids, and polycythemia vera.[34] Polycythemia vera is thought to be a myeloproliferative disorder that results from a clonal proliferation of red blood cell precursors.

Erythrocytosis of paraneoplastic origin can be distinguished from polycythemia vera by the absence of pancytosis or splenomegaly and from secondary polycythemia by the absence of de-

creased arterial oxygen saturation.[35] Surgical removal of the erythropoietin-producing tumor is the treatment of choice. Phlebotomies may be of assistance in temporarily reducing the red blood cell load. The chemotherapeutic agent, hydroxyurea (40–50 mg/kg divided BID PO) can be used to induce reversible bone marrow suppression by inhibiting DNA synthesis without inhibiting RNA or protein synthesis.[34]

OTHER SYNDROMES OF ECTOPIC HORMONE PRODUCTION

One of the best characterized and most frequently encountered ectopic hormone syndromes in human medicine is the syndrome of inappropriate secretion of antidiuretic hormone. Although recognized in a variety of cancers in man, it is largely unrecognized in veterinary oncology. The diagnostic criteria for the syndrome of inappropriate secretion of antidiuretic hormone include hypo-osmolality and hyponatremia of extracellular fluids, urine that is less than maximally dilute, absence of volume depletion, sustained renal excretion of sodium, and normal renal and adrenal function.[21] The clinical signs result from the excess retention of water. They include weakness and lethargy that may progress to seizures, coma, and death.

The ectopic production of adrenocorticotropic hormone (ACTH) or related polypeptides has been described for a variety of cancers in man, including small-cell lung cancer, bronchial carcinoids, islet cell tumors of the pancreas, medullary cancer, and pheochromocytoma.[21] This condition has been reported to occur in a primary lung tumor in a dog.[36] This syndrome results from excessive production of steroids from normal adrenal glands that are under the influence of the ectopic production of ACTH or ACTH-like substances. Clinical signs that may be seen are similar to those of Cushing's disease; in addition, muscle weakness, lethargy, weight loss, pronounced hypokalemia, metabolic alkalosis, glucose intolerance, and mild hypertension may be identified. The tumors are rarely suppressible with dexamethasone.[21]

HYPERTROPHIC OSTEOPATHY

Hypertrophic osteopathy is a bony disease of dogs and cats that is often associated with primary and metastatic lung tumors. Other extrathoracic tumors such as the esophageal sarcoma and rhabdomyosarcoma of the urinary bladder have also been identified with this paraneoplastic syndrome.[36-39] Pneumonia, heartworm disease, congenital and acquired heart disease, and focal lung atelectasis have also been implicated in this condition.[37] The disease results in an increase in peripheral blood flow and a periosteal proliferation of new bone along the shafts of long bones, often beginning with the digits and extending as far proximally as the femur and humerus. Initially, there is soft-tissue proliferation followed by a production of osteophytes that tend to radiate from the cortices at 90 degrees (Fig. 5-1).[37] The cause of this unique syndrome is unknown; however, the successful treatment by vagotomy suggests a neurovascular mechanism that may involve a reflex emanating from the tumor and the nearby pleura which is carried through afferent vagal fibers.[40] Prednisone offers temporary improvement in clinical signs; the glucocorticoid may also reduce the extent of swelling. Other factors incriminated include hyperestrogenism, deficient oxygenation, and increased blood flow.[41] Removal of the tumor can result in a resolution of clinical signs and a regression of the bony changes. Other treatments such as unilateral vagotomy on the side of the lung lesion, incision through the parietal pleura, subperiosteal rib resection, or bilateral cervical vagotomy, and the use of analgesics have been suggested.[42]

HEMATOLOGIC-HEMOSTATIC ABNORMALITIES

ANEMIA

One of the most common hematologic abnormalities associated with cancer is anemia. The disorder is found in at least 20% of human cancer patients and has been identified as a significant problem in cancer-bearing companion animals.[43] The mechanisms associated with the development of anemia are numerous (Table 5-3).[43]

Anemia of chronic inflammatory disease is commonly seen in animals with metastatic or disseminated tumors. A shortened erythrocyte life-span, disordered iron metabolism, depressed bone marrow response, and disordered iron storage characterize this type of anemia.[43]

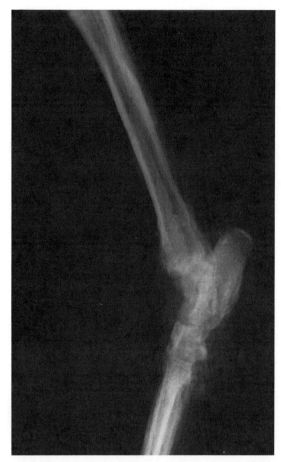

Figure 5-1. Hypertrophic osteopathy in the hind limb of a dog with a primary lung tumor. Note marked periosteal reaction typical of hypertrophic osteopathy.

Clinically, anemia of chronic inflammatory disease is recognized by normocytic and normochromic blood cells, normal bone marrow cellularity, depressed iron metabolism, and

Table 5-3. Types of Anemias in Cancer-Bearing Small Animals

Anemia of chronic inflammatory disease
Blood loss anemia
Leukoerythroblastic anemia
Microangiopathic hemolytic anemia
Immune-mediated hemolytic anemia
Hematopoietic dysplasia
Chemotherapy-induced nonregenerative anemia
Hypersplenism
Histiocytic medullary reticulosis
Megaloblastic anemia
Red cell aplasia

reticuloendothelial iron sequestration. The treatment is directed at elimination of the neoplastic condition.

Blood-loss anemia is seen in many types of cancer and may be recognized when the red blood cells are microcytic and hypochromic due to decreased hemoglobin synthesis. Poikilocytosis, microleptocytosis, inadequate reticulocytosis, increased total iron-binding capacity, decreased serum iron concentrations, and elevated platelet counts may also be seen in this condition.[44,45] The blood loss may be obvious, such as what is seen in bleeding superficial tumors, or inapparent, such as with bladder or gastrointestinal tumors. The marked decrease in serum iron concentration may be treated with ferrous sulfate (10–20 mg daily PO), accompanied by appropriate steps to eliminate the tumor.[45]

Microangiopathic hemolytic anemia can be secondary to hemolysis in the arteriolar circulation resulting from damage to arteriolar endothelium or from fibrin deposition within the artery.[43] An important cause of this type of anemia is cancer-induced disseminated intravascular coagulation. Hemolysis and schistocytosis are the hallmark of microangiopathic hemolytic anemia. A variety of tumors, including hemangiosarcoma, have been associated with this condition. Removal of the tumor and appropriate supportive care (intravenous fluids) may be useful in this type of anemia.

Immune-mediated hemolytic anemia is sometimes triggered by tumors in animals. It results in premature destruction of red blood cells by immune mechanisms.[46,47] The diagnosis is based on finding antibody or complement on the surface of the patient's red blood cells through a Coomb's test or slide agglutination test, spherocytosis, and nonregenerative anemia. Medical management with prednisone ($\leq$ 2 mg/kg daily PO) and azathoprine (2 mg/kg daily for 4 days, then 0.5–1 mg/kg every other day PO) may be indicated if a rapid resolution of the underlying neoplastic condition is not possible.[46] Contrary to some reports, cyclophosphamide may be of limited value in treating immune-mediated hemolytic anemia and associated conditions in the dog.[48]

Chemotherapy-induced nonregenerative anemia is seen in animals with bone marrow hypoplasia of the erythroid or other cell lines. It results in a decreased red cell mass, normal erythrocytic indices, and an inadequate reticu-locytosis.[43] Chemotherapeutic agents frequently cause a reduction of white blood cells and platelets. The degree of anemia associated with the administration of chemotherapeutic agents is generally mild and not associated with clinical signs.

Other less likely causes of cancer-induced anemia include leukoerythroblastic anemia, hematopoietic dysplasia, hypersplenism, erythrophagocytosis, megaloblastic anemia, and red cell aplasia.[43] Many of the mentioned mechanisms work alone or in concert to induce a decrease in red blood cell numbers. Clinical signs relating to the anemia may be overshadowed by the manifestations of the underlying neoplastic condition, but they can limit the quality of life of the cancer-bearing animal.

LEUKOCYTOSIS

An elevation in the white blood cell count has been seen in a variety of people with cancer and in dogs with lymphoma.[49,50] The mechanism of the elevated white blood cell count is obscure; it may involve a granulopoietic factor of the tumor or result from tissue necrosis and granulocyte breakdown with a positive feedback initiating an increase in the production of neutrophils.[50] The condition is not generally of clinical significance.

THROMBOCYTOPENIA

The incidence of thrombocytopenia in tumor-bearing dogs has been reported to be as high as 36%.[47] Mechanisms associated with the decrease in platelet numbers in dogs with cancer include decreased platelet production from the bone marrow, sequestration of platelets in capillaries, increased platelet consumption as in disseminated intravascular coagulation (DIC), and increased platelet destruction. One investigator reported that platelet consumption was the most significant hemostatic abnormality in tumor-bearing dogs.[51] In addition, decreased platelet numbers and elevated plasma fibrinogen concentrations were most often seen in animals with extensive tumors involving spleen or marrow.[51] DIC, a common cause of platelet consumption, is seen in 39% of all dogs with the condition.[30] If DIC is suspected, prolongation of clotting times (activated coagulation time, one step prothrombin time, and activated partial

sultant impaired concentrating ability caused by increased serum viscosity.[53] Neurologic signs (*e.g.*, seizures, ataxia, nystagmus) occur secondary to CNS tissue hypoxia due to altered blood flow and diminished delivery of O_2 to neural tissue. A hypertrophic cardiomyopathy-like state may occur, followed by generalized cardiac failure because of the excessive cardiac workload secondary to the high volume of hyperviscous blood. Myocardial hypoxia may also occur. The treatment of M-component disorders revolves around appropriate antitumor and supportive therapies. Multiple myeloma has been reported to respond to melphalan (0.1 mg/kg daily for 10 days, then 0.05 mg/kg daily PO) and prednisone (0.5 mg/kg daily PO) therapy with a median survival time of 18 months.[53] Radiation therapy and surgery may also be of value in select cases. Lymphoma may be best treated with doxorubicin as a single agent, or with combination chemotherapy using cyclophosphamide, vincristine, prednisone and doxorubicin.[55] The hyperviscosity syndrome may require immediate therapy directed to the reduction of the protein levels in the blood. Plasmaphoresis has been shown to be effective in rapidly reducing protein levels in patients exhibiting signs associated with the hyperviscosity syndrome.[56] Supportive care involves fluid therapy to treat dehydration. Antibiotics are often indicated because myeloma cells are thought to secrete an immunosuppressive substance that suppresses macrophage and lymphocyte function.

FEVER

Fever that is not associated with infection may be a manifestation of malignant disease. The increase body temperature may be mediated by a tumor-produced lymphokine (*e.g.*, interleukin 1) or reactive macrophages that release lymphokines in response to the tumor. Although the incidence of cancer-associated fever is not known in animals, in humans up to 40% of fevers of unknown origin will be found to be caused by cancer.[21] Fever that is directly related to malignant disease can be treated symptomatically with antipyretics or nonsteroidal anti–inflammatory agents. A resolution of the underlying malignant condition will usually result in a disappearance of the fever.

NEUROLOGIC ABNORMALITIES

The remote effects of cancer on the nervous system result in a wide variety of clinical signs. To constitute a true paraneoplastic syndrome, these conditions must not result from tumors directly involving the nervous system. The cause of these neurologic syndromes is not well understood. There are several reports in the veterinary literature of cancer-induced peripheral neuropathies, including a case of trigeminal nerve paralysis and Horner's syndrome in the dog.[57–61] Animals also exhibit neurologic signs secondary to endocrine, fluid, and electrolyte disturbances that result from neoplasia. Hypercalcemia, hyperviscosity syndrome, and hepatoencephalopathy are common examples. The neurologic syndromes of myasthenia gravis (*e.g.*, megaesophagus, acetyl cholinesterase-responsive neuropathy) secondary to thymoma are well described in the literature. The elimination of the neoplastic condition may result in a resolution of these neurologic syndromes.

REFERENCES

1. Hall TC: Paraneoplastic syndromes. Ann NY Acad Sci 230:1–577, 1974
2. Odell WD, Wolfsen AR: Hormonal syndromes associated with cancer. Ann Rev Med 29:379–406, 1978
3. Blackman MR, Rosen SW, Weintraub BD: Ectopic hormones. Ann Intern Med 23:85–113, 1978
4. Landel AM, Hammond WG, Megiud MM: Apsects of amino acid and protein metabolism in cancer-bearing states. Cancer 55:230–237, 1985
5. Chory ET, Mullen JL: Nutritional support of the cancer patient: Delivery systems and formulations. Surg Clin North Am 66:1105–1120, 1986
6. Dorn CR: Epidemiology of canine and feline tumors. J Am Anim Hosp Assoc 12:307–312, 1976
7. Crowe SE, Oliver J: Cancer cachexia. Compend Contin Educ Pract Vet 3:681–690, 1981
8. DeWys WD, Begg C, et al: The impact of malnutrition on treatment results in breast cancer. Cancer Treat Rep (suppl) 65:87–91, 1981
9. Harvey KB, Moldawer LL, et al: Biological measures for the formulation of a hospital prog-

nostic index. Am J Clin Nutr 34:2013–2022, 1981

10. Herber D, Byerly LO, et al: Pathophysiology of malnutrition in the adult cancer patient. Cancer 58:1867–1873, 1986

11. Fields ALA, Cheema-Dhadli S, et al: Theoretical aspects of weight loss in patients with cancer. Cancer 50:2183–2188, 1982

12. Daly JM, Copeland EM, Dudrick SJ: Effects of intravenous nutrition on tumor growth and host immunocompetence in malnourished animals. Surgery 44:655–659, 1978

13. Chlebowski RT, Heber D: Metabolic abnormalities in cancer patients: Carbohydrate metabolism. Surg Clin North Am 66:957–968, 1986

14. Landel AM, Hammond WG, Meguid MM: Aspects of amino acid and protein metabolism in cancer-bearing states. Cancer 55:230–237, 1985

15. Tayek JA, Bristrian BR, et al: Improved protein kinetics and albumin synthesis by branched chain amino acid-enriched total parenteral nutrition in cancer cachexia. Cancer 58:147–157, 1986

16. Dempsey DT, Mullen JL: Macronutrient requirements in the malnourished cancer patient. Cancer 55:290–294, 1985

17. McAndrew PF: Fat metabolism and cancer. Surg Clin North Am 66:1003–1012, 1986

18. Crowe DT: Enteral nutrition for critically ill or injured patients. Pt II. Compend Contin Educ Pract Vet 10:719–732, 1986

19. Hodgkins E: Metabolic alterations and nutritional support in the small animal cancer patient, pp. 1–24 (monograph). Topeka, Kansas, Hill's Pet Products, Inc, 1987

20. Meuten DJ: Hypercalcemia. Vet Clin North Am 14:891–910, 1984

21. Griffin TW, Rosenthal PE, Costanza ME: Paraneoplastic and endocrine syndromes. In Cady B (ed), Cancer Manual, 7th ed, pp. 373–390. Boston, American Cancer Society, 1986

22. Cryer PE, Kissane JM: Clinicopathologic conference: Malignant hypercalcemia. Am J Med 65:486–494, 1979.

23. Kruger JM, Osborne CA, Polzin DJ: Treatment of hypercalcemia. In Current Veterinary Therapy IX, Kirk RW (ed), p. 75–90. Philadelphia, WB Saunders, 1986

24. Brennan MD: Hypoglycemia in association with non-islet cell tumors. In Service FJ (ed), Hypoglycemic Disorders: Pathogenesis, Diagnosis, and Treatment, pp. 143–151. Boston, G K Hall Medical Publishers, 1983

25. Leifer CE, Peterson ME, Matus RE, Patnaik AK: Hypoglycemia associated with nonislet cell tumors in 13 dogs. J Am Vet Med Assoc 186:53–55, 1985

26. Strombeck DR, Krum S, Meyer D, et al: Hypoglycemia and hypoinsulinemia associated with hepatoma in the dog. J Am Vet Med Assoc 169:811–812, 1976

27. DiBartola SP, Reynolds HA: Hypoglycemia and polyclonal gammopathy in a dog with plasma cell dyscrasia. J Am Vet Med Assoc 180:1345–1349, 1982

28. deSchepper J, Vandestock J, deRick A: Hypercalcemia and hypoglycemia in a case of lymphatic leukemia in the dog. Vet Rec 94:602–603, 1974

29. Allen TA: Canine hypoglycemia. In Kirk RW (ed), Current Veterinary Therapy VIII, pp. 845–850. Philadelphia, WB Saunders, 1983

30. Feldman EC: Disease of the endocrine pancreas. In Ettinger SJ (ed), Textbook of Veterinary Internal Medicine, pp. 1615–1649. Philadelphia, WB Saunders, 1983

31. Leifer CE, Peterson ME: Hypoglycemia. Vet Clin North Am 14:873–889, 1984

32. Scandellari C, Zaccaria M, de Palo C, et al: The effect of propranolol on hypoglycemia: Observation in five insulinoma patients. Diabetologia 15:279–302, 1978

33. Giger U, Gorman NT: Acute complications of cancer and cancer therapy. In Gorman NT (ed), Oncology, pp. 147–168. New York, Churchill Livingstone, 1986

34. Peterson ME, Randolph JF: Diagnosis and treatment of polycythemia vera. In Kirk RW (ed), Current Veterinary Therapy VIII, pp. 406–408. Philadelphia, WB Saunders, 1983

35. Hammond D, Winnick S: Paraneoplastic erythrocytosis and ectopic erythropoietins. Ann NY Acad Sci 230:219–226, 1974

36. Ogilvie GK, Haschek WM, Weigel RM, Withrow SJ, et al: Canine primary lung tumors: Prognostic factors for remission and survival after surgery. J Am Vet Med Assoc (in press)

37. Brody RS: Hypertrophic pulmonary osteoarthropathy in the dog: A clinicopathologic survey of 60 cases. J Am Vet Med Assoc 178:1242–1256, 1971

38. Halliwell WH, Ackerman N: Botryoid rhabdomyosarcoma of the urinary bladder and hypertrophic osteoarthropathy in a young dog. J Am Vet Med Assoc 165:911–913, 1974

39. Wandera JG: Further observations on canine spirocircosis in Kenya. Vet Rec 99:348–351, 1976

40. Daly PA, Chang P, Goodman L, Wiernik PH: Hypertrophic pulmonary osteoarthropathy and metastases from a malignant fibrous histiocytoma. Cancer 45:595–598, 1980

41. Holing HE: Hypertrophic pulmonary osteopathy. J Thorac Cardiovasc Surg 46:310–321, 1963

42. Brodey RS: Hypertrophic osteoarthropathy. In Spontaneous Animal Models of Human Disease, pp. 23–54. New York, Academic Press, Inc, 1980

43. Madewell BR, Feldman BF: Characterization of anemias associated with neoplasia in small animals. J Am Vet Med Assoc 176:419–425, 1980

44. Beck WS: Hypochromic anemias. Iron deficiency and excess. In Beck WS (ed): Hematology, pp. 127–151. Cambridge, MA, MIT Press, 1977

45. Feldman BF: Management of the anemic dog. In Kirk RW (ed): Current Veterinary Therapy VIII, pp. 395–400. Philadelphia, WB Saunders, 1983

46. Dodds WJ: Autoimmune hemolytic disease and other causes of immune-mediated anemia: An overview. J Am Anim Hosp Assoc 13:437–441, 1977

47. Madewell BR, Feldman BF, O'Neil S: Coagulation abnormalities in dogs with neoplastic disease. Thromb Haemost 44:35–38, 1980

48. Ogilvie GK, Felsberg PJ, Harris SW: Short term effect of cyclophosphamide and azathioprine on the selected aspects of the canine immune system. J Vet Immunol Immunopathol 18:119–127, 1988

49. MacEwen EG, Patnaik AK, Wilkins RJ: Diagnosis and treatment of canine hematopoietic neoplasms. Vet Clin North Am 7:107–119, 1977

50. Robinson WA: Granulocytosis in neoplasia. Ann NY Acad Sci 230:212–217, 1974

51. O'Donnell MR, Stichter SJ, Weiden PL, Storb R: Platelet and fibrinogen kinetics and canine tumors. Cancer Res 41:1379–1383, 1981

52. Helfand SC, Couto CG, Madewell BR: Immune-mediated thrombocytopenia associated with solid tumors in dogs. J Am Anim Hosp Assoc 21:787–794, 1985

53. MacEwen EG, Hurvitz AI: Diagnosis and management of monoclonal gammopathies. Vet Clin North Am 7:119–132, 1977

54. Dewhirst MW, Stump GL, Hurvitz AI: Idiopathic monoclonal (IgA) gammopathy in a dog. J Am Vet Med Assoc 170:1313–1316, 1977

55. Cotter SM, Goldstein MA: Comparison of two protocols for maintenance of remission in dogs and lymphoma. J Am Anim Hosp Assoc 23:495–499, 1987

56. Matus RE, Leifer CE: Immunoglobulin-producing tumors. Vet Clin North Am 15:741–753, 1985

57. Presthus J, Teige J: Peripheral neuropathy associated with lymphoma in a dog. J Small Anim Pract 27:463–469, 1976

58. Carpenter JL, King NW, Abrams KL: Pheochromocytoma in dogs: 13 cases. J Am Vet Med Assoc 191:1594–1596, 1987

59. Cardinet GH, Holliday TA: Neuromuscular diseases of domestic animals: A summary of muscle biopsies from 159 cases. Ann NY Acad Sci 317:290–313, 1979

60. Shahar R, Rosseau C, Steiss J: Peripheral polyneuropathy in a dog with functional islet B-cell tumor and widespread metastases. J Am Vet Med Assoc 187:175–177, 1985

61. Sorjonen DA, Braund KG, Hoff EJ: Paraplegia and subclinical neuromyopathy associated with a primary lung tumor in a dog. J Am Vet Med Assoc 180:1209–1211, 1982

6

CYTOLOGIC TECHNIQUES IN CANCER DIAGNOSIS

Peter S. MacWilliams

Diagnosis and clinical management of malignant tumors in animals involve frequent use of laboratory tests. In addition to hematology, clinical chemistry, and radiographic studies, veterinarians frequently collect samples for microscopic evaluation of cellular detail as a part of the diagnostic process. Diagnostic cytology, exfoliative cytology, and cytopathology are similar terms used to describe the microscopic examination of cells that either exfoliate freely from epithelial surfaces or that are removed from tissues by mechanical means such as aspiration, scraping, or flushing.

This chapter summarizes the advantages, limitations, and applications of diagnostic cytology in cancer diagnosis. Collection, slide preparation, and staining of cytologic specimens are emphasized along with general principles of microscopic examination and interpretation. Chapters on specific tissues or locations should be consulted for detailed descriptions of specific tumors. Several books and publications contain color photomicrographs of the cytologic appearance of neoplasia.[1–9]

ADVANTAGES AND LIMITATIONS

In general, collection and processing of cytology specimens are simple procedures that require minimal equipment and provide results rapidly at a low level of risk to the animal.[3,10] Specimens that are examined frequently in the diagnosis of cancer, such as bone marrow, fine-needle aspirates of tissue masses and lymph nodes, or fluids from body cavities, can be collected and examined microscopically in less than half an hour. Collection requires appropriate needles, syringes, glass slides, and aseptic technique. Most specimens can be collected with only manual restraint of the animal. Tranquilization or infiltration of the skin overlying the sampling site with a local anesthetic is usually unnecessary. Simplicity of collection and avoidance of general anesthesia minimize patient risk. Studies in human beings and the experience of veterinary oncologists and pathologists indicate that chances of spreading a malignant tumor as a result of cytologic collection are remote.[11,12]

Diagnostic cytology offers significant time savings in the differential diagnosis of cancer.[13] For example, a Wright-stained slide of a fine-needle aspiration of an ulcerated skin lesion on the hind limb of an old dog may reveal a homogeneous population of round cells with single, round to oval nuclei and numerous small, fine basophilic cytoplasmic granules (see Fig. 17-2). In this case, inflammatory disease could be eliminated from consideration and a diagnosis of mast cell tumor could be made in a few minutes. The client can be informed, and prognosis and avenues of treatment can be discussed immediately. A surgical biopsy and examination of a histologic section would require hospitalization, anesthesia, surgery, and a delay of a few days or weeks for mailing, processing, and interpretation. By shortening the time between presentation and diagnosis, client anxiety is minimized, significant cost savings can be achieved, and treatment can be initiated more rapidly.[3,8,13,14] All of these factors contribute to more effective client relations.

Cytopathology serves several purposes in cancer diagnosis. During the initial phase of examination, specimens from affected tissues, organs, or body cavities can be examined to differentiate between neoplasia and inflammation.[3] Such differentiation is one of the most important and frequent uses for diagnostic cytology in clinical oncology. If a diagnosis of cancer is confirmed, cytologic findings can provide information for staging, prognosis, and detection of metastasis; selection and assessment of treatment; and detection of recurrence.[3,10] Surgical biopsy is necessary when the cytology reveals suspicious but inconclusive evidence of malignancy.

Limitations of a diagnostic procedure must be recognized when results are interpreted. Observations and conclusions in diagnostic cytology are based on the morphology of individual cells, cell clusters, and tissue fragments. Collection and slide preparation destroy tissue architecture. Histologic features that are lost or obscured in cytologic preparations include infiltration of surrounding tissue, invasion of vessels and lymphatics, and stromal characteristic such as palisading, whorling, fibroplasia, or mineralization.

Several factors determine the contribution or success of diagnostic cytology in cancer diagnosis. The person examining the specimen needs the complete history, clinical findings, location and description of lesion, and a definition of the question to be answered as a result of the submission.[3] Specimen quality is a major determinant of success and is affected by method of collection, preparation of smears, preservation or shipment of samples, and staining technique.[10] There is a definite advantage in having the same person collect the specimen, make the smears, and examine the slides microscopically.[13] An adequate well-stained specimen that is representative of the lesion can reveal valuable information when examined by an astute observer. Caution is necessary when applying cytologic findings to major clinical decisions. Considering the limitations and variables, a surgical biopsy with histologic confirmation is recommended when expensive therapy, radiation, radical surgery, or euthanasia is a possible decision.

TYPES OF SPECIMENS

A variety of specimens can be useful in cancer diagnosis. Major categories include fluid specimens, needle aspirations, impression smears, and scrapings, washes, or brushings of epithelial surfaces.[1,6] Abdominal or thoracic fluid is frequently evaluated when clinical or radiographic evidence indicates an effusion.[15] Other examples of liquid specimens that can be examined for cancer cells include urine and fluids collected from the prostate, subarachnoid space, and chambers of the eye.[6] Bone marrow aspirations and fine-needle aspiration of lesions, tissue masses, lymph nodes, and other organs represent an important category.[16] Palpable lesions are especially amenable to fine-needle aspiration, but with roentgenographic localization, deep, nonpalpable lesions or organs can be aspirated. Some lesions, because of their location or texture, require brushing, scraping, coring, or surgical biopsy to obtain representative samples. Impression smears of excised tissues or biopsy specimens prior to formalin fixation provide rapid, timely information.[1] Cytologic material can be washed from epithelial surfaces as occurs with a nasal flush, transtracheal or bronchial wash, and lavages of organ lumens and body cavities.[4,17]

SPECIMEN COLLECTION

An important aspect of diagnostic cytology is to have the necessary equipment and supplies available for collection and preparation. Specific requirements vary with the type of specimen. For general purposes, a cytology tray should contain needles, syringes, glass slides, specimen tubes, pencil, scalpel blades, fine forceps, formalin-filled jars, and paper towels.[12] Specialized instruments include bone marrow needles, Tru-Cut* needle for core biopsy, and spinal needles (Fig. 6-1). Glass slides should be of high quality, precleaned, and frosted on one end for marking. Unforseen events can occur during collection, such as clotting of fluid samples from body cavities or from tissue masses that were thought to be solid but, in fact, contained fluid-filled cystic areas. Not having the correct specimen tube within quick reach can render a specimen useless and necessitate recollection. In addition to plain tubes, the tray should have sterile tubes and tubes containing ethylenediaminetetraacetic acid (EDTA).[6] Spray fixative or 95% ethanol are necessary for some staining techniques that require wet fixation.

Collection and slide preparation are major determinants of diagnostic success in the fine-needle aspiration of lesions or organs.[4,10,11,14] For most aspirates, a 22-, 23-, or 25-gauge needle and a 6- or 12-cc syringe are adequate.[1,6,13] Larger-bore needles are sometimes necessary for fibrotic lesions, but their routine use is discouraged because they cause more hemorrhage and contaminate the specimen with blood.[13] Needle length is determined by the size, depth, and location of the target site, but for the majority of procedures, a 1- or 1.5-inch needle is preferred. Careful palpation of the target lesion or organ is an important first step to detect variations in consistency, define margins, and identify surrounding structures.[12] The site should be clipped of hair and washed, and a surgical disinfectant should be applied. Surgical gloves are usually unnecessary; they interfere with tactile sensation. The lesion is localized and fixed in position with one hand. The needle is inserted briskly through the skin and into the target area. The syringe plunger is withdrawn to produce suction while the needle tip is moved within the tissue along several axes. This is

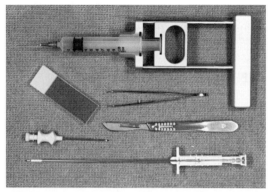

Figure 6-1. Materials for slide preparation and specialized instruments for sample collection. Franzen syringe holder *(top)* allows one-handed control of needle angle and syringe for fine-needle aspirations. Cores of soft-tissue masses can be obtained with a Tru-cut biopsy needle *(bottom)*. Large hub and stylet of a Rosenthal needle *(bottom left)* are advantageous for aspiration of bone marrow.

accomplished by withdrawing the needle slightly without leaving the target lesion and reinserting at a different angle. Redirecting the needle within the tissue while maintaining suction collects cells and tissue fragments in the needle bore from different locations. Very little material will appear within the syringe barrel unless fluid is encountered or hemorrhage occurs during collection. The syringe plunger is released to relieve suction before the needle is withdrawn from the target lesion. This step is very important because removing the needle with negative pressure in the syringe will draw cellular material from the needle into the syringe, where it usually adheres to the barrel or plunger and is irretrievably lost. A second complication is specimen contamination with hemorrhage by aspiration of blood vessels in surrounding tissue during withdrawal. Immediately after removal from the site, the needle is separated from the syringe, air is drawn into the syringe, and the needle is reconnected. Small amounts of needle contents are applied to glass slides for preparation of smears by forcing air through the needle. Most clinicians prefer plastic syringes with plain Luer tip rather than those with Luer-Lok tip because the latter frequently hinder the rapid removal and reattachment of needles. A Franzen syringe holder* (Fig. 6-1) is an option

---

* Tru-Cut, Travenol Laboratories, Deerfield, IL 60015.

* Cameco Syringe Pistol, Precision Dynamic Corp., 3031 Thornton Avenue, Burbank, CA 91504.

that gives the operator single-handed control of aspiration and needle angle and frees the other hand for palpation and fixation of the lesion.[12,13]

PREPARATION OF SLIDES

The consistency of the aspirated material determines the method of smear preparation. Smears of cavity fluids or fine-needle aspirates with the consistency of blood are prepared in the same manner as blood films.[4,6] For either specimen, the film of cells should occupy two-thirds of the glass surface and have the shape of a thumbprint. Cytology films that go to the end of the slide are too long; they are a disadvantage because cell clusters significant to the diagnosis may be lost or carried to the extreme edges, where staining and visibility are poor. The length of the film depends on the size of the drop, the viscosity of the fluid, and the angle and speed of the slide used for spreading.[5] Thick, tenacious specimens require a low spreading angle and slower speed. The opposite is necessary for thin, watery fluids.

Additional procedures are sometimes indicated if a milliliter or more of fluid is obtained from a tissue space or body cavity. Enumeration of erythrocytes and nucleated cells along with measurement of total protein and specific gravity provide information that is useful in cancer diagnosis.[15] Fluids with low cell numbers require some form of concentration before slides are made.[5] Thoracic and abdominal fluids can be sedimented by allowing cells to settle undisturbed in a vertical tube for 10 to 30 minutes. Centrifugation at a moderate force (800 g for 5 min.) is the usual method of concentration. Supernatant is removed after sedimentation or centrifugation. Smears are made from drops of sediment or cell button that has been resuspended in a small amount of supernatant. The cytocentrifuge* is a specialized instrument for preparing consistent films of fluid specimens, especially those with low cell count and limited volume.[5]

Red blood cells may obscure the microscopic examination of cells or cell aggregates on smears of hemorrhagic fluids. This problem can be alleviated by making smears from the upper layers of sedimented or centrifuged cells. The

* Cytospin, Shandon Southern Instruments, Sewickley, PA 15143.

upper layers contain higher numbers of nucleated cells, which can be removed with a microhematocrit tube or pipette. Alternatively, a capillary tube of bloody fluid can be spun in a microhematocrit centrifuge. Smears of nucleated cells concentrated in the buffy coat are made by breaking the capillary tube at the erythrocyte-leukocyte interface.

The squash method of slide preparation (Fig. 6-2) produces a cellular monolayer by dislodging cells from tissue fragments.[4] Squash preparations are suited for making smears of thick, semisolid material or of macroscopic particles observed in fluid samples and fine-needle aspirates.[6] Pasteur pipettes or capillary tubes can be used to retrieve particles from fluid specimens. Discrete fragments in fine-needle aspirates can be isolated with thin forceps after the syringe contents have been expressed onto a glass slide. A small drop of material or tissue fragment is placed on a glass slide at one end. The specimen is gently compressed by placing a second slide on top. The cellular material is spread by pulling the two slides apart.

Impression smears of excised tissues provide immediate information to the clinician and augment the histopathologic findings by revealing cellular details not visible in histologic sections.[4] For tissues with the consistency of lymph node, a flat, fresh-cut surface is exposed by trimming the tissue with a blade (Fig. 6-3). Blotting the cut surface on a paper towel removes excess blood and tissue juice. Cells are exfoliated by gently pressing the blotted tissue surface to a glass slide.[6] Firm tissues require mincing or scraping with a blade to dislodge cells (Fig. 6-3). With a technique similar to the one for collecting a skin scraping, the fresh-cut surface is scraped with the flat edge of a scalpel. Cellular material that accumulates on the blade edge is smeared on a glass slide using the blade as a spreader.[6]

FIXATION AND CYTOLOGIC STAINS

Slides should be labeled with a pencil or permanent marker before being stained or submitted to a laboratory. This is especially important if more than one site or more than one location within a site is sampled. The choice of stain determines the method of fixation.[4] Wright stain and new methylene blue (NMB) use air-dried

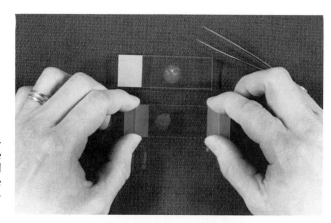

Figure 6-2. Squash method of slide preparation. Small tissue fragment from fine-needle aspirate *(top slide)* is placed on one slide and covered with a second slide. Drawing the two slides apart in opposite directions produces an even film of cells.

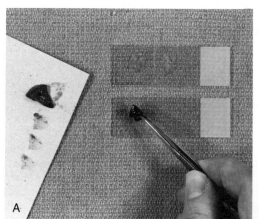

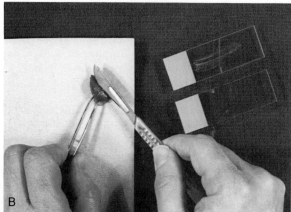

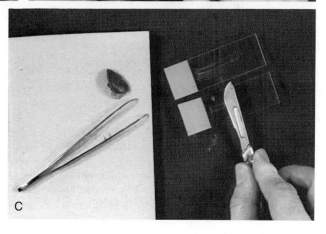

Figure 6-3. Preparation of impression smears. Fresh surface is exposed by cutting with a blade. Cut surface of tissue is blotted on a paper towel to remove excess blood and then touched to a glass slide *(A)*. Firm tissues require a different technique. Fresh-cut surface is scraped with a blade *(B)*. Cellular material on blade edge is spread on a slide *(C)*.

smears. Once slides are made and dried, they should be stained within one or two days. Air-dried smears should not be refrigerated. Stains such as Papanicolaou and Sano trichrome require immediate fixation in 95% ethanol before the cellular material dries.[1,8,18]

NMB, Wright stain, and other Romanovsky stains similar to Wright, such as Diff-Quik,* Geimsa, Leishman, or May-Grunwald, are the

* Diff-Quik, American Scientific Products, McGraw Park, IL 60085.

stains used most frequently in veterinary cytology.[1,4,5] Most veterinarians are familiar with the microscopic appearance of cells stained with Wright and Diff-Quik because both stains are used for routine examination of blood films. These stains produce a rainbow of color resulting from varying shades of pink, red, blue, and purple. Definition of cytoplasmic texture, granules, and vacuoles is excellent, but the nuclear chromatin pattern is course and smudged and therefore obscures nucleolar morphology (Fig. 6-4).[1,7] Users of Diff-Quik are cautioned that cytoplasmic granules of mast cells sometimes fail to stain.[4,7] Staining times need to be increased for cytology smears that are more dense than blood films. For staining cellular smears, exposure times are frequently increased two- or threefold above those required for blood films.[4] Papanicolaou, Wright, and other Romanovsky stains can be decolorized by dipping in acid-alcohol* if the cells are overstained or if it is necessary to remove stain so that other more specialized stains can be applied.[19]

New methylene blue has the advantage of being a rapid stain that allows immediate viewing, but slides are not permanent.[4] A small drop of NMB applied directly to an air-dried smear is covered with a coverslip for viewing as a wet mount. Colors produced by NMB are limited to varying shades of blue and purple. Erythrocytes do not stain with NMB. This feature allows examination of cells in bloody specimens that would be obscured if stained with Wright or Diff-Quik. Fat and cholesterol crystals are not dissolved because NMB is water soluble. Compared to Wright stain, NMB enhances nuclear detail by producing a clear, distinct image of nuclear membrane, chromatin pattern, and nucleolus.[5] Because it is a wet mount, NMB allows three-dimensional visualization of cells and depth perception of cell clumps, but the slide will dry out within an hour unless the edges are sealed with mounting glue. A permanent slide can be made if the coverslip is removed gently while the slide is wet. The slide is immersed carefully in water to remove NMB, air-dried, and then restained with Wright. When the advantages and limitations of Wright and NMB are considered, it is not surprising that these stains are often used in conjunction.

* 1% solution of HCl in 70% ethanol (10 ml of concentrated HCl in 990 ml of 70% ethanol).

Papanicolaou stain is the standard method used in human cytopathology.[19] The Sano trichrome method produces similar results, and modifications of it have been developed for animal specimens.[1,8,18] Both stains require that slides be fixed immediately before drying by immersion in 95% ethanol or sprayed with cytologic fixative or unscented hair spray. A few seconds' delay in fixation will induce air-drying artifacts in the cells. Cells and tissue fragments prepared with Papanicolaou or Sano trichrome stain bear close resemblance to their counterparts in histologic sections.[5] Anatomical pathologists usually prefer wet-fixed slides stained with either stain for cytologic evaluation. These staining procedures require multiple reagent baths, constant replenishment, and filtration of some components.[7] Cells stained by these methods have superb nuclear detail and the added advantage of transparency, which allows a three-dimensional view of nuclear and cellular configurations. Features that are especially well-defined include nuclear chromatin, nucleolus, and the shape and thickness of the nuclear membrane (Fig. 6-4). Granules, vacuoles, and other cytoplasmic details are poorly defined. Table 6-1 summarizes a rapid, predictable, and easy to maintain modification of Papanicolaou stain suitable for animal specimens. Reagents for this method are more readily available than some of those required for Sano trichrome.

Additional diagnostic information can be obtained by fixing appropriate portions of cytology samples for preparation of histologic sections. Tissue fragments and clots from fine-needle aspirations, lavages, and washes can be separated and placed in 10% buffered formalin.[4,10,12] The cellular button resulting from sedimentation and centrifugation can be similarly fixed by removing supernatant and gently layering formalin on top of the sediment. After fixation, the pellet of cells is submitted to a diagnostic laboratory. Examination of these sections by a pathologist may provide information on tissue architecture to supplement or confirm the cytologic evaluation.

Cytology specimens are frequently submitted to outside laboratories for primary diagnosis or for a second opinion.[4] All too often, the condition of the sample on arrival precludes a thorough assessment. The outside laboratory should be consulted for specific mailing and fixation requirements. For general purposes, several air-

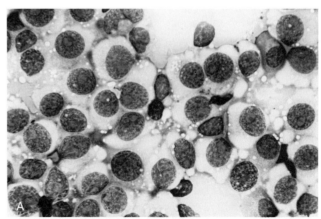

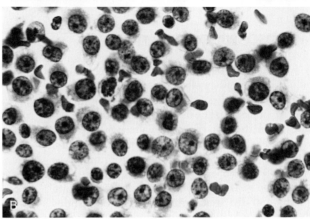

Figure 6-4. Microscopic comparison of neoplastic cells stained with Wright and with modified Papanicolaou (850 ×). Wright stain slide *(A)* of a canine transmissible venereal tumor reveals a uniform population of round cells with round to oval eccentric nuclei, granular chromatin, and prominent nucleoli. Cell margins are distinct, and small, round, sharply defined cytoplasmic vacuoles are obvious. Cells from the same tumor on the Papanicolaou-stained slide *(B)* appear smaller because of alcohol fixation. Cell margins and cytoplasmic features are difficult to see. Details of nuclei that are especially visible with this stain include size, shape, and number of nucleoli, shape and configuration of nuclear membranes, and characteristics and distribution of chromatin.

dried, unstained smears should be made and labeled. Fluids with low cell count should be centrifuged and smears of sediment prepared. For excised tissues, slides should be made by impression and by scraping the cut surface. Stained slides can be submitted, but by including several unstained slides, the pathologist has the option of slide selection and choice of stain. Some laboratories supply mailing containers. Most laboratories prefer rigid plastic or foam containers for mailing slides (Fig. 6-5). Glass slides in cardboard slide mailers usually break when mailed in an envelope. Exposure of air-dried slides to formalin vapors interferes with the staining process and renders the slides useless for cytologic examination. Slides mailed in the same package as formalin-fixed specimens should be put in an air-tight container or plastic bag.[4]

Table 6-1.   Modified Papanicolaou Stain*

1. Wet fixation in 95% ethanol for minimum of 15 minutes
2. Gill hematoxylin,† 2–5 minutes
3. Distilled water changed repeatedly until water is clear
4. Ammonia water, 2 dips (2 ml conc. NH₄OH in 1 l water)
5. Distilled water, 2 dips
6. 95% Ethanol, 5 dips
7. 95% Ethanol, 5 dips
8. Orange G-6 (OG-6),† 2–3 minutes
9. 95% Ethanol, 5 dips
10. 95% Ethanol, 5 dips
11. Eosin-alcohol 50 (EA-50),† 2–3 minutes
12. 95% Ethanol, 5 dips
13. 95% Ethanol, 5 dips
14. Xylene, 5 dips
15. Xylene, 5 dips
16. Permanent coverslip applied without allowing slide to dry

* Montgomery JL: Personal communication, 1987.
† Harleco, Gibbstown, NJ 08027, or American Scientific Products, McGraw Park, IL 60085.

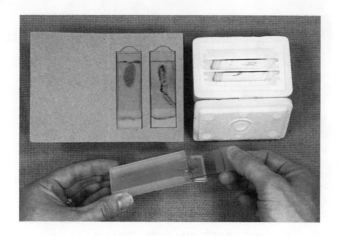

Figure 6-5. Mailing containers for glass slides. Containers made with foam *(right)* or plastic *(bottom)* minimize slide damage. Cardboard slide flats *(left)* are not rigid enough to prevent breakage unless they are boxed prior to mailing.

MICROSCOPIC EXAMINATION

A systemic approach to the microscopic examination of a cytology slide that is representative and well stained contributes valuable information in cancer diagnosis.[5] Elements to be considered in the microscopic evaluation are individual cells, cell aggregates, tissue fragments, and background.[3,20] Using low power objectives (4× and 10×), several slides from the site should be scanned to assess cellularity, stain quality and distribution of cells. The best slides should be selected for examination at higher magnifications. Low-power scanning usually reveals the location of cell aggregates, tissue fragments, or giant cells. These elements frequently collect along the feather edge of the film. Higher magnifications are used to identify cells and background features and to study nuclear and cytoplasmic details of individual cells and those in groups or clusters.

Assessment of the general characteristics and composition of the cell population is an important part of the microscopic evaluation.[3] These observations require knowledge of the history, clinical signs, source and description of the sample, and of any specimen contamination with blood during collection.[12] A composite of the cytologic features is used to differentiate between inflammatory and neoplastic disease. A predominance of neutrophils or a mixed population of neutrophils and macrophages with fewer and variable numbers of lymphocytes, plasma cells, or giant cells indicates an inflammatory process.[5,7] Benign or malignant neoplasms are characterized by the absence of inflammation and the presence of a monomorphic population of cells with general features that are similar (Figs. 6-4, 6-8).[7] If neoplasia is confirmed, cellular features may indicate (1) benign or malignant status, (2) epithelial, mesenchymal, or discrete cell origin, (3) specific cell type (*e.g.*, squamous cell, fibroblast, lymphoblast), and (4) degree of differentiation.[1,3] Necrosis or secondary sepsis of a neoplasm may produce a cytologic picture of acute or chronic inflammation (Fig. 6-6).[1]

Microscopic features frequently reveal the origin of the neoplasm.[1, 5–7] The cytologic appearance of epithelial tumors includes a highly cellular smear containing cohesive sheets, clusters, or clumps of round to oval cells with intact cell membranes and round to oval nuclei (Fig. 6-6). Neoplasms of glandular epithelium may contain acinar or ductular formations or cytoplasmic secretory products. Mesenchymal neoplasms, such as fibromas and their malignant counterpart, exfoliate poorly and yield slides that are sparsely cellular. Scrapings are usually necessary to obtain a representative specimen. Mesenchymal neoplasms exfoliate as individual cells rather than cell clusters or cohesive sheets. The cells are spindle-shaped or polyhedral and contain oval nuclei (Fig. 6-7). Cell membranes are often indistinct. Smears of discrete or round-cell tumors (histiocytoma, mast cell tumor, lymphosarcoma, transmissible venereal tumor) are very cellular with noncohesive cell clusters and numerous individual, round to oval cells (Fig. 6-8). Cell membranes are usually intact and surround a round to oval nucleus.[7]

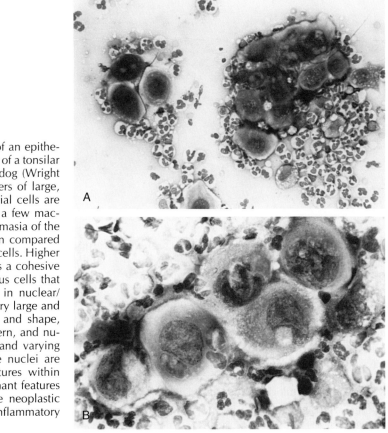

Figure 6-6. Cytologic features of an epithelial neoplasm: impression smear of a tonsilar squamous cell carcinoma in a dog (Wright stain). Two variable-sized clusters of large, pleomorphic, squamous epithelial cells are surrounded by neutrophils and a few macrophages (*A*, 340 ×). Hyperchromasia of the malignant cells is obvious when compared with the adjacent inflammatory cells. Higher magnification (*B*, 850 ×) reveals a cohesive cluster of pleomorphic squamous cells that vary in size (anisocytosis) and in nuclear/cytoplasmic ratio. Nuclei are very large and have extreme variation in size and shape, course irregular chromatin pattern, and nucleoli that are large, multiple, and varying in size and shape. Two of the nuclei are molded around adjacent structures within the cells. Recognition of malignant features is important to differentiate the neoplastic process from the confounding inflammatory response.

CRITERIA OF MALIGNANCY

Cytologic determination of benign or malignant status is of paramount importance. A cytologic diagnosis of malignancy may influence subsequent decisions such as additional procedures to detect metastases, selection of chemotherapeutic agent, need for exploratory or radical excisional surgery, or consideration of euthanasia.[1] Table 6-2 summarizes the cytologic fea-

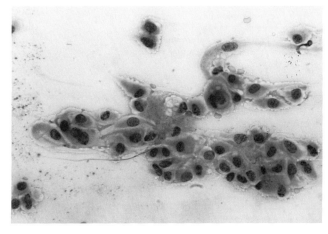

Figure 6-7. Cytologic features of a mesenchymal neoplasm: impression smear of a neurofibrosarcoma (Wright stain, 340 ×). The mass was attached to the dura of the cervical spinal cord in a dog. A uniform population of spindle-shaped cells with single, oval, or round nuclei indicates a mesenchymal neoplasm. Malignant features are not especially prominent.

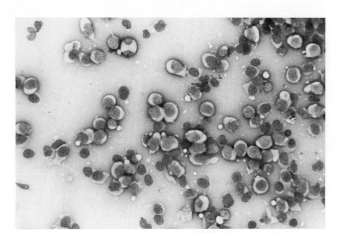

Figure 6-8. Cytologic features of a discrete cell or round-cell tumor: impression smear of a canine histiocytoma (Wright stain, 340 ×). A homogeneous population of round discrete cells and the absence of cohesive clusters are compatible with a round-cell tumor. These cells have variable amounts of pale cytoplasm and nuclei that are round, oval, or indented. Granules are not present in the cytoplasm or background.

tures of malignant tumors.[1,3,6,7,9,10,12] Irregularity, angularity, extremes, and lack of consistency are general terms that encompass many of the listed criteria.[20,21] Examples would include irregular nuclear shapes, sharp angular nucleoli, extreme variability in nuclear to cytoplasmic ratio, and inconsistent nuclear morphology among cells in a cluster or among nuclei within the same cell (Figs. 6-6, 6-9, 6-10). Only cells that

Table 6-2. Cytologic Features of Malignancy

CELLULAR
  Monomorphism: composed of the same cell type
  Pleomorphism: variation in cell morphology within the same population
  Hyperchromasia
  Anisocytosis ± giant cells
  Irregular cell clusters: prominant overlapping and molding of cells

NUCLEAR
  Variation in size (anisokaryosis) and shape
  Irregular shapes: lobulation, indentation, projections, folding
  Nuclear/cytoplasmic ratio increased and variable
  Course, irregular chromatin pattern*
  Uneven distribution of chromatin*
  Variation in thickness of nuclear membrane*
  Enlarged, multiple nucleoli
  Variation in size and shape of nucleoli
  Variation in number of nucleoli among cells
  Molding around adjacent structures or cells
  Cells with multiple nuclei exhibiting other malignant characteristics
  Abnormal mitotic figures

CYTOPLASMIC
  Irregular cell margins
  Vacuolation
  Cytoplasmic contents: granules, secretory product, phagocytosed material

* Papanicolaou or Sano trichrome stain needed for visualization.

are intact and well preserved are inspected for malignant characteristics. Broken cells or cells with degenerative alterations should be excluded. Morphologic alterations in the nucleus provide the most numerous and definitive criteria, and stains that enhance nuclear detail, such as Papanicolaou, Sano trichrome, and NMB, are advantageous.[8,18,20] There is no single morphologic feature that determines malignancy. A positive diagnosis is based on identifying at least four or more nuclear features of malignancy.[7]

Cytoplasmic features are not especially useful for establishing benign or malignant status. They are more valuable for assessing degree of differentiation and identifying cytoplasmic granules and secretory products that can suggest a specific cell or tissue origin (Figs. 17-2, 6-4).[3,20] For these purposes, the cytoplasmic detail of a slide stained with Wright or Diff-Quik is preferred.[7] Algorithmic approaches to the identification of specific cutaneous neoplasms have been developed; they use features of the nucleus, cytoplasm, background, and cell aggregates.[2,6a]

Specimens yielding equivocal findings should be reported as suspicious or inconclusive. A second collection or a surgical biopsy with histologic evaluation is indicated in these instances. Histologic confirmation is also recommended in most situations before clinical decisions of major consequence are effected. Correlations between cytologic findings and the subsequent histologic diagnoses are generally good and improve as the experience of the observer increases. Studies with human specimens indicate that cytologic diagnosis of cancer has a high degree of diagnostic accuracy and low numbers of false posi-

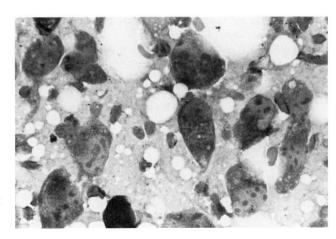

Figure 6-9 Cytologic features of malignancy with Wright stain (850×). Fine-needle aspirate of an undifferentiated sarcoma in the pelvis of a dog reveals individual polyhedral cells that are very pleomorphic. Variation in cell size and shape are extreme. Nucleoli are prominent and are extremely variable in size, shape, and number. Hyperchromasia of the cytoplasm with Wright stain does not allow visualization of nuclear margins and shapes.

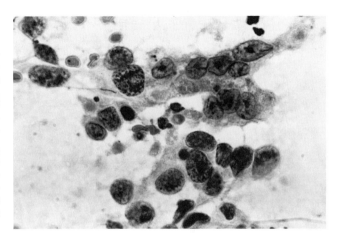

Figure 6-10. Cytologic features of malignancy with Papanicolaou stain (850×). Fine-needle aspirate of a deep mass within the hindleg of a cat reveals evidence of an undifferentiated sarcoma. Enhancement of nuclear detail with this stain allows clear visualization of irregular, angular nuclear shapes, coarse irregular chromatin pattern, variation in nucleolar size and shape, and uneven thickening of the nuclear membrane. Crowding, overlapping, and molding of nuclei to adjacent structures within clusters is also evident because of transparent nature of Papanicolaou stain.

tives.[11] A study with canine mammary tumors revealed low numbers of false positives (0–3%), high percentage of predictive positive values (90–100%), but a low level of sensitivity (17–25%)[22] These studies and an increasing level of clinical experience indicate that careful specimen collection and preparation combined with deliberate microscopic evaluation of malignant features provide reliable information that is immediate to the diagnosis of cancer.

REFERENCES

1. Allen SW, Prasse KW: Cytologic diagnosis of neoplasia and perioperative implementation. Compend Contin Educ Pract Vet 8:72–80, 1986
2. Barton CL: Cytologic diagnosis of cutaneous neoplasia: An algorithmic approach. Compend Contin Educ Pract Vet 9:20–33, 1987
3. Cardozo PL: Atlas of Clinical Cytology, pp. 13–52. Netherlands, Targa bv'S-Hertogenbosch, 1976
4. Meyer DJ: The management of cytology specimens. Compend Contin Educ Pract Vet 9:10–17, 1987
5. Perman V, Alsaker RD, Riis RC: Cytology of the Dog and Cat. South Bend, IN, American Animal Hospital Association, 1979
6. Rebar AH: Handbook of Veterinary Cytology, St. Louis, Ralston Purina Co., 1979
6a. Cowell RL, Tyler RD: Diagnostic Cytology of the Dog and Cat. Goleta, CA, American Veterinary Publications, 1989
7. Rebar AH, Boon GD, DeNicola DB: A cytologic comparison of Romanovsky stains and Papanicolaou-type stains. II. Cytology of inflammatory and neoplastic lesions. Vet Clin Pathol 11(2):16–26, 1982
8. Roszel JF: Exfoliative cytology in diagnosis of malignant canine neoplasms. Vet Scope 12:14–20, 1967

9. Takahashi M: Color Atlas of Cancer Cytology, ed 2. pp. 32–56. Tokyo, Igaku-Shoin, 1981

10. Schumann GB, Colon VF: The Clinician's Guide to Diagnostic Cytology. Chicago, Year Book Medical Publishers, 1982

11. Kline TS: Handbook of Fine Needle Aspiration Biopsy Cytology, pp. 1–7. St. Louis, CV Mosby, 1981

12. Koss LG, Woyke S, Olszewski W: Aspiration Biopsy: Cytologic Interpretation and Histologic Bases, pp. 3–21. Tokyo, Igaku-Shoin, 1984

13. Lowhagen T, Willems J: General comments on aspiration biopsy cytology. In Weid GL, Koss LG, Reagen JW (eds): Compendium on Diagnostic Cytology, ed. 5, pp. 506–511. Chicago, Tutorials of Cytology, 1983

14. Linsk JA, Franzen S: Clinical Aspiration Cytology, pp. 1–8. Philadelphia, JB Lippincott, 1983

15. Meyer DJ, Franks PT: Effusion: Classification and cytologic examination. Compend Contin Educ Pract Vet 9:123–129, 1987

16. Thrall MA: Cytology of lymphoid tissue. Compend Contin Educ Pract Vet 9:104–111, 1987

17. French TW: The use of cytology in the diagnosis of chronic nasal disorders. Compend Contin Educ Pract Vet 9:115–121, 1987

18. Roszel JF: Genital cytology of the bitch. Vet Scope 19:2–15, 1975

19. Koss LG: Diagnostic Cytology and Its Histopathologic Bases, ed. 3. pp. 1187–1227. Philadelphia, J B Lippincott, 1979

20. Frost JK: Examination of the cell. In Weid GL, Koss LG, Reagen JW (eds): Compendium on Diagnostic Cytology, ed. 5, pp. 13–14. Chicago, Tutorials of Cytology, 1983

21. Frost JK: Concepts Basic to General Cytopathology, ed. 4. Baltimore, Johns Hopkins Press, 1972

22. Allen SW, Prasse KW, Mahaffey EA: Cytologic differentiation of benign from malignant mammary tumors. Vet Pathol 23:649–655, 1986

7

BIOPSY PRINCIPLES

Stephen J. Withrow

One of the most important steps in the management of the cancer patient is the procurement and interpretation of an accurate biopsy specimen. Not only will the biopsy afford a diagnosis; it will also help to predict biologic behavior of a tumor and thus determine the type and extent of treatment that should be afforded. A casually done or omitted biopsy may have serious implications for patient management. Virtually all masses should be histologically evaluated before or after removal. If a mass warrants surgical removal, it warrants tissue analysis!

Many variations in technique and equipment for biopsy procedures are described in the veterinary literature. The common goal is to procure enough neoplastic tissue to establish an accurate diagnosis. Certainly many biopsy techniques could be used on any given tissue mass. Which procedure to use will often be determined by the goals for the case, the site of the mass, the equipment available, the general status of the patient, and the veterinarian's personal preference and experience. Specific techniques unique to specific tumors or locations will be discussed in chapters about those tumors or locations.

When should the surgeon know what he is treating *before* the actual treatment? The answer to this question is all too often overlooked. An accurate tissue diagnosis should be attained before treatment in most situations for the following reasons:

1. The type of treatment (surgery, radiation, chemotherapy, or something else) or the extent of treatment (conservative or aggressive resection) may be altered by knowing the tumor type. Certain cancers (*e.g.*, soft-tissue sarcomas, oral fibrosarcomas, or mast cell tumors) have high local recurrence rates and therefore require removal with wider margins than benign lesions. Several studies in animals and humans have shown a positive correlation between permanent local disease control (perferably after first surgery) and survival. In other words, do the resection correctly the first time. A biopsy is particularly important if the surgery is in a difficult location for reconstruction (*e.g.*, distal

extremity, tail, or head and neck) or if the proposed procedure carries significant morbidity (*e.g.*, maxillectomy or amputation). Virtually all externally accessible masses beyond benign skin tumors should be subjected to tissue biopsy prior to operative intervention.

On the other hand, if knowledge of tumor type would not change the treatment (lung lobectomy for solitary lung mass or splenectomy for splenic mass) or if the biopsy is as difficult or dangerous as the curative treatment (brain biopsy), then the biopsy information should be attained after surgical removal.

2. The owner's willingness to submit the pet to treatment might be altered by knowledge of the tumor type and therefore prognosis. For example, some owners would be willing to do a mandibulectomy for an acanthomatous epulis (benign oral tumor) with an excellent prognosis but not for a melanoma with a potentially poor prognosis.

GENERAL GUIDELINES FOR TISSUE PROCUREMENT AND FIXATION

1. The proper performance of an incisional or needle biopsy does *not* negatively influence survival, even though a short-lived increase in cancer cells can be measured in draining vessels and lymphatics. The advantages of an accurate diagnosis far outweigh the theoretical disadvantage of enhancing tumor metastasis. On the other hand, cancer cells may be allowed to contaminate the tissues surrounding the mass, making resection more difficult. Careful hemostasis and obliteration of dead space will minimize local contamination of the biopsy site. Furthermore, the biopsy site should be chosen so that it may be subsequently removed along with the entire mass. In particular, care should be taken not to "spill" cancer cells during a biopsy within the thoracic or abdominal cavities, where they may seed pleural or peritoneal surfaces.
2. The juncture of normal and abnormal tissue is frequently the best area for the pathologist to see differences in tissues as well as invasiveness. Avoid biopsies that contain only ulcerated or inflamed tissues.
3. The larger the sample, the more likely it is to be diagnostic. Tumors are not ho-

mogeneous; they usually contain areas of necrosis, inflammation, and reactive tissue. Several samples from one mass are more likely to yield an accurate diagnosis than a single sample.

4. Biopsies should not be obtained with electrocautery, which tends to deform (through autolysis or polarization) the cellular architecture. Electrocautery is better used for hemostatis after blade removal of a diagnostic specimen or not at all.
5. Care should be taken not to unduly deform the specimen with forceps, suction, or other handling methods prior to fixation.
6. If evaluation of margins of excision is desired, it is best for the surgeon to mark the specimen (fine suture on questionable edges) or submit margins in a separate container.
7. Proper fixation is extremely important. Tissue is generally fixed in 10% buffered neutral formalin with 1 part tissue to 10 parts fixative.
8. Tissue thicker than one centimeter will not fix deeply. Large masses can be cut into appropriate-size pieces and representative sections submitted or sliced like a loaf of bread, leaving one edge intact, to allow fixation. After fixation (2–3 days), tissue can be mailed with a 1:1 ratio of tissue to formalin.
9. A *detailed* history should accompany all biopsy requests. Interpretation of surgical biopsies is a combination of art and science. Without all the vital diagnostic information (signalment, history of recurrences, invasion in bone, rate of growth, and so on) the pathologist's ability to deliver accurate and clinically useful information will be significantly compromised.
10. A pathologist trained in veterinary medicine is preferred over a pathologist trained in human diseases. Although many cancers are histologically similar across species lines, enough differences exist to result in interpretive mistakes.

BIOPSY METHODS

The more commonly used methods of tissue procurement are needle punch biopsy, incisional biopsy, and excisional biopsy.

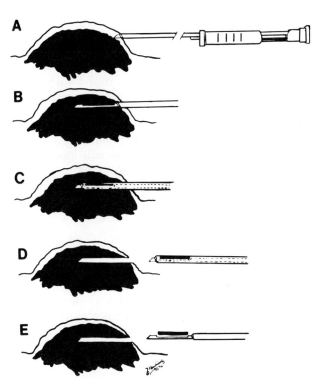

Figure 7-1. Mechanism of action of Tru-Cut biopsy needle for typical nodular tumor: *(A)* A small skin incision is made with a Number 11 blade to allow insertion of the instrument. With the instrument closed, the outer capsule is penetrated. *(B)* The outer cannula is fixed in place and the inner cannula with specimen notch is thrust into tumor. Tissue then protrudes into notch. *(C)* Inner cannula is now held steady while outer cannula is moved forward to cut off the biopsy specimen. *(D)* Entire instrument is removed closed with tissue contained within. *(E)* Inner cannula is pushed ahead to expose tissue in specimen notch.

NEEDLE PUNCH BIOPSY

This method uses various types of needle-core instruments* to obtain tissue.[1,2] The most common instrument used in our hospital is the Tru-Cut® needle. Students practice using the instrument on apples prior to biopsy of an actual tumor. If you cannot biopsy an apple, you won't have much luck on a tumor. These instruments, generally 14 gauge in diameter, procure a piece of tissue that is about the size of the lead in a lead pencil and 1 to 1.5 cm long. Even though the sample size is small, the pathologist can usually visualize the structural relationship of the tissue and tumor cells. Virtually any accessible mass can be sampled by this method. It may be used for externally located lesions or for deeply seated lesions (of the kidney, liver, or prostate, for example) by means of closed methods or at the time of open surgery.

The most common usage of the needle punch biopsy is for externally palpable masses. Except for highly inflamed and necrotic cancers (espe-

cially in the oral cavity) where incisional biopsy is preferred, most biopsies can be done on an outpatient basis with local anesthesia and only rarely sedation. The area to be biopsied is clipped and cleaned. The skin or overlying tissue is prepared as for minor surgery. If the overlying tissue (usually skin and muscle) is intact, it is blocked with local anesthetic in the region the biopsy needle will penetrate. Tumor tissue is very poorly innervated and generally does not require local anesthesia.

The clinician fixes the mass in place with one hand or has an assistant. A small 1 to 3 mm stab incision is made in the overlying skin with a scalpel blade to allow insertion of the biopsy instrument (Fig. 7-1). The tissue is gently removed from the instrument with a scalpel blade or hypodermic needle and placed in formalin. Through the same skin hole, several needle cores of tissue are removed from different sites to get a "cross section" of tissue types within the mass. Samples may be gently rolled on a glass slide for cytologic preparations before fixation. Sutures in the skin hole are generally not required. Needle biopsy tracts are probably a minimal risk for tumor seeding; in any event

---

* Franklin Modified Vim-Silverman Needle, V. Mueller Co., Chicago, IL or Tru-Cut biopsy needles, Travenol Laboratories, Deerfiled, IL, among others.

they are, if possible, removed intact with the tumor at subsequent resection.

The Tru-Cut needle with plastic casings is "disposable" and therefore cannot be steam sterilized. It may, however, be sterilized with gas (ethylene oxide) and used repeatedly until it becomes dull.

Needle-core biopsies are fast, safe, easy, and cheap, and usually they can be performed as outpatient procedures. They are generally more accurate than cytology but not as accurate as incisional or excisional biopsy.

INCISIONAL BIOPSY

Incisional biopsy is used when neither cytology nor needle-core biopsy has yielded diagnostic material. Additionally, it is preferred for ulcerated and necrotic lesions because more tissue can be obtained with this method. Under sterile conditions, a wedge of tumor tissue is removed from the mass. Ideally, a composite biopsy of normal and abnormal tissue is obtained from a location that will not compromise subsequent curative resection (Fig. 7-2). Care should be taken not to widely open uninvolved tissue

planes that could become contaminated with released tumor cells. Small incisions through muscle bellies are preferred to contaminating intramuscular compartments. The incisional biopsy tract is always removed in continuity with the tumor at subsequent resection.

EXCISIONAL BIOPSY

This method is used when the treatment would not be altered by knowledge of tumor type (*e.g.*, "benign" skin tumors, solitary lung mass, splenic mass, and others). It is more frequently performed than indicated, but when used on properly selected cases, it can be both diagnostic and therapeutic as well as cost effective.

INTERPRETATION OF RESULTS

The pathologist's job is to determine whether a tumor is present or not and, if one is present, whether it is benign or malignant and its histologic type, grade (if available) and margins (if excisional). Making an accurate diagnosis is not as simple as putting a piece of tissue in formalin

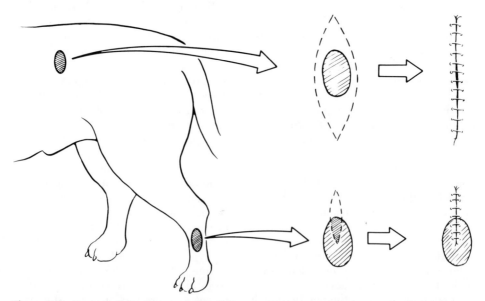

Figure 7-2. Excisional *(top)* contrasted with incisional *(bottom)* biopsy. The top tumor may be as easy to remove as to biopsy, and removal may not negatively influence other possible treatments (more surgery, radiation, and so on). The bottom tumor, however, requires knowledge of tumor type prior to excision because inappropriate removal could compromise subsequent aggressive excision (short of amputation). Note that biopsy incision is in a plane that would be included in a subsequent resection.

and waiting for results. Many pitfalls must be avoided if the end result is to be accurate. Potential errors can take place at any level of diagnosis, and it is up to the clinician in charge of the case to interpret the full meaning of the biopsy result. As many as 10% of biopsy results may be inaccurate in a clinically significant sense.

If the biopsy result does not correlate with the clinical scenario, several options are possible. The veterinarian can call the pathologist and express concern over the biopsy result. An exchange of information should be helpful for both parties and not looked upon as an affront to the pathologist's authority or expertise. The conversation may lead to resectioning of available tissue or paraffin blocks, use of special stains for certain possible tumor types (*e.g.*, toluidine blue for mast cells), or a second opinion by another pathologist. If the tumor is still present in the patient, and particularly if options for therapy widely vary, a second (or third) biopsy should be performed.

A carefully performed, submitted, and inter-preted biopsy may be the most important step in management and subsequent prognosis of the patient with cancer. All too often tumors are not submitted for histologic evaluation after removal because "the owner didn't want to pay for it." Biopsies should not be an elective owner decision. Instead, they should be as automatic as closing the skin after ovariohysterectomy (do you okay that with the owner?). The charge for submission and interpretation of the biopsy should be included in the surgery fee if need be, but the biopsy must be done. With increasing medicolegal concerns, it is not medical curiosity alone that mandates knowledge of tumor type.

REFERENCES

1. Osborne CA: Symposium on biopsy techniques. Vet Clin North Am 4:2, 1974
2. Withrow SJ, Lowes N: Biopsy techniques for use in small animal oncology. J Am Anim Hosp Assoc 17:889–902, 1981

8

SURGICAL ONCOLOGY

Stephen J. Withrow

Complete surgical removal of localized cancer cures more patients (humans and animals) than any other form of treatment.[1] Before this hope for cure can be realized, surgeons must have a thorough understanding of anatomy, physiology, resection and reconstruction options for all organs, expected tumor behavior, and the various alternatives or adjuvants to surgery. Surgical oncologists should not only be good technicians (cancer carpenters) but dedicated tumor biologists. Surgery will play a role at one point or another in the management of most cancer patients. This surgery may include any of the following: diagnosis (biopsy), resection for cure, palliation of symptoms, debulking, and a wide variety of ancillary procedures to enhance and compliment other forms of treatment.

Most patients with cancer are "old." Old is a relative term. It is much more important to know the physiologic age of the patient than its chronologic age. An "old" dog or cat with normal measurable organ function should not be denied treatment simply on the basis of age. I am aware of no cancer where the age of the patient has any bearing on tumor-related prognosis. "Old" animals will tolerate aggressive surgical intervention as well or as poorly as "young" patients.

SURGERY FOR DIAGNOSIS

Although biopsy principles are covered in another chapter (Chapter 7), it bears emphasizing that properly timed, performed, and interpreted biopsies are one of the most critical steps in the management of the cancer patient. Not only does the surgeon need to procure adequate tissue to establish a diagnosis, but the biopsy must not compromise subsequent surgical resection.

SURGERY FOR CURE

To be in a position to provide the optimal operation for the patient with cancer, the surgeon should be able to answer the following questions:

1. What is the type, stage, and grade (if available) of cancer to be treated?
2. What are the expected local and systemic effects of this tumor type and stage?
3. Is a cure possible?
4. Is an operation indicated at all?
5. What are the options for alternative treatment?

A recurring theme in surgical management of cancer is that the first surgery has the best chance of cure. Several mechanisms for this finding have been advanced. Untreated tumors have had less time to metastasize than recurrent cancer. Untreated tumors have near normal anatomy, which facilitates operative maneuvers. In recurrent disease, previously noninvolved tissue planes may have been seeded and wider resection may be required than for the initial tumor. An ill-defined negative aspect of recurrent cancer is reported to be related to changes in vascularity and local immune responses. Regardless of the mechanism, curative surgery is best performed at the first operation.

The surgical technique chosen will obviously vary with the site, size, and stage of the tumor. Some general statements about cancer surgery that need to be emphasized follow:

All incisional biopsy tracts should be excised in continuity with the primary tumor, since tumor cells are capable of growth in these wounds. Fine-needle aspiration cytology tracts are of little concern, while punch biopsy tracts are of intermediate concern. With this in mind, all biopsies should ideally be positioned in such a manner that the tracts they create can be removed at surgery.

Early vascular ligation (especially venous) should be attempted to diminish release of large tumor emboli into the systemic circulation. This is probably only clinically meaningful for tumors with a well-defined arterial and venous supply,

such as splenic tumors, retained testicles, and lung tumors. Small numbers of cancer cells are constantly being released into the venous circulation by most tumors. Larger, macroscopic cell aggregates may be more dangerous, however, and they may be prevented from vascular escape with early venous ligation.

Local control of malignant cancer requires that variable margins of normal tissue be removed around the tumor. Resection can and should be classified in more detail than simply radical or conservative (Table 8-1).[2] Tumors with high probability of local recurrence (soft-tissue sarcoma, malignant mast cell tumors, feline mammary adenocarcinoma, among others) should have 2- to 3-cm margins removed three-dimensionally. Tumors are not flat, and wide removal in one plane does not insure complete excision. Fixation of malignant cancer to adjacent structures mandates removal of the adherent area in continuity with the tumor (Fig. 8-1). This is commonly seen with oral cancer that is firmly adherent to the underlying mandible or maxilla. Invasive cancer should not be peeled out, shelled out, enucleated, curetted, or whittled on if a cure is expected. Some malignant cancers are surrounded by a pseudocapsule. This capsule is almost invariably composed of compressed tumor cells, *not* healthy reactive host cells. If a malignant tumor is opened at the time of resection, that procedure is often no better than a large biopsy. The aim should be a level of dissection that is one tissue plane away from the mass. Invasion of cancer into the medullary cavity of a bone requires subtotal or total bone resection and not curettage.

Tumors should be handled gently to avoid the risk of breaking off tumor cells into the operative wound, where they may grow. Copious lavage of all cancer wound beds will mechanically remove small numbers of exfoliated tumor cells, but this procedure should not

Table 8-1. Classification of Resection and Wound Margins[2]

TYPE OF SURGERY	PLANE OF DISSECTION	RESULT
Intracapsular	Tumor removed in pieces or curetted; "debulking"	Macroscopic disease left behind
Marginal	Removal just outside or on pseudocapsule or reactive capsule, "shelled out"	Usually leaves microscopic disease
Wide	Tumor and capsule never entered, normal tissue surrounds specimen	Possible skip lesions
Radical	Entire compartment or structure removed (e.g., amputation)	No local residual cancer

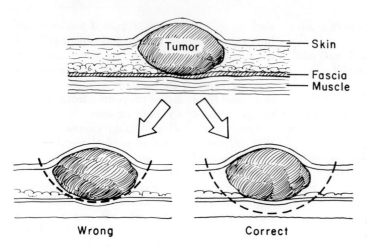

Figure 8-1. Typical soft-tissue cancer is in proximity to skin and underlying fascia. Inappropriate removal is to "peel it off" the deeper fascia, where microscopic extension is probable. Correct removal entails wide margins three-dimensionally, including overlying skin and underlying fascia.

replace gentle tissue handling and wide removal.

The aggressiveness of resection should only rarely by tempered by fears of wound closure. It is better to leave a wound partially open with no cancer than closed with residual cancer.

LYMPH NODE REMOVAL

A great deal of controversy surrounds the surgical management of regional lymph nodes draining the primary tumor site. As a general rule, epithelial cancers are more likely to metastasize to lymph nodes than are mesenchymal cancers. However, any enlarged regional lymph node requires investigation. Lymphadenopathy may be from metastasis of cancer (firm, irregular, and sometimes fixed to surrounding tissue) or from hyperplasia and reactivity to various tumor factors, infection, or inflammation. The former cause is a poor prognostic sign, and the latter may be a beneficial host response. Enlarged lymph nodes as a result of cancer metastasis and invasion are generally uniformly effaced by tumor cells and can often be diagnosed by fine-needle aspiration. Positive lymph nodes usually are a sign of impending systemic metastasis. Lymph nodes should be removed under two general circumstances.

If the lymph node is positive for cancer and not fixed to surrounding normal tissues, it may be possible to remove the node with some therapeutic intent. Frequently, however, several lymph nodes drain a primary tumor site

(e.g., the oral cavity) and lymphadenectomy is incomplete (e.g., neck dissection). Although it is usually not practical, removal of the primary tumor, intervening lymphatic ducts, and draining lymph node has been recommended (en bloc resection). En bloc resection may be possible for a malignant toe tumor with metastasis to the popliteal lymph node, but it is usually only accompanied with amputation. Few other anatomic sites are routinely amenable to this therapy.

Normal-appearing lymph nodes that are known to drain a primary tumor site can be randomly sampled (by biopsy or cytology) to gain further staging information. This is particularly important if adjuvant therapy decisions (irradiation or chemotherapy) would be predicated on confirmation of residual cancer. Intrathoracic or intra-abdominal lymph nodes are perhaps most critical since they are not readily accessible to follow-up examination.

Lymph nodes are *not* removed under two general circumstances. Lymph nodes in critical area (retropharyngeal, hilar, mesenteric) which have eroded through the capsule and become adherent (fixed) to surrounding tissues cannot be curatively removed without serious harm to the patient. They are best biopsied and left alone or treated with other modalities. The occasional exception is metastasis of limb and foot tumors to prescapular and popliteal lymph nodes, which can be removed with amputation (radical en bloc resection).

Prophylactic removal of "normal" draining lymph nodes or chains of lymph nodes (as opposed to sampling for stage) is of no benefit and may be harmful.[3] Regional lymph nodes may in fact be the initiator of favorable local and systemic immune responses, and elective removal has been associated with poor survival in certain human cancers.[4,5]

PALLIATIVE SURGERY

Palliative surgery is an attempt to improve the quality of the patient's life (to relieve pain or improve function), but not necessarily the length of the patient's life. This type of surgery requires very careful consideration of the expected operative morbidity of the procedure as opposed to the expected gain to the patient and the client. In essence, it comes down to a decision of when to give up. One of the most difficult decisions in surgical oncology is the decision *not* to operate. Treatment of any kind should never be worse than no treatment.

Certain situations exist, however, where palliative surgery may be beneficial. If an infected and draining mammary tumor in a patient with asymptomatic lung metastasis is the limiting factor in the patient's life, mastectomy may still be a logical procedure. Splenectomy for hemangiosarcoma is commonly performed but probably has little impact on survival and can be considered palliative, since it stops the threat of immediate hemorrhage but not preexisting metastasis.

DEBULKING SURGERY

Incomplete removal of a tumor (planned or unplanned) is referred to as debulking or cytoreductive surgery. It is commonly performed but rarely indicated.[6] Its theoretical indication is to enhance the efficacy of other treatment modalities. Debulking is a practical consideration prior to cryosurgery to decrease the amount of tissue to freeze and the time freezing will take. It may also help the treatment planning and dosimetry with certain forms of irradiation, but the improved cancer control achieved with subsequent irradiation is more a result of geometric considerations than removal of a few logs of tumor cells. Removing 99.9% of a 1-cm tumor (1×10^9 cells) still leaves a million cancer cells behind. Immunotherapy and chemotherapy could

theoretically be helped by tumor volume reduction,[7] but no well-controlled clinical trials have shown a benefit to date in veterinary medicine. If deep-seated tumors are debulked with the anticipation of postoperative radiation therapy, the margins of known tumor or the operative field should be marked with radiopaque metal clips to allow proper treatment planning from radiographs.

SURGERY AND CHEMOTHERAPY

The combined use of chemotherapy and surgery is becoming more commonplace in veterinary oncology. Many chemotherapy agents will impede wound healing to some extent. In spite of this risk, few clinically relevant problems occur when surgery is performed on a patient receiving chemotherapy.[8,9] General recommendations are to wait 7 to 10 days after surgery to begin chemotherapy, especially for high risk procedures.[10] The use of intraoperative or perioperative chemotherapy is receiving increased attention.[11,12] It could have a greater possibility for complicating wound healing.

SURGERY AND RADIATION

Theoretical advantages can be argued for both pre- and postoperative radiation.[13] Either way, some impairment of wound healing potential will exist. Radiation damage to normal tissues (stem cells, blood vessels, and lymphatics) is more permanent than chemotherapy damage. As radiation dose and field size increase, the potential complications (with or without surgery) increase. If radiation therapy is given preoperatively, surgery can be performed after acute radiation reactions have resolved. Postoperative radiation is recommended to start immediately after surgery or after a 2- to 3-week delay. In spite of the theoretical problems, surgery can be safely performed on irradiated tissues. The complications that may occur are not prohibitive.

PREVENTION OF CANCER

Certain common cancers in dogs and cats can be prevented. It is well known that early (< 1 yr) oophorectomy reduces the risk of breast cancer 200-fold in the dog and to a lesser degree in the cat. Castration of the male dog will help prevent perianal adenomas, prostatic adenocarcinoma, and obviously, testicular cancer. Elective removal of cryptorchid testes is another example of preventive surgery.

MISCELLANEOUS ONCOLOGIC SURGERY

With greater use of regional and intra-arterial chemotherapy, surgeons may be called upon to place long-term vascular access catheters.

Surgeons and radiotherapists may work together for the operative exposure of nonresectable cancer so that large doses of irradiation may be delivered to the tumor or tumor bed after exclusion of radiosensitive structures (Chapter 10).

DISCUSSION

It is clear that surgery will be the mainstay of cancer treatment in veterinary medicine for many years to come. It is also clear that a surgical procedure should not be performed just because it is possible. Although rhinotomy and curettage of the canine nasal cavity can be performed, the procedure does not improve survival over untreated patients.[14] Likewise, in selected patients, simple and radical mastectomies have the same influence on survival in dogs and humans, but they may have different results in the cat.[15,16] More surgery is not always better surgery. Long-term follow-up of well-staged and -graded tumors with defined surgical technique is necessary to demonstrate the true value of any operation. A great deal of progress in surgical technique and surgical thinking needs to take place before the use of surgery can be optimized. It is to be hoped that a better understanding of expected tumor biology and more precise staging methods (angiograms, CT scans, and so forth) will facilitate more precise surgical operations. In spite of these anticipated advances in technology and biology, the most difficult aspect of surgical intervention to acquire is judgment.

REFERENCES

1. Chabner BA, Curt GA, Hubbard SM: Surgical oncology research development: The perspective of the National Cancer Institute. Cancer Treat Rep 68:825–829, 1984
2. Enneking WF: Musculoskeletal Tumor Surgery. New York, Churchill-Livingstone, 1983
3. Panel report on the colloquium on clinical immunology. J Am Vet Med Assoc 181:973–976, 1982
4. Olson RM, Woods JE, Soule EH: Regional lymph node management and outcome in 100 patients with head and neck melanoma. Am J Surg 142:470–473, 1981
5. Veronesi U, Adamus J, Bandiera DC, Brennhovd IO, et al: Delayed regional lymph node dissection in Stage I melanoma of the skin of the lower extremities. Cancer 49:2420–2430, 1982
6. Moore GE: Debunking debulking. Surg Gynecol Obstet 150:395–396, 1980
7. Morton DL: Changing concepts of cancer surgery: Surgery as immunotherapy. Am J Surg 135:367–371, 1978
8. Ferguson MK: The effect of antineoplastic agents on wound healing. Surg Gynecol Obstet 154:421–429, 1982
9. Graves G, Cunningham P, Raaf JH: Effect of chemotherapy on the healing of surgical wounds. Clin Bull 10:144–149, 1980
10. van Zuidewijn DBWD, Wobbes T, Hendriks T, et al: The effect of antineoplastic agents on the healing of small intestinal anastomoses in the rat. Cancer 58:62–66, 1986
11. Fisher B, Gunduz N, Saffer EA: Influence of the interval between primary tumor removal and chemotherapy on kinetics and growth of metastases. Cancer Res 43:1488–1492, 1983
12. Fisher B: Cancer surgery: A commentary. Cancer Treat Rep 68:31–41, 1984
13. Tepper J, Million RR: Radiation therapy and surgery. Cancer Treat Symp 1:111–117, 1984
14. MacEwen EG, Withrow SJ, Patnaik AK: Nasal tumors in the dog: Retrospective evaluation of diagnosis, prognosis, and treatment. J Am Vet Med Assoc 170:45–48, 1977
15. MacEwen EG, Hayes AA, Harvey HJ, Patnaik AK, Mooney S, Passe S: Prognostic factors for feline mammary tumors. J Am Vet Med Assoc 185:201–204, 1984
16. Golinger RC: Breast cancer controversies: Surgical decisions. Semin Oncol 7:444–459, 1980

9

CHEMOTHERAPY

Robert C. Rosenthal

Chemotherapy has become a major treatment modality in veterinary oncology. Unlike surgery or radiation therapy, it is usually intended to have a systemic effect. Chemotherapy may be employed with a number of goals in mind. The ultimate goal of chemotherapy is to cure the patient of cancer. With the exception of canine transmissible venereal tumors, whether cure from chemotherapy occurs in veterinary medicine is debatable.[1] Nonetheless, chemotherapy has other benefits. It may help control generalized rapidly progressive disease not amenable to surgery or radiation therapy, and it may help increase the disease-free interval after such initial therapy. It may help prevent spread of the neoplasm by controlling early metastases that are proliferating rapidly and have a relatively small likelihood of containing resistant cells. Chemotherapy may also benefit the patient by symptomatic relief of related problems and temporary restoration of deteriorated function.[2]

Of the three major types of therapy—surgery, radiation therapy, and chemotherapy—only chemotherapy is intended to deal with systemic or undetected metastatic disease. Metastatic disease is the primary cause of death in patients with neoplasia regardless of the mode of therapy. Clearly, the more effective the chemotherapy in controlling the distant spread of the disease, the longer the comfortable survival of the patient. An understanding of the basic principles of chemotherapy can help provide a basis for sensible, effective chemotherapy and prolonged survival.

BIOLOGIC BASIS

Three aspects of cell kinetics must be considered in discussions of the biologic basis of chemotherapy: cell cycle kinetics, growth classes of tissues, and Gompertzian growth of tumors.[1,3–5]

Both normal and neoplastic cells proceed around the cell cycle in an orderly progression from mitosis to mitosis. Mitosis (M phase) marks the beginning of the cell cycle. Cell division in mammalian cells takes an average of 30 to 90 minutes. The G_1 (gap 1) phase is the period of greatest temporal variability. Days to weeks may be involved in this period of RNA and protein synthesis, depending on the tissue type. From G_1, cells may enter a G_0 phase, which is a resting, nonproliferating state. Cells may remain in G_0 for long periods or return to G_1 and proceed in the cell cycle. The period of DNA synthesis (S phase) follows G_1 and generally lasts about two hours. This is followed by the G_2 (gap 2) phase, another period of RNA and protein synthesis, which generally lasts about six to eight hours. Various chemotherapeutic agents affect the cell cycle at different phases. A knowledge of the cell cycle is fundamental to the establishment of a sensible chemotherapeutic plan.

Not all tissues behave in the same manner with respect to growth and renewal characteristics. Tissues may be grouped as static, expanding, or renewing. This classification separates highly differentiated tissues (static tissues such as nerves or striated muscle) in which cells no longer undergo mitosis from those whose cells retain the capacity for mitosis. Cells comprising tissues in the expanding group (organs and glands) can undergo mitosis with the proper stimulus. The renewing tissues are those with mitotically active cell populations such as leukocytes, erythrocytes, megakaryocytes, mucosa, epidermis, and gametes. This group of tissues made up of cells with short half-lives is precisely the group of tissues most susceptible to the effects of drugs intended to kill neoplastic cells.[1]

Just as tissues can be grouped, cells within tissues can also be categorized. A cell may have stem cell potential, may be maturing, or may be functional. A stem cell is an undifferentiated cell found in tissue undergoing renewal. Stem cells can synthesize DNA and divide. One daughter cell remains a stem cell, whereas the other differentiates more fully.[6] Stem cells respond to stimuli such as hormones or possibly to chemical feedback from mature cells, which may stimulate or inhibit division. The loss of mature cells may cause the stem cell compartment to become more active. Neoplastic cells may be dividing, temporarily nondividing, or permanently nondividing. In malignant neoplastic tissue, only a small proportion of cells are differentiated. The remainder are dividing or retain the capacity to do so. In normal tissues, only a small proportion of the cells are dividing.[4]

In both normal and neoplastic cell populations, there are relatively more dividing cells in a small population and relatively fewer dividing cells in a large population. Gompertzian growth refers to a growth pattern exhibiting increased doubling time and decreased growth fraction as a function of time.[2] The increase in doubling time is related to both the decreased proportion of proliferating cells and the increased cell loss from exfoliation, metastasis, and cell death. It is evident that the cytoreductive effects of surgery or radiation therapy can induce a renewed level of proliferative activity within a tumor and render the tumor more susceptible to chemotherapeutic attack as its constituent cells proceed around the cell cycle.

PHARMACOLOGIC FACTORS

To affect a tumor, the chemotherapeutic agent must reach the site of action. Its effectiveness is measured in terms of its concentration and exposure time at the site. The effective contact time, the product of drug concentration multiplied by drug exposure time, is affected by a number of important factors.[2] Route of administration and absorption may influence the efficacy of an administered drug. Chemotherapeutic agents may be administered orally, subcutaneously, intravenously, or intramuscularly for systemic effect. Local effect may be obtained by intralesional injection, topical administration, or introduction of the drug into the pleural cavity, peritoneal cavity, urinary bladder, or cerebrospinal fluid. Chemotherapeutic drugs may be given intra-arterially or by inhalation, but these routes are not often employed for animal patients. Biotransformation of the drug also needs to be considered. Prednisone, frequently included in chemotherapeutic protocols, must undergo hepatic conversion to prednisolone before it becomes an active drug.[7] Cyclophosphamide is likewise metabolized by the liver to an active form and is therefore effective orally or parenterally but not when locally instilled.

Distribution of a drug partially determines its effectiveness. If the drug does not reach the tumor, its exposure will be nil and the neoplastic cells will be unaffected. The blood-brain barrier represents such a problem in distribution. Most chemotherapeutic agents will not gain access to the brain. The effect of tumors on decreasing the integrity of the blood-brain barrier is still open to question. Drugs normally excluded from the brain may enter the cancer-afflicted brain because of a disrupted blood-brain barrier.

Once a drug has been properly administered, adequately absorbed, and biologically transformed into an active form, the potential for interaction with other drugs must be considered. Patients may be receiving multiple drug therapy, including therapies directed at problems other than the tumor. Drug interactions can occur in several ways. Direct chemical or physical interactions, interference with absorption or receptor binding, or altered metabolism or excretion might have an impact on a drug's net effect. For example, antibiotics might alter gastrointestinal absorption by affecting microbial flora; aspirin may interfere with binding of drugs to serum albumin.[2] The chemotherapeutic protocol itself may call for multiple drugs given simultaneously or sequentially. The potential for drug interaction is great. Possibly harmful interactions may either decrease the effectiveness of a drug to nonbeneficial levels or increase its toxicity.[8]

A final pharmacologic factor influencing chemotherapy is excretion. Most antineoplastic drugs are excreted by the kidneys or liver; if these organs are not functioning adequately to rid the body of the drug, rapid accumulation may result in severe, perhaps unmanageable, toxicity. The amount of drug given or the dosage interval may need to be adjusted to compensate for impaired excretion.[9,10]

TOXICITY

Chemotherapy treads a narrow path between efficacy and toxicity. In fact, chemotherapeutic protocols are most often limited not by the ability of drugs to kill tumor cells but by their toxicity to the patient. Recalling one of the biologic bases for chemotherapy—i.e., that the proliferating neoplastic cells can be attacked most effectively as they pass around the cell cycle—will help explain some of the more commonly noted toxicities related to renewing tissue classes. The most commonly encountered problems relate to gastrointestinal toxicity, bone marrow suppression, and immunosuppression.[8,11] Vomiting and anorexia may be noted as the gastrointestinal epithelium is affected or as

the result of effects on the central nervous system. Although these problems are usually not life-threatening, they can be detrimental to the patient. Antiemetics may or may not be helpful. Other gastrointestinal toxicities seen less frequently include diarrhea, stomatitis, esophagitis, and gastrointestinal ulceration.[12] Organ-specific dose adjustments may need to be considered for individual drugs such as doxorubicin, vincristine, and cis-platinum.[13]

Bone marrow toxicity leading to leukopenia and immune suppression affecting both humoral and cell-mediated immunity are two very serious problems associated with chemotherapy. Bone marrow toxicity may affect all the cellular components of the blood. Anemia and thrombocytopenia can be life threatening; however, because of the shorter life-span and smaller reserve of white blood cells, leukopenia and the associated risk of infection are the primary and more common problems. Different chemotherapeutic agents cause different patterns of myelosuppression; some are more profound and persistent than others. Chemotherapy may need to be postponed until acceptable numbers of white blood cells return to the peripheral blood. Recommended leukocyte counts at which to postpone therapy have been published.[2,6,14,15] One such guideline is 4000 total white blood cells per microliter with at least 2500 granulocytes per microliter. Clearly, the number of granulocytes is the most important consideration. At the present time, there is no consensus regarding the use of prophylactic antibiotics in this setting. Although infection may be difficult to document in the myelosuppressed patient, the clinician should be aware of the possibility of urinary or respiratory tract infection or septicemia and be prepared to culture and identify the organism and to treat the condition as needed. The prophylactic use of antibiotics may make specific microbial culturing more difficult and encourage the emergence of resistant strains of bacteria. Because of the increased risk of infection as granulocyte counts fall, prophylactic therapy with broad-spectrum bactericidal antibiotics, such as trimethoprim-sulfa or the third generation cephalosporin ceftazidime, may be necessary when there are fewer than 1200 granulocytes per microliter.

As veterinary oncologists use more intensive chemotherapy in the future, protocols will almost certainly be amended to reflect both the acceptance of more myelosuppression (to gain an increased likelihood of control) and improved methods of dealing with myelosuppression. Generally, chemotherapy can be reinstituted in one to two weeks, after a return to normal white blood cell parameters. When resuming chemotherapy, it may be advisable to decrease the amount of the offending drug by 25%, although it is always important to keep in mind the close relationship of toxicity and efficacy.

The problems of immunosuppression relate closely to bone marrow toxicity and myelosuppression. There is great variation in the amount of immunosuppression encountered with chemotherapy, and the clinician must be constantly aware of its dangers. The combination of reduced nonspecific immunity (myelosuppression) and impaired humoral and cell-mediated immunity can render the patient prone to serious, life-threatening infection with little or no means of defense. Fortunately, immunosuppression associated with chemotherapy usually does not last long beyond the time of drug administration. Nonetheless, chemotherapies should include as few immunosuppressive drugs as feasible without compromising the treatment.

Less common toxicities involve other body systems and vary with the drug given. For example, hemorrhagic cystitis associated with cyclophosphamide is a well-known complication that limits the prolonged use of that drug in dogs.[16] Cyclophosphamide has also been associated with the development of bladder carcinoma in dogs.[17] The bladder is not the only susceptible organ of the genitourinary system. The canine kidney is subject to damage from methotrexate, streptozotocin, and platinum compounds; doxorubicin is potentially nephrotoxic in cats.[18] Sterility in males and congenital malformations are also possible complications. Skin reactions and alopecia are less frequent in veterinary medicine than in human medicine, but they occur.[19] Clipped hair may not regrow or may regrow a different color. Wire-haired and curly-coated breeds (*i.e.*, Old English sheepdogs, poodles, pulis, Afghan hounds, and some terriers) seem more likely to develop alopecia. The lung, liver, heart, and central nervous system are all subject to toxicity from various chemotherapeutic agents, although manifestations at these sites are seen far less often than at the others. Anticancer drugs themselves may be mutagenic. Some drugs may actually enhance the metastatic potential of cancer cells.[10] Increased use of anticancer compounds may reveal them to be more serious offenders than is currently appreciated.

Dogs and cats differ in their toxic reactions to a number of chemotherapeutic agents. Both dose and dose-limiting toxicity must be considered in light of the species being treated. Important differences are noted in the sections on doxorubicin, *cis*-platinum, 5-fluorouracil, and cyclophosphamide.

DRUG RESISTANCE

A major problem confronting the chemotherapist has been drug resistance, which may be temporary or permanent.

Temporary drug resistance is based on pharmacologic or kinetic considerations. Pharmacologic resistance may be related to (1) the inaccessibility of some agents to some body compartments, and to (2) the nature of the blood supply in a tumor and poor diffusion of the drug to the neoplastic cells. Kinetic considerations are also important. Within the tumor, growth fraction decreases with increased mass and distance from the blood supply. Late in the natural course of a tumor, the majority of cells are in G_0 phase and thus resistant to drugs that are only effective against actively cycling cells. In neither of these situations are the cancer cells inherently resistant to the drugs.[20]

Permanent drug resistance is a greater problem. Important aspects of the problems of emerging permanent drug resistance relate to the natural history of tumor growth and the ability to detect a neoplasm clinically. Consider a tumor arising from a single transformed cell. This cell undergoes 30 doublings to become an approximately 1-g mass of 10^9 cells, generally considered the smallest clinically detectable mass. The mass will increase to 10 grams (10^{10} cells) after another 3.25 doublings. At this point it is more likely to be detected, but the metastatic process may already have begun.[21]

Once metastases have been established, localized forms of therapy (surgery, radiation) will be ineffective; systemic therapy will be required. The next 6.75 doublings will result in a tumor mass of 10^{12} cells, about 1 kg of tumor, the maximum compatible with life in most instances. Of a total of 40 doublings in the natural history of a tumor, 30 or more occur before any mass is detected. Therefore, every malignant tumor noted clinically is late in its course. The genetic instability of cancer cells and the selection of variant subpopulations are hallmarks of tumor progression. The result is that the tumor mass is heterogenous in several characteristics including resistance to drugs.[21,22]

It was demonstrated experimentally over 40 years ago that microbial drug resistance develops spontaneously, not as the result of drug treatment. Similarly, cancer cells develop resistance spontaneously. With time, both the number and proportion of resistant cells increase regardless of the mutation rate. Once resistance emerges, the probability of attaining cure falls rapidly from 95% to 5% in just 1.77 logs of growth (5.9 doublings).[23,24]

Spontaneous drug resistance in the cancer cell may occur by several mechanisms relating to the presence of the active form of the drug in a cancer cell or other biochemical responses by the cell to avoid drug toxicity. A cancer cell may develop resistance to a drug by more than one mechanism.

Antineoplastic drugs act intracellularly. If they are unable either to gain access to or to remain within the cancer cell, their cytotoxic effect will be decreased. Resistance to methotrexate may be based on decreased carrier-mediated uptake into the cell; resistance to doxorubicin may be based on increased removal of the drug from the cancer cell. Resistance related to decreased uptake may be overcome by giving greater amounts of the drug. The resultant increases in serum concentrations might alter uptake kinetics sufficiently to allow the drug to enter the cell efficiently. Of course, this tactic carries with it the probability of increased toxicity and can only rarely be employed.

Once within the cancer cell, some anticancer drugs still need to be activated. Defective drug activation occurs in neoplastic cells that have decreased concentrations of deoxycytidine kinase, leading to resistance to cytosine arabinoside. Doxorubicin is ineffectively activated in the presence of decreased concentrations of cytochrome p-450. Resistance to methotrexate has been associated with defective polyglutamation. The polyglutamated form of methotrex-ate is retained in the cell for long periods of time even in the absence of extracellular drug, thus increasing the effective contact time between the drug and the cancer cell.[20]

It is also reasonable to anticipate that increased drug inactivation in the cancer cell will lead to resistance. Increased concentrations of cytidine deaminase in resistant cancer cells favor a pathway for cytosine arabinoside, which yields the inactive product, ara-U, rather than the active product, ara-CTP. Doxorubicin and alkylating agents are inactivated by increased concentrations of glutathione in resistant cancer cells. Cis-platinum is inactivated by increased concentrations of metallothionein. Alterations in both activation and inactivation of anticancer drugs decrease the cytotoxicity by decreasing the intracellular concentration of active drug.[20]

Some cancer cells acquire resistance through other intracellular responses. Enhanced DNA repair related to the increased excision of damaged bases or increased ligation of intact DNA segments has been associated with resistance to the alkylating agents doxorubicin and cis-platinum. By gene amplification, neoplastic cells are able to increase the amount of an intracellular target and thus diminish the efficacy of an anticancer drug.[20]

The neoplastic cell may not necessarily produce greater concentrations of intracellular products but may rather slightly alter the targets. Altered dihydrofolate reductase effectively reduces folate cofactors from di- to tetrahydrofolate forms but is not successfully inhibited by methotrexate. Alterations in tubulin and membrane lipids are associated with resistance to vincristine and doxorubicin respectively. These structural components are vital for successful cell replication. Altered steroid receptors provide a means of resistance to steroids in cases where these drugs have an antineoplastic effect.[20]

Pleiotropic drug resistance (PDR) may develop after exposure to a single dose of an antitumor antibiotic or a plant alkaloid, usually doxorubicin or vincristine. Tumor cells that develop PDR become cross resistant to unrelated compounds, even those that have different mechanisms of action. Such resistant cells have high concentrations of enzymes important in membrane glycoprotein synthesis and low concentrations of enzymes that catabolize membrane glycoproteins. The membranes of cells with PDR are characterized by the presence of a specific moiety called "P-glycoprotein." This component seems to provide these cells a degree of impenetrability like that offered by the glycoprotein capsules of antibiotic-resistant bacteria.[24] Cells exhibiting PDR may also have an effective efflux pump that lowers intracellular drug concentrations. It has been suggested that PDR represents one example of a general mechanism that protects the organism (here, the tumor) against naturally occurring toxins.[25] In the future, it may be possible to overcome PDR by directing monoclonal antibodies tagged with cellular toxins to specific antigenic determinants of "P-glycoprotein."

The concept of drug resistance is an important one for the chemotherapist to understand because it carries with it implications for therapy. By cytoreducing a tumor mass it is theoretically possible to turn back the resistance clock by removing a large mass of cells, leaving a small non resistant population. It is also apparent that early treatment, even in the face of a theoretically late disease, is beneficial. There is nothing to be gained from a "wait and see" approach if metastasis is likely and effective drugs are available. Additionally, it is clear that the best chance of cure accompanies the first therapy. It is well recognized that second and third therapies tend to be less effective in inducing and maintaining remissions.[24] In responsive diseases such as lymphosarcoma, the use of alternating combinations of non-cross-resistant drugs may help delay this emergence of resistance and result in longer first remissions and survivals.[26] On the other hand, maintenance therapy has not been proven to be beneficial, and its role remains undefined. Such therapy may theoretically encourage the emergence of highly resistant clones. Clearly, more attention must be paid to the design of all cancer therapy with the question of drug resistance in mind.

PRINCIPLES AND GUIDELINES

The clinician must understand what can realistically be expected of a chemotherapeutic protocol. This understanding will lay the groundwork for reasonable guidelines for chemotherapy.

Although patients may benefit from the use of a single chemotherapeutic drug, more often there are advantages in the use of multiple drugs

in combination. Chemotherapeutic drugs kill a constant fraction of tumor cells, and the fraction killed by one drug is independent of that killed by another. Drugs can be used in combination to attack different portions of the cell cycle specifically. Drugs can be chosen that have different major toxicities in order to limit any one toxicity and to allow each drug to be used in full dosage. It is toxicity of drugs and not their ability to kill cancer cells that limits chemotherapy. Combination chemotherapy also helps to avoid both inherent drug resistance and the emergence of resistant subpopulations due to acquired resistance.[27] Intermittent treatment schedules allow intensive attack on the neoplasm and a rest period for recovery of normal cells before the next treatment. In theory, there should be added benefit from intensifying the chemotherapeutic attack when very small numbers of neoplastic cells remain. At the biochemical level, combinations of drugs may act by sequential, concurrent, or complementary inhibition, and it may be possible to design protocols based on such interactions. To date, however, it appears that the most successful combined regimens have been empirical in nature, employing drugs ideally known to be individually active against the tumor in question.[28] There are many unanswered questions concerning not only the most efficacious individual drugs for any particular cancer but also the most efficacious combinations and how best to schedule chemotherapy in relation to surgery, radiotherapy, immunotherapy, and hyperthermia. Although the list of considerations governing the use of chemotherapy is long and seems to be growing, the following are some basic principles:[14,29,30]

1. Use drugs known to be effective as single agents.
2. Use drugs with different mechanisms of action.
3. Use drugs with different toxicities.
4. Use an intermittent treatment schedule.

To use the principles of chemotherapy previously discussed safely and effectively, the clinician must satisfy certain guidelines.[31] A thorough history and physical examination along with an appropriate biochemical, hematologic, and radiographic data base are necessary for chemotherapy. In all cases, a histological diagnosis of malignancy is imperative. An understanding of the biological behavior of the specific tumor aids in both prognosis and selection of drugs. The clinician must also understand the drugs and their toxicity among species. Human dosages can only rarely be given to pet animals without modification. Indeed, dogs and cats differ in their responses to some chemotherapeutic agents, including doxorubicin, *cis*-platinum, and 5-fluorouracil. Appropriate drugs and safe dosage schedules for the species being treated should be used. Both monitoring the toxicities associated with the treatment and evaluating patient response are important to the proper management of the patient receiving chemotherapy. Monitoring toxicity to alter or limit treatment is needed for the well-being of the patient, but the patient should also be evaluated to judge the effect of the treatment on the disease. No chemotherapy should be undertaken without the full understanding and cooperation of the owner concerning the goals of the therapy as well as the potential toxicity, the costs, and the necessary commitment to regular follow-up. Certainly not all owners will elect chemotherapy; some will opt for no therapy with or without euthanasia. Chemotherapy can, however, help extend the patient's happy, comfortable life in many instances. This is the primary consideration in offering chemotherapy as a realistic treatment in the management of neoplasia.

DRUGS USED IN CHEMOTHERAPY

Chemotherapeutic agents can be placed into broad classifications that help make them more easily understood, yet each drug has its own characteristics and pecularities. Table 9-1 comments on the mechanisms, indications, and toxicities of selected drugs commonly used in veterinary oncology and should help the clinician provide effective, rational chemotherapy. Table 9-1 is not intended to provide a comprehensive summary of all possible agents. Note that many dosages are expressed as mg/m² (body surface area) rather than mg/kg. This physiologically accurate method of dosing chemotherapeutic drugs allows precise comparison of dosages among species.[32,33] See Table 9-2 for conversions from weight in kilograms to body surface area in square meters for dogs. The table is also applicable to domestic cats but is not appropriate for

larger nondomestic cats. The species-specific constant used in the fractional logarithmic formula for calculating body surface area from body weight is slightly different for dogs and cats. At low body weights, however, the difference is not of practical importance. In fact, whether to use mg/m² or mg/kg for prescribing anticancer agents may depend on the dose-limiting toxicity of the drug in question. For drugs with dose-limiting myelosuppression, mg/kg may prove to be better than mg/m²; for drugs with dose-limiting toxicity of nonhematopoietic tissues, mg/m² may be better.[34a]

The drugs discussed are those most commonly used by veterinary oncologists, but it is important to remember that their efficacy is not proven in all cases. The reader is referred to the specific discussions of the various tumors for details of response and impact on survival.

ALKYLATING AGENTS

Alkylating agents are compounds that substitute an alkyl radical ($R—CH_2—CH_2^+$) for a hydrogen atom on some organic compounds. Alkylation causes breaks in the DNA molecule and cross-linking of the twin strands of DNA and thereby interferes with DNA replication and RNA transcription.[1,8] Most alkylating agents contain more than one alkylating group and are considered polyfunctional. These drugs are nonspecific to cell cycle phases.

Cyclophasphamide is the most widely used alkylating agents in veterinary medicine. It has been employed for lymphoreticular neoplasia, various sarcomas and carcinomas, mast cell tumors, and transmissible venereal tumors both as a single agent and in combination with other drugs.[14] Cyclophosphamide requires hepatic activation and thus must be given by oral or intravenous routes. Its major dose-limiting toxicities are hematologic and gastrointestinal. Leukopenia may be most severe within a week or two of administration; recovery usually follows within 10 days. Anemia and thrombocytopenia are less common but may be seen with chronic use.[8,31]

A unique and important toxicity associated with cyclophosphamide is sterile hemorrhagic cystitis. Active metabolites of cyclophosphamide cause mucosal ulceration, necrosis of smooth muscle and small arteries, and hemorrhage and edema in the urinary bladder. The renal pelvis

(Text continues on p. 72)

Table 9-1. Chemotherapeutic Agents Used in Veterinary Medicine

NAME	BRAND NAME (MANU-FACTURER)	CELL CYCLE SPECIFICITY*	POSSIBLE INDICATIONS	SUGGESTED DOSAGES	TOXICITY
ALKYLATING AGENTS					
Cyclophosphamide	Cytoxan (Mead Johnson)	CCNS	Lymphoreticular neoplasms, various sarcomas and some carcinomas	50 mg/m² PO 4 consecutive days/wk; 250 mg/m² IV weekly	Leukopenia, anemia, thrombocytopenia (less common), nausea, vomiting, sterile hemorrhagic cystitis
Chlorambucil	Leukeran (Burroughs Wellcome)	CCNS	Chronic lymphocytic leukemia, lymphoreticular neoplasms	2–8 mg/m² PO 2–4 days/wk	Mild leukopenia, thrombocytopenia, anemia, nausea, vomiting (not common)
Nitrogen mustard	Mustragen (Merck Sharp & Dohme)	CCNS	Lymphoreticular neoplasms	5 mg/m² IV	Leukopenia, thrombocytopenia, nausea, vomiting, anorexia
Melphalan	Alkeran (Burroughs Wellcome)	CCNS	Multiple myeloma, monoclonal gammopathies, lymphoreticular neoplasms	1.5 mg/m² PO for 7–10 days, repeat cycle	Leukopenia, thrombocytopenia, anemia, anorexia nausea, vomiting
Busulfan	Myleran (Burroughs Wellcome)	CCNS	Chronic granulocytic leukemia	4–6 mg/m² PO daily until WBC count approaches normal	Leukopenia, thrombocytopenia, anemia, pulmonary fibrosis (rare in animals)
Dacarbazine	DTIC (Dome Laboratories)	CCNS	Malignant melanoma, various sarcomas	200 mg/m² IV for 5 days every 3 weeks	Leukopenia, thrombocytopenia, anemia, nausea, vomiting, diarrhea (often decreases with later cycles)
ANTIMETABOLITES					
Methotrexate	Methotrexate (Lederle)	S	Lymphoreticular neoplasms, myeloproliferative disorders, various carcinomas and sarcomas	2.5 mg/m² PO daily, or 20 mg/m² IV weekly	Leukopenia, thrombocytopenia, anemia, stomatitis, diarrhea, hepatopathy, renal tubular necrosis
6-Mercaptopurine	Purinethol (Burroughs Wellcome)	S	Lymphosarcoma, acute lymphocytic leukemia, granulocytic leukemia	50 mg/m² PO daily until response or toxicity	Leukopenia, nausea, vomiting, hepatopathy
5-Fluorouracil	Fluorouracil (Roche Laboratories)	S	Various carcinomas and sarcomas	200 mg/m² IV weekly	Leukopenia, thrombocytopenia, anemia, anorexia, nausea, vomiting, diarrhea, stomatitis, CNS (dog and cat)
	Efudex Cream (Roche Laboratories)		Cutaneous tumors	Apply twice daily for 2–4 weeks	DO NOT USE IN CATS BY ANY ROUTE
Cytosine arabinoside	Cytosar-U (Upjohn)	S	Lymphosarcoma, myeloproliferative disorders	100 mg/m² SQ or IV drip for 4 days, repeat q 3–4 wk; 600 mg/m² over 48 hr, repeat in 3–4 wk	Leukopenia, thrombocytopenia, anemia, nausea vomiting, anorexia, bone marrow toxicity

(Continued)

Table 9-1. Chemotherapeutic Agents Used in Veterinary Medicine (continued)

NAME	BRAND NAME (MANU-FACTURER)	CELL CYCLE SPECIFICITY*	POSSIBLE INDICATIONS	SUGGESTED DOSAGES	TOXICITY
PLANT ALKALOIDS					
Vincristine	Oncovin (Eli Lilly)	M	Transmissible venereal tumor, lymphosarcoma	0.75 mg/m^2 IV weekly	Peripheral neuropathy, paresthesia, constipation
Vinblastine	Velban (Eli Lilly)	M	Lymphosarcoma, various carcinomas	2.0 mg/m^2 IV weekly	Leukopenia, nausea, vomiting
ANTIBIOTICS					
Doxorubicin	Adriamycin (Adria Laboratories)	CCNS	Lymphosarcoma, various sarcomas, thyroid carcinoma	30 mg/m^2 IV every 3 wk (do not exceed 240 mg/m^2 total)	Leukopenia, thrombocytopenia, nausea, vomiting, cardiac toxicity, reactions during administration
Bleomycin	Blenoxane (Bristol Laboratories)	CCNS (G$_1$, S, and M)	Squamous cell carcinomas, other carcinomas	10 mg/m^2 IV or SQ for 3–9 days, then 10 mg/m^2 IV weekly (do not exceed 200 mg/m^2 total)	Allergic reactions following administration, pulmonary fibrosis
HORMONES					
Prednisolone		NA	Lymphoreticular neoplasms, mast cell tumors, CNS tumors	Vary widely depending on indication: 60 mg/m^2 PO daily to 20 mg/m^2 PO every 48 hr	Hyperadrenocorticism, secondary adrenocortical insufficiency
Diethylstilbestrol		NA	Perianal adenomas, prostatic neoplasms (adjunctively)	1.1 mg/kg IM once	Bone marrow toxicity, feminization
MISCELLANEOUS					
L-Asparaginase	Elspar (Merck Sharp & Dohme)	NA	Lymphoreticular neoplasms	10,000–12,000 units/m^2 IM weekly	Anaphylaxis, coagulation abnormalities
o,p′-DDD	Lysodren (Calbiochem)	NA	Adrenocortical tumors	50 mg/kg PO daily to effect, then 50 mg/kg PO every 7–14 days PRN	Adrenocortical insufficiency
cis-platinum	Platinol (Bristol)	CCNS	Squamous cell carcinoma, osteosarcoma, other carcinomas	60–70 mg/m^2 IV drip q 3–5 weeks; saline diuresis before and after treatment required. DO NOT USE IN CATS.	Nausea, vomiting bone marrow, renal
Hydroxyurea	Hydrea (Squibb)	NA	Chronic myelogenous leukemia	40–50 mg/kg PO div. BID until WBC count returns to normal	Anemia, leukemia, altered nail growth

* CCNS = cell cycle phase nonspecific; S = S phase specific; M = M-phase specific; NA = not applicable.

Table 9-2. Conversion Table of Weight in Kilograms to Body Surface Area in Square Meters for Dogs

KG	M²	KG	M²
0.5	0.06	26.0	0.88
1.0	0.10	27.0	0.90
2.0	0.15	28.0	0.92
3.0	0.20	29.0	0.96
4.0	0.25	30.0	0.96
5.0	0.29	31.0	0.99
6.0	0.33	32.0	1.01
7.0	0.36	33.0	1.03
8.0	0.40	34.0	1.05
9.0	0.43	35.0	1.07
10.0	0.46	36.0	1.09
11.0	0.49	37.0	1.11
12.0	0.52	38.0	1.13
13.0	0.55	39.0	1.15
14.0	0.58	40.0	1.17
15.0	0.60	41.0	1.19
16.0	0.63	42.0	1.21
17.0	0.66	43.0	1.23
18.0	0.69	44.0	1.25
19.0	0.71	45.0	1.26
20.0	0.74	46.0	1.28
21.0	0.76	47.0	1.30
22.0	0.78	48.0	1.32
23.0	0.81	49.0	1.34
24.0	0.83	50.0	1.36
25.0	0.85		

may also be affected. The patient may show signs of hematuria, pollakiuria, and stranguria. Although both dogs and cats may be affected, the problem appears to be much less common in cats,[16] owing either to inherent species differences or differences in the dosage and schedule employed. Early recognition of signs, diuresis, and cessation of cyclophosphamide administration help limit the problem in most cases. Some cases may be persistent and require more aggressive therapy, such as the instillation of 1% formalin solution into the bladder.[35] Measures helpful in avoiding cyclophosphamide-associated sterile hemorrhagic cystitis include:

1. Not administering cyclophosphamide to a patient with concurrent cystitis or hematuria
2. Administering the daily dose in the morning and providing free access to fresh water at all times as well as ample opportunity to urinate
3. Being certain the patient urinates before the owners retire for the night

The concomitant use of prednisone would usually not be contraindicated and might help diminish the inflammatory response in the blad- der wall as well as decrease the concentration of cyclophosphamide metabolites in residual urine by encouraging polyuria.

Chlorambucil is often used in chemotherapy of canine lymphosarcoma as a replacement for cyclophosphamide, either in maintenance regimens or when myelosuppression or sterile hemorrhagic cystitis has been a problem. Chlorambucil has also been used effectively as induction and maintenance therapy for canine chronic lymphocytic leukemia.[36] Although chlorambucil acts more slowly than cyclophosphamide and seems to have less myelosuppressive toxicity, regular monitoring of white blood cell parameters is warranted.[1,14]

Nitrogen mustard and melphalan are two other classical alkylating agents sometimes used in veterinary medicine but less frequently than cyclophosphamide or chlorambucil. Topical nitrogen mustard may be efficacious in the management of canine cutaneous T-cell-like lymphoma (cutaneous lymphosarcoma, mycosis, fungoides), but the drug must be handled with great caution owing to the significant potential for contact dermatitis among those applying it as well as its potential mutagenic and carcinogenic effects.[37,38]

Dacarbazine (DTIC) is a nonclassical alkylating agent that has been used alone and in combination for malignant melanoma and various sarcomas. Its use appears to result in relatively short responses in a limited number of cases. It has the advantage of being relatively nonmyelosuppressive, and the associated gastrointestinal toxicity seems to diminish rather than increase with continued therapy.[39]

ANTIMETABOLITES

The antimetabolites are structural analogues of normal metabolites required for cell function and replication and interfere with these processes by substitution for or competition with a metabolite. The antimetabolites are highly schedule-dependent S-phase-specific drugs. Many questions remain unanswered regarding their best use.[8,31]

Methotrexate inhibits dihydrofolate reductase competitively and interferes with both purine and pyrimidine synthesis. It has been used most often in combination with other drugs in the therapy of lymphoreticular neoplasms and myeloproliferative disorders. Its use has also been reported in metastatic transmissible venereal tumor, Sertoli cell tumor, and osteogenic sarcoma.[40] Methotrexate toxicity to the bone marrow and gastrointestinal tract can be severe; with high-dose regimens appropriately timed "rescue" may be achieved by administering citrovorum factor (folinic acid), the specific antidote. More commonly in veterinary medicine, methotrexate is given in a low-dose regimen that is far less toxic and does not require "rescue."[1,8,14,40]

Other antimetabolites used less frequently include the purine analogue 6-mercaptopurine and the pyrimidine analogues 5-fluorouracil and cytosine arabinoside. The dose-limiting toxicity of these drugs is primarily hematologic in dogs. 5-Fluorouracil is severely neurotoxic in cats and should not be used topically or systemically in that species.[41–44]

PLANT ALKALOIDS

Vincristine and vinblastine are alkaloids extracted from the periwinkle plant, *Vinca rosea*. They act specifically in M phase by binding with the microtubular protein tubulin and blocking mitosis by interfering with chromosomal separation in metaphase. Although vincristine and vinblastine share a common mechanism of action, resistance to one does not imply resistance to the other. They also have different major toxicities. Vincristine affects the nervous system. The toxicities of paresthesia, loss of deep tendon reflexes, and sensory neuropathy are more easily recognized in human patients than animal patients. Constipation secondary to autonomic neuropathy is sometimes noted.[45] Vinblastine toxicity is primarily hematologic. Myelosuppression may be a severe problem. Both drugs have been used in the treatment of lymphoreticular neoplasms. Vincristine is the treatment of choice for transmissible venereal tumor and has been used for various sarcomas and carcinomas.[46,47] Vinblastine has been used in the treatment of mast cell tumors and carcinomas.[8,47]

ANTIBIOTICS

The antitumor antibiotics are natural products derived from various strains of the soil fungus *Streptomyces*. They are cytotoxic drugs that are nonspecific to cell cycle phase and that act by binding (intercalating) DNA and inhibiting DNA

or RNA synthesis.[8] Bleomycin has been used occasionally in veterinary oncology, but doxorubicin has been the most frequently used member of this class in veterinary medicine. Doxorubicin has important hematologic, gastrointestinal, and cardiac toxicities in dogs; in cats, renal toxicity is important.[48,49] Although signs of gastrointestinal upset, vomiting, and diarrhea can usually be managed symptomatically and supportively, myelosuppression may be a dose-limiting problem in the short term. Cumulative cardiac toxicity results in a dose-related cardiomyopathy.[50] The true role of electro- and echocardiograms in predicting cardiomyopathy is not known, but these procedures have not proven to have predictive value to date. The evaluation of serial endomyocardial biopsies and electron-microscopic evaluation would be an ideal approach but is not generally practical in veterinary medicine. Because doxorubicin undergoes hepatic metabolism, dosages should be reduced if hepatic damage is present. Doxorubicin must be administered slowly (over at least 10 to 15 minutes) through a free-flowing intravenous line. Patient restlessness, facial swelling, or head shaking may signal excessively rapid administration or anaphylaxis. If these signs are seen, administration should be stopped temporarily and started at a slower rate when signs abate. Pretreatment with antihistamines or corticosteroids may help avoid some of these complications. Despite its apparently numerous drawbacks, doxorubicin has had wide application in the treatment of canine lymphosarcoma as both a first-line and a salvage drug.[51,52] It has also been used for various carcinomas and sarcomas with limited success.[1,14,40]

HORMONES

Unlike other chemotherapeutic agents, hormones are not primarily cytotoxic drugs. Hormonal agents are more selective than cytotoxic drugs in their actions.[53] Peptide hormones interact with cell membrane-bound nucleotide cyclase systems such as those that convert adenosine triphosphate (ATP) to cyclic adenosine monophosphate (cAMP), which acts as a "second messenger" to deliver and amplify regulatory signals to intracellular sites. Steroid hormones enter the cells and bind to a specific receptor protein. "Transformation" ("activation") of this newly formed complex allows it to pass the nuclear membranes, where it binds to DNA. This binding alters the transcription of the cell's messenger RNA, resulting in synthesis of new protein. Steroid-induced increases in free fatty acids may cause dissolution of the nuclear membrane, leading to cell death, although this does not appear to be their primary effect in chemotherapy.[28,54] It has also been suggested that glucocorticoids may kill lymphosarcoma cells by disrupting the usual balance between chromatin fragmentation and DNA repair, in addition to their antiproliferative effect.[54a]

Adrenal corticosteroids have important clinical uses in the therapy of lymphosarcoma and mast cell tumors. They may be of benefit in the therapy of central nervous system neoplasms because of their ability to cross the blood-brain barrier and reduce cerebral edema.[55] Their beneficial actions in other solid tumors probably relate more to anti-inflammatory effects than to direct antitumor effects.[7]

Sex hormones have been used in the treatment of hormone-dependent tumors of mammary, prostatic, or perianal gland origin. As for cytotoxic therapies, the benefit of these drugs in this setting remains largely unproven. With increasing availability of estrogen and progesterone receptor analysis, rational hormonal therapy of mammary gland tumors will become likely. Currently, antiestrogenic therapy remains experimental.

Some hormones may also have a valuable role as replacement therapy following ablative surgery or in the management of some metastatic problems (T_3/T_4 supplementation in canine thyroid carcinoma) or in dealing with paraneoplastic syndromes such as hypercalcemia (corticosteroids) and anemia (anabolic steroids).[53]

MISCELLANEOUS AGENTS

Other drugs that do not easily fall into any of the previously mentioned categories have also been used to treat animal cancers.

L-asparaginase in an enzyme preparation derived from a variety of bacteria. By hydrolyzing asparagine to aspartic acid and ammonia, L-asparaginase deprives neoplastic cells that lack the ability to synthesize L-asparagine of extracellular sources, thereby rapidly inhibiting protein synthesis. L-asparaginase acts against cells in G_1. It has been used in the therapy of canine lymphoreticular neoplasms.[40] Anaphylaxis has been the most dangerous side-effect. Other toxicities include gastrointestinal disturbances, hepatotoxicity, hemorrhagic pancreatitis, and coagulation defects.[1,8,31] After conjugation with polyethylene glycol, L-asparaginase has a prolonged serum half-life and is less toxic. This form of L-asparaginase (PEG-asparaginase) has been used in cases of canine lymphosarcoma alone and in combination with other drugs.[56]

The cell-cycle-nonspecific drug o,p'-DDD directly suppresses both normal and neoplastic adrenocortical cells.[31] With proper management, o,p'-DDD may be beneficial in patients with inoperable adrenocortical carcinoma as well as patients with adrenocortical hyperplasia secondary to a pituitary neoplasm. In addition to careful monitoring for impending hypoadrenocorticism, the clinician must be aware of toxic manifestations, including vomiting, diarrhea, and depression.[31]

Platinum complexes have been shown to have tumoricidal activity; *cis*-diaminedichloroplatinum (CDDP) is a cell-cycle-nonspecific drug that inhibits DNA synthesis and has some alkylating activity. It has been used in human medicine for testicular, ovarian, and bladder carcinoma; its true indications in veterinary medicine are still uncertain, but CDDP may be helpful in the therapy of some lung tumors, squamous cell carcinomas, and osteosarcomas.[57–60,60a,60b] CDDP causes nausea and vomiting, which may be severe and prolonged. Renal insufficiency is usually the dose-limiting toxicity in dogs, but myelosuppression may also be a problem. Canine dosages of CDDP should not be used in cats because of its extreme pulmonary toxicity.[61] Lower dosages may be useful, but no safe schedule is currently in use. CDDP is rapidly finding its way into use in veterinary medicine.[62]

MULTIMODALITY THERAPY

Chemotherapy for human cancers has progressed tremendously in the past 40 years, but in veterinary medicine it is still in its infancy. An understanding of the biologic and pharmacologic principles underlying chemotherapy, the chemotherapeutic agents, and the potentials and limitations of drug therapy will enhance the delivery of appropriate therapy. The near future will present promising new therapeutic and prognostic options for a very challenging clinical problem.

The classical approach to cancer therapy has been to use a local therapy, usually surgery but sometimes radiation, first and alone. The patient has been observed until the disease recurred. At the time of relapse, chemotherapy might be attempted. This approach, of course, lessens the likelihood of a good response to drug therapy because of the late and recurrent nature of the disease. Now it is common practice to plan adjuvant chemotherapy as part of the initial treatment for cancers with a high metastatic rate, such as canine osteosarcoma and thyroid carcinoma and feline mammary carcinoma. While local therapy is still very important in reducing the total tumor burden by removing or reducing the bulk of the primary tumor, the known biologic behavior of many of the commonly encountered tumors indicates that cure is not attained by these means. It is here that chemotherapy, planned and conducted in conjunction with other therapies, is likely to be most beneficial. When applied to the much smaller tumor burdens left after surgery, chemotherapy may have a better chance of working. Whether adjunctive chemotherapy will bring about a cure seems to depend at least in part on the metastatic burden at the time of the primary therapy.[63]

Another means of combining modalities is neoadjuvant chemotherapy, the use of drugs before the definitive treatment (surgery or radiation) for the primary tumor. As with adjuvant chemotherapy, the prospects for "cure" seem to vary with the metastatic burden at the time therapy is undertaken, but there are some advantages to the neoadjuvant approach. By moving chemotherapy "up front," it may be possible to reduce the size of the surgical or radiation field, even if the chemotherapy is not itself curative. Noncurative cytoreduction (by surgery or radiation) leads to increased proliferation, which in turn leads to increased resistance, increased shedding of tumor cells, and increased protection in sanctuaries. Neoadjuvant chemotherapy should help diminish these problems. Also, early chemotherapy may have an effect on undetected micrometastatic disease, which theoretically is kept somewhat in check by a suppressive effect from the primary tumor.[64,65] Some implications for surgery are obvious; any significant decrease in the size of the primary tumor will make the surgical procedure easier and less deforming. In addition, even if tumor cells are dislodged at the time of surgery, they may have been sterilized by chemotherapy and therefore be less likely to cause spread by direct implantation. Neoadjuvant chemotherapy is not without its potential disadvantages. There is always the possibility that the tumor will be totally unresponsive to the chosen drugs. In that case, the patient will have had suffered unwarranted toxicity, immunosuppression, and delay in more effective therapy.

The concepts of combined or multimodality therapy are still relatively new to veterinary medicine. More thought should be given to planning the entire course of cancer treatment in order to present a client with a fully developed plan that includes whatever modalities might benefit the patient. It is worthwhile, then, to have in mind the indications for and problems with various combinations of surgery, radiation, and chemotherapy. In general, in combined modality treatments, chemotherapy and biologic therapy can be considered useful to combat micrometastatic disease, radiation to sterilize local disease, and surgery to remove the gross tumor. The true role of either local or systemic hyperthermia is not known yet but most likely lies in an adjunct setting. Probably the most common combination considered presently is surgery followed by chemotherapy. Local treatment rids the patient of the primary disease, and chemotherapy eliminates the micrometastatic burden. For diseases with a high likelihood of not being cured by surgery alone, the consideration of postoperative drugs is an attractive one but has not been fully evaluated. Tumors that might benefit from such therapy (but have not yet been proven to do so) include osteosarcomas, hemangiosarcomas, oral malignant melanomas, and large thyroid carcinomas in dogs and mammary adenocarcinomas in cats. In any case, adjuvant chemotherapy should not be undertaken unless there is some evidence that the tumor being treated is at least somewhat responsive to the drug or drugs used. A significant problem is evaluation of the efficacy of adjunctive treatment intended to treat micrometastatic (and, therefore, unmeasureable) disease. If surgery were, in fact, curative, adjunctive therapy would appear to have been beneficial, the owner would have assumed unwarranted expense, and the patient would have suffered unnecessary toxicity when chemotherapy really had no role. The evaluation of adjunctive chemotherapy will be a complex issue for veterinary oncologists.

REFERENCES

1. Madewell BR, Theilen GH: Chemotherapy. In Theilen GH, Madewell BR (eds): Veterinary Cancer Medicine, pp. 157–196. Philadelphia, Lea & Febiger, 1987

2. Haskell CM: Principles of cancer chemotherapy. In Haskell CM (eds): Cancer Treatment, pp. 27–52. Philadelphia, WB Saunders, 1980

3. Schabel FM: The use of tumor growth kinetics in planning "curative" chemotherapy of advanced solid tumors. Cancer Res 29:2384, 1969

4. Yoxall AT, Hind JER (eds): Veterinary Applications of the Pharmacology of Neoplasia: In Pharmacological Basis of Small Animal Medicine. London, Blackwell Scientific Publications, 1975

5. Hess PW, MacEwen EG, McClelland AJ: Chemotherapy of canine and feline tumors. J Am Anim Hosp Assoc 12:350, 1976

6. Pierce GB, Fennell RH, Jr: Pathology. In Holland JF, Frei E, III (eds): Cancer Medicine, 2nd ed, pp. 149–167. Philadelphia, Lea & Febiger, 1982

7. Rosenthal RC, Wilcke JR: Glucocorticoid Therapy. In Kirk RW (ed): Current Veterinary Therapy, VIII, pp. 854–862. Philadelphia, WB Saunders, 1983

8. Haskell CM: Drugs used in cancer chemotherapy. In Haskell CM (ed): Cancer Treatment. Philadelphia, WB Saunders, 1980

9. Bennett WM, Singer I, Golper T, et al: Guidelines for drug therapy in renal failure. Ann Intern Med 86:754, 1977

10. Takenaga K: Modification of the metastatic potential of tumor cells by drugs. Cancer Metastasis Rev 5:67–75, 1986

11. MacEwen EG: Cancer chemotherapy. In Kirk RW (ed): Current Veterinary Therapy, VII. Philadelphia, WB Saunders, 1980

12. Harris JB: Nausea, vomiting and cancer treatment. CA 28:194, 1977

13. Sulkes A, Collins JM: Reappraisal of some dosage adjustment guidelines. Cancer Treat Rep 71(3):229–233, 1987

14. Hess PW: Principles of cancer chemotherapy. Vet Clin North Am 7:21, 1977

15. Giger U, Gorman NT: Acute complications of cancer and cancer therapy. In Gorman NT (ed): Oncology, pp. 147–168. New York, Churchill Livingston, 1986

16. Crow SE, Theilen GH, Madewell BR, et al: Cyclophosphamide-induced cystitis in the dog and cat. J Am Vet Med Assoc 171:259, 1977

17. Weller RE, Wolf AM, Oyejide A: Transitional cell carcinoma of the bladder associated with cyclophosphamide therapy in a dog. J Am Anim Hosp Assoc 15(6):733–736, 1979

18. Cotter SM, Kanki PH, Simon M: Renal disease in five tumor-bearing cats treated with adriamycin. J Am Anim Hosp Assoc 21(3):405–409, 1985

19. Conroy JD: The etiology and pathogenesis of alopecia. Compend Cont Ed Pract Vet 1:806, 1979

20. Curt GA, Clendeninn NJ, Chabner BA. Drug resistance in cancer. Cancer Treat 68(1):87–98, 1984

21. Fidler IJ, Hart IR: Biological diversity in metastatic neoplasms: Origins and implications. Science 217:998–1003, 1982

22. DeVita VT: The relationship between tumor mass and resistance to chemotherapy. Cancer 51(7):1209–1220, 1983

23. Goldie JN, Coldman AJ: A mathematic model for relating the drug sensitivity of tumors to their spontaneous mutation rate. Cancer Treat Rep 63(11–12):1727–1733, 1979

24. Goldie JH: New thoughts on resistance to chemotherapy. Hosp Pract 18(5):165–177, 1983

25. Myers C, Cowan K, Sinha B, et al: The phenomenon of pleotropic drug resistance. In DeVita VT, Hellman S, Rosenberg SA (eds): Important Advances in Oncology, pp. 27–38. Philadelphia, JB Lippincott, 1987

26. Goldie JH, Coldman AJ, Gudauskas GA. Rationale for the use of alternating non-cross-resistant chemotherapy. Cancer Treat Rep 66(3):439–449, 1983

27. Chabner BA: The role of drugs in cancer treatment. In Chabner, BA (ed): Pharmacologic Principles of Cancer Treatment, pp. 3–14. Philadelphia, WB Saunders, 1982

28. Carter SK, Livingston RB: Principles of cancer chemotherapy. In Carter SK, Glatstein E, Livingston RB (eds): Principles of Cancer Treatment, pp. 95–110. New York, McGraw-Hill, 1981

29. Rosenthal RC: Chemotherapy. In Slatter, DH

(ed): Textbook of Small Animal Surgery, pp. 2405–2417. Philadelphia, WB Saunders, 1985

30. Damon LE, Cadman EC: Advances in rational chemotherapy. Cancer Invest 4(5):421–444, 1986

31. Carter SK, Livingston RB: Drugs Available to Treat Cancer. In Carter SK, Glatstein E, Livingston RB (eds): Principles of Cancer Treatment, pp. 111–145. New York, McGraw-Hill, 1981

32. Freireich EJ, Gehan EA, Rall DP, et al: Quantitative comparison of toxicity of anticancer agents in mouse, rat, hamster, dog, monkey, and man. Cancer Chemother Rep 50(4):219–244, 1966

33. Henness AM, Theilen GH, Madewell BR, et al: Use of drugs based on square meters of body surface area. J Am Vet Med Assoc 171:1076, 1977

34. Vriesendorp HM: Optimal prescription method for cancer chemotherapy. Exp Hematol 13(suppl 16):57–63, 1985

34a. Page RL, Macy DW, Thrall DE, et al: Unexpected toxicity associated with use of body surface area for dosing melphalan in the dog. Cancer Res 48:288–290, 1988

35. Weller RE: Intravesical instillation of dilute formation for treatment of cyclophosphamide-induced hemorrhagic cystitis in two dogs. J Am Vet Med Assoc 172:1206, 1978

36. Leifer CE, Matus RE: Chronic lymphocytic leukemia in the dog: 22 cases (1974–1984). J Am Vet Med Assoc 198(2):214–217, 1986

37. McKeever PJ, Grindem CB, Stevens JB, et al: Canine cutaneous lymphoma. J Am Vet Med Assoc 180(5):531–536, 1982

38. Ackerman L: Cutaneous T cell-like lymphoma in the dog. Compend Cont Ed Sm Anim Pract 6(1):37–42, 1984

39. Chabner BA: Nonclassical alkylating agents: In Chabner BA (ed): Pharmacologic Principles of Cancer Treatment, pp. 340–362. Philadelphia, WB Saunders, 1982

40. Gorman NT: Use of Cytotoxic Drugs in the Management of Neoplasia. In Gorman NT (ed): Oncology, pp. 121–146. New York, Churchill Livingston, 1986

41. Chabner BA: Pyrimidine antagonists. In Chabner BA (ed): Pharmacologic Principles of Cancer Treatment, pp. 183–212. Philadelphia, WB Saunders, 1982

42. McCormack JJ, Hohns DG: Purine Antimetabolites. In Pharmacologic Principles of Cancer Treatment, pp. 213–228. Philadelphia, WB Saunders, 1982

43. Harvey HJ, MacEwen EG, Hayes AA: Neurotoxicosis associated with use of 5-fluorouracil in five dogs and one cat. J Am Vet Med Assoc 171:277–278, 1977

44. Hennes AM, Theilen GH, Madewell BR, et al: Neurotoxicosis associated with use of 5-fluorouracil. J Am Vet Med Assoc 171:692, 1977

45. Couto CG: Toxicity of anticancer therapy. Proceedings of the 10th Kal Kan Symposium, 1987, pp. 37–46. Vernon, California, Kal Kan Foods, Inc, 1987

46. Calvert CA, Leifer CE, MacEwen EG: Vincristine for treatment of transmissible venereal tumor. J Am Vet Med Assoc 181:163–164, 1982

47. Rosenthal RC: Clinical applications of vinca alkaloids. J Am Vet Med Assoc 179:1084, 1981

48. Susaneck SJ: Doxorubicin therapy in the dog. J Am Vet Med Assoc 182(1):70–73, 1983

49. Cotter SM, Kanki PJ, Simon M: Renal disease in five tumor-bearing cats treated with adriamycin. J Am Anim Hosp Assoc 21(3):405–409, 1985

50. Loar AS, Susaneck SJ: Doxorubicin-induced cardiotoxicity in five dogs. Semin Vet Med Surg (Sm Anim) 1(1):68–71, 1986

51. Calvert CA, Leifer CE: Doxorubicin for treatment of canine lymphosarcoma after development of resistance to combination chemotherapy. J Am Vet Med Assoc 179(10):1011–1012, 1981

52. Postorino NC, Susaneck SJ, Withrow SJ, et al: Single agent therapy with adriamycin for canine lymphosarcoma. Proc Vet Cancer Soc 7:37, 1987

53. Rosenthal RC: Hormones in cancer therapy. Vet Clin North Am 12:67, 1982

54. Meyers FH, Jawetz E, Goldfein A: The adrenocortical steroids. In Meyers FH, Jawetz E, Goldfein A (eds): Review of Medical Pharmacology, 6th ed. Los Altos, CA, Lange Medical Publications, 1978

54a. Wielckens K, Delfs T, Muth A, et al: Glucocorticoid-induced lymphoma cell death: The good and the evil. J Steroid Biochem 27(1–3):413–419, 1987

55. Franklin RT: The use of glucocorticoids in treating cerebral edema. Compend Cont Ed Sm Anim Pract 6(5):442–447, 1984

56. MacEwen EG, Rosenthal RC, Matus R, et al: A preliminary study on the evaluation of asparaginase: Polyethylene glycol conjugate against canine malignant lymphoma. Cancer 59(12):2011–2015, 1987

57. Mehlhaff CJ, Leifer CE, Patnaik AK, et al: Surgical treatment of primary pulmonary neo-

plasia in 15 dogs. J Am Anim Hosp Assoc 20(5):799–803, 1984

58. Himsel CA, Richardson RC, Craig JA: Cisplatin chemotherapy for metastatic squamous cell carcinoma in two dogs. J Am Vet Med Assoc 189(12):1575–1578, 1986

59. Shapiro W, Kitchell B, Theilen G: Clinical evaluation of cisplatin for advanced canine malignancies. Proc Vet Cancer Soc 6:5, 1986

60. Withrow SJ, LaRue SM, Wrigley RH, et al: Limb sparing treatment for canine osteosarcoma. Proc Vet Cancer Soc 6:12–13, 1986

60a. Shapiro W, Fossum TW, Kitchell BE et al: Use of cisplatin for treatment of appendicular osteosarcoma in dogs. J Am Vet Med Assoc 192(4):507–511, 1988

60b. Knapp DW, Richardson RC, Bonney PL, et al: Cisplatin therapy in 41 dogs with malignant tumors. J Vet Int Med 2:41–46, 1988

61. Knapp DW, Richardson RC, DeNicola DB, et al: Cis-plastin toxicity in cats. J Vet Intern Med 1(1):29–35, 1987

62. Page R. Cis-plastin, a new antineoplastic drug in veterinary medicine. J Am Vet Med Assn 186(3):288–290, 1985

63. Griswold DP: Body burden of cancer in relationship to therapeutic outcome: Consideration of preclinical evidence. Cancer Treat Rep 70(1):81–86, 1986

64. Sugarbaker EV, Thornwaite J, Ketcham AS: Inhibitary effect of a primary tumor on metastasis. In Day SB, Myers WPL, Stansly P, et al (eds): Cancer Invasion and Metastasis: Biologic Mechanisms and Therapy, pp. 227–240. New York, Raven Press, 1977

65. Gorelik E, Segal S, Feldman M: Growth of a local tumor exerts a specific inhibitory effect on progression of lung metastases. Int J Cancer 21:617–625, 1978

10

RADIATION THERAPY

Donald E. Thrall
Mark W. Dewhirst

Radiation therapy is available to many private practitioners on a referral basis. Radiation therapy is conducted in most schools of veterinary medicine and is also available on a limited basis in some private veterinary practices and in collaboration with physician radiation oncologists. The animal-owning public is becoming more knowledgeable about the various types of cancer treatment and many owners expect radiation therapy to be available if it is indicated for their pets. The purpose of this chapter is to familiarize practicing veterinarians with the principles of radiation therapy so that they can discuss this treatment intelligently with animal owners and be able to identify patients that might benefit from irradiation.

RATIONALE

Radiation kills cells; it is this property of ionizing radiation that renders it useful in cancer therapy. One hopes by irradiating a tumor to sterilize the tumor and preserve adjacent normal tissue. Preservation of normal tissue must be the goal in every irradiated patient because so-called late radiation damage to normal tissue may be an unacceptable, often progressive, and even life-threatening result of radiation therapy. The dose of radiation that can be given to a tumor is therefore limited by the tolerance of adjacent normal tissue. Administration of the maximum dosage of radiation tolerated by adjacent normal tissue does not always result in tumor cure. Tumor cells are generally not more sensitive to radiation than the surrounding normal tissue cells. In fact, tumor cells may be more radioresistant than adjacent normal tissue cells because of tumor cell hypoxia, which develops as a result of poor perfusion in the tumor. Hypoxic cells are more radioresistant than fully oxygenated cells, possibly by a factor of 2.5 to 3.0 (Fig. 10-1). Nevertheless, tumors are often controlled by radiotherapy, and the way in which the radiotherapy is given can greatly influence tumor curability. For example, the dose per fraction (each radiation treatment is called a fraction), number of fractions, and total time over which

79

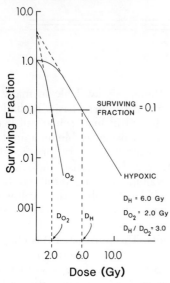

Figure 10-1. Radiation cell survival curves illustrating the effect of oxygenation on radiosensitivity. Survival curves are shown for two populations of cells, one fully oxygenated and the other hypoxic. The slope of the survival curve for fully oxygenated cells is much steeper than the slope of the curve for hypoxic cells. In this example, the ratio of radiation doses necessary to reduce survival by a factor of 0.1 is 3.0. Thus, there is a direct relationship between hypoxia and radioresistance. The practical significance of this phenomenon is that tumor cells rendered hypoxic as a result of vascular deficiency are more radioresistant than oxygenated tumor cells and adjacent normal tissue cells.

radiation therapy is delivered are known to influence the tolerance of the normal tissue and tumor control. Judicious treatment planning, whereby a minimum of normal tissue is irradiated, can allow for a higher tumor dose, thus increasing the probability for cure. Alternatively, multiple treatments from different ports, chosen so that radiation overlaps from different directions at the target volume, can help to reduce the overall dose to adjacent normal tissue, even though a relatively large volume of normal tissue receives a relatively small dose. Finally, shrinking-field techniques can be used wherein some initial number of fractions are delivered to a large tissue volume, in order to sterilize microscopic foci extending into normal tissue. Then for subsequent fractions the field is reduced to the primary tumor volume.

The radiation dose for humans and animals has evolved empirically, and attempts are being made to refine it further. Results from investigations in progress will not be available for many years. In the radiation treatment of human cancer, it is common to give daily irradiation for 6–7 weeks. Usually this involves daily fractions of 1.8–2.0 Gray (Gy) (1 Gy = 100 rads) with a resulting total dose of 60–70 Gy. At present, radiation therapy is routinely given to animals in 10–12 fractions of 4.0–5.0 Gy each, usually three times per week. Radiation is routinely given to animals and humans in several smaller fractions rather than one large fraction in part because radioresistant hypoxic tumor cells become reoxygenated during the course of radiation therapy and their radiosensitivity increases. More oxygen becomes available for use by hypoxic cells as more radiosensitive fully oxygenated cells are killed. Another reason why fractionating the radiation dose is more effective relates to a homeostatic change in proliferation rate that occurs in normal tissue after radiation begins. Normal cells compensate for the injury they receive by shortening their division time and increasing their relative number. Because this same phenomenon may also occur in tumors, overall treatment must not be protracted, or the tumor cells may compensate also.

EVALUATION OF POTENTIAL PATIENTS

In most instances, radiation therapy is of greatest value for treatment of localized solid tumors that cannot be excised completely, or that cannot be excised without resulting in an unacceptable cosmetic or functional defect.

Before radiation therapy is considered for any patient, a pretreatment data base must be compiled. This should include information from a complete physical examination, urinalysis, routine blood tests such as CBC, and a chemical screening profile. The purpose of this data base is to assure that the patient has no preexisting medical condition that would make it difficult to complete the treatment or would limit survival after treatment. The primary tumor should be examined carefully and should be radiographed in order to determine more completely the extent of its local involvement. Regional lymph nodes must be examined carefully. If it is unclear whether a lymph node contains metastatic cancer, lymph node biopsy or fine-needle aspirate should be examined prior to initiation of therapy.

Thoracic radiographs should be made to search for distant metastases. Radiographs should also be made of other sites where metastasis is likely—*e.g.*, abdominal radiographs to evaluate possible iliac lymph node metastasis from a malignant perianal tumor.

Once a histologic diagnosis is obtained and it agrees with the signalment, history, and clinical findings, the biology of the tumor must be considered carefully. Tumor site must be given equal consideration as tumor type because tumors of identical histologic type but in different locations often vary in biologic behavior and response to therapy. A good example of this phenomenon in the dog is squamous cell carcinoma of the external nose, gingiva, and tonsil. Gingival squamous cell carcinoma has a low metastatic potential and a high likelihood of being controlled with local radiation therapy. Squamous cell carcinoma of the external nose has a moderate rate of distant metastasis and does not respond as well to radiation therapy. Squamous cell carcinoma of the tonsil has a very high rate of distant metastasis and only a fair response to local radiation therapy. Not only histologic type and site but also stage must be considered because response to treatment and biologic behavior are related to these variables in combination.

Radiation therapy should be considered as the sole treatment modality only for tumors that are likely to remain localized. For tumors characterized by a high incidence of systemic metastasis, radiation therapy should not be the only method of treatment since it is a local therapy much like surgery. Additional treatment methods aimed at distant disease, such as chemotherapy, whole body hyperthermia, or biologic response modifiers, should also be considered.

COMBINATION OF RADIATION THERAPY WITH SURGERY

Surgery always has been and probably always will be the treatment method employed first in animals with localized solid tumors. In many instances this is justified. Unfortunately, limitations of tumor removal generally seem to be unappreciated by practicing veterinarians, and substandard types of excision are frequently employed. Often, surgery is followed by a sense of well-being because all physical evidence of

tumor has been removed; yet tumor recurrence is often noted weeks or months later. When tumors recur after surgery, they are usually more difficult to manage than if more aggressive therapy had been implemented originally. The histopathology report describing excised specimens should always be read carefully since the histopathologist often comments on whether tumor cells extend to the periphery of the sample. If they do, recurrence of the tumor is eminent and additional therapy should be instituted immediately rather than waiting until the tumor recurs. In addition, incomplete excision should be assumed if dissection into the tumor is required to remove it. Only aggressive wide excisions should be considered potentially complete for invasive cancers.

Radiotherapy can be used preoperatively, postoperatively or intraoperatively.[1a] The basic rationale for use of preoperative irradiation is to sterilize tumor cells at the periphery of the volume of tissue that is to be removed. Preoperative irradiation is useful when surgical removal of the tumor is planned but it is doubtful that the entire tumor can be removed because tumor-free tissue margins cannot be achieved. Preoperative irradiation is not routinely used in animals although its use is indicated in specific situations. One such situation is in dogs with soft tissue sarcomas. Surgery alone is often ineffective in controlling these tumors. Preoperative irradiation in this disease is likely to improve the rate of local tumor control.[1a]

The rationale behind the use of postoperative irradiation is to sterilize residual tumor cells after incomplete tumor removal. Use of radiation therapy postoperatively should not be routine practice, except in a few specific situations. All tissues handled during surgery, including sites of wound drainage, must be irradiated. This often leads to large radiation fields, which increases the chance of complications. In addition, routine use of postoperative radiotherapy may tend to promote less aggressive attempts to control the tumor surgically. Radiation therapy can be used postoperatively in situations where the size of the tumor limits the homogeneity of radiation dose distribution that can be achieved. This preirradiation cytoreductive procedure is an intentionally incomplete tumor resection performed for the purpose of increasing the effectiveness of radiotherapy. One such example in the dog is the use of surgery to remove the majority of nasal cavity tumors prior to ortho-voltage radiotherapy. Because of the relatively low energy of orthovoltage x-rays, homogeneous irradiation of bulky nasal cavity tumors is nearly impossible without exceeding normal tissue tolerance. Surgical cytoreductive procedures followed by irradiation could be supported for all tumors because the procedure leaves fewer tumor cells to kill with radiation, but based on results from treatment of cancer in people, surgical procedures must result in disease being reduced to microscopic levels before any therapeutic gain is achieved.

A relatively new method of combining radiation and surgery is intraoperative irradiation. Intraoperative irradiation involves administration of radiation during operative exposure of a tumor and is usually used for treatment of deeply seated tumors in the thoracic and abdominal cavities. The advantage of intraoperative irradiation is that some of the normal tissues can be retracted outside of the radiation field and a large dose of radiation can be administered directly to the tumor. Because of the likelihood of producing necrosis in normal tissue, which cannot be retracted outside of the radiation field, with one large potentially tumoricidal intraoperative radiation dose, the dose of intraoperative radiation is usually less than the expected dose required for tumor cure. Typical intraoperative doses are in the range of 15 to 25 Gy. The intraoperative dose is then supplemented with conventional external-beam irradiation.

TECHNICAL FACTORS OF RADIATION THERAPY

Once a tumor has been identified for which radiation therapy has been deemed an acceptable treatment, a dosage prescription or treatment plan is formulated. This involves planning the size and number of radiation fields in order to maximize tumor irradiation while sparing normal tissue, or limiting normal tissue irradiation as much as possible. The treatment plan must result in the most aggressive, potentially effective treatment prescription possible since reirradiation of recurrent disease will be associated with a high likelihood of necrosis. Aggressive radiotherapy results in fibrosis and decreased blood supply. Affected tissue remains

compromised for life and is generally incapable of withstanding even moderate doses of later radiation without undergoing necrosis.

Simple radiation therapy plans can be calculated without computer assistance; the dose on the central beam axis at the surface and at selected depths in tissue can be estimated. Such calculations, however, assume that tissue is homogeneous, having the physical characteristics of water. Of course in practice this is not true, and any tissue heterogeneity introduces errors in the dose estimation. The greater the tissue heterogeneity, the greater the error. Error is particularly great when low-energy radiation is used. In formulating the treatment plan, the geometry of the patient and the tumor must be taken into consideration. In complex arrangements, where the patient surface is not flat or there is extreme tissue heterogeneity, the treatment plan must be calculated with a radiation therapy planning computer (Fig. 10-2).[1b]

In general, radiation dose per fraction, total radiation dose, and treatment time do not vary. In veterinary medicine, a commonly used dose scheme is 12 fractions of 4 Gy each given on a Monday, Wednesday, Friday schedule for a total dose of 48 Gy. As stated previously, this dose scheme has been derived empirically and is basically the maximum tolerable dose for most normal tissues. If the patient lives a convenient distance from the treatment facility, radiation therapy can be done on an outpatient basis. In other instances, the patient remains hospitalized for the duration of treatment. Each treatment requires sedation or anesthesia. For the sake of complete relaxation and ease of setting up multiple and repeatable fields, general anesthesia is preferred.

The source of radiation used in veterinary medicine is usually one of three types. The first is x-rays generated from a therapeutic x-ray machine. These machines operate at low milliampere values (5–20) and high kilovolt peak values (150–300) relative to diagnostic x-ray machines. This type of radiation therapy machine is called an orthovoltage x-ray machine, and the radiation is called orthovoltage radiation or orthovoltage x-rays. Because orthovoltage x-rays have relatively low energy, their absorption in bone is much greater than in soft tissue. This creates a problem when it is necessary to irradiate heterogeneous tissue volumes containing tissue of varying physical density. In addition,

Figure 10-2. *(A)* Computed tomographic image of a canine brain in which an enhancing mass, subsequently diagnosed as a neurofibrosarcoma, can be seen on the floor of the cranial vault. The decision was made to irradiate this tumor. Note the extensive temporal muscle atrophy that has altered the surface contour of the patient. This surface alteration makes calculation of tissue radiation dose difficult without computer assistance because some areas of the patient's surface will be closer to the radiation source than others. *(B)* Computer-generated radiation therapy plan of the same patient in which 100% of the dose is given through one lateral field. Radiation isodose lines are shown. Isodose lines give a visual representation of the dose at various positions across the radiation field. The paths of these curves trace all points within the treated volume where the radiation dose is equal to the indicated value. In other words, the 60 isodose line indicates all points where the tissue dose equals 60% of the maximum dose. It is apparent that the temporal muscle atrophy has caused the upper aspect of the isodose lines to shift deeper into the head. This results in a higher brain radiation dose than estimated when central axis dose is estimated without computer assistance. Also, when the tumor region is examined, it can be seen that there is approximately a 10% variation in dose across the tumor. In some instances, this magnitude of tumor dose variation is acceptable, but in this situation it is not because this particular treatment configuration would result in a higher radiation dose to the normal brain than to the tumor. *(C)* Computer-generated radiation therapy plan for the same patient where 50% of the radiation dose is given through each of parallel opposed fields. In addition, a wedge-shaped compensating filter had been added to Field 1 in order to compensate for the surface contour alteration produced by the temporal muscle atrophy. As can be seen, the distribution of radiation within the brain and tumor is now much more homogeneous. Even though by using plan C more of the brain will receives a larger radiation dose than if plan B were used, the treatment plan in C is more appropriate because it will allow a larger radiation dose to be given to the tumor relative to the normal brain, the tumor dose is homogeneous, and no portion of brain receive a higher radiation dose than the tumor.

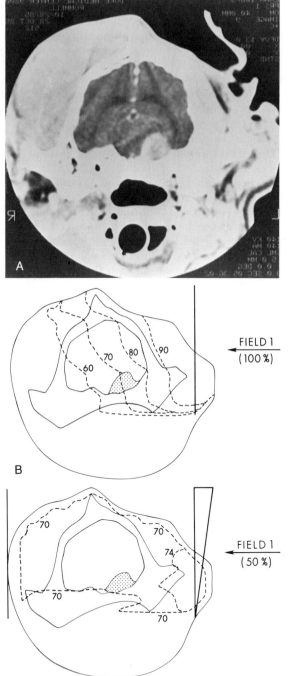

it is difficult to treat deeply seated tumors with low-energy radiation without exceeding the tolerance dose of skin. Orthovoltage x-rays were once commonly used to treat cancer in people, but they have now been replaced by equipment capable of producing higher energy radiation. Nevertheless, orthovoltage x-ray machines continue to be used for treatment of tumors in animals and are effective for treating small, superficially located, soft-tissue tumors.

The second source of radiation used to treat cancer in animals is radioactive cobalt. ^{60}Co emits gamma rays with energy approximately 10 times greater than the energy of orthovoltage x-rays. ^{60}Co teletherapy (distant therapy) machines were once the workhorse of human cancer radiotherapy. They have now been largely replaced by linear accelerators. The major advantage of ^{60}Co in comparison to orthovoltage x-rays is its greater penetrability, which allows for more homogeneous irradiation of large tumors and tissue volumes containing bone and soft tissue. In addition, because of the high energy of ^{60}Co gamma rays, the maximum dose from any field is not on the surface of the skin but 5 mm below the surface. This "skin-sparing" phenomenon of high-energy radiation has resulted in less severe skin responses to radiation therapy than when orthovoltage x-rays were in use routinely.

The third source of radiation used to treat cancer in animals is a linear accelerator. Linear accelerators produce x-rays by bombarding a metallic target with high-energy electrons. This is the same mechanism used to produce x-rays in an orthovoltage x-ray machine, with the major difference being that the energy of electrons bombarding the target is much higher. Linear accelerators produce x-rays with an energy similar to that of ^{60}Co and ranging upward to approximately 20 times greater than cobalt. This is one reason why linear accelerators have replaced cobalt machines for human cancer radiation therapy. Additional reasons are that the dose rate from a linear accelerator is much greater than the dose rate from a cobalt machine, making it possible to treat more patients per day, and the edge of the treatment field, the penumbra, is sharper, making the actual treatment field more distinct. Also, the depth of maximum dose (skin-sparing effect) ranges from 5 mm to as deep as 1.5 cm.

TUMOR RESPONSE TO RADIATION THERAPY

Selection of patients for radiation therapy should be based on the physical condition of the patient and related likelihood of successfully completing treatment as well as on tumor site and type. The size of the tumor, regardless of histologic type, is another important factor; size is inversely related to likelihood of control and directly related to likelihood of complications. As stated previously, the biologic behavior of the tumor can be predicted from its site and type. Radiation therapy should not be used as the sole treatment modality for tumors characterized by a high propensity for systemic metastasis.

Unfortunately, few prospective studies have evaluated response of animal tumors to radiation therapy. There is therefore a temptation to place too much significance on anecdotal reports or unfounded statements about radiation response of animal tumors. This is dangerous practice and should be avoided. Because new information regarding treatment response may not yet be available in the literature, consultation with a specialist should be sought before making firm recommendations to an animal owner for radiation therapy.

Often, one is tempted to base prognosis on the gross change in tumor volume during or immediately after irradiation. This practice is inaccurate because change in tumor volume is influenced by such factors as extent of stromal component and cell proliferation kinetics in addition to radiosensitivity. Thus, in some patients radiotherapy is accompanied by a decrease in tumor volume, and in others with essentially the same prognosis it is not. It is also important to recognize that for months after radiotherapy it may be possible to identify tumor cells that look active in biopsy specimens from tumors that have not completely regressed. This must not be taken as evidence of recurrence because it is impossible to determine by histologic means whether these cells are clonogenic. The most reliable sign of tumor recurrence is gross evidence of active tumor growth.

In Table 10-1, we present our evaluation of the available literature on radiation response of some of the more common canine tumors. These evaluations should be considered only as a guide because treatment modifications are continually

Table 10-1.   Radiation Response of Selected Canine Tumors

TUMOR TYPE*	SITE	RADIATION RESPONSE	REFERENCE
SCC	Gingiva	Good–Excellent	1c
SCC	External nose	Poor	2
SCC†	Tonsil	Fair–Good	3
SCC	Nasal cavity	Poor–Fair	4
ACA	Nasal cavity	Fair–Good	4, 5
FSA	Gingiva	Poor	6
FSA	Nasal cavity	Fair–Poor	4, 5
CSA	Nasal cavity	Fair–Poor	4, 5
AE	Gingiva	Good–Excellent	7
TVT	Variable	Excellent	8
HPC	Extremities	Fair–Poor	9
MCT§	Cutaneous	Poor–Excellent	10
OMM†	Gingiva, lips	Fair–Good	11
PAA	Perianal	Good	12

* SCC, squamous cell carcinoma; ACA, adenocarcinoma; FSA fibrosarcoma; CSA, chondrosarcoma; AE, acanthomatous epulis; TVT, transmissible venerial tumor; HPC, hemangiopericytoma; MCT, mast cell tumor; OMM, oral malignant melanoma; PAA, perianal adenoma.
† High tendency for distant metastasis but fair local control.
§ Response to therapy seemingly adversely affected by degree of undifferentiation.

being developed. Equally important, poor response of a tumor type to conventional therapy should not be taken as evidence that new types of therapy should not be tried in those tumors. Investigation of new types of cancer treatment in animals with spontaneous tumors will affect tumor treatment in humans as well as animals and, we hope, will lead to improvement in tumor control.

Cats are not included in Table 10-1 because, in general, less is known about radiation response of feline tumors. Radiation therapy is nonetheless a reasonable treatment choice for localized nonresectable feline tumors. Through experience in treating feline tumors, more information will be gained concerning the overall response of a variety of feline tumor types.

COMPLICATIONS OF RADIATION THERAPY

Most animals develop some effects in normal tissue as a result of being irradiated. The effects observed are limited to the treated area. Since most animal tumors treated with radiotherapy are external, the side-effects observed are largely in the skin, mucous membranes, and surrounding soft tissues or bone. Nausea and vomiting, which are often encountered in human patients, are not seen in animals unless the abdomen is irradiated. Effects in normal tissue can be divided into changes occurring during the last portion of irradiation or the first few weeks after irradiation has been completed (acute effects) and those occurring after months or years (late effects).

The rate of development of effects for a given dose and fractionation scheme is related largely to the rate of cell turnover in the target tissue. For example, commonly encountered acute effects for more rapidly dividing tissues include mucositis, moist desquamation, and hair loss in the treated area (Fig. 10-3). These effects occur because of damage inflicted to proliferating stem cells. The rate of repair of this tissue injury is dependent on the rate of repopulation of the damaged stem cells. Typically, mucositis and moist desquamation will last 2–4 weeks from onset, after which healing will ensue. Hair loss requires a longer period for replacement, often several months. Radiation will often permanently alter the function of the hair follicles, the new hair may be coarser and of a different color. For example, white or gray hair regrowth is common in black-haired patients. As long as the time–dose schemes described in this chapter are used, there is every reason to believe that acute effects will heal spontaneously within the time frame described. Although acute effects may be painful to the patient and distressing to the owner, they do not represent a serious threat to the health of the patient.

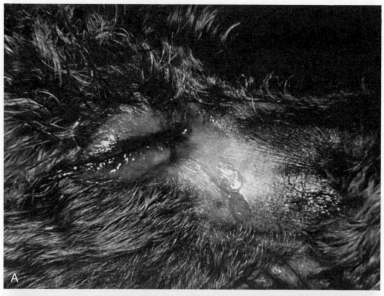

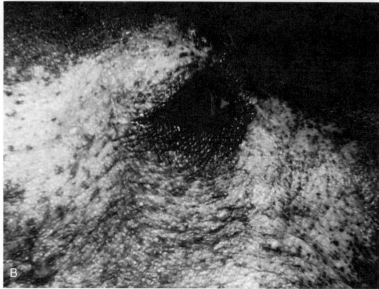

Figure 10-3. *(A)* Blepharospasm, epiphora, and moist desquamation are apparent in this dog shortly after completion of radiotherapy for a maxillary gingival tumor. These changes are called acute changes and are usually not dose-limiting. *(B)* Four weeks later the acute effects have subsided. There is now hair loss and skin depigmentation in the treated area. The skin also appears fibrotic.

Clinical signs associated with mucositis (which often accompanies irradiation of oral tumors) include drooling, difficulty in chewing, loss of appetite, and halitosis. Examination of the affected mucous membranes will reveal intensely inflamed mucosa and superficial ulceration. These signs can usually be partially ameliorated with a soft or liquid diet. The excessive salivation and drooling can be aided through the use of mouthwash diluted 1:1 with water. Occasionally, systemic administration of broad-spectrum antibiotics will help to reduce oral flora and alleviate the intensity of the reaction.

Moist desquamation is often seen when intact skin is included in the radiotherapy field. Denudation of the superficial keratinized layer of skin leaves a moist, erythematous, edematous dermis (Fig. 10-3). Moist desquamation can lead to a variety of clinical signs depending on its location. On a limb, it can lead to temporary lameness. In many sites it can lead to self-mutilation, which will require appropriate methods of restraint to prevent the animal from prolonging the healing process. The pain and tenderness of moist desquamation can be aided with the use of perfume-free water-based creams. Creams containing corticosteroids should not be used as they tend to prolong the healing process. Use of warm-water compresses to remove dried exudate are also beneficial. Full-thickness skin necrosis rarely occurs with radiation doses suggested in this chapter.

Acute effects can be seen in other tissues as well. Owners should be informed of these prior to initiation of radiotherapy in order to prevent misunderstanding later. Commonly encountered acute effects are listed in Table 10-2.

Late radiation effects occur much more slowly than acute effects; they may develop after a period of several months or years during which no abnormal clinical signs are observed. Late effects occur because of damage to blood vessels and connective tissue in the tumor bed. Tissues in which late effects are seen have a slow proliferative rate as compared with tissues that respond early. Contraction and fibrosis of muscles and joints may be associated with restriction of limb motion. The most serious late complication encountered is necrosis, which is extremely difficult to manage because the vascular supply of the surrounding tissue that was in the radiation field is often also compromised. Surgical treatment of necrosis is often not successful.

The most common site of radiation necrosis in animals is the mandible. If the time–dose scheme recommended in this chapter is used, the probability of necrosis is small—i.e., <5%.

The type of late effects encountered is related to the tissues irradiated, as was the situation for acute effects. Some types of late effects are listed in Table 10-3. Again, the likelihood of producing one of these effects with the radiation dose scheme described here is extremely low.

Some deeply seated normal tissues are particularly sensitive to late effects. It is not recommended that radiotherapy be administered to these tissues without consulting a qualified specialist. Those tissues include kidney, lung, spinal cord, brain, and bowel. The eye is also particularly sensitive to late radiation damage. For example, a dose of more than 2–3 Gy to the lens may result in cataract formation.

Irradiated tissue is much more susceptible to trauma because one long-term effect of irradiation is reduced blood flow in the tissue, which renders the tissue less able to repair itself after injury. Extreme care must be taken when manipulating irradiated tissue. Very simple procedures, such as punch biopsy, may result in tissue necrosis. Dental procedures, particularly extractions, should be done with extreme caution in regions of prior radiotherapy. It is recommended that all dental procedures or extractions be done prior to commencement of

Table 10-2. Commonly Encountered Acute Normal Tissue Effects in Radiation Therapy

REGION IRRADIATED	EXPECTED ACUTE EFFECT
Skin	Moist desquamation
	Hair loss
Mouth	Mucositis
	Salivation
	Bad odor
Nasal cavity	Nasal discharge
	Mucositis
	Moist desquamation
Eye	Blepharitis
	Blepharospasm
	Conjunctivitis
	Corneal ulceration
Foot	Loss of foot pad
	Moist desquamation
	Loss of nail
Neck	Moist desquamation
	Pharyngitis, esophagitis
	Tracheitis
Pelvis	Cystitis, colitis

Table 10-3. Possible Late Effects Resulting from Irradiation of Various Normal Tissues

REGION IRRADIATED	LATE EFFECT
Skin	Fibrosis/contraction
	Necrosis
	Nonhealing ulcer
	Contraction
	Hair color change
Limb	Neuropathy
	Fibrosis/contraction
	Contraction
Neck	Hypothyroidism
Oral cavity	Bone necrosis
	Periodontal disease
	Xerostomia
Bowel	Stricture
Spinal cord	Myelopathy
Kidney	Fibrosis
	Dysfunction
Lung	Fibrosis
Brain	Encephalopathy
Eye	Cataract
	K. Sicca

radiotherapy to minimize the chances for bone necrosis at a later time. Irradiated tissue should not be traumatized surgically unless absolutely necessary. As stated previously, reirradiation of tissue is generally not tolerated because of the fibrosis and decreased vascularity induced by the initial irradiation.

CAUSES OF RADIOTHERAPY FAILURES

Even when a seemingly ideal patient is selected and what is thought to be optimal radiotherapy is given, failure can be encountered: the tumor recurs or continues to grow. In these instances it is very important to consider all possible causes of treatment failure so that future treatment can be more efficacious. A review of some possible causes of radiotherapy failure is given below. These basic concepts have been previously described.[13]

HISTOLOGIC TUMOR TYPE

As can be seen from Table 10-1, the probability of tumor control is related to tumor type. It is tempting to draw strict conclusions from data such as those in Table 10-1 estimating response to treatment on the basis of histologic tumor type. Although such generalizations can be made, strict conclusions should not be drawn. For example, in a published review of *in vitro* radiation survival of cultured human tumor cells expressed as a function of predicted clinical radioresponsiveness, a wide range of results were found within each tumor category (Fig. 10-4).[14] Thus, there may be a wide range of tumor responses encountered among tumors of the same histologic type in similar anatomic sites, possibly reflecting actual differences in inherent cellular radiosensitivity. The predictive value of this observed difference in radiosensitivity could be exploited in individual patients by direct assay of cellular radiosensitivity *in vitro* of biopsy specimens.[15]

TUMOR VOLUME

It can be assumed that the volume of the tumor at the time of radiotherapy is inversely related to the likelihood of tumor control. This assumption is supported by clinical investigation[11] and is probably based on the direct relationship between the number of clonogenic tumor cells present and tumor volume. Therefore, any delay in administering radiotherapy is likely to result in a lower probability of tumor control because of increased tumor volume. This concept also reinforces the potential value of postoperative radiotherapy and of beginning it as soon after incomplete tumor excision as possible rather than waiting for clinical evidence of recurrence.

TUMOR CELL HYPOXIA

As stated previously, tumor cells in regions of inefficient blood supply may become hypoxia. These cells are more radioresistant than fully oxygenated tumor cells and adjacent normal tissue cells by a factor of as much as 3.0 (Fig. 10-1). Their radioresistance probably results from lack of oxygen fixation of radiation damage in DNA under hypoxic conditions. Hypoxic cells have been thought responsible for failure of radiation therapy to control some tumors. One likely benefit of fractionation of the radiation dose is reoxygenation of hypoxic tumor cells in the interval between fractionations.[16] If reoxygenation is not complete by the end of radiotherapy, however, surviving radioresistant hypoxic tumor cells might subsequently become oxygenated and cause tumor recurrence. On the other hand, it has been suggested that when doses of 2 Gy per fraction are used, the tumor may be sterilized without complete reoxygenation.[16] Nevertheless, hypoxic tumor cells have been the stimulus for many new approaches to modifying radiotherapy, including use of hyperbaric oxygen, hypoxic cell sensitizers, radioprotective agents, and hyperthermia. Discussion of these modifiers of radiotherapy is beyond the scope of this book, except for hyperthermia, which is covered in another chapter. It is sufficient to note here that hypoxia may be a significant cause of radiotherapy failure.

INSUFFICIENT TUMOR RADIATION DOSE

Failure to control a tumor with radiotherapy will clearly be the result of radiation doses less than what is needed for tumor sterilization. Delivery of a nontumoricidal dose may be unavoidable if adjacent normal tissues are not capable of withstanding a tumoricidal dose. On the other hand, delivery of a nontumoricidal dose may result from selection of a suboptimal

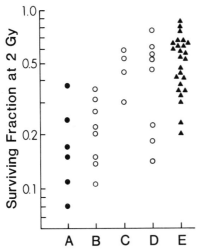

A: neuroblastoma, lymphoma, myeloma

B: medulloblastoma, small-cell lung carcinoma

C: breast, bladder, cervix carcinoma

D: pancreas, colorectal, squamous lung carcinoma

E: melanoma, osteosarcoma, glioblastoma,

      renal carcinoma

Figure 10-4. Available data concerning *in vitro* survival of cultured human tumor cells following one 2-Gy dose were reviewed. Tumors were divided into five groups ranging from those considered clinically radiosensitive, group A, to those considered clinically radioresistant, group E. Although there is a trend of increased survival following 2 Gy as clinical impression of radioresistance increases, there is extreme variability within each group. Thus, survival of cultured tumor cells *in vitro* may have value as a predictor of clinical radiosensitivity; however, variability within each tumor grouping is so great that histologic diagnosis alone should not be used as a predictor of response. (Reprinted from Deacon J, et al: The radioresponsiveness of human tumours and the initial slope of the cell survival curve. Radiother Oncol 2:317–323, 1984, with permission)

dose prescription or from an error in treatment planning that causes part of the tumor to receive less than the planned dose. It is the nature of radiation dose-response curves that a slight change in radiation dose may result in a dramatic change in tumor control probability. The exact relationship between radiation dose and tumor control probability depends on the exact shape of the dose-response curve (Fig. 10-5).[17] Examination of the dose-response curves in Fig. 10-5, reveals that their general shape is sigmoidal, meaning that up to a certain dose there is little likelihood of tumor control. After this dose is reached, tumor control increases rapidly as radiation dose is increased. After the upper plateau region of the curve is reached, there is no additional gain from increase of dose; additional dose will only serve to increase normal tissue complications.

It is desirable to deliver the prescribed radiation dose with an accuracy of ±2%. This can be achieved under ideal conditions, but in many instances the actual dose delivered varies from the prescribed dose by more than 2%. Under these circumstances, the observed change in tumor control will depend on the exact shape

of the tumor dose-response curve and the region of the curve at which one is operating. For example, consider the situation where one is operating at the ascending portion of the dose-response curve with a total delivered dose 5 Gy lower than the total prescribed dose of 60 Gy as a result of treatment planning error. If the tumor dose-response curve is steep, as for Tumor A, a 50% difference in tumor cure probability could result from the 5-Gy error. If the curve is not so steep, a less pronounced effect will probably be observed, but a significant reduction in likelihood of tumor control could still result (Fig. 10-5).[17] The major point of this discussion is to emphasize the importance of prescribing the absolute best radiation dosage and to administer it as accurately as possible. Nonchalance toward the dose and the effect of tumor location and tissue heterogeneity on its distribution will ultimately result in lack of control of potentially controllable tumors. For a more complete discussion of this phenomenon see reference 1b.

One last cause of delivery of a suboptimal radiation dose is geographic miss, where a por-

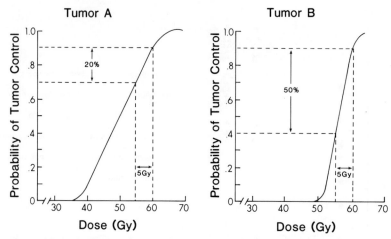

Figure 10-5. Radiation dose–response curves for two groups of tumors. The dose–response curve for the group of tumors identified as Tumor A is relatively shallow in comparison to the curve for the group of tumors identified as Tumor B. Slight changes in dose will have less of an effect in tumors with shallower dose-response curves than in tumors with steep dose-response curves. However, it is important to recognize that the sigmoidal shape of dose-response curves means that slight changes in dose may result in dramatic changes in probability of tumor control.

tion of the tumor is not included in the radiation field or is outside of the volume of tissue receiving the prescribed dose. The effect of this error is failure to cure the tumor. Meticulous treatment planning is necessary in order to avoid geographic miss. This includes determining the extent of the tumor as accurately as possible. Computed tomography has facilitated this process, particularly in dogs with tumors in complex anatomic regions (Fig. 10-2).

SUMMARY

Radiation therapy has become a sophisticated part of cancer treatment in animals. It can be given effectively and safely, and it is available to practitioners on a referral basis in many parts of this country. Radiation therapy should be considered for use in patients with localized solid tumors, where surgical treatment is unlikely to result in tumor control, or where the associated defect is unacceptable to the animal owner. Depending on tumor type, site, and stage, tumor control or long-term palliation with the use of radiation is possible in many animals with cancer.

REFERENCES

1a. McLeod DA, Thrall DE: The combination of surgery and radiation in the treatment of cancer: A review. Vet Surg (in press)

1b. Thrall DE, McLeod DA, Bentel GC, Dewhirst MW: A review of treatment planning and dose calculation in veterinary radiation oncology. Vet Radiol (in press)

1c. Gillette EL: Hyperthermia effects in animals with spontaneous tumors. Natl Cancer Inst Monograph No. 61:361–364, 1982

2. Thrall DE, Adams WM: Radiotherapy of squamous cell carcinomas of the canine nasal plane. Vet Radiol 23:193–196, 1982

3. MacMillan R, Withrow SJ, Gillette EL: Surgery and regional irradiation for treatment of canine tonsillar squamous cell carcinoma. Retrospective review of eight cases. J Am Anim Hosp Assoc 18:311–314, 1982

4. Adams WM, Withrow SJ, Walshaw R, et al: Radiotherapy of malignant nasal tumors in 67 dogs. J Am Vet Med Assoc, 191:311–315, 1987

5. Thrall DE, Harvey CE: Radiotherapy of malignant nasal tumors in 21 dogs. J Am Vet Med Assoc 183:663–666, 1982

6. Thrall DE: Orthovoltage radiotherapy of gingival fibrosarcomas in dogs. J Am Vet Med Assoc 179:159–162, 1981

7. Thrall DE: Orthovoltage radiotherapy of acanthomatous epulides in 39 dogs. J Am Vet Med Assoc 184:826–829, 1984

8. Thrall DE: Orthovoltage radiotherapy of canine transmissible venereal tumors. Vet Radiol 23:217–219, 1982

9. Evans SM: Canine hemangiopericytoma: A retrospective analysis of response to surgery and orthovoltage radiation. Vet Radiol 28:13–16, 1987

10. Thrall DE, Dewhirst MW: Use of radiation and/or hyperthermia for treatment of mast cell tumors and lymphosarcoma in dogs. Vet Clin North Am 15:835–844, 1985

11. Dewhirst MW, Sim DA, Forsyth K, et al: Local control and distant metastases in primary canine malignant melanomas treated with hyperthermia and/or radiotherapy. Int J Hyperthermia 1:219–234, 1985

12. Gillette EL: Radiation therapy of canine and feline tumors. J Am Anim Hosp Assoc 12:359–362, 1976

13. Fletcher GH, Peters LJ: Causes of failures in the radiation therapy of head and neck cancer. Paper presented at the 27th Annual Meeting of the American Society for Therapeutic Radiology and Oncology, Miami, FL, Sept 29–Oct 4, 1985

14. Deacon J, Peckham MJ, Steel GG: The radioresponsiveness of human tumors and the initial slope of the cell survival curve. Radiother Oncol 2:317–323, 1984

15. Peters LJ, Brock W, Johnson T: Predicting radiocurability. Cancer 55:2118–2122, 1985

16. Withers HR, Peters LJ: Biologic aspects of radiation therapy. In Fletcher GH (ed): Textbook of Radiotherapy, 3rd ed., pp. 103–180. Philadelphia, Lea & Febiger, 1980

17. Williams MV, Denekamp J, Fowler JF: Dose-response relationships for human tumors: Implications for clinical trials of dose-modifying agents. Int J Radiat Oncol Biol Phys 10:1703–1707, 1984

11

IMMUNOLOGY AND BIOLOGIC THERAPY OF CANCER

E. Gregory MacEwen

IMMUNITY TO TUMORS

Malignant transformation may be associated with phenotypic changes in the involved cells, including the loss of normal antigenic components from cell surfaces, the induction of neoantigens, and other membrane changes. Some of these phenotypic changes may evoke an immune response. In addition to antigenic phenotypic changes, malignant cell membranes may develop structural differences that will further render them susceptible to natural effector cells.

Solid tumors removed at surgery are sometimes characterized by a marked mononuclear cell infiltrate, unrelated to tissue necrosis, which is suggestive of host resistance of an immunologic nature. These mononuclear cells represent a mixture of cells such as lymphocytes, macrophages, plasma cells, and mast cells. In some situations the presence of infiltrative mononuclear cells is associated with a better prognosis.

INDUCED CELL-MEDIATED IMMUNITY

Induced cell-mediated immunity is primarily directed to tumors expressing strong tumor-associated (specific) antigens (TAA) sometimes referred to as tumor-specific transplant antigens (TSTA). Even though T cells may be quite effective in mediating potent antitumor immunity, they do not appear to play a major role in immune surveillance against malignant cells.

T cell activation includes the generation of helper (T_H) and suppressor (T_S) subsets as well as cytotoxic T-lymphocytes (T_c). Amplification of these responses requires interleukins and various lymphokines. T_H cells generate lymphokines that are important for the recruitment and activation of macrophages and natural killer (NK) cells (Fig. 11-1). The lymphokines or cytokines have a specific ability to regulate certain components of the immune response, which may be useful in altering the growth and metastasis of cancer.[1]

The important lymphokines and cytokines are:

1. Migration inhibition factor (MIF), which functions to arrest macrophages at the (antigenic) tumor site

Figure 11-1. Effective antitumor immune response depends on a variety of cells, including macrophages, T cells, B cells, and natural killer cells. Macrophages can be activated by tumor-associated antigens (TAA) to release various monokines such as interleukin-1 (IL-1) and other factors, including tumor necrosis factor (TNF), hydrogen peroxides (H_2O_2), and lysosomal enzymes. Macrophages may also contain receptors (R) that may "fix" antigens to their cell surface for "presentation" to lymphocytes. Progenitor T cells can be activated by antigens or IL-1 to proliferate and release lymphokines such as macrophage-activating factor (MAF), interferon (IFN), and migration inhibition factor (MIF), which inhibits macrophage mobility. Interleukin-2 (IL-2) released from T helper (T_H) cells further augments the generation of cell-mediated cytotoxic T-lymphocytes (T_c) and natural killer (NK) cells. Suppressor T (T_S) cells inhibit responses of other lymphocytes. B-lymphocytes can produce antibody (Ab) that may be directly cytotoxic (in the presence of complement) or necessary for lymphocyte (K cell) antibody-dependent cytotoxicity. See text for further details.

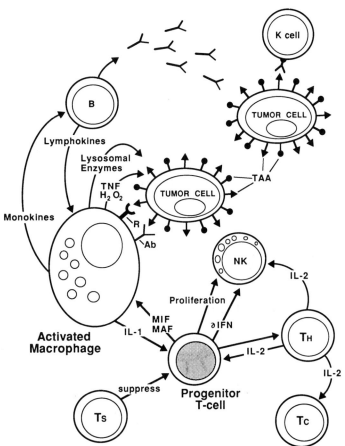

2. Macrophage activity factor (MAF), which is very similar to γ-IFN (see below) and will "activate" the macrophage
3. Chemotactic factor for macrophages (CFM), which will recruit other phagocytic cells to the tumor cell
4. Lymphotoxins (LT), which will lyse tumor cells *in vitro*
5. Transfer factor (TF), which will transfer the specific immune response to other lymphocytes
6. Interferons (IFN), which have many immunoregulatory and antiproliferative functions. They may suppress or enhance antibody production, express cell surface antigens, modulate T cell function, and regulate natural killer cell and macrophages function.
7. Interleukin-1 (Il-1), which is a cytokine derived from macrophages and can enhance T cell proliferation. IL-1 may also augment the release of B cell growth factor. IL-1 causes fever and stimulates the liver to secrete acute-phase proteins.
8. Interleukin-2 (IL-2), a mitogenic factor (MF) that amplifies the proliferation of other T cells. IL-2 is produced by T_H cells and helps to generate and control the proliferation of T_c cells.
9. Interleukin-3 (IL-3) or colony-stimulating factor (CSF), which can stimulate the production of granulocyte-macrophage progenitor cells.

NATURAL CELL-MEDIATED IMMUNITY

Some cells are capable of lysing tumor cells without prior recognition or sensitization to specific antigens. These effector cells include killer cells, NK cells, macrophages, and to some extent polymorphonuclear leukocytes.

Killer Cells

Killer cells (K cells), believed to be members of the monocyte-macrophage lineage, destroy target cells that have reacted with antibody. This is referred to as antibody-dependent cellular cytotoxicity (ADCC). It is postulated that IgG antibody serves to bridge the K cell to the target cell. The K cell bonds the fragment crystallizable (F_c) portion of the antibody (IgG) molecule. The antigen and the target cell are bound by the antigen-binding site of the antibody. The result is target cell death of the target cell.[1]

Macrophages

When associated with different tissues, macrophages are given different names. In connective tissue they are histiocytes, in the lining of the liver they are Kupffer cells, in the brain they are microglia, and in the lung they are called alveolar macrophages.

As effectors, macrophages generally express little cytotoxicity unless "activated" by lymphokines, bacterial substances, or interferon.[2] Activated macrophages are considered cytotoxic to most tumor cells regardless of their phenotypic expression. An important property of an activated macrophage is its ability to differentiate tumor cells from normal cells. The recognition process requires cell-to-cell contact and involves interaction of surface glycoproteins of both the macrophage and the tumor cell. Tumor cell destruction results predominantly from a nonphagocytic, contact-mediated secretion of substances that are cytotoxic.[3] There is controversy regarding the substances responsible for cytotoxicity.

Tumor necrosis factor (TNF) or cachectin is one substance that may participate in the *in vivo* destruction of tumor cells. TNF can cause both hemorrhagic necrosis of tumors *in vivo* and selective lysis of some tumor cells *in vitro*.[4] A proposed mechanism of action is that TNF acts as a protease, enzymatically destroying some surface protein vital to the integrity of the cell.[5]

Another substance that may contribute to the lysis of cells is a cytolytic protease. This protease is only released when macrophages bind to tumor cells and not when they bind to normal cells. Macrophages can also express a cytotoxic factor (CF) that has been proposed to cause damage to cell membranes.[6]

A second major mechanism of macrophage cytotoxicity that has been identified is the release of superoxide anions (O_2^-) and hydrogen peroxide (H_2O_2). H_2O_2 is considered by some to be an important effector molecule in macrophage cytotoxicity.[2]

Macrophages can also mediate inhibiting effects on immune functions. Prostaglandins (PGE_2) elaborated by macrophages will inhibit some lymphoproliferative responses.[7]

NK Cells

The NK cells, also termed the large granular lymphocyte (LGL) in humans, account for 2% to 5% of peripheral blood lymphocytes.[1] The target cell structure(s) recognized by NK cells have yet to be defined. They do not correlate with any of the well-characterized cell surface antigens, such as major histocompatibility complex (MHC) products. Some evidence suggests that the transferrin receptor present on all dividing cells may be implicated.[7] The determinants recognized by NK cells seem to be more prevalent on tumor cells in tissue culture than in the body. Susceptibility of a target cell to lysis by NK cells depends on the degree of differentiation of the target and its capacity to repair membrane damage.

NK activity can be regulated by interferon, by IL-2 in a stimulating way, and by PGE_2 in an inhibitory way. IFN will transform noncytolytic NK precursors into a lytic state and enhance the cytolytic capacity of already active cells.[8]

The biologic role of NK cells is not clearly defined. There is evidence from experimental systems that NK cells participate in the rejection of transplanted tumor cells, in the prevention of metastases, and in graft-versus-host reactions. Their role in killing established tumors is most likely minimal. NK activity is probably more pronounced against lymphoreticular tumors than solid tumors.[7]

INTERACTION BETWEEN INDIVIDUAL EFFECTOR CELL MECHANISMS

It is unrealistic to attribute the complex tumor–immune system interactions to a function of one cell population. Antitumor activity is a result of interactions among various effector cell populations. Such interaction may be mediated through direct cell-to-cell contact or through biologic factors produced by lymphocytes.

B Cell Responses

The role of antibodies against tumor expressed antigens is unclear. Antibodies may be involved in the direct lysis of tumor cells or in the recruitment of cells carrying F_c receptors, such as NK cells and macrophages. In addition, antibodies may form soluble immune complexes that may subvert the cellular immune responses.[9,10]

The effector cell of B-lymphocytes is called a plasma cell. Plasma cells are very active in antibody production, synthesizing and secreting many thousands of antibody molecules per minute, but the cells live only 3 to 6 days. In the initial or primary response to antigen, IgM is the predominant product secreted, and IgG usually predominates in the secondary response. Not all B cells mature into plasma cells. Some revert back to small lymphocytes called memory cells. These long-lived cells are responsible for what is termed the secondary immune response.

Immune Complexes

The nature of the immune complexes detected in cancer patients in unknown, and precise immunochemical characterization is lacking. Immune complexes may suppress or augment immunologic functions.[11] B cell function can be suppressed when the B cells' F_c-receptor is cross-linked to its antigen receptor by an antigen-antibody complex. This results in inhibitory antibody synthesis. When antibody-antigen complexes interact with antigen-presenting cells (macrophages) through the F_c-receptor, the net result can be stimulation of B cell function.

In addition, these complexes may bind directly to T_c cells and thus prevent their recognition of the tumor cell, or they may bind to T_H cells and prevent them from recognizing the tumor and from recruiting T_c cells.[7]

Immunosurveillance

Immunosurveillance is one form of host surveillance that might help limit tumor development. Immunosurveillance is most likely mediated by more than one component of the immune system (*e.g.*, T cells, NK cells, and macrophages). The most convincing evidence for T cell-mediated immunosurveillance is seen in the studies in nude mice and immunocom-petent normal mice. These two groups of mice have the same incidence of spontaneous tumors, chemically induced tumors, and tumors caused by RNA tumor viruses. But the incidence of tumors produced by DNA tumor viruses is increased in the nude (T cell-deficient) mice. This indicates that only in the case of DNA virus-induced tumors is there evidence of T cell-mediated surveillance.[12]

In children with primary immunodeficiency disease, there is an increase in malignancies of lymphoreticular origin only. In adults with viral or iatrogenic immunosuppression, there is also an increased risk of lymphoreticular neoplasms and some skin tumors.[12] It has been postulated that immunosuppression may result in the release of ubiquitous viruses with oncogenic potential, leading to the increase in tumors seen.

Immunologic Escape Mechanisms[7,12]

Immunologic escape occurs when the balance between factors that control tumor growth is subverted and the tumor progresses. The following factors may contribute to this phenomenon:

1. "Sneaking through"—In animals previously immunized by tumor cells, and then challenged with a dose of cells optimal for tumor rejection, the tumor cells "sneak through" and are not recognized and a tumor develops.
2. Antigen modulation—Antibody modulates antigens on the cell surface by producing antigen shedding, endocytosis, and redistribution of the antigen within the cell membrane. This facilitates escape by removing target antigens.
3. Antigen masking—Antigens on the cell surface may be hidden or "masked" by such glycoproteins as sialomucins. Methods to remove these glycoproteins use neurominidase, which can restore expression of the antigens and thus render the cell susceptible to attack by the immune system.
4. Antigen shedding—Saturation of antigen binding sites on the T cell, especially in the tumor microenvironment, may interfere with local T cell-mediated immunity.
5. Tolerance—Exposure to either very large amounts of antigens or repeated low amounts of antigen can produce tolerance. Tolerance has best been seen experimentally when

previous exposure to antigens, such as is seen in the murine mammary tumor virus system, results in a more progressive tumor growth. Experiments in which congenitally virally infected mice were given milk infected with the mouse mammary tumor virus showed no tumor development. The mice had developed a tolerance of the virus due to exposure to low amounts of tumor antigens.

6. Lymphocyte trapping—Lymphocytes in the tumor vicinity, such as a local lymph node, may become fixed to the node and the level of tumor antigen may induce tolerance.

7. Blocking factors—Antigen-antibody complexes tend to be immunosuppressive and thus have a "protective" effect on tumor development.

8. Tumor products—Prostaglandins can be elaborated from tumors and can inhibit NK and K cell functions. Similarly, other factors, such as glycoprotein subunits, can suppress surrounding T cell functions.

9. Tumor heterogeneity—Tumor cells tend to be genetically unstable and capable of generating clonal variants with increasing malignant properties during progression.

Immune Response Cascade[1,7]

The immune response cascade can proceed as follows. Antigens are first presented (free or associated with target cells, such as tumor cells) to tissue-fixed macrophages. A small percentage of the antigen will find its way to the surface of the macrophage and become associated with the Class II MHC antigen. IL-1 is then secreted from the macrophage. Antigen-specific, mature, "committed" lymphocytes (either T or B cells) bind to the antigen. Certain T cells are stimulated and proliferate with the help of T_H cells. The antigen-specific B-lymphocytes interact with the T_H cells and develop into plasma cells that secrete antibody.

The effector T_H cells, stimulated by IL-1, also secrete lymphokines such as IL-2, B cell growth factor (BCGF) and interferon γ. IL-2 stimulates development of T cells and activates NK cells. Further, T_S may suppress some T and B cells. Thus, the immune response is regulated (Fig. 11-1).

Potential for Therapy

Most studies have shown that immunotherapy or biologic therapy will be most effective in removing tumor foci inaccessible to conventional treatment or may enhance specific or nonspecific antitumor activity. The primary task of immunotherapy is the heightening of any anti-TAA responses that are mounted by the host and the modulation of cytotoxic effector functions.

BIOLOGIC THERAPY

NONSPECIFIC IMMUNOSTIMULATION— BACTERIAL PRODUCTS

Bacterial products exert their major effect on the activation of B- and T-lymphocytes, NK cells, and macrophages.[13] They intensify antibody-dependent cellular cytotoxicity (ADCC), induce IFN, and elaborate TNF. *Corynebacterium parvum* is one bacterial substance that has been studied quite extensively. Most studies in humans using *C. parvum* alone or in combination with surgery have been unremarkable. A few studies have shown some positive effects in pulmonary carcinoma patients and melanoma patients. With others, I recently completed a study of canine oral melanoma treated with combined *C. parvum* therapy and surgery.[14] Forty-two dogs were treated with *C. parvum* plus surgical excision, and 47 were treated with surgery alone. All melanomas were clinically staged by the World Health Organization clinical staging system before treatment was begun. All dogs underwent complete surgical removal of the primary tumor by blade excision. Dogs with enlarged regional (submandibular) lymph nodes underwent lymphadenectomy. The *C. Parvum* therapy (0.1–0.5 mg/kg IV weekly) was started no later than 1 month after surgery. The median survival times were 228 days for dogs treated by surgery alone and 370 days for those treated by surgery and *C. parvum*. When the dogs with stage 1 disease (primary tumor less than 2 cm in diameter) were excluded from the analysis, the median survival for the dogs that had surgery alone was 121 days and 288 days for dogs treated with the combined therapy (Fig. 11-2). This study indicates that *C. parvum* retarded disease in dogs with malignant melanoma and further indicates that *C. parvum* may be more effective in the treatment of dogs with advanced oral melanoma.

A biologic response modifier that has received quite extensive study is the attenuated live mycobacterium, Calmette-Guerin bacillus

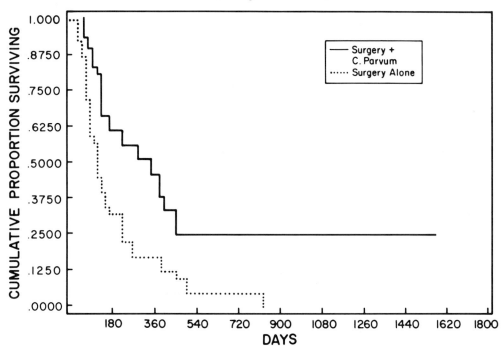

SURVIVAL TO TREATMENT
(Stage II and III)

Figure 11-2. A survival curve of 89 dogs with oral melanoma treated by surgery alone (*n* = 47) or by surgery plus *C. parvum* (*n* = 42). Dogs treated with the *C. parvum* had a significant prolongation in survival time (*p* = 0.01).[14]

(BCG).[15,15a] Its use is based on its effect in augmenting immune effector cell function and antitumor activity in animal models, and its ability to induce partial or complete regression when inoculated into cutaneous metastases of human patients with malignant melanoma. In an attempt to circumvent potential toxicity associated with the use of a viable organism, the methanol-extractable residue (MER) of BCG has also been evaluated in both animals and humans for clinical trials.[16,17] In a recent trial, MER was evaluated in dogs with osteosarcoma after amputations as a prevention of distant metastasis. In 21 dogs treated with intradermal MER, no appreciable beneficial effect on decreasing incidence of metastasis and enhancing survival time was found.[17]

A major drawback to the further study of these bacterial agents is the lack of definition of their chemistry and the inability to produce a pure pharmaceutical product. With fractionation of the BCG organism and its cell wall into components, it has been shown that these compo-

nents induce delayed hypersensitivity. When injected interlesionally they induce regression of injected lesions and the development of specific systemic tumor immunity. Cell wall skeletons of BCG and trehalose dimycolate have been used in clinical trials in humans and are undergoing study in animals. These BCG cell wall preparations have been used to successfully treat bovine ocular squamous cell carcinoma and equine sarcoids.[18,19]

An active component of the BCG cell wall is a substance termed muramyl dipeptide (MDP). In experimental models MDP and its analogue muramyl tripeptide (MTP) have been shown to increase the immune response against viral, bacterial, parasitic, or other vaccines, including whole or split influenza virus. In addition, antitumor activity of MDP has been observed in a variety of experimental models.[20,20a]

Nonspecific antitumor immunity has also been demonstrated after administration of liposomes containing MDP. In a murine metastatic melanoma model, Fidler and co-workers have reported that following primary tumor excision, repeated injections of liposome-encapsulated MDP decreased the number of lung metastases and increased the survival time.[21] MDP encapsulated within liposomes is readily phagocytized by monocytes and activates macrophages to a higher degree than free MDP (Fig. 11-3). A combination of MDP and macrophage-activating factor (MAF) in liposomes has also been shown to stimulate synergistic tumoricidal activity in rat alveolar macrophages. In studies in our laboratory, we have found that dogs with osteosarcoma treated with liposome-encapsulated muramyl peptides and amputation have a longer survival time than dogs treated with amputation alone. To date we have treated 27 dogs in our study; 13 dogs have received surgery alone, and 14 dogs have received surgery plus liposome-encapsulated MTP. The median survival time for the dogs treated by surgery alone is 77 days and for the dogs treated with the combined immunotherapy and surgery, it is 222 days. These results of our study encourage us to believe that liposome-encapsulated immune stimulants have clinical potential as antitumor agents.[21a,21b]

Another bacterial product that has received extensive study is a mixture of *S. marcescens* and *S. pyogenes*.[22] This combination has been termed a mixed bacterial vaccine (MBV). MBV is composed of bacterial cell walls, peptidoglycans, endotoxins, and exotoxins. We have shown antitumor activity in dogs and cats[22] and MBV also has been reported to have antitumor activity in humans.[22a] We have also evaluated the effect of MBV on the eosinophilic granuloma complex in 42 cats.[23] Eight of these cats had a primary untreated eosinophilic granuloma, and 34 of them were diagnosed as having recurrent granulomas after failing corticosteroid therapy. Of the 42 cats that we treated, 16 had a complete regression of disease and 13 had a partial regression of at least 50%. The overall response rate—complete regression plus partial regression for the 33 evaluable cases—was 87%. The results of this study indicate that mixed bacterial vaccines may have activity not only in tumors but in the feline eosinophilic granuloma complex.

S. aureus (Staph A, Cowan I strain) has been found to contain a cell wall protein called Protein A which binds the F_c portion of certain immunoglobulins. Based on the fact that Protein A

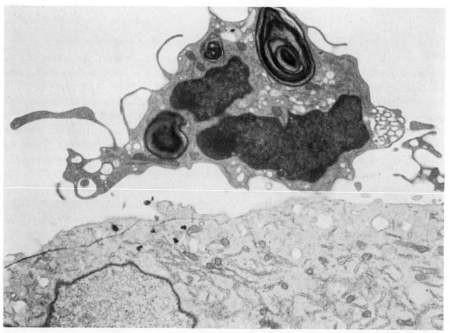

Figure 11-3. Transmission electromicrograph of a macrophage showing 3 liposomes within the cytoplasm. The liposomes are slowly degraded, releasing the MDP into the cell and "activating" the macrophage to become tumoricidal. (Courtesy of I.J. Fidler.)

will absorb IgG from the serum, a number of studies have evaluated Staph A and purified Protein A for its ability to remove so-called "blocking factors." The removal of these blocking factors is supposed to allow for immunologic modulation and resultant antitumor activity. The results, using Staph A or purified Protein A, have been generally unpredictable.

Studies of canine mammary adenocarcinoma and of human patients with colonic carcinoma have shown that extracorporeal immunoabsorption of plasma over Staph A (with Protein A) has resulted in tumoricidal activity.[24,25] Similar antitumor activity has been seen in dogs and cats with lymphosarcoma after extracorporeal immunoabsorption over Staph A. The mechanism of the antitumor activity might include removal of circulating immune complexes, activation of plasma factors such as complement, and release into the plasma of bacterial products that may have immunomodulatory activity.[25]

NONSPECIFIC IMMUNOSTIMULATION— CHEMICAL IMMUNOMODULATORS

Several chemically defined nonspecific immunostimulants either have been or are currently available for clinical study. The agent that has received the most attention during the past few years is levamisole, an anthelmentic with immunorestorative capacities. In human patients positive effects have been seen in non-oat-cell lung carcinoma and colon-rectal carcinoma.[16] In addition a large trial evaluating levamisole as maintenance therapy in patients with myeloma has demonstrated an increase in the duration of response to chemotherapy. Additional trials using levamisole as an adjuvant to surgery in human patients with melanoma or head and neck cancer have shown no benefits.[16] Attempts to demonstrate immunorestorative effects with levamisole in human patients undergoing therapy have produced inconsistent results and have not clearly shown that levamisole has immunomodulatory activity.

In a recent study of canine mammary tumors, 144 dogs with untreated malignant mammary tumors were clinically staged and randomly treated after mastectomy with either a placebo or levamisole.[26] There was no significant difference in either survival time or cancer-free survival time between the two groups. A similar study also failed to show any effectiveness in 64 cats with malignant mammary cancer when levamisole was combined with radical mastectomy.[27] Finally, in a study of canine lymphosarcoma, 98 dogs with previously untreated lymphosarcoma were treated with a combination chemotherapy protocol and then randomly assigned either levamisole or a placebo group. There was no significant difference either in remission or survival time between the levamisole and placebo groups.[28]

Most recently the antihistamine agents that block the H_2 receptor, cimetidine and ranitidine, have been shown to enhance a variety of immunologic functions both in vivo and in vitro.[29] Human patients receiving cimetidine have exhibited enhanced cell-mediated immunity as evaluated by increased response to skin test antigens, restoration of sensitivity following development of acquired tolerance to 1-chloro-2,4-dinitrobenzene (DNCB), and increased responses of peripheral blood lymphocytes to mitogen stimulation. Although the mechanisms of this enhancement have not been clearly defined, most studies suggest that cimetidine functions by inhibiting suppressor cell activity.[30] It has been suggested that suppressor cell activity may be mediated through the histamine-induced release of a soluble factor. The release of this factor can be blocked by H_2 receptor antagonists. Other evidence of the role of the H_2 blockers as immunomodulators is based on the finding that they enhance graft-versus-host reactions and potentiate the effects of interferon. The potential of the H_2 antagonists as biologic response modifiers awaits further in vitro and in vivo studies.

SPECIFIC ACTIVE IMMUNOTHERAPY—TUMOR CELL VACCINATION

Tumor cell vaccines are used to enhance specific mechanisms associated with antitumor resistance. Modified cancer vaccines may offer a means whereby the immunogenicity of tumor cells may be artificially enhanced for use in active immunization protocols. Modification of the cancer cell can comprise (1) infection with certain viruses, (2) chemical attachment of foreign determinants, (3) introduction of foreign determinants by somatic cell hybridization, and (4) isolation and purification of relevant tumor-specific antigens.

In veterinary medicine most of the recent studies using modified tumor vaccines have been performed by Dr. Jeglum at the University of Pennsylvania. She has performed studies in both canine lymphoma and feline mammary adeno-carcinoma.[31,32] Fifty-eight dogs with lymphomas were treated with combination chemotherapy (vincristine, cyclophosphamide, L-asparaginase, doxorubicin) followed by intralymphatic autoch-thonous tumor cell vaccine. Thirty dogs received chemotherapy alone. Dogs treated with the tumor cell vaccine had a significantly longer median remission time (98 days) than those treated by chemotherapy alone (28 days). There was, however, no significant difference in the survival times, 308 days and 204 days, in the vaccine and chemotherapy groups respectively.[31]

In the study of feline mammary tumors, the tumor cell vaccine did not enhance survival over the use of surgery alone.[32]

Lymphokines and Cytokines[7,12,16]

Many of the specific biologicals potentially available for therapy are cell products of lymphocytes (lymphokines) or of cells in general (cytokines). Many lymphokines have the function of regulating various components of the immune response, and their use to manipulate the system may be helpful in altering growth and metastasis of cancer. Lymphokines may have augmenting effects on T and B cells. Additionally, lymphokines may also decrease suppressive functions of the immune system and, in doing that, may enhance immune responses in animals with cancer. Few studies have been performed in veterinary medicine to evaluate lymphokines for activity as biologic response modifiers.

Interferon. The interferons are a family of proteins produced by a number of cells with different origins. Type I alpha- and beta-interferons are produced, respectively, by induced leukocytes and fibroblasts, and Type II gamma-interferon is produced by lymphocytes in response to antigenic or mitogenic stimulation. The interferons have now been identified and purified for therapeutic studies. They were initially thought to have only antiviral activity, but multiple other functions previously thought related to impurities in the preparations have now been documented as effects of interferon itself.[33,34,35] Relatively low doses of interferon have been shown to enhance antibody formation and lymphocyte blastogenesis, while higher doses have inhibited both of these functions and have delayed hypersensitivity while enhancing macrophage phagocytosis and cytotoxicity, lymphocyte cytotoxicity, NK cell activity, and surface antigen expression.

The future of interferon therapy in animals probably depends on the availability of genetically produced, recombinant DNA interferon. Interferons tend to be species specific; however, studies are underway with alpha-interferon, which has been shown to have cross-species specificity. For example, bovine alpha-interferon has been used to treat feline leukemia.[35a]

The antitumor action of interferon occurs either through a direct antiproliferative effect or through a stimulatory action on the immune system. In addition, interferon prolongs the cell cycle and inhibits cell multiplication by increasing the various phases of the cell cycle.[8]

Alpha-interferon has been shown to have objective antitumor activity in a number of human tumors.[16,33-36] Objective responses have been noted in over 50% of patients with non-Hodgkin's lymphoma with favorable histology and in 20% to 25% in patients with five other types of tumors. A tumor that has been considered highly responsive to interferon treatment is the hairy-cell leukemia in humans. The favorable response rate using interferon in this disease currently is around 75%.[37] In humans, tumors sharing an intermediate response to alpha-interferon have been malignant melanoma, renal cell carcinoma, Kaposi's sarcoma, and myeloma. The immunomodulatory capabilities of this cytokine have been demonstrable, and effects on NK cell and macrophage activity have been documented. Two other interferons undergoing extensive evaluation are the beta- and gamma-interferons.

Other cytokines of particular interest are interleukin-1, interleukin-2,[37] and interleukin-3 or granulocyte-macrophage colony-stimulating factor (GM-CSF). Interleukin-1 plays an essential role in the initiation and augmentation of specific T cell cytotoxicity and helper stimulation of antibody production. It may also induce inflammatory mediators, acute phase reactants, and fever.[7,37a] Recent evidence indicates that the monocyte is the major source of interleukin-1. Interleukin-2, also termed T cell growth factor, is produced by helper T cells. Interleukin-2 is necessary for the growth of T cells and K cells and potentiates their cytotoxic activity.[37] It is currently being evaluated in human cancer patients, used both alone and in combination with cultured cytotoxic or helper T cells.[37] IL-3, also known as granulocyte–macrophage colony-stimulating factor, will stimulate the production of monocyte and macrophage progenator cells.[37b]

Another cytokine that is receiving interest for its potential antitumor activity is the macrophage-activating factor (MAF).[16] Activated macrophages have the capacity to nonspecifically but selectively kill tumor cells. MAF nonspecifically activates macrophages. Encapsulating macrophage activators into liposomes has been one way to induce in vivo activation with resultant regression of systemic metastasis in a murine melanoma model.[38]

Thymosin. Another group of cytokines with demonstrable effect on the immune system is the thymosins.[16] A number of recent studies have demonstrated both an in vivo and in vitro immune restorative effect in immunodeficient children. Further, two studies have demonstrated both an in vitro and in vivo stimulatory effect of thymosin on T cell function in patients with malignancy. Additionally, two prospectively randomized clinical trials evaluating thymosin in patients with oat cell carcinoma of the lung and squamous cell carcinoma of head and neck have demonstrated an improved disease-free interval and survival.[16] In humans, two thymosin products are available for clinical study. Fraction 5, the material used in the above-mentioned studies, is extracted from the thymus gland of fetal calves. A thymosin product termed alpha-1 is a polypeptide with lymphokine functions several times more potent than Fraction 5. To date no studies of these products have been performed in animals with spontaneous tumors.

Tumor Necrosis Factor. Another cytokine that is under intense study is termed tumor necrosis factor (TNF). TNF is thought to be released from the macrophage after exposure to bacterial agents such as lipopolysaccharides.[39] It is preferentially cytotoxic for transformed cells and was originally named for its ability to cause hemorrhagic necrosis of transplanted subcutaneous tumors in mice. TNF may be most effective when combined with cytotoxic drugs. Current studies are underway to evaluate TNF in canine malignancies.

Tuftsin. Tuftsin is an integral part of the heavy chain of the IgG molecule.[40,41] Two enzymes are required to release tuftsin from its carrier molecule. Tuftsin has been shown to have specific stimulating effects on the granulocyte and macrophage functions—e.g., phagocytosis, pinocytosis, motility, chemotaxis, immunogenic stimulation, and bacterial and tumoricidal activities.

An antineoplastic effect of tuftsin in vivo has been shown in several tumor lines. In L-1210 murine leukemia, tuftsin-treated mice have shown prolonged survival. In a murine melanoma model and a sarcoma model tuftsin has been found to have antineoplastic activity. In human patients, responses have been documented in acute myeloblastic leukemia and in a nasopharyngeal and alveolar cell carcinomas.[41]

PASSIVE IMMUNOTHERAPY

Passive immunotherapy entails the transfer of antitumor antibody to cancer patients in order to cause tumor regression or prevent tumor recurrence. The current interest in antibody therapy is based on the ability to produce large quantities of antibodies to specific antigens. These antibodies are termed monoclonal antibodies since they arise from one clone cell and are essentially identical antibodies with respect to antigen recognition. They can be coupled to chemotherapeutic agents, radioactive materials, and also toxins and can be used to target these highly selective toxic agents. The potential for monoclonal antibody therapy appears to be enormous. The use of antibody in animal tumor models and in humans has recently been reviewed and the results summarized.[42] This approach appears to offer the best possibilities of tumor-specific therapy for the next few years.

Another form of passive immunotherapy has been the use of nonspecific serum factors. Selective destruction of malignant lymphocytes has been observed in leukemic mice, cats, and dogs following infusions of normal serum, plasma, whole blood, and plasma cryoprecipitate.[43-46] A dog with acute lymphoblastic leukemia remained in complete remission for 19 months after 2 months of plasma therapy.[47] The occasional but well-documented remissions in human leukemia patients after transfusion of normal blood or plasma might represent the human counterpart of this phenomenon. A heparin precipitate from plasma that has antileukemic activity in mice bears resemblance to a fraction of plasma called cold-insoluble globulin (CI_g) or fibronectin (F_N). F_N is a major glycoprotein of blood and tissue. It has been shown to enhance macrophage-mediated tumoricidal activity *in vitro*[48] and to stimulate T cell blastogenesis by macrophage activation.[49] F_N has also been shown to decrease metastasis in a murine melanoma model.[50]

In an unpublished study of 18 cats with lymphoma or leukemia treated with fibronectin infusions, 9 (50%) had a response—7 a partial response and 2 a complete response. We also have treated a dog with acute lymphoblastic leukemia. The dog developed a partial response to F_N. More recently we have treated a cat with erythroleukemia with infusions of F_N (Fig. 11-4). The potential of F_N will depend upon further studies in either experimental animal models or in spontaneous tumors in animals.

CONCLUSIONS

The use of biologic response modification as a treatment of cancer is attractive because it makes use of the host's natural defenses. The success of this therapy may depend on the presence of tumor-associated antigens on tumor cells that are capable of eliciting a rejection response, as in organ transplantation rejection. Biologic therapy is still faced with the presence of heterogeneity of tumor cell populations and with the fact that tumor cells will undergo clonal diversification. In addition, the antigenic and immunosusceptibility properties of primary and metastatic tumor foci are individually changeable. Host immune capacity can fluctuate widely, and immunologic idiosyncracies could be of determinant significance; for instance, the point at which specific or nonspecific immune stimulation will lead to suppressor activation cannot be predicted in advance, and individual monitoring over time appears to be needed to prevent the stimulation of counterproductive effects.

Tumor debulking, either surgically or by radiation or chemotherapy, may in itself facilitate host immune responsiveness and could further the impact of extrinsic immunologic intervention.

The use of biologic therapy is still under investigation. It is already clear that highly purified biologic substances can be effective in the tumor-bearing host. Clinical studies with alpha-interferon have now demonstrated the responsiveness of drug-resistant lymphoma, melanoma, and renal carcinoma in humans. These results, along with the early clinical results using monoclonal antibody, confirm the concept that we need not think of biologic therapy as a tool that can be used only in patients with undetectable and minimal tumor burdens. While

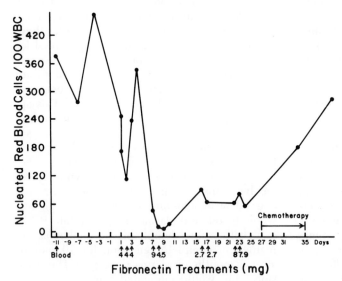

Figure 11-4. Graph showing the results of fibronectin treatments on the number of nucleated red blood cells (nRBC) in a cat with erythroleukemia. After five treatments the count has been reduced from > 420 nRBC/100 WBC to 10 nRBC/100 WBC.

this modality may work best with minimal tumor burdens—a situation that is true for chemotherapy—biologic therapy can be useful as a single modality in clinically apparent disease. However, new and exciting responses are now being reported using IL-2 combined with lymphokine-activated killer (LAK) cells or tumor derived activated killer (TDAK) cells in humans with advanced renal carcinoma and melanoma.[51,52] The future of biologic therapy will depend upon the availability of newer agents and the evaluation of these agents in well-designed prospective clinical trials.

REFERENCES

1. Johnston MI: Basic concepts of immunity. In Torrence PF (ed): Biological Response Modifiers, pp. 21–55. New York, Academic Press, 1985

2. Adams DO, Nathan CF: Molecular mechanisms in tumor-cell killing by activated macrophages. Immunol Today 4:166, 1983

3. Fidler IJ, Kleinerman ES: Lymphokine-activated human blood monocytes destroy tumor cells but not normal cells under cocultivation conditions. J Clin Oncol 2:937–943, 1984

4. Helson L, Helson C, Green S: Effects of murine tumor necrosis factor on heterotransplanted human tumors. Exp Cell Biol 17:53–60, 1979

5. Flick DA, Gifford GE: Tumor necrosis factor. In Torrence PF (ed): Biological Response Modifiers, pp. 171–218. New York, Academic Press, 1985

6. Espervick T, et al: The role of monocyte cytotoxic factor in monocyte-mediated lysis of tumor cells. Immunology 57:255–259, 1986

7. Roitt I, Brostoff J, Male D: Immunity to tumors. In Immunology Roitt I, Brostoff J, Male D (eds): Immunology, pp. 18.1–18.16. St. Louis, CV Mosby, 1985

8. Borden EC, Ball LA: Interferon: Biochemical, cell growth inhibitory, and immunological effects. In Brown ER (ed): Progress in Hemology, Vol. 12, pp. 299–399. New York, Grune & Stratton, 1981

9. Hellstrom I, Hellstrom K, Evans CA, et al: Serum mediated protection of neoplastic cells from inhibition by lymphocytes immune to their tumor-specific antigens. Proc Natl Acad Sci USA 62:362–368, 1969

10. Baldwin RW, Price MR, Robins RA: Blocking of lymphocyte-mediated cytotoxicity for rat hepatoma cells by tumor-specific antigen-antibody complexes. Nature (New Biol) 238:185–186, 1972

11. Williams RC Jr: Immune Complexes in Clinical and Experimental Medicine, pp. 250–300. Cambridge, MA, Harvard University Press, 1980

12. Bast RC Jr: Principles of cancer biology: Tumor immunology. In DeVita VT Jr, Hellman S, Rosenberg SA (eds): Cancer: Principles and Practice of Oncology, 2nd ed, pp. 125–150. Philadelphia, JB Lippincott, 1985

13. Baldwin RW, Byers VS: Immunoregulation by bacterial organisms and their role in the immunotherapy of cancer. In Chedid L, Miescher PA, Muller-Eberhard HJ (eds): Immunostimulation, pp. 73–94. New York, Springer-Verlag, 1980

14. MacEwen EG, Patnaik AK, Harvey HJ, et al: Canine oral melanoma: Comparison of surgery versus surgery plus *Corynebacterium parvum*. Cancer Invest 45:397–402, 1986

15. MacEwen EG: Approaches to therapy using biological response modifiers. In Brown NO (ed): The Veterinary Clinics of NA. Clinical Veterinary Oncology, pp. 667–688. Philadelphia, WB Saunders, 1985

15a. Bostock DE, Gorman NT: Intravenous BCG therapy of mammary carcinoma in bitches after surgical excision of the primary tumor. Eur J Cancer 14:879–886, 1978

16. Oldham RK, Smalley RV: Biologicals and biological response modifiers. In DeVita VT Jr, Hellman S, Rosenberg SA (eds): Cancer: Principles and Practice of Oncology, 2nd ed, pp. 2223–2245, Philadelphia, JB Lippincott, 1985

17. Meyer JA, Dueland RT, MacEwen EG, et al: Canine osteogenic sarcoma treated by amputation and MER. Cancer 49:1613–1616, 1982

18. Kleinschuster SJ, Rapp HJ, Green SB, et al: Efficacy of intratumorally administered mycobacterium cell wells in the treatment of cattle with ocular carcinoma. J Natl Cancer Inst 67:1165–1171, 1981

19. Murphy JM, Severin GA, Lavach JP, et al: Immunotherapy of ocular equine sarcoid. J Am Vet Assoc 174:269–272, 1979

20. Leclerc C, Morin A, Chedid L: Potential use of synthetic muramyl peptides as immunoregulating molecules. In Thompson RA and Rose NR (eds): Recent Advances in Clinical Immunology, No. 13, pp. 187–204. New York, Churchill Livingstone, 1982

20a. Smith BW, Kurzman ID, Schultz KT, et al: Muramyl dipeptide augments the activity of canine plastic-adherent mononuclear cells for canine osteosarcoma cells. Vet Immunol Immunopathol (in press)

21. Fidler IJ, Sone S, Fogler WE: Efficacy of liposomes containing a lipophilic muramyl dipeptide derivative for activating the tumoricidal properties of alveolar macrophages in vivo. J Biol Response Mod 1:43–55, 1982

21a. MacEwen EG, Kurzman ID, Smith BW, et al: Therapy of metastasis in canine osteosarcoma. In Lopez-Berestein G, Fidler IJ (eds): Liposomes in the Therapy of Infectious Diseases and Cancer, UCLA Symposium on Molecular and Cellular Biology, New Series, Vol. 89. New York, Alan R Liss (in press)

21b. MacEwen EG, Kurzman ID, Rosenthal RC, et al: Therapy of osteosarcoma in dogs with intravenous injection of liposome-encapsulated muramyl tripeptide. J Natl Cancer Ins (in press)

22. MacEwen EG: General concepts of immunotherapy of tumors. J Am Anim Hosp Assoc 12:363–373, 1976

22a. Nauts HC: Bacterial products in the treatment of cancer: Past, present and future. In Jeljaszewicz J, Pulverer G, Roszkowski W (eds): Bacteria and Cancer, pp. 1–26. New York, Academic Press, 1982

23. MacEwen EG, Hess PW: Evaluation of effect of immunomodulation of the feline eosinophilic granuloma complex. J Am Anim Hosp Assoc 23:519–526, 1987

24. Terman DS, Young JB, Shearer WT: Preliminary observations on the effects on breast adenocarcinoma of plasma perfused over immobilized protein A. N Engl J Med 306:935–936, 1982

25. Gordon BR, Matus RE, Hurvitz AI, et al: Perfusion of plasma over *Staphylococcus aureus:* Release of bacterial products is related to regression of tumor. J Biol Response Mod 3:266–270, 1984

26. MacEwen EG, Harvey HL, Patnaik AK, et al: Evaluation of effect of levamisole and surgery on canine mammary cancer. J Biol Response Mod 4:418–426, 1985

27. MacEwen EG, Hayes AA, Mooney S, et al: Evaluation of effect of levamisole on feline mammary cancer. J Biol Response Mod 5:541–546, 1984

28. MacEwen EG, Hayes AA, Mooney S: Levamisole as adjuvant to chemotherapy for canine lymphosarcoma. J Biol Response Mod 4:427–433, 1985

29. Ershler WB, Hacker MP: Pharmacologic modulation of the immune response in mice by cimetidine. Int J Immunopharmacol 4:352, 1982

30. Jin Z, Kumar A: Inhibition of suppressor cell function by cimetidine in a murine model. Clin Immunol Immunopathol 38:350–356, 1986

31. Jeglum KA, Young KM, Barnsley K, et al: Chemotherapy versus chemotherapy with intralymphatic tumor cell vaccine in canine lymphoma. Cancer 10:2042–2050, 1988

32. Jeglum KA, Hanna MG, Hoover HC, et al: A prospective randomized trial of adjuvant active specific immunotherapy in feline breast cancer. Am J Vet Res (in press)

33. Gressler I, Tovey MG: Antitumor effects of interferon. Biochim Biophys Acta 516:231–247, 1978

34. Taylor-Papadimitriou J: Effects of interferons on cell growth and function. In Gressler I (ed): Interferon 2, pp. 13–76. Orlando, FL, Academic Press, 1980

35. Foon KA, Sherwin SA, Abrams PG, et al: Treatment of advanced non-Hodgkin's lymphoma with recombinant leucocyte A interferon. N Engl J Med 311:1148–1152, 1984

35a. Cummins JM, Tompkins MB, Olsen RG, et al: Oral use of human alpha interferon in cats. J Biol Resp Modif 7:513–523, 1988

36. Quesada JR, Swanson DA, Trindale A, et al: Renal cell carcinoma: Antitumor effects of leukocyte interferon. Cancer Res 43:940–947, 1983

37. In vivo effects of interleukin-2. National Cancer Institute Biological Response Modifiers Program Workshop. J Biol Response Mod 3:455–527, 1984

37a. Durum SK, Schmidt JA, Opperheim JJ: Interleukin-1—An immunological perspective. Ann Rev Immunol 3:263–287, 1985

37b. Clark SC, Kamen R: The human hematopoietic colony-stimulating factors. Science 263:1229–1237, 1987

38. Fidler IJ: Therapy of spontaneous metastases by intravenous injection of liposomes containing lymphokines. Science 208:1469–1470, 1980

39. MacEwen EG: Biological therapy and chemotherapy. Semin Vet Med Surg (Small Anim) 1:5–16, 1986

40. Fridkin M, Gottlieb P: Tuftsin, Thr-Lys-Pro-Arg. Anatomy of an immunologically active peptide. Mol Cell Biochem 71:73–97, 1981

41. Najjar VA: Tuftsin: A natural activation of phagocytic cells with antibacterial and antineoplastic activity. In Torrence PF (ed): Biological Response Modifiers, pp. 141–169. New York, Academic Press, 1985

42. Oldham RK: Monoclonal antibodies in cancer therapy. J Clin Oncol 9:582–590, 1983

43. Kassel RL, Old LJ, Carswell EA, et al: Serum-

mediated leukemia cell destruction in AKR leukemia. J Exp Med 138:925–938, 1983

44. Kassel RL, Old LJ, Day NR, et al: Plasma-mediated leukemia cell destruction current status. Blood Cells 3:605–621, 1977

45. Hardy WD Jr, Hess PW, MacEwen EG, et al: Treatment of feline lymphosarcoma with blood constituents. In Clemsen J, John DS (eds): Comparative Leukemia Research, pp. 518–521. Basel, Switzerland, Kargen, 1976

46. Hayes AA, MacEwen EG, Matus RE, et al: Antileukemic activity of plasma cryoprecipitate therapy in the cat. In Hardy WD Jr, Essex M, McClelland AJ (eds): Feline Leukemia Virus, pp. 235–251. New York, Elsevier, 1980

47. MacEwen EG, Patnaik AK, Hayes AA, et al: Temporary plasma-induced remission of lymphoblastic leukemia in a dog. Am J Vet Res 42:1450–1452, 1981

48. Perri RT, Kay NE, McCarthy J, et al: Fibronectin enhances in vitro monocyte-macrophage-mediated tumoricidal activity. Blood 60:430–435, 1982

49. Lause DB, Beezhold DH, Doran JE: Induction of lymphocyte blast transformation by purified fibronectin in vitro. J Immunol 132:1294–1299, 1984

50. Terranova VP, William LE, Liotta LA, et al: Modulation of the metastatic activity of melanoma cells by laminin and fibronectin. Science 226:982–985, 1984

51. Rosenberg SA, Lotze MT, Muul LM, et al: A progress report on the treatment of 157 patients with advanced cancer using lymphokine-activated killer cells and interleukin-2 or high dose interleukin-2 alone. N Engl J Med 316:889–897, 1987

52. West WH, Tauer KW, Yannelli JR, et al: Constant-infusion recombinant interleukin-2 in adoptive immunotherapy of advanced cancer. N Engl J Med 316:898–905, 1987

12

CRYOSURGERY

Stephen J. Withrow

Cryosurgery is the controlled use of cold temperature to induce cellular death. Initially it was used enthusiastically for a variety of neoplastic and nonneoplastic conditions, but today it is chosen only for a few conditions at selected sites.[1] Cryosurgery is not absolutely essential to proper treatment of animals with cancer. Yet, because it is fast and predictable and in many settings does not require general anesthesia, it can be a useful addition to conventional therapy.

SOURCE OF CRYOGEN AND EQUIPMENT

Many types of cryogens can be used to induce cold temperature in tissue. The most commonly used are nitrous oxide (N_2O) and liquid nitrogen (N_2). The advantages and disadvantages of these cryogens are summarized in Table 12-1.

Liquid nitrogen is a little more difficult than nitrous oxide to work with because it evaporates slowly and usually requires transfer from the Dewar flask (storage container) to the applicator. Nitrous oxide uses the same blue tank employed for anesthesia purposes and does not evaporate between uses. The costs per procedure for the two cryogens are comparable.

Nitrous oxide is suitable for small lesions (<1 cm.), but it is somewhat restricted by its inferior temperature, speed of freezing, depth of penetration, and lack of spray capabilities. On the other hand, it is acceptable for the more common small benign lesion (of the skin and eyelid, for example) that is frequently treated. For larger lesions (diameters > 1 cm) having a rich blood supply or invading bone, N_2 is a superior cryogen in spite of its more difficult handling properties.

Nitrous oxide machines are usually portable on wheels with the tank attached and have a variety of probe sizes and configurations. Some models have a spray orifice, but N_2O sprays very ineffectively compared to N_2. Certain machines also have a thermister incorporated into the probe head which documents the probe temperature (not tumor temperatures). A device that rewarms the probe tip is also available on

Table 12-1. Comparison of Liquid Nitrogen and Nitrous Oxide

	LIQUID NITROGEN (N_2)	NITROUS OXIDE (N_2O)
Lowest temperature	$-196°C$	$-89°C$
Availability	Welding firms, medical supply firms, artificial insemination stations	Medical supply firms
Storage	Requires a Dewar flask (storage container) and evaporates at 1% per week	Contained in standard blue tank (as for anesthesia purposes)
Probe freezing	Yes	Yes
Spray freezing	Yes	Poor
Depth of freezing	Deep	Shallow

some models to allow more rapid detachment of the probe from the tumor after freezing.

Liquid nitrogen machines may be small and portable in a brief case,* or they can be purchased with a combination of a Dewar flask and applicator.† N_2 may be applied with various probes or with a fine mist or spray. Spray freezing is capable of faster and deeper penetration of tissue than is probe freezing. Additionally, it has advantages in treating lesions that are not spherical.

Regardless of the cryogen used, it is advisable to purchase a temperature monitoring device with thermocouple needles to monitor temperature in the tumor and normal tissues to be protected. Monitoring is especially important as one is learning the technique and is always used in monitoring temperatures of critical normal tissue (nerves, rectal mucosa, joint capsule, and so forth).

MECHANISM OF CELL DEATH

Much literature exists on the mechanism of cell death after freezing.[2] In summary, two basic events lead to death of a cell after freezing:

1. Direct cellular death. This occurs in the first few minutes after freezing and results from ice crystal disruption of cellular membranes, electrolyte changes, alteration of cellular proteins, and thermal shock.
2. Vascular collapse. Small blood vessels and particularly capillaries are irreversibly damaged after freezing and subsequently col-

* Cryogun, Brymill Corp., Vernon, CT 06066.

† CS-76, Frigitronics, Shelton, CT 06484.

lapse, inducing hypoxia and infarction of frozen tissue. Large and medium-sized arteries, and to a lesser extent veins, are resistant to permanent injury.

The most important factors that influence cell death or survival after freezing are the speed of freezing and thawing, the number of freezes applied, and the coldest temperature reached throughout the tumor.

Fast freezing and slow thawing are most lethal to mammalian cells. The time taken to reach the coldest temperature is influenced by many factors, including type of cryogen (liquid nitrogen is fastest) and tumor and host variables. Local factors that slow down the freezing process are high vascularity, density (bone is harder to freeze than soft tissue), and large volume.

The number of freezes applied per treatment session is important. Most small benign tumors are treated twice at the same sitting (freeze-thaw, freeze-thaw), while malignant, vascular, dense, or large tumors are generally treated three times. Little advantage in cell kill is gained by more than three freezes of the same volume of tissue at the same sitting.

A general lethal temperature for most mammalian cells is stated to be $-20°C$. This temperature should be reached throughout the tumor. Colder temperatures are desirable when possible. The length of time the tissue is maintained at low temperature is not a critical factor in cell death

GENERAL TECHNIQUE[1,3]

Externally accessible tumors (*e.g.*, skin and anus) may be treated under local anesthesia only.

Treatment of other tumor sites may require sedation (eyelid) or general anesthesia (oral cavity) for adequate restraint of the patient.

Surrounding hair is clipped minimally, and an antiseptic is applied. The tumor is then biopsied and debulked of redundant tissue. Exposed hemorrhagic tumor tissue may be coagulated with silver nitrate or a suture ligature applied to the base of pedunculated lesions. Sterile placement of this ligature is not necessary because it will slough with the frozen tumor tissue. The ligature has the additional advantage of acting as a "tourniquet" to decrease rewarming by the host. If convenient, debulking can be performed; it will decrease the freezing time and allow colder temperatures to reach the tumor margins. Freezing large tumor to depth has no advantage over freezing the margins to depth after debulking.

Once the tumor has been biopsied, it can be frozen by probe or spray. Probe freezing is adequate for smaller lesions that are more or less spherical because the ensuing ice ball is spherical. A ratio of probe size to tumor that approaches 1 facilitates a faster freeze of tumor tissue. Warm probes are applied to a warm, moist tumor surface, and freezing is begun. A bond of the probe to the tumor (cryoadhesion) rapidly ensues and is maintained throughout the freeze (30 seconds to a few minutes). A probe will not adhere to dry, intact epithelium. If the probe prematurely detaches from the tumor, both probe and tumor should be allowed to thaw, and the process begun again. Once the desired depth of freezing has been achieved, active freezing is stopped. The probe may take several minutes to detach and should not be forcibly detached in order to avoid tissue injury. Once the tumor surface is moist again, the tumor is refrozen.

I prefer spray freezing with liquid nitrogen to probe freezing since it is faster, more lethal to depth, and more easily applied to nonspherical lesions. Various sized spray orifices are provided with most machines. Practice is required to learn how to control the fine spray of N_2 to just cover the tumor or desired tissue and prevent "run-off." Careful observation and palpation of surrounding tissue is necessary to avoid inadvertent freezing of normal tissue. Insulation (styrofoam cups, vaseline, and so forth) is only rarely employed and, in fact, may be dangerous because it may act as a "cryoprobe" when frozen and cover up frozen tissue below it. Sufficient practice with spraying will virtually eliminate the need for insulators. Practice on gelatin molds or necropsy material should be gained before patients are treated.

Regardless of probe or spray freezing, adequate margins of normal tissue should be frozen outside the lesion. This may be several millimeters for benign lesions or as much as a centimeter for malignant lesions. Although thermocouples are ideal for monitoring temperatures in tissue, visual observation and palpation of the "ice ball" suggest what temperature has been reached. The ice ball is anything below 0°C, and since mammalian cells are reliably killed only at −20°C, the entire volume of the ice ball will not die. Approximately 70% to 80% of the frozen tissue will slough. If you "guess" correctly and freeze the entire tumor to −20°C, the lesion should not recur. If you "guess" wrong, tumor recurrence is likely.

EXPECTED TISSUE RESPONSE

Immediately after freezing the patient may experience mild discomfort. This rarely requires pain relief and is absent within 12 hours. The frozen tissue will swell slightly and turn a darker color owing to death and collapse of blood vessels. If exposed tissue is present (ulcerated tumor or biopsy surface), it may ooze a small amount of serum or blood. This usually forms a dry scab within several days. Mucous membranes sites (oral, eyelid, anus) may have a moist discharge for a week or longer.

Even though the tissue may "look" infected by standard criteria, antibiotics are not necessary. In essence, the frozen and dead tissue acts like a biologic bandage while the body is producing bacteria-resistent granulation tissue at the deep juncture of dead to living cells.

Within 10 to 21 days the scab will fall off, exposing a pink bed of epithelium (small lesions) or a reddish bed of granulation tissue that will contract or epithelialize, leaving a small hairless area.

Superficial layers of frozen dead bone will generally be adherent and may require debridement 2 or 3 months after freezing. Hair regrowth may be white or gray on the periphery of the lesion owing to death of melanocytes and preservation of hair follicles.

Owners are instructed to leave the area alone, to afford only minimal general hygiene, and to keep the pet from licking or rubbing the area. Most animals leave the site alone, presumably owing to death of sensory nerves. A routine recheck is requested at 2 to 3 weeks and subsequent rechecks are determined by the histologic tumor type and its biologic behavior.

SPECIFIC TUMOR SITES

Although many tumor types and sites have been frozen, experience has suggested four specific sites that may be treated by cryosurgery with predictably successful results: eyelid, perianal region, oral cavity, and skin. As a general rule, large, malignant cancers should be frozen only as a last resort because cryosurgery does not afford evidence of surgical margins for pathologic review, and further appropriate treatment must be delayed until recurrence. Additionally, large lesions (> 2.5 cm) take longer to heal after cryosurgery than after surgery. With this in mind, tumor types recommended for cryosurgery are generally benign (or only locally invasive) and small (< 2.5 cm).

EYELID[4-6]

Benign tumors of the eyelid (meibomian gland adenoma, papilloma, and so forth) are common in older dogs. Although not life-threatening, they may cause problems from local irritation or corneal ulceration. Surgical excision and reconstruction of the eyelid often require general anesthesia and longer treatment time than cryosurgery.

Most patients require light sedation or anesthesia prior to treatment. The base of the tumor is usually anesthetized locally. A chalazion forcep is then applied around the tumor and eyelid to allow the lid to be held steady and remove it from contact with the globe. Additionally the forcep acts as a tourniquet, reducing blood flow to the tumor, thus speeding the freezing process.

The excised portion of the tumor is submitted for biopsy purposes. Silver nitrate should be used with caution to prevent exposure of the conjunctiva to irritation. A cryo probe (for small lesions) or a cryo spray is then applied to the tumor and a few millimeters of surrounding eyelid. This is generally a full-thickness freeze. Any length of eyelid may be frozen.

The eyelid is unique in its property of maintaining near normal cosmetics and function after freezing. The eyelid is supported by a circumferential array of connective tissue called the tarsal plate. After freezing, the tarsal plate remains intact to allow epithelialization while adnexal structures (eyelashes, sebaceous glands, and tumor) die and are removed. Most cryosurgery sites are covered with pink epithelium within two weeks and have a minimal recession of the eyelid margin. The area will slowly repigment over 3 to 6 months, though cilia will not regrow.

Recurrence rates are less than 5%, which is at least as good as surgery with less anesthesia, shorter surgery time, and comparable cosmetics. Large, malignant tumors or tumors fixed to the orbit should generally be excised, and enucleation and orbitectomy may be indicated.

PERIANAL REGION[7]

Perianal tumors are most commonly seen in the older intact male dog (Chapter 19) and are usually perianal adenomas. Cryosurgery can be an effective treatment for isolated and defined lesions that do not encompass more than 180° of the anal circumference.

Since most dogs are under general anesthesia for castration, freezing can be performed at the same time. The top of the tumor or a wedge of tissue is removed with a blade and a suture (ligature or mattress) is applied at the base for hemostasis. The tumor is then frozen with care to avoid extensively freezing the anal and rectal mucosa. No more than 180° of the anal circumference should be frozen to avoid anal stenosis resulting from fibrosis. Multiple lesions may be frozen as long as they are separated by normal unfrozen tissue.

The resulting eschar may be more moist than most haired skin cryosurgery sites but still does not require antibiotics. Elizabethan collars may be utilized if perineal licking is severe (rare).

Local recurrence rates when combined with castration have been less than 5%. The advantages of cryosurgery over blade excision are speed, economy, and lack of infection. Deeply invasive, 360°, and malignant cancers should generally not be frozen.

ORAL CAVITY[8]

Cancer of the oral cavity may invade bone. Eradication of tumor in bone can be accomplished with a variety of methods, including cryosurgery. Freezing is generally applicable to low-grade tumors that are adherent or minimally invasive into one cortex. Full-thickness freezing of maxilla or mandible will usually result in an oronasal fistula or fracture, respectively. Freezing of normal bone will significantly reduce its breaking strength for a year or more.[9] If the bone can be protected from stress and infection (impossible in the mouth), the full-thickness frozen bone can act as an autograft and become revascularized and viable.

The advantage that cryosurgery has in minimally invasive bone lesions is destruction of tumor cells within the bone and maintenance of a bony framework for preservation of function. Tumors with extensive bone fixation or invasion should generally be surgically removed. Freezing of pharyngeal or tonsillar lesions may result in life-threatening edema and swelling.

Under general anesthesia, regional radiographs will help determine the extent of bony invasion. Tumors adherent to underlying bone without evidence of radiographic bone involvement must be considered invasive of the underlying bone. If the extent of bone invasion does not preclude freezing, the tumor is aggressively debulked and biopsied. The underlying bone with at least a 5-mm margin is frozen three times. Depth of freezing can only be determined by placing a thermocouple into underlying bone through a small drill hole. Depth of freezing in bone will not be as easily accomplished as in soft tissues.

After freezing, the tissue will slough off rapidly owing to abrasion by food and the tongue. A superficial area of dead bone 2 to 3 mm in depth will become necrotic. This will form a sequestra that may take several months to fall off or can be electively removed when it becomes loose to the touch. Once the sequestra is removed, healing progresses rapidly.

A rare reported complication is nitrogen embolization.[10] This problem is induced when nitrogen is sprayed under pressure into exposed cancellous bone and expands intravenously. The nitrogen emboli then travel to the right atria and cause cardiovascular compromise and death. Theoretically, cardiocentesis and removal of nitrogen could be beneficial.

Control rates for oral malignancy in the published literature are generally poor, largely because of poor case selection (tumors are malignant, advanced, or large), rather than inherent resistance to cryosurgery.

SKIN[11]

Benign skin tumors, particularly in the dog, are perhaps the most common tumor condition in pet animals. Most of these tumors are not life-threatening and treatment is for cosmetic, inflammatory, and occasionally functional reasons. Freezing these tumors is fast, easy, safe, and economical.

A small area around the tumor is clipped of hair to prevent it from matting on the ensuing eschar. The skin and subcutaneous tissue are then infiltrated with a local anesthetic. The top of the tumor or a wedge of tissue is removed for biopsy purposes, and the tumor is frozen twice.

Healing may produce white hair on the periphery of the frozen area and small areas of hairless epithelium in the center. Most cryosurgery sites are cosmetically normal.

Large mast cell tumors should not be frozen because rapid degranulation may result in a release of histamine, heparin, and other vasoactive substances that may induce hypotensive shock. Small mast cell tumors (< 1 cm) may be safely frozen but may have a marked local response due to degranulation of tumor cells.

DISADVANTAGES OF CRYOSURGERY

Several factors make cryosurgery less desirable than conventional surgery:

1. **Equipment expense.** Initial equipment expense for cryoinstrument, thermocouples and Dewar flask (if using liquid nitrogen) can run from $500 to several thousand dollars. This investment can be made up in savings of anesthesia, surgical expenses

(sterilization, suture, and so forth), and time.

2. **Evaporation of N₂.** Depending on how many cases are treated per week, evaporation of N_2 can be an inconvenience. Since most cases treated by cryosurgery are elective and benign, they can be "stored up" and treated every 2 to 3 weeks to coincide with delivery of N_2.

3. **Aesthetics of dead tissue.** Cryosurgery is not as "clean" as blade excision, but if owners are advised in advance of expected responses and the advantages of cryosurgery, few complaints will arise.

4. **False hopes for cryosurgery.** Contrary to some published reports, a systemic immunologic response to released or altered tumor antigens killed *in vivo* has not been clinically documented.

   Cryosurgery is also not a panacea for untreatable conditions. If a tumor could not be excised and expected to granulate or epithelialize (*e.g.*, tumors more than one-third the circumference of a limb or tail), freezing will not change those conditions.

5. **Lack of surgical margins.** Because the deeper levels of tumor invasion are left *in situ*, the margins of tumor destruction cannot be determined. For most conditions treated with cryosurgery (small, benign, and not life-threatening), this is not crucial but may allow an undesirable time lapse between incomplete treatment and recurrence of malignancies.

ADVANTAGES OF CRYOSURGERY

Cryosurgery has some advantages over conventional surgery:

1. **Speed.** Most lesions can be frozen faster than they can be surgically excised.

2. **Expense per treatment.** Although initial equipment expense can be substantial, the cost per treatment for consumable (liquid nitrogen or nitrous oxide) is usually less than $1 or $2.

3. **Ease of treatment.** Once some experience has been gained, cryosurgery will be considered easier than surgical excision for most surgeons.

4. **Safety.** Because of the ability to avoid general anesthesia in many cases, the usual risk of general anesthesia is avoided.

CONDITIONS IN WHICH CRYOSURGERY SHOULD NOT BE PERFORMED

Certain tumors, conditions, or sites should not be frozen:

1. **Osteosarcoma of long bones.** Although local tumor control may be achieved, secondary fracture through further weakened bone will invariably occur when full-thickness freezing of a long bone is performed.[9]

2. **Intranasal tumors.** Aggressive freezing of intranasal tumors frequently results in serious loss of palatine bone and large oronasal fistulas.[12]

3. **Circumferential anus.** The anus (or any body orifice) should not be frozen 360° for fear of inducing a fibrotic stricture of the lumen.[7]

4. **Large mast cell tumors.** Rapid degranulation of killed mast cells may lead to profound hypotensive shock.

5. **Large, aggressive tumors.** Tumors with life-threatening potential are better treated surgically when possible.

REFERENCES

1. Withrow SJ (ed): Symposium on Cryosurgery. Vet Clin North Am 10(4), 1980
2. Hoyt RF Jr, Seim HB III: Veterinary cryosurgery: Mechanisms of cell death, cryosurgical instrumentation, and cryogens, Pt I. Compend Cont Educ 3(5):426–436, 1981
3. Seim HB III, Hoyt RF Jr: Veterinary cryosurgery, Pt II. Principles of application. Compend Cont Educ 3(8):695–702, 1981
4. Holmberg DL, Withrow SJ: Cyrosurgical treatment of palpebral neoplasms: Clinical and experimental results. Vet Surg 8(3):68–73, 1979
5. Holmberg DL: Cryosurgical treatment of canine eyelid tumors. Vet Clin North Am 10(4):831–836, 1980
6. Roberts SM, Severin GA, Lavach JD: Prevalence and treatment of palpebral neoplasms in the dog: 200 cases (1975–1983). J Am Vet Med Assoc 189:1355–1359, 1986

7. Liska WD, Withrow SJ: Cryosurgical treatment of perianal gland adenomas in the dog. J Am Anim Hosp Assoc 14(4):457–463, 1978

8. Harvey HJ: Cryosurgery of oral tumors in dogs and cats. Vet Clin North Am 10(4):821–830, 1980

9. Withrow SJ: Application of cryosurgery to primary malignant bone tumors in dogs (phase I study). J Am Anim Hosp Assoc 16:493–495, 1980

10. Harvey HJ: Fatal air embolization associated with cryosurgery in two dogs. J Am Vet Med Assoc 173(2):175–176, 1978

11. Krahwinkel DJ Jr: Cryosurgical treatment of skin diseases. Vet Clin North Am 10(4):787–801, 1980

12. Withrow SJ: Cyrosurgical treatment for nasal tumors in the dog. J Am Anim Hosp Assoc 18:585–589, 1982

13

HYPERTHERMIA

Mark W. Dewhirst
Rodney L. Page
Donald E. Thrall

Hyperthermia is an exciting, relatively new cancer treatment modality. It can be defined as raising tissue temperatures above normothermia, to perhaps as high as 42–50°C, for specified periods of time in order to produce an antitumor effect. This chapter will provide a concise summary of the biologic rationale for the use of hyperthermia in cancer therapy, a review of the methods used for producing it, and a discussion of recent clinical results. Readers interested in further details about this form of therapy are referred to several recent books and monographs.[1-17]

BIOLOGIC EFFECTS OF HEAT

Heat has been noted to produce several biologic effects on both tissues and cells. This provides a strong rationale for its potential as an anticancer treatment modality:

1. Temperatures above 41.5°C are cytotoxic; the rate of cell kill is exponential and dependent on temperature (Fig. 13-1).[18]
2. Cytotoxicity is more prominent in cells that are at low pH or nutritionally deprived. This type of environment is often observed in tumors but is uncommon in normal tissues.[19]
3. Tumor blood vessels appear to be more sensitive to heat damage than their normal tissue counterparts.[20]
4. Tumor microcirculation is often vasodilated and is generally unable to respond to hyperthermia. However, normal tissues can vasodilate with increases in blood flow and cooling of tissue. Thus, when tumor tissue is subjected to equal power deposition rates, its temperature tends to be higher than that of normal tissue.[20]
5. Hyperthermia is also known to interact synergistically with radiation and a number of chemotherapeutic drugs.[5]

INTERACTION WITH RADIOTHERAPY

When hyperthermia is combined with radiotherapy, synergism is observed in terms of cell

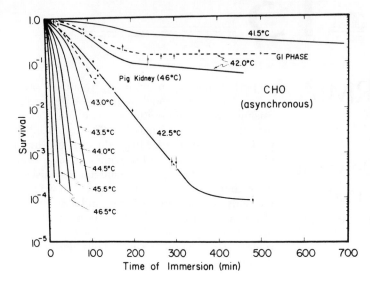

Figure 13-1. Cell survival curves for Chinese hamster ovary cells heated *in vitro* at temperatures between 41.5 and 46.5°C. The rate of cell kill is dependent upon temperature, with increasing rates as temperature increases. The flattening of the curves at 41.5, 42.0, and 42.5°C is due to thermotolerance induction (acquired resistance to further heat killing). The cell survival curve shown with the dashed lines is a relatively resistant pig kidney line at 46°C. (Dewey WC, Hopwood LE, Sapareto SA, et al.: Cellular responses to combinations of hyperthermia and radiation. Radiology 463–474, 1977)

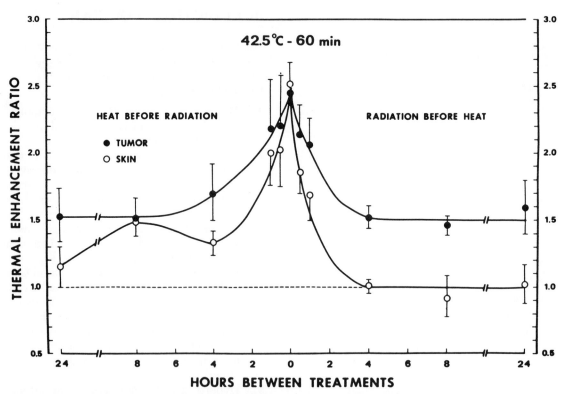

Figure 13-2. Hyperthermic modification of radiation effects on tumor and normal tissue (skin). The thermal enhancement ratio refers to the reduction in radiation dose needed to achieve an isoeffect, relative to radiation alone. The maximum enhancement is seen when the two modalities are given simultaneously. The greatest differential in effect, however, is seen when hyperthermia follows radiation by 3–4 hours. With this sequence, relatively little enhancement is seen in skin, while the enhancement in tumor is significant. (Overgaard J.: The biological basis for clinical treatment with combined hyperthermia and radiation pp. 415–423. In Karcher KH (ed): Progress in Radio-Oncology II, New York, Raven Press, 1982)

kill. The greatest amount of synergism is seen when the two treatments are given simultaneously, although interactive effects are observed even when they are separated by several hours (Fig. 13-2). Most studies indicate that administration of radiotherapy 2–3 hours before heat tends to reduce the enhancement in normal tissues relative to tumor. Thus, in situations where substantial volumes of normal tissue will be heated, sequential therapy with a 2–3 hour delay might be most advantageous.[21,22]

INTERACTION WITH CHEMOTHERAPEUTIC AGENTS AND OTHER DRUGS

When hyperthermia is combined with some chemotherapeutic agents, synergistic interactions are again produced (Table 13-1). In addition, a number of agents that are not cytotoxic at normothermia become quite cytotoxic at elevated temperatures. Hahn[5] has categorized drugs according to their temperature interaction relationships. Alkylating agents, nitrosoureas and cis-platinum show temperature-dependent enhanced cytotoxicity starting at 39°C. Bleomycin and doxorubicin, on the other hand, show relatively little synergism at 41°C but marked enhancement at 43°C. Some drugs have been shown to have no synergism with heat. They include antimetabolites such as methotrexate and vinca alkaloids such as vincristine.

THERMAL ISOEFFECT DOSE

Since the rate of cell kill is dependent on temperature, it is theoretically possible to convert any time–temperature combination to an equivalent number of minutes at an index temperature.[23,24] Clinically, this type of conversion is desirable because temperatures are not easily controllable during local or regional therapy and duration of heating varies from one institution to the next. Thus, this type of approach would allow therapy to be prescribed with some predictability.

Numerous studies in vitro and in vivo have demonstrated that the relationship between cell kill rate and temperature undergoes a change at 43°C (sometimes referred to as the "break point".) Above this temperature a 1°C increase is equivalent to doubling the heating time at the lower temperature. Below the break point, a 1°C drop is equivalent to reducing the heating time by a factor of 4–6. A number of investigators have studied the clinical usefulness of the isoeffect dose.[23–25] It has been shown to have clinical validity in that it can be used to predict clinical outcome in terms of tumor control and normal tissue damage. In spite of these correlations, however, a number of modifiers of the relationship make its true validity questionable without appropriate modifications.[25]

PHYSICAL METHODS OF HYPERTHERMIA

It is convenient to categorize the physical methods of hyperthermia delivery into three classes, depending upon how much of the body is targeted for heating. Methods designed to heat small regions are referred to as local hyperthermia. Regional hyperthermia generally refers to methodologies designed to heat whole limbs or body cavities, such as the abdomen or pelvis. Systemic or whole body hyperthermia has also been studied. A variety of techniques have been used to achieve local and regional heating, although the basic concept is similar for both (Fig. 13-3). A power supply is needed to power an applicator (microwave, radiofrequency, or ultrasound). The applicator is the device that actually deposits power into the tissue, which results in temperature rise. Tissue temperature is measured with invasive procedures using thermistors, thermocouples, or other so-called noninteractive thermometers that do not heat selectively or interfere with microwave fields.

Table 13-1. Drugs with Demonstrated Supra-Additivity with Hyperthermia

NAME	EFFECT OF HYPERTHERMIA
Cyclophosphamide	Enhanced cytotoxicity
Thiotepa	Enhanced cytotoxicity
Melphalan	Enhanced cytotoxicity
Cis-platinum	Enhanced cytotoxicity
Nitrosoureas	Enhanced cytotoxicity
Bleomycin	Threshold effect, most prominent above 42–43°C
Doxorubicin	
Cysteamine	No cytotoxicity at 37°C; cytotoxic above 42°C
Amphotericin B	
Lidocaine	Temperature-dependent cytotoxicity above 40°C
Thiopental	Temperature-dependent cytotoxicity above 40°C

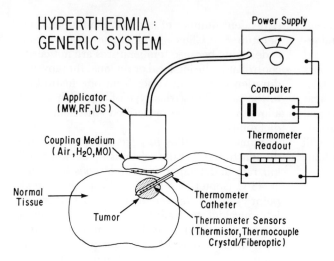

HYPERTHERMIA:
GENERIC SYSTEM

Power Supply

Applicator
(MW, RF, US)

Computer

Coupling Medium
(Air, H₂O, MO)

Thermometer
Readout

Normal
Tissue

Thermometer
Catheter

Tumor

Thermometer Sensors
(Thermistor, Thermocouple
Crystal/Fiberoptic)

Figure 13-3. Figurative representation of the essential components of most local and regional hyperthermia systems. Applicators, which deposit power into tissue, can deposit energy via radiofrequency waves (RF), microwaves (MW), or ultrasound (US). Coupling media can consist of either air, water, or mineral oil (MO). Thermometers are inserted into the tissue and provide feedback to a power supply that controls the power deposited.

LOCAL HYPERTHERMIC TECHNIQUES

Local hyperthermic techniques can be subcategorized into external and interstitial techniques. *External hyperthermia* uses either microwaves, ultrasound, or radiofrequency to deposit energy into the tissue through the body surface from an external applicator at a depth limited to 3–4 cm. Ultrasound can penetrate further into tissue, perhaps to depths of 6–7 cm, or greater if focusing techniques are used.[12] Both radiofrequency and microwave techniques have been employed for *interstitial hyperthermia*. For this application, the hyperthermic sources are inserted directly into tissues.

REGIONAL HYPERTHERMIC TECHNIQUES

Current studies show that deep-seated sites are more difficult to heat than superficial locations. Storm and collaborators studied magnetic induction techniques, operating at 13.56 MHz.[26] A second technique that has been studied extensively is the cophasic microwave array (annular phased array).[27] The physical principle is straightforward, in that it is possible to deposit power at significant depths if two opposed microwave antennae are driven in phase, even though the depth of penetration from a single antenna at the same frequency would be considerably less. In comparative trials, this device has been shown to be superior to magnetic induction techniques, in that greater volumes of tumor appear to be heated with the cophasic arrays.[28]

THERMOMETRY FOR LOCAL AND REGIONAL HYPERTHERMIA

As will be discussed in the clinical results section, measurement of tissue temperature is critically important for assessment of the therapeutic value of a given treatment. Because temperature distributions are typically quite nonuniform, multiple temperature measurements should be obtained whenever possible. Currently, several centers are investigating the combination of heat transfer modeling with limited invasive temperature measurements as a "compromise" to achieve more detailed knowledge of the heated field.[25,29] Clearly, this or similar approaches are necessary to achieve a dosimetry that has enough detail to provide adequate assessment of the efficacy of treatment.

METHODS OF ACHIEVING WHOLE-BODY HYPERTHERMIA

Many methods of inducing whole-body hyperthermia have been evaluated. The earliest was injection of bacterial pyrogens.[30] Even though it produced several intriguing responses, this method was extremely unpredictable and fell into disfavor. Methods developed in the last 10 to 15 years have provided more reproducible results. All devices currently used typically heat at a rate of 0.05–0.1°C/min. The target temperature (41.8–42.0°C) is maintained as a "plateau phase" for a variable time period (1.5–6 hours). A "cooling phase" is then actively induced to return body temperature to normal.[31]

Whole-body heating can be accomplished in many ways. Currently, direct heat transfer across the skin surface is the most common method.[32] Extracorporeal heating of blood has also been used to provide direct heat delivery to regional or systemic circulation.

The optimal means of inducing whole-body hyperthermia has not yet been identified because no suitable direct comparison between comparable devices has been made. A potential advantage of whole-body hyperthermia over other forms of hyperthermia is the possibility of achieving more uniform temperature distribution in all tissues of the body, including tumor tissue. However, sites that receive inadequate heating are potential sanctuary sites for neoplastic cells. With the devices currently being used, completely uniform heating is not possible, although uniformity is probably better with whole-body than with local or regional techniques.[31]

CLINICAL RESULTS

HYPERTHERMIA ALONE

The use of hyperthermia alone has been shown in dogs and humans to result in a low proportion of complete responses and even fewer long-term controls. The general conclusion reached in most studies is that hyperthermia alone is of relatively little value for treatment of malignancy.[33,34]

HYPERTHERMIA AND RADIOTHERAPY

Several studies in pet animals and humans have shown that adjuvant hyperthermia is capable of improving response rates and long-term control of tumors over radiotherapy alone. Brewer and Turrel observed a long-term (1-year) control rate of 50% in dogs with oral or facial sarcomas.[35] This represented an apparent improvement over reported control rates with radiotherapy alone, which were no better than 10% to 15%. Gillette el al. observed a reduction in radiation dose needed for control of oral squamous cell carcinomas, with a therapeutic gain factor of 1.1, for adjuvant hyperthermia at a 50% probability for tumor control.[36] More important, the steepness of the radiation dose-effect curve was increased with heat, and the probability of higher percentages of tumor control was increased while

the probability of late complications from radiotherapy did not increase.

Richardson et al. studied the combination of radiotherapy and hyperthermia for the treatment of canine hemangiopericytomas.[37] Nine of 11 animals thus treated achieved a complete response, although five recurrences were noted at 60 to 340 days after treatment. The total radiation dose delivered ranged from 8.0 to 30.0 Gy, delivered in weekly fractions of 4.0 to 8.0 Gy. Examination of the pattern of recurrences suggested that a minimum of 20.0 Gy was necessary to achieve a high probability of long-term control. A comparison of these data with reported series from other institutions indicated that this approach might be superior to the use of radiotherapy alone. However, because of the unusual radiation fractionation scheme, it is not possible to know whether the radiotherapy or the heat was responsible for the difference.

In a prospective randomized study, Dewhirst et al. examined the initial and long-term control rates for a variety of histological types for radiotherapy alone and for heat plus radiotherapy.[38–40] An improvement in complete and long-term control rates was noted for all histologic types studied, which included squamous cell carcinomas, fibrosarcomas, mast cell sarcomas, malignant melanomas, and mammary carcinomas. Overall, the probability for complete response and local control at two years post-therapy was better by a factor of 2 for adjuvant hyperthermia.

Prognostic Factors

Dewhirst et al. examined a variety of potentially important prognostic factors in their series. Histologic tumor type was not statistically important for achievement of complete response, although considerable variability among types was observed (Table 13-2). Histology was important, however, in determining length of response. Mammary carcinomas had the most significant improvement in long-term control with adjuvant heat.

Tumor volume had a significant influence on the probability of complete response, which decreased as volume increased. The volume effect was less profound for heat plus radiotherapy, providing a potential rational for expecting improved results for the combined therapy on large tumors (i.e., > 10 cm³) relative to that achievable with radiotherapy alone. Temperature nonuniformities were also shown to have a

Table 13-2. Comparison of Treatment Responses to Histology and Volume of Tumor: Radiotherapy Alone vs. Hyperthermia Plus Radiotherapy

	COMPLETE RESPONSE RATES (%)			RESPONSE DURATION PROBABILITY, RELATIVE
	XRT	Δ + XRT	n§	XRT alone ‖
HISTOLOGY				
Mast cell sarcoma*	33.0	77.0	46	1.23
Mammary adenocarcinoma*	12.0	57.0	32	7.82
Fibrosarcoma*	33.0	43.0	19	1.15
Squamous cell carcinoma*	44.0	62.0	82	1.88
Melanoma†	21.0	76.0	34	3.09
VOLUME (CM³)‡				
<1.8	60.0	85.0	52	1.6
1.8–8.3	61.0	55.0	57	1.6
8.3–49	15.0	48.0	54	1.0
>49	7.0	46.0	54	2.0

* Data abstracted from Dewhirst et al., Cancer Res 43:5735–5741, 1983.
† Data abstracted from Dewhirst et al., Int J Hyperthermia 1:219–234, 1985.
‡ Data abstracted from Dewhirst and Sim, Cancer Res 44:4772s–4780s, 1984
§ Each histologic or volume group had about ½ n in each treatment arm.
‖ Relative relapse rate: for example, a mammary adenocarcinoma receiving Δ + XRT was 7.82 times as likely not to have local regrowth as one treated with XRT alone, given that they were followed for the same length of time post-therapy.

significant influence on tumor response and long-term control rates. In general, measured tumor temperature minima were highly correlated with the probabilities for complete response and long-term control (Fig. 13-4).

Recently, several studies in humans have confirmed the importance of the prognostic factors described above.[41–44] Furthermore, multivariate analyses have repeatedly pointed to the fact that tumor temperature minimum is the most important factor influencing complete response and long-term control probabilities.

Normal Tissue Effects

In the assessment of any new form of therapy it is necessary to evaluate the frequency of normal tissue complications. In the case of hyperthermia and radiotherapy, both direct thermal injuries and the potential of heat enhancement of radiation effects have been assessed.

Hyperthermic injury to overlying skin has been a common problem in studies of pet animals. The frequency of skin burns and infarcts has been reported to be as high as 45%.[38,45] Conservative management achieved healing in 85% of such cases. An analysis of temperature distributions of these cases revealed a strong correlation between the probability of serious thermal injury and maximum intratumoral temperature (Fig. 13-5). Thus, a potential method for avoiding thermal injury would be to prevent

intratumoral temperature maxima from exceeding 46–48°C during a 30-minute heating period.

The studies by Gillette et al. and Dewhirst and Sim indicate that hyperthermia does not seem to enhance the frequency of either early or late radiation complications although further study is indicated.[36,45]

WHOLE-BODY HYPERTHERMIA

Whole-body hyperthermia has only recently been tested clinically in veterinary oncology. Initial studies have been conducted on laboratory animals and normal dogs to determine physiologic compensation and potential toxicities to systemic thermal stress as well as the extent of temperature nonuniformity encountered during whole-body hyperthermia.

Toxicity reported during uncontrolled hyperthermia (experimental heat stroke) in dogs includes coagulation abnormalities, neurological dysfunction, and hepatic necrosis.[46,47] Elevation of body temperature for therapeutic purposes must be rigidly monitored to prevent such toxicity; it should not exceed 42.0°C. Increased liver enzymes have been reported in normal dogs undergoing whole-body hyperthermia; hemostatic or neurologic toxicity was not observed. Cardiovascular response to elevated temperature is characterized by an increase in heart rate, cardiac output, and systolic blood pressure secondary to sympathetic nervous system stim-

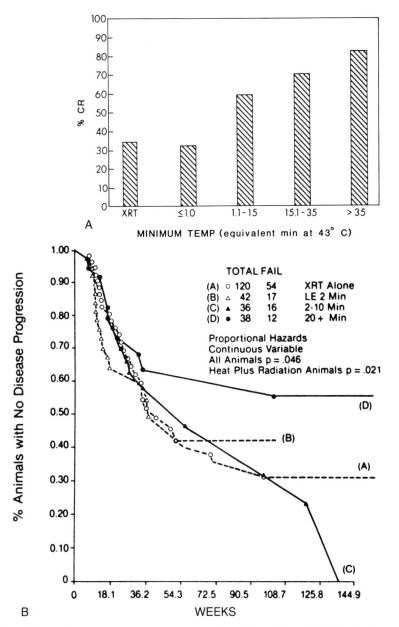

Figure 13-4. *(A)* Influence of minimum tumor temperature on complete response (CR) rates of canine and feline tumors treated with heat and radiotherapy. The probability for achieving a CR was 35% for radiotherapy alone (*n* = 110). When measured intratumoral temperatures were less than 1 equivalent minute at 43°C, there was no improvement in CR rate. When measured intratumoral minima exceeded 35 equivalent minutes at 43°C, the CR rate was increased substantially, to >80%. The number of animals in each of the subgroups that received hyperthermia and radiotherapy was between 20 and 30. *(B)* Influence of minimum temperature on response duration. As in *A,* the minimum intratumoral temperature influenced the duration of tumor response. When intratumoral temperature minima exceeded 20 equivalent minutes at 43°C, the percentage of animals achieving long-term control was 55%, compared with 30% for radiotherapy alone. (Dewhirst MW, Sim DA: The utility of thermal dose as a predictor of tumor and normal tissue responses to combined radiation and hyperthermia. Cancer Res (suppl) 44:4772s–4780s, 1984)

ulation. Normal, healthy dogs have been shown to tolerate this physiologic strain without toxicity. When patients are judiciously selected, older animals with solid tumors also tolerate the procedure well.[52]

WHOLE-BODY HYPERTHERMIA AND CHEMOTHERAPY

The combination of hyperthermia and chemotherapy has not been studied in pet animals to date, except in Phase I studies of whole-body hyperthermia. There is tremendous potential for such studies and it is hoped that work will begin in this area.

Thrall *et al.* have recently documented significant temperature nonuniformity in dogs during whole-body hyperthermia induced by a radiant heat device.[31] While rectal temperature was found to be an accurate reflection of systemic arterial temperature during the plateau phase of heating, temperatures at several tissue sites

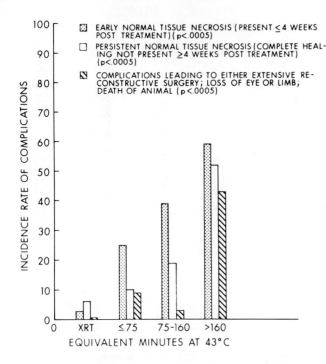

Figure 13-5. Influence of intratumoral temperature maxima on the frequency of thermal injury to adjacent normal tissue. When intratumoral temperature maxima exceeded 160 equivalent minutes at 43°C, the frequency of serious thermal injuries was significantly higher than the rate of injuries for radiotherapy alone or for lower temperature maxima. (Dewhirst MW, Sim DA: Estimation of therapeutic gain in clinical trials involving hyperthermia and radiotherapy. Int J Hyperthermia 2:165–178, 1986)

varied significantly from rectal temperature during the plateau phase. Some of the variations below rectal temperature could be explained by lack of adequate insulation in superficial sites, while variations above rectal temperature were thought to be due to metabolic heat production.

The altered pharmacokinetic disposition of antineoplastic agents at elevated temperature is currently under clinical investigation. Pilot studies of *cis*-platinum pharmacokinetics have been reported in normal dogs during whole-body hyperthermia.[49] The results suggest that *cis*-platinum metabolites are produced at a higher rate when *cis*-platinum is incubated *in vitro* at 43°C rather than 37°C. *In vivo*, a dramatic increase in *cis*-platinum clearance suggests that these metabolites are more readily bound to tissue macromolecules during whole-body hyperthermia. Thus, greater tumor concentrations of reactive *cis*-platinum would be expected at elevated temperatures.[5] Enhanced cytotoxicity of *cis*-platinum at elevated temperatures in addition to altered pharmacokinetic disposition of the drug at 42°C suggest potential therapeutic advantages if normal tissue toxicity can be reduced relative to tumor toxicity.

A limited number of studies on dogs with spontaneous neoplasia undergoing whole-body hyperthermia have been reported.[50,51] Fourteen

of 21 dogs with long bone osteosarcoma tolerated fractionated whole-body hyperthermia treatments well (water bath technique). The remaining 7 experienced treatment-limiting toxicity. Transient depression and neuromuscular weakness was observed in 3 of these 7 dogs and 4 dogs died (3 of gastric torsion and 1 of unknown causes). Five of the 7 dogs were Great Danes, the other 2 were Irish wolfhounds. Stress is considered a causative factor in dilation and the pathogenesis of torsion in dogs. In addition, general anesthesia and positioning during whole-body hyperthermia (dorsal recumbency) may have increased the likelihood of torsion.

Physiologic and metabolic stress of whole-body hyperthermia in normal and tumor-bearing dogs has been recently evaluated (hyperthermic cabin and radiant heating technique).[48,52] No clinical signs of persistent toxicity were observed in any dog as a result of whole-body hyperthermia. Substantial increases in heart rate and blood pressure occur in older, tumor-bearing dogs during whole-body hyperthermia, but the increases are well tolerated if no cardiac abnormalities are detected on preclinical evaluation (physical examination and auscultation, as well as radiographic, electro- or echocardiographic evaluation). Subclinical alterations in liver enzymes and platelet numbers following whole-body hyperthermia in dogs with neoplasia further support the need for thorough pretreatment evaluation. In general, laboratory abnormalities observed following whole-body hyperthermia resolve within 1 week of treatment.

Tumor response to whole-body hyperthermia alone or in combination with other modalities has been reported very infrequently in veterinary literature. Combined radiation therapy and fractionated whole-body hyperthermia (water bath technique) were reported in 7 dogs with long bone osteosarcoma.[50,51] Complete response of the tumor was achieved in all dogs, and recurrence was noted in 6 of the dogs between 65 and 195 days (1 dog had no local recurrence). The initial metastatic lesions were first observed in skeletal sites at 56–310 days (one dog showed pulmonary metastasis initially). This is an atypical pattern of metastasis for this tumor type and may represent an alteration in biologic behavior induced by whole-body hyperthermia or emergence of tumor at sanctuary sites. Nearly simultaneous recurrence of disseminated malignant melanoma at multiple distal extremity sites following a complete response to whole-body hyperthermia combined with *cis*-platinum treatments has been observed by these authors.* These sites remained cooler than rectal temperature during the hyperthermia treatments and thus represented potential sanctuary sites.

Dewhirst reported on 9 dogs treated with whole-body hyperthermia alone (water blanket technique).[2] Seven of these dogs had Stage IIIa mast cell tumors. Four of the 7 had complete or partial responses. Three complete responses were obtained; two of these failed at less than 7 months, but one persisted at least 4 years post-therapy.

Klein *et al.* reported a pilot study of 13 dogs, 9 with lymphoproliferative disorders, treated with whole-body hyperthermia (magnetic induction technique) in combination with hyperthermic sensitizers.[53] Fatal complications in 3 of 8 dogs treated with hyperthermia were associated with excessive tumor burden, elevated liver enzymes, and thrombocytopenia prior to treatment (along with neoplastic invasion of the liver and bone marrow). Death was attributed to acute tumor necrosis and secondary systemic toxicity. Three of the 8 dogs had partial or complete responses. The conclusion from this

study was that modification of treatment protocols and proper identification of eligible patients are necessary if whole-body hyperthermia is to be useful in lymphoproliferative disorders.

The appropriate application of whole-body hyperthermia remains to be defined. The fact that disseminated neoplasia is poorly controlled by chemotherapy alone provides justification for clinical research of additional therapeutic modalities. A great deal of investigation is needed to answer questions related to the correct combination of heat, radiation, and cytotoxic drugs. In addition, tumor types must be identified that are more sensitive to treatment protocols involving whole-body hyperthermia than to chemotherapy alone if any therapeutic benefit is to be achieved.

REFERENCES

1. Dethlefsen LA (ed): Third International Symposium: Cancer therapy by hyperthermia, drugs, and radiation. Natl Cancer Inst Monograph No. 61, 1982
2. Dewhirst MW, Connor WG: Hyperthermia. In Slatter D (ed): Textbook of Small Animal Surgery, pp. 2427–2440. Philadelphia, WB Saunders, 1985
3. Dewhirst MW, Connor WG: Hyperthermia. In Gourley IM and Vasseur PB (eds): Textbook of Soft Tissue Surgery, pp. 941–960. Philadelphia, JB Lippincott, 1983
4. Frizzell LA, Dunn F: Biophysics of ultrasound. In Lehman JF (ed): Therapeutic Heat and Cold, pp. 353–385. Baltimore, Williams & Wilkins, 1982
5. Hahn GM: Hyperthermia and Cancer, 285 pp. New York, Plenum Press, 1982
6. Hornback N, Shupe R: Hyperthermia and Cancer: Human Clinical Trial Experience, 2 vols, 336 pp. Boca Raton, FL, CRC Press, 1984
7. Jain RK, Gullino PM (eds): Thermal Characteristics of Tumors: Applications in Detection and Treatment, 542 pp. New York, New York Academy of Sciences, 1980
8. Lehmann JF (ed): Therapeutic Heat and Cold, 641 pp. Baltimore, Williams & Wilkins, 1982
9. Lowenthall JP (ed): Hyperthermia in cancer treatment. Cancer Res (suppl) 44:1984
10. Milder JW (ed): Conference on hyperthermia in cancer treatment. Cancer Res 39:2232–2340, 1979
11. Nussbaum CH (ed): Physical Aspects of Hyper-

* Page RL: Unpublished data.

thermia, 645 pp. New York, American Institute of Physics, 1982

12. Oleson JR, Dewhirst MW: Hyperthermia: An overview of current progress and problems. Curr Probl Cancer 8:1–62, 1983

13. Overgaard J (ed): Hyperthermic Oncology, Vol. 1. London, Taylor & Francis, 1984

14. Overgaard J (ed): Hyperthermic Oncology, Vol. 2. London, Taylor & Francis, 1985

15. Storm FK (ed): Hyperthermia in Cancer Therapy, 566 pp. Boston, GK Hall Medical Publishers, 1983

16. Streffer C (ed): Cancer Therapy by Hyperthermia and Radiation, 341 pp. Baltimore, Urban & Schwarzenberg, 1978

17. Vaeth JM (ed): Hyperthermia and radiation therapy/chemotherpy in the treatment of cancer. Front Radiat Ther Oncol 18:1–196, 1984

18. Dewey WC, Hopwood LE, Sapareto SA, Gerweck LE: Cellular responses to combinations of hyperthermia and radiation. Radiology 123:463–474, 1977

19. Gerweck LE, Richards B: Influence of pH on the thermal sensitivity of cultured human glioblastoma cells. Cancer Res 41:845–849, 1981

20. Reinhold HS, Endrich B: Tumour microcirculation as a target for hyperthermia. A review. Int J Hyperthermia 2:111–137, 1986

21. Overgaard J: The biological basis for clinical treatment with combined hyperthermia and radiation. In Karcher KH (ed): Progress in Radio-Oncology II, pp. 415–423. New York, Raven Press, 1982

22. Overgaard J, Overgaard M: A clinical trial evaluation of the effect of simultaneous or sequential radiation and hyperthermia in the treatment of malignant melanoma. In Overgaard J (ed): Hyperthermic Oncology, Vol. 1. London, Taylor & Francis, 1984

23. Field SB, Morris CC: The relationship between heating time and temperature: Its relevance to clinical hyperthermia. Radiother Oncol 1:179–186, 1983

24. Sapareto SA, Dewey WC: Thermal dose determination in cancer therapy. Int J Radiol Oncol Biol Phys 10:787–800, 1984

25. Dewhirst MW, Winget JM, Edelstein-Keshet L, Sylvester J, Engler MJ, Thrall DE, Page RL, Oleson JR: Clinical application of thermal isoeffect dose. Int J Hyperthermia, 3:307–318, 1987

26. Storm FK, Harrison WH, Elliott RS, Morton DL: Normal tissue and solid tumor effects of hyperthermia in animal models and clinical trials. Cancer Res 39:2245–2251, 1979

27. Turner PF: Deep heating of cylindrical or elliptical tissue masses. Natl Cancer Inst Monograph No. 61:493–495, 1982

28. Oleson JR, Sim DA, Conrad J, Fletcher AM, Gross EJ: Results of a Phase I regional hyperthermia device evaluation: Microwave annular array vs. radiofrequency induction coil. Int J Hyperthermia 2:327–336, 1986

29. Roemer RB, Cetas TC: Applications of bioheat transfer simulations in hyperthermia. Cancer Res (suppl) 44:4788s–4798s, 1984

30. Coley WB: The treatment of malignant tumors by repeated inoculations of erysipelas with a report of ten original cases. Am J Med Sci 105:488–511, 1893

31. Thrall DE, Page RL, Dewhirst MW, Meyer RE, Hoopes PJ, Kornegay JN: Temperature measurements in normal and tumor tissue in dogs undergoing whole body hyperthermia. Cancer Res 46:6229–6235, 1986

32. Robins HI: Role of whole-body hyperthermia in the treatment of neoplastic disease: Its current status and future prognosis. Cancer Res (suppl) 44:4878–4883, 1984

33. Dewhirst MW, Connor WG, Sim DA: Preliminary results of a phase III trial of spontaneous animal tumors to heat and/or radiation: Early normal tissue response and tumor volume influence on initial response. Int J Radiol Oncol Biol Phys 8:1951–1961, 1982

34. Meyer JL: The clinical efficacy of localized hyperthermia. Cancer Res 44:4745–4751s, 1984

35. Brewer WG, Turrel JM: Radiotherapy and hyperthermia in the treatment of fibrosarcomas in the dog. J Am Vet Med Assoc 18:146–150, 1982

36. Gillette EL, McChesney SL, Dewhirst MW, Scott RJ: Response of canine oral carcinomas to heat and radiation. Int J Radiol Oncol Biol Phys 13:1861–1867, 1987

37. Richardson RC, Anderson VL, Voorhees WD, Blevins WE, Inskeep TK, Janás W, Shupe RE, Babbs CF: Irradiation-hyperthermia in canine hemangiopericytomas: Large-animal model for therapeutic response. J Natl Cancer Inst 73 (5):1187–1194, 1984

38. Dewhirst MW, Sim DA: The utility of thermal dose as a predictor of tumor and normal tissue responses to combined radiation and hyperthermia. Cancer Res (suppl) 44:4772s–4780s, 1984

39. Dewhirst MW, Sim DA, Sapareto S, Connor WG: The importance of minimum tumor temperature in determining early and long term responses of pet animal tumors to heat and radiation. Cancer Res 44:43–50, 1984

40. Arcangeli G, Arcangeli G, Guerra A, Lovisolo G, Cividallie A, Marino C, Mauro F: Tumor response to heat and radiation: Prognostic variables in the treatment of neck node metastases from head and neck cancer. Int J Hyperthermia 1:207–217, 1985

41. Dunlop PRC, Hand JW, Dickinson RJ, Field SB: An assessment of local hyperthermia in clinical practice. Int J Hyperthermia 2:39–50, 1986

42. Luk KH, Pajak TF, Perez CA, Johnson RJ, Conner N, Dobbins T: Prognostic factors for tumor response after hyperthermia and radiation. In Overgaard J (ed): Hyperthermic Oncology, Vol. 1, pp. 353–356. London, Taylor & Francis, 1984

43. Oleson JR, Sim DA, Manning MR: Analysis of prognostic variables in hyperthermia treatment of 163 patients. Int J Radiol Oncol Biol Phys 10:2231–2239, 1984

44. van der Zee J, van Rhoon GC, Wike-Hooley JL, Faithfull NS, Reinhold HS: Whole body hyperthermia: A report of a phase I–II study. Eur J Cancer Clin Oncol 19:1189–1200, 1983

45. Dewhirst MW, Sim DA: Estimation of therapeutic gain in clinical trials involving hyperthermia and radiotherapy. Int J Hyperthermia 2:165–178, 1986

46. Kew M, Bershoh I, Seftel H: Liver damage in heatstroke. Am J Med 49:192–202, 1979

47. Rosenthal T, Shapiro Y, Seligsohn U, Ramot B: Disseminated intravascular coagulation in experimental heatstroke. Thromb Diath Haemor 26:417–425, 1971

48. Macy DW, Macy CA, Scott RJ, Gillette EL, Speer JF: Physiological studies of whole-body hyperthermia of dogs. Cancer Res 45:2769–2773, 1985

49. Riviere JE, Page RL, Dewhirst MW, Tyczkowska K, Thrall DE: Effect of hyperthermia on cisplatin pharmacokinetics in normal dogs. Int J Hyperthermia 2:351–358, 1986

50. Kapp DS, Lord PF: Tolerance of dogs to fractionated systemic hyperthermia. Natl Cancer Inst Mongraph 61:391–394, 1982

51. Lord PF, Kapp DS, Morrow D: Increased skeletal metastases of spontaneous canine osteosarcoma after fractionated systemic hyperthermia and local x-irradiation. Cancer Res 41:4331–4334, 1981

52. Page RL, Meyer RE, Thrall DE, Dewhirst MW: Cardiovascular and metabolic response of tumor-bearing dogs to whole body hyperthermia. Int J Hyperthermia 3:513–526, 1987

53. Klein MK, Dewhirst MW, Fuller DJM: Whole body hyperthermia and heat sensitizing drugs: A pilot study in canine lymphoproliferative disease. Int J Hyperthermia 3:187–198, 1987

14

PHOTODYNAMIC THERAPY

Richard E. Thoma

Photodynamic therapy (PDT), also known as photoradiation therapy (PRT) or phototherapy (PT),[1-4] uses photosensitizing chemicals that have a propensity for partial concentration in tumor tissue. When proper wavelengths of light penetrate the tumor, these chemicals cause a photochemical reaction involving oxygen that destroys cells containing the photosensitive chemical. Since normal tissue surrounding the tumor generally has a lower concentration of the chemical, it should be spared from damage, leading to a relatively tumor-specific necrosis.

The phenomenon of photosensitization was first reported by Raab in 1900.[5] No practical application was attempted until Dr. Thomas Dougherty, a chemist at Roswell Park Memorial Institute in Buffalo, New York, observed that tissue cultures in fluorescein exhibited cell death on exposure to light. He then investigated this phenomenon and used hematoporphyrin derivative (HPD) as a photosensitizer in laboratory animals.[6] This was followed by clinical trials in human patients with advanced cancer[7] and in naturally occurring animal tumors.[4] PDT is now undergoing clinical evaluation aimed at approval by the United States Food and Drug Administration. HPD is a mixture of well-known porphyrins and some unknown compounds. Dihematoporphyrin ether (DHE) was identified as the active component and further studies were launched to understand and use this new compound.[8] DHE (Photofrin II®) is the primary chemical being studied for antitumor activity, but other types of agents, notably phthalocyanines and chlorines, are also under active investigation.

The mechanism of PDT involves the generation of singlet oxygen, a short-lived, highly reactive form of oxygen. When DHE is photoirradiated at specific wavelengths of light, it becomes electronically excited. The electron energy of the excited porphyrin is transferred to the ambient tissue oxygen, elevating the oxygen from the ground state triplet form to the excited singlet state. Singlet oxygen is unstable and must oxidize nearby structures to restabilize itself. DHE molecules are particularly concentrated in the plasma and mitochondrial membranes, and they damage these structures when exposed to light. No damage (no photochemical reaction) occurs in the absence of light. When damage occurs faster than the cell's ability to repair itself, cell death occurs. DHE concentration in tissue is particularly high along the microvascular beds, where it causes further injury by microvascular collapse.

Edema, tissue discoloration (darkening), and swelling are visible as the process takes place, usually within a few minutes of initiation of photoirradiation. Optimum dosage for DHE, tissue concentration times, and light doses are continually being evaluated.

The dosage of HPD used in dogs and cats has been determined to be 5 mg/kg. DHE is currently being administered at 1–2 mg/kg. Either drug is administered intravenously, followed by a waiting period of 72 hours before phototherapy, to allow drug concentration in the tumor and serum clearance. An ideal photosensitizer for cancer therapy would be one that has little or no systemic toxicity, is taken up and retained only by tumor tissue, and is efficiently activated by wavelengths of light that are not absorbed by the surrounding tissues. DHE has an LD_{50} in mice of 30 times therapeutic dosage. At current drugs dosages used, it appears safe.

While malignant and certain benign tumors tend to concentrate these drugs, reticuloendothelial organs, which also retain these drugs, need to be protected from light during intra-abdominal procedures. DHE can be activated at several wavelengths. The longest wavelength absorbence of 630 nanometers (nm) is generally used because it is least absorbed by skin and other tissues. Biologic effect in tissue can be obtained at depths of up to 1 cm from the point of light application.

Light sources are varied. An argon ion laser coupled with a dye laser is used with fiberoptics for delivery of light. Insertion of the fibers into the tissues (interstitial) allows for delivery of the light source and has been used in animal studies.[4]

Argon lasers of 5–19 watts (W) produce the quantity of light needed to pump the dye lasers. The blue-green light from the argon laser penetrates tissue only fractionally compared to red light—thus the need for dye lasers. Dye lasers need a light source (*e.g.*, argon laser) to activate an internal jet stream of dye (rhodamine B) that can be tuned to the desired wavelength. This exit light goes through a series of concave reflecting mirrors that make it a coherent (laser) beam in the wavelength desired. Optic beam splitters divide this red beam from the dye laser into four equal smaller beams and focus each beam into fiberoptic cords. About 20% of the light is lost to reflection and normal divergence. Therefore, 1 watt into the coupler (splitter) at 80% efficiency would give four beams at 200 mW each. The fibers generally used are Teflon-coated quartz silica 400 microns in diameter. They are flexible and can efficiently transmit light from the laser to the patient. Fibers can be obtained with various delivery tips to emit light forward, or laterally and forward (spherical or cylindrical). Spherical light dispersion is used for intraluminal lesions in, for example, bladder. Cylindrical dispersion is used in tubular organs such as the esophagus, trachea or bronchus. The placement of fibers via needles directly into tumors is called interstitial treatment. This allows the total amount of light to be delivered directly into the tumor, thus minimizing the effects to or from surrounding tissues.

The fibers can be introduced into the tumor (interstitial) with 16- to 18-gauge hypodermic needles. The needles are placed into the tumor approximately 1 cm apart in a tetrahedonal pattern. The fiber is introduced from the hub end into the tumor. The needle can then be withdrawn slightly to fully expose the fiber tip for uninhibited light delivery. The fibers also fit

Table 14-1.   Remission Status (93 Cases)

	COMPLETE		PARTIAL		NONE		NFU*	
	1	2	1	2	1	2	1	2
Protocol†								
Number of patients	32	20	21	10	6	1	3	
Percentage of total	34	22	23	11	6	1	3	
Percentage of protocol	50	67	35	30	9	3	5	

* No followup
† Protocol 1 was using only one photoirradiation session 48–72 hours after injection of HPD. Protocol 2 is our current protocol of 2 photoirradiation sessions at Day 3 and Day 10 after injection of HPD.

Table 14-2. Summary of 93 dogs and cats treated with photodynamic therapy

NO. OF CASES	DIAGNOSIS	SITES†	REMISSION STATUS Complete‡ 1	2	Partial 1	2	None 1	2	No Follow-up	FOLLOW-UP TIMES (months)/RESPONSE* Complete	Partial	None	No Followup
5	Acanthomatous epulus	1, 1, 1, 1, 1	1							36, 36, 18, 40, 42			
2	Undifferentiated adenocarcinoma	5, 3	1		1					1§	1		
1	Basosquamous carcinoma	2				1					1		
1	Anal gland carcinoma	5	1							36			
1	Eosinophilic granuloma	5			1								
1	Fibroma	2	1								1		
3	Fibromatous epulus	1, 1, 2	1		1				1	55, 7			x
9	Fibrosarcoma	1, 2, 2, 5, 6, 2, 3, 3, 5		3	3	1	1	1		60	3, 1, 87‖, 54‖, 6, 1	1, 1	
3	Hemangiopericytoma	6, 6, 6	1		1		1				3, 8, 1		
1	Hemangiosarcoma	6	1							12			
1	Leiomyoma	2			1						1		
1	Liposarcoma	2	1							18			
7	Mammary adenocarcinoma	4, (all)	3	3					1	8, 36, 4, 4, 12	2		x
14	Mast cell (malignant)	1, 6, 6, 1, 6, 6, 6, 2, 4, 6, 2, 6, 5, 1	5	6	1	1			1	3, 12, 36, 36, 6, 6, 72, 6, 2, 2, 12	3, 6		x
3	Melanoma (malignant-amelanotic)	5, 2, 1	1	1	1					18, 12	2		
7	Melanoma (Malignant-melanotic)	1, 1, 1, 1, 2, 2, 2	2	2	2	1				8, 6, 36	1, 1, 6, 1		
1	Myxofibrosarcoma (hamster)	2					1				1		
2	Myxoma	5, 5			1		1				1	1	
1	Nasal carcinoma	2				1					1		
1	Odontoma	1		1							7		
7	Osteosarcoma-head	2 (all)	4		2		1			48, 18, 117	1, 3, 2	1	
3	Osteosarcoma-limb	6 (all)			1			2				1, 4, 1	
3	Undifferentiated sarcoma	2, 2, 2	2	1						12, 1§, 2§			
2	Sebaceous adenocarcinoma	2, 6	2							36, 12			
10	Squamous cell carcinoma	1, 1, 1, 2, 2, 6, 6, 2, 2	2	1	3	4				3§, 16, 2§, 12	5, 1, 1, 16, 1, 1, 1		x
3	Synovial cell sarcoma	6, 6, 6			1	2				36	1, 24		
TOTAL PERCENT RESPONSES			52		31		7						

* Response definitions:
    complete remission—tumor gone from site treated
    partial remission—at least 50% reduction in volume but not complete, or a complete that recurred on same site as treatment
    no response—less than 50% reduction
    no followup—no followup of case
† Site codes:
    1—oral, 2—head, skull, maxilla, mandible, 3—soft tissue neck, head, 4—mammary, 5—subcutaneous tissues, 6—legs, paws
‡ Protocol 1 was using only one photoirradiation session 48–72 hours after injection of HPD. Protocol 2 is our current protocol of two photoirradiation sessions at Day 3 and Day 10 after injection of HPD.
§ Died, no tumor found on necropsy
‖ Tumor gone; surgery and PDT used together

easily into the working channel of most endoscopes.

In general, light doses are expressed in terms of delivered light. A retrospective study of 75 tumors in cats and dogs that I treated showed a direct correlation of response to delivered light dosage. Light dosage is expressed in Jouyles (J) per cc (J/cc), which is 1 Watt for 1 second per unit volume of tumor. This study showed the optimal light dose to be 410–420 J/cc of tumor volume.

GENERAL OVERVIEW OF TREATMENT

1. **Day 0.** Inject DHE or HPD intravenously. Direct sunlight should then be avoided for a period of 3 to 5 weeks. However, sunlight has not been a major problem with dogs and cats because they have fur and pigmented skin.
2. **Day 3.** Photoirradiation:
   a. Administer general anesthesia.
   b. Do surgical preparation over area to be treated (after determination of tumor volume).
   c. Tune laser, measure fiber output, cold sterilize fiber tips.
   d. Calculate required light dose and administer the light.
3. **Day 10.** Repeat photoirradiation procedure.

This can be done on an outpatient basis, hospitalizing the patient only for the anesthesia/ photoirradiation session. The patient is discharged and rechecked weekly for 1 month, monthly for 6 months, then semiannually as needed. Complete remissions have lasted as long as 9 years (Table 14-1, 2). Repeat therapy on the same patient can be done as needed for recurrences or new tumors.

Photodynamic therapy (PDT) appears to have several very distinct advantages:

1. Very low toxicity (transient generalized photosensitivity persists a few weeks).
2. Repeatability. This therapy can be repeated on recurrent tumors as often as needed.
3. Efficacy. Several very resistant tumors have responded well, as outlined in Table 14-1.
4. Ease of administration (technology easily learned and applied).
5. Safety for clinical staff. There are no radiation or drug toxicity exposure problems. Minor laser precautions are necessary but are quite easy to comply with.

The main disadvantages are:

1. Lasers are expensive and can be technically difficult to maintain. Technology is progressing toward less expensive and complicated light sources that will be a major breakthrough for enhancing this therapy as a clinical reality.
2. Depth of penetration of external light sources is 1 to 2 cm; interstitial implants may be impossible or too invasive for large, deep-seated tumors.
3. Not all tumors absorb photosensitizers at the same rate or to the same concentration.

REFERENCES

1. Dougherty TJ, Weishaupt KR, Boyule DG: Photoradiation therapy of malignant tumors. In DeVita V, Hellman S, Rosenberg (eds): Principles and Practice of Oncology, pp. 1836–1844. Philadelphia, JB Lippincott, 1982
2. Thoma RE, Stein RM, Weishaupt KR, et al: Phototherapy: A promising cancer therapy. Vet Med Clin Small Anim, Nov:1693–1700, 1983
3. Thoma RE: Phototherapy. In Kirk R (ed): Current Veterinary Therapy, pp. 438–441. Philadelphia, WB Saunders, 1983
4. Dougherty TJ, Thomas RE, Boyule DG, et al: Interstitial photoradiation therapy for solid primary tumors. Cancer Res 41:401–404, 1981
5. Raab C: Uber die wirkung fluoreszirenden stoffe auf infusoria. Z Biol 39:524, 1900
6. Dougherty TJ, Grindley GB, Fiel R, et al: Photoradiation therapy. II. Cure of animal tumors with hematoporphyrin and light. J Natl Cancer Inst 55:115, 1975
7. Dougherty TJ, Kaufman JE, Goldfarb A, et al: Photoradiation therapy for the treatment of malignant tumors. Cancer Res 38:2628, 1978
8. Dougherty TJ, Potter WR, Weishaupt KR: The structure of the active component of hematoporphyrin derivative. In Doiron DR, Gomer CJ (eds): Porphyrin Localization and Treatment of Tumors, p. 301. New York, Alan R. Liss, 1984
9. Weishaupt KR, Gomer CJ, Dougherty TJ: Identification of singlet oxygen as the cytotoxic agent in photoactivation of a murine tumor. Cancer Res 36:2326, 1976
10. Henderson BW, Dougherty TJ: Studies on the mechanism of tumor destruction by photoradiation therapy (PRT). In Doiron DR, Gomer CJ (eds): Porphyrin Localization and Treatment of Tumors, p. 601. New York, Alan R. Liss, 1984
11. Svaasand LO, Doiron DR, Dougherty TJ: Temperature rise during photoradiation therapy of malignant tumors. Med Phys 10:10, 1983

15

NEW DEVELOPMENTS IN CANCER THERAPY

Ilene Kurzman

E. Gregory MacEwen

Advancement in veterinary oncology has been limited in part because most of the available therapeutic agents are associated with significant toxicity at optimal doses. Improvement in therapy requires agents that more specifically kill tumor cells while sparing normal cells. Most recently, the search for a treatment for acquired immunodeficiency syndrome in humans has led to the development of antiretroviral drugs that may be useful in the treatment of diseases associated with feline leukemia virus. In the last decade, new developments have allowed drugs to be targeted directly to the site of a tumor or metastasis, preferential interference with the proliferation of tumor cells by drugs that are not toxic to normal cells, and extension of the half-life of drugs in the body. Bone marrow transplantation will soon be available in the clinical setting to rescue animals from high-dosage treatments that would otherwise be lethal.

Many of the new developments in cancer therapy will be discussed in this chapter. Knowledge in veterinary oncology and in the treatment of cancer in all species is increasing rapidly. We must remain alert to upcoming developments in the war against cancer.

ANTIRETROVIRAL AGENTS

Research over the last three decades has provided evidence to support the theory that leukemia, lymphoma, and related neoplastic diseases are caused in many animal species by transmissible oncogenic viruses. In most instances these viruses remain latent and harmless to their hosts, but they can be activated and subsequently can induce disease. More recently, attention has been focused on retroviruses as causative agents of leukemia and lymphoma. Research on acquired immunodeficiency syndrome (AIDS) and AIDS-related complex has spawned development of a number of antiretroviral agents. Many of these drugs are inhibitors of reverse transcriptase, which is essential to the replication of retroviruses.

Suramin is the first drug that has been shown to completely inhibit reverse transcriptase.[1] The mechanism of the inhibition is unknown at this time. In one study, two cats infected with feline leukemia virus were treated with weekly intravenous injections of 20 mg/kg of suramin. Within 14 days after the start of treatment, infectious virus was undetectable in the serum of both cats; after cessation of suramin treatment, virus infection returned within 14 days. The major adverse side-effects of suramin in these cats were transient vomiting and anorexia.[2]

Another recently developed antiretroviral drug is 3'-azido-3'-deoxythymidine (AZT), which is a potent inhibitor of the *in vitro* replication and cytopathic effect of human T cell leukemia virus III (HTLV-III). AZT acts as a chain terminator of DNA synthesis. Cellular DNA-polymerase alpha is 100 times less susceptible to inhibition by AZT than is HTLV-III reverse transcriptase. It is suggested that this difference in sensitivity accounts for the selective antiviral activity of AZT.[3]

In 1987, AZT was approved for clinical use. AZT is produced by the Burroughs Wellcome Company under the name of Retrovir. In a placebo-controlled clinical trial of AZT, reported by Burroughs Wellcome, in a total of 281 patients infected with human immunodeficiency virus, the most frequent adverse reactions were granulocytopenia and anemia. Significant anemia occurred after 4 to 6 weeks of therapy, and required a dosage adjustment or cessation of therapy and, in some cases, blood transfusions.[4] Experiments are now underway to evaluate the effect of AZT therapy on cats infected with feline leukemia virus, with or without leukemia. Preliminary testing shows AZT to be well tolerated in the cat.

It is doubtful that the antiretroviral agents alone will be very beneficial in the treatment of cancer. However, if one could halt the replication of the causative agent—the virus—while the animal is being treated with chemotherapy or immunotherapy, response to treatment could be enhanced as well as sustained.

TARGETED DRUG DELIVERY

One of the strategies currently being employed in the fight against cancer is improving the effectiveness of existing agents by altering such features as drug disposition, kinetics, and dose-response ratios. Various drug delivery systems are being investigated for their ability to target drugs to specific tumor sites and to specific cell types. Of these, liposomes, magnetic microspheres, and monoclonal antibodies appear to be the most promising.

LIPOSOMES

Liposomes are closed lipid-bilayer vesicles. They are either small, sonicated unilamellar vesicles or large multilamellar vesicles. Water-soluble drugs can be encapsulated within the aqueous interior, and hydrophobic drugs can be incorporated into the lipid bilayer(s) (see Fig. 15-1). The proposed advantages of liposomes are:[5]

1. prolonged drug effect due to longer half-life than the free nonencapsulated drug
2. the possibility that liposomes will be sequestered in the site of the tumor
3. reduction of toxicity in those tissues that do not tend to accumulate liposomes, such as the heart or kidneys
4. protection of a drug from attack by host enzymes and the immune system until it reaches its target
5. direction of liposomes to their natural target, the phagocytic cells of mainly the liver, spleen, and lung, and the blood monocytes, or direction by altering the surface of the liposome
6. amplification of therapeutic effect by incorporation of numerous drug molecules in each target-directed liposome
7. selective release of drug from liposomes in the desired location as a function of physical factors such as local temperature or pH
8. delivery of drugs designed to be active after endocytic uptake

It seems that the most logical approach to the use of liposomes is to take advantage of their natural tendency to be taken up by the reticuloendothelial cells of the liver, spleen, and lung and by the blood monocytes (some investigators believe that it is the blood monocyte that phagocytoses the liposome and then the monocyte migrates into the liver, spleen, or lung). It is well accepted that augmentation of immune functions performed or mediated by blood monocytes has significant antitumor effects. It has been shown *in vitro* and *in vivo* that activated monocytes are important effector cells against tumors and against metastases. The localization

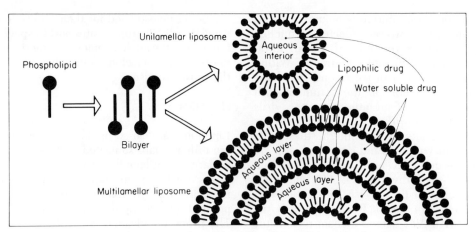

Figure 15-1. Schematic structure of a unilamellar and multilamellar liposome with incorporated drug. Water-soluble drugs are encapsulated within the aqueous interior and lipophilic drugs are encapsulated within the lipid bilayers.

of liposomes within macrophages or monocytes provides a highly efficient method of targeting immunopotentiators to these cells. We have recently completed a randomized study in which we evaluated liposome-encapsulated muramyl tripeptide-phosphatidylethanolamine (liposome/MTP-PE), a potent nonspecific monocyte activator, as treatment for metastasis in dogs undergoing amputation for osteosarcoma.[5a,5b] The median metastasis-free interval for 14 dogs treated with liposome/MTP-PE was 168 days, significantly longer than the 58 days for the 13 dogs treated by surgery alone; p = 0.002. The median survival time for dogs treated with liposome/MTP-PE was 222 days, as compared to 77 days for dogs treated by surgery alone; p <0.002. In the liposome/MTP-PE-treated group, there are still 4 dogs alive at greater than one year postamputation (17, 19, 26, and 32 months), however, in the surgery alone group, all dogs had died by 15 months. This study shows that liposome/MTP-PE is more effective than surgery alone. Further studies are now underway to evaluate liposome/MTP-PE treatment in combination with other therapeutic agents.

A major limitation in the use of available chemotherapeutic agents is their association with significant toxicity when used at optimal doses. Encapsulating such drugs in liposomes markedly reduces their toxicity. In a study that compared the toxicity of free doxorubicin and liposome-encapsulated doxorubicin in mice, it was found that at a dose of 7.5 mg/kg, every 2 weeks for up to 16 weeks, 100% of the mice receiving liposome/doxorubicin survived the cumulative dosage of 60 mg/kg, while only 2% of mice receiving free doxorubicin survived this dosage. The reduced toxicity of the liposome/doxorubicin included reduction in body and organ weight loss, reduced severity of pathologic changes, and fewer blood biochemical changes. Nephrotoxicity, which was severe among the free doxorubicin-treated mice, was insignificant among the liposome-treated mice. The antitumor activity of doxorubicin when encapsulated in liposomes is fully preserved and in some animal models it is enhanced.[6]

Another area of liposome and cancer therapy that is being investigated is the use of hyperthermia and pH sensitivity as modalities for targeting the liposome. The composition of liposomes can be adjusted so that the particular liposome is either more or less sensitive to heat or pH. Because of their increased vascularity, tumors are generally maintained at a higher temperature than normal tissue. By designing the liposome to be more permeable at this increased temperature, there is the potential that release of drug can be enhanced in the area of the tumor. A similar logic applies to the use of pH-sensitive liposomes. In a number of human and animal tumor interstitial fluids, the pH is found to be considerably lower than in normal tissue. This difference is potentially useful if liposomes could be constructed so that they release encapsulated drug when passing through a region of lower pH.[7]

The use of liposomes as a vehicle in targeted drug delivery has very real potential for use in cancer therapy as well as in the treatment of many other diseases. Evidence that encapsulation in liposomes reduces the toxicity of chemotherapeutic drugs without altering their efficacy suggests that liposomes may soon play a significant role in cancer therapy. The fact that liposomes naturally accumulate in liver, spleen, and lung makes such a vehicle of particular interest for the treatment of metastasis.

MAGNETIC MICROSPHERES

Iron particles (1–3 μm in diameter) can be directed through blood vessels to selectively targeted tissues by an external magnetic field. This ability led to the idea for the use of such particles as a drug delivery system. Microspheres, made by combining Fe_3O_4 and denatured human albumin through a water-in-oil phase-separation emulsion polymerization, are capable of carrying water-soluble drugs. These spheres are small enough to prevent microembolization, biodegradable, minimally reactive with blood components, and nontoxic; they can accommodate a wide variety of water-soluble drugs.[8] As with liposomes, the use of microspheres potentially would allow for a higher concentration of a chemotherapeutic drug in the targeted site than could be achieved by systemic administration owing to the toxic side-effects of such drugs.

Response to therapy with magnetic microspheres has been seen in rodent models. Twenty-two rats with Yoshida sarcoma implants in their tails were treated with doxorubicin-bearing microspheres. All demonstrated marked tumor regression, and 17 (77%) showed complete remission. No deaths or metastases occurred in the experimental group, while all rats receiving free doxorubicin or placebo microspheres had widespread metastases and all died. In addition, animals receiving free doxorubicin showed a decrease in weight suggestive of doxorubicin toxicity, while those receiving doxorubicin microspheres had no decrease in weight.[9] In another study, rats with AH7974 lung metastases were treated with doxorubicin-bearing micros-

pheres. Histopathologic examination of the lungs revealed that the rats treated with microspheres showed greater antitumor drug effects than those treated with free doxorubicin.[10]

Microspheres are most easily delivered to extremities by intra-arterial routes; selective catheterization can be used for delivery to other sites, such as the liver or lungs. In a study of dogs with spontaneously occurring soft-tissue and osteogenic sarcomas of the extremities, preferential methods of access were found for both sites; extra-osseous tumors were perfused by the intra-arterial route, and osseous tumors were perfused by the intramedullary method. Primary bone tumors with significant soft-tissue components required a combination of intra-arterial and intramedullary administration. In 36 dogs with osteogenic sarcoma, magnetic microspheres were infused while the target site was exposed to an external magnetic field created by a 5-kw electromagnet. By labeling the microspheres with ^{99m}Tc, it was found that those that did not localize in the tumor were trapped in the reticuloendothelial system (lung, liver, and spleen). Of the 36 dogs, 27 had received doxorubicin-bearing microspheres. Four of the 27 showed regression, but relapse was observed in all the dogs.[8] An adverse reaction seen in some of the dogs in this study was a severe vasculitis at the site of the localized spheres, resulting in necrosis and limb death. The investigators thought this was due to the doxorubicin since none of the dogs receiving empty spheres had this reaction. Another complication noted was the escape of some of the spheres into the circulation and into the cerebral hemisphere. The investigators thought that the placement of the magnetic field (which was close to the head in these cases) contributed to the escape of the spheres.*

It is clear that the study of magnetic microspheres as carriers of chemotherapeutic agents is in its earliest phase. Much research needs to be done on routes of administration, dosage of drugs, and other questions. The results of rodent studies suggest that magnetic microspheres may potentially be an effective drug delivery system for use in cancer treatment.

* Richardson R, Elliot G: Personal communication.

MONOCLONAL ANTIBODIES[11]

The discovery of a method to produce antibodies of selected specificity by a clone of cells derived from a single cell had immediate impact on cancer diagnosis and therapy. Monoclonal antibodies (MAb) can be used to detect tumor antigens in serum, to distinguish between normal and malignant cells in histologic studies of tumors, and when radiolabeled, to scan for sites of tumors or metastases that are undetected by other means. As a therapeutic modality, MAb can be used to target tumor cells. MAb can also be used as vehicles to carry toxins, drugs, or radionuclides. Drugs or toxins that exhibit toxicity for tumor cells when conjugated with MAb would result in more specific targeting to tumor cells. An advantage of such therapy is that by specific delivery to tumor cells, it is possible that a dosage that has less systemic toxicity could be administered with the same effect as the higher, nonconjugated dosage.

One limitation to therapy with MAb is that killing of the tumor cell is dependent on internalization by that cell of the bound drug or toxin. One way around this is to use radionuclides. It is possible to design the radionuclide to deposit its energy within a few cell diameters. This would eliminate the need for the tumor cell to internalize the antibody-bound agent and would protect the nonmalignant cells that are more than a few cell diameters from the targeted tumor cell. Another problem with the MAb-bound drug or toxin therapy is that the quantity of drug that can be bound to the antibody is limited. A way to increase it is to encapsulate the drug in a liposome and then couple the liposome to the MAb.

Most of the work with MAb has been done in experimental animal model systems. Although many MAb have been produced for human tumors and human trials have begun, the development of MAb to companion animal tumors is just now underway. A few MAb have already been developed for animal tumors and they will probably be in use in detection and therapy when this book is printed.

RETINOIDS

Retinoids are the group of molecules that consists of Vitamin A and its natural and synthetic derivatives. These agents have been shown to have effect on the prevention and therapy of cancer in animals and in humans. In particular, retinoids prevent experimentally induced cancer of the bladder, breast, and skin, and there is evidence suggesting their potential for the prevention of cancers of the pancreas, prostate, lung, esophagus, and colon.[12] Although only limited human clinical trials have been conducted thus far, certain retinoid derivatives have shown therapeutic activity in preleukemic syndromes, squamous carcinoma of the head and neck, carcinoma of the lung, malignant melanoma, kerato-acanthoma, oral leukoplakia, and breast adenocarcinoma.[13]

One study of the effect of 13-*cis*-retinoic acid on the development of spontaneous thymic lymphomas in AKR mice (this mouse strain has a very high incidence of lymphomas) showed that mice fed a diet supplemented with 13-*cis*-retinoic acid had a 15% incidence of lymphoma, compared to a 45% incidence in those fed a normal diet. These results suggest that 13-*cis*-retinoic acid may be useful in the prevention of neoplasia originating from the lymphoid tissue.[14] In a recent study, cats with a total of 15 cancerous (squamous cell carcinoma) and precancerous (epidermal dysplasia) lesions were treated with 13-*cis*-retinoic acid at a dose of approximately 3 mg/kg/day for an average of 68 days. Side-effects were readily controlled with frequent application of topical anti-inflammatory medication. At the completion of treatment, only 1 of the 15 lesions showed partial clinical and microscopic improvement. This study indicates that 13-*cis*-retinoic acid at the dose and duration of administration used was not effective in the treatment of these lesions.[15] The findings of this study are less promising than those of studies on humans and various animal models.

The specific mechanism of action of retinoids is not known. Theories have included restoration of cell membrane integrity, normalization of cellular gap junctions, effects on cell surface glycoconjugates, prevention of cell cycles from entering S phase, blockage of ornithine decarboxylase activity, and stimulation of the immune system, particularly the cytotoxic effects of killer T cells and the tumoricidal effects of macrophages.[16,17]

With regard to immunity, there is evidence to suggest that *in vivo* enhancement of cell-mediated immunity by retinoids and the subsequent increase in tumor resistance is the mechanism by which retinoids inhibit the growth and development of certain types of tumors. It is of interest that inhibition of growth by retinoids is primarily seen with tumors that are strongly immunogenic or in immunocompetent mice. Vitamin A has been repeatedly shown to stimulate T cell mitogenic response. Retinoic acid stimulates cell-mediated immunity, as has been shown by enhancement of skin graft rejection and by induction of cytotoxic T cells in mice fed high dosages. It has also been reported that high dosages of Vitamin A enhanced immune function in burn and surgical trauma cases.[18]

Cancer prevention and therapy is potentially the most significant clinical use of retinoids. Based on the results of preliminary animal and clinical studies, chronic maintenance therapy may be needed for successful chemoprevention of cancer with retinoids.[19] The observed toxicities have been well tolerated and no chronic toxicities have been noted. One must conclude that the future of retinoids, both in the clinic and in the laboratory, is most promising, particularly with the development of new synthetic retinoids.

INHIBITORS OF POLYAMINE BIOSYNTHESIS

Interest in polyamines has grown steadily in the past few years because of increasing recognition of their essential role in cellular growth, multiplication, and differentiation, and their apparent role in stabilization of DNA. Polyamines have been found to stabilize cell-free DNA, thus inhibiting enzyme degradation and denaturation by x-ray and heat. The effects of polyamines on the structural integrity of DNA suggests a possible role for polyamine depletion in cancer chemotherapy.

Ornithine decarboxylase (ODC) is the first enzyme in the polyamine biosynthetic pathway. ODC activity is markedly increased, as is the concentration of polyamines, in rapidly growing tissues. D,L-α-Difluoromethylornithine (DFMO) is a potent and irreversible inhibitor of ODC. DFMO is relatively nontoxic and has been found to exhibit significant antitumor activity in murine tumor models, including EMT6 mammary sarcoma,[20] 1-methyl-1-nitrosourea-induced mam-

mary gland carcinoma,[21] B16 melanoma,[22] and Lewis lung carcinoma.[22,23] It is of particular interest that, in the study of the 1-methyl-1-nitrosourea-induced tumors, it was found that in mammary gland tissue analyzed for polyamine concentration, tumor-bearing rats treated with DFMO had a significantly decreased polyamine concentration as compared with tumor-bearing rats that did not receive DFMO. DFMO did not affect the polyamine concentration in the mammary gland tissue of non-tumor-bearing rats, suggesting that the inhibition of polyamine biosynthesis by DFMO is specific to tumor tissue and does not affect normal tissue.

Studies evaluating the antitumor effects of DFMO have reported that mice and rats tolerate the drug extremely well; the only side-effect noted was diarrhea, which completely resolved when the drug was stopped.[24] A toxicity study of DFMO in the dog reported that a dose of >200 mg/kg/day resulted in diarrhea that resolved on stopping the drug.[25] In addition, Phase I tolerance studies in humans with DFMO have been completed in the Untied States and abroad. The initial data indicate that in humans, DFMO is well tolerated with no serious toxicity. Thrombocytopenia, anemia, and hearing loss have been reported, but these effects were completely reversible on stopping the drug.[26,27]

In the search for a therapeutic approach to cancer that is relatively nontoxic to the host, there is sufficient evidence to warrant the evaluation of DFMO as an antitumor agent in animals. Recent studies show that both interferon and interferon inducers significantly potentiate the antitumor activity of DFMO in laboratory animals. The combination of DFMO and an interferon inducer should be investigated for effectiveness in the control of cancer in companion animals.

MEMBRANE TRANSPORT INHIBITORS

The mechanism of action of most of the antineoplastic drugs available today is their ability to damage DNA directly or impair its synthesis. Such cytotoxic agents are associated with severe toxicities because of their attack on any cell undergoing rapid DNA synthesis—both normal (e.g., skin, bone marrow) and tumor cells. The development of drugs that affect other cellular components may lead to therapeutic agents that are less toxic or for which toxicities may be more easily controlled. Cellular membranes have a significant function in the regulation and organization of intracellular activities. New agents that impair the function of membranes in tumor cells are being investigated. Below are the findings thus far regarding two such agents.

LONIDAMINE

Lonidamine causes an inhibition of tumor growth that is accompanied by characteristic changes in tumor cell mitochondria. Such mitochondrial disruption is thought to be related to decreased oxygen consumption.[28] Restriction of oxygen consumption alters energy metabolism. Tumor cell metabolism is characterized by an increase in the pentophosphate pathway, which is accompanied by high rates of lactate production when glucose is the substrate under aerobic conditions. In turn, conversion of glucose-6-phosphate is linked to a higher amount of mitochondrial-bound hexokinase, and it is this enzyme that is particularly sensitive to Lonidamine.[29] The result is an increase in anaerobic glycolysis, mediated through the inhibition of mitochondrial-bound hexokinase. Cells under the influence of Lonidamine tend to accumulate lactate owing to a selective inhibition of lactate transport.[30] This results in a steady reduction in the intracellular pH. The low pH of the cells makes them particularly more sensitive to certain treatments, such as hyperthermia.[31]

When tested against transplantable tumor systems, Lonidamine demonstrated antitumor activity in experiments using subcutaneously implanted Lewis lung tumor cells. When Lonidamine was given at a dose of 100 mg/kg intraperitoneally 24 hours after tumor implant, an increase in life-span of 106% was seen.[32] This activity against Lewis lung cancer is of interest in view of the relative resistance of this tumor to standard chemotherapy agents. On the other hand, Lonidamine has shown no antitumor activity against L1210 lymphoid leukemia, P388 leukemia, B16 melanoma, or implanted ependymoblastoma.[28,32,33]

Studies in humans have shown that Lonidamine does have a modest degree of antitumor activity in certain selected tumors. Responses have been seen in sarcomas, a very resistant small-cell lung carcinoma, and a poorly differentiated adenocarcinoma of the lung.[33] It is hypothesized that Lonidamine may have more activity in certain tissues that in others. The lung has a considerably higher oxygen tension than other tissues, which perhaps makes lung metastases more sensitive to effects of oxygen consumption.[33] In addition, in human patients with chronic lymphocytic leukemia, a 20% response rate has been detected.[34]

Lonidamine may be of benefit in combination with radiation therapy. Published evidence suggests that Lonidamine does not possess a direct synergistic effect on radiation, but rather prevents repair of potentially lethal damage of cancer cells.[35]

Since Lonidamine "recognizes" the energy metabolism of tumors rather than their histogenetic features or their morphologic type, it must be expected that response depends solely on the thermodynamic state of the cancer cells. The thermodynamic condition is, however, inconsistent; it fluctuates with the function of the cells and the variations in the microenvironment. Lonidamine will most likely be more effective in the microenvironment of cells that are heavily dependent on aerobic glycolysis. Its use as a single agent in cancer chemotherapy will depend on further evaluation in selected tumor systems. The results thus far would indicate that Lonidamine is most likely to have antitumor activity when combined with other cancer treatments, such as chemotherapy, radiation therapy, and hyperthermia.[36]

BENZALDEHYDE

Benzaldehyde is an aromatic aldehyde that has been shown to inhibit the growth of transformed mouse and simian cells.[37] It has also been shown to have antitumor activity in human carcinoma patients.[38] The mechanism of action is not fully known. Benzaldehyde affects the membrane transport system of cells transformed by cultured simian virus 40 and blocks thymidine, glucose, and other nucleosides in transformed cells, but not in normal cells.[39] A reduction in intracellular adenosine-5-triphosphate (ATP) has also been observed in cells transformed by simian virus 40.[39] The low ATP concentration affects the uptake of nucleosides because this uptake requires the phosphorylation process that is dependent on ATP.[40,41] Thus, benzaldehyde may affect the phosphorylation process, resulting in a membrane transport inhibition of essential energy sources.

In a recent study, 14 dogs and 11 cats with various malignancies were treated daily with benzaldehyde at a dose of 10 mg/kg, orally, divided into 4 doses. A partial response—greater than 50% regression—was observed in animals with an oral squamous cell carcinoma and an oral melanoma. A minimal response—less than 50% regression—was observed in a dog with a sweat gland adenocarcinoma and a cat with mast cell sarcoma. One dog with an oral melanoma had stabilization of tumor growth for 8 weeks. Another dog with a recurrent melanoma had a greater than 50% response that lasted for approximately 18 months.[42]

Although some antitumor activity has been observed with benzaldehyde, the optimal dosage has not been fully established in the dog or the cat. Thus, further evaluation of the effects of benzaldehyde at various dosages and in various tumor types needs to be done.

POLYETHYLENE GLYCOL CONJUGATES

A problem often encountered in chemotherapy is the rapid excretion or inactivation of the agent. Covalent modification with polyethylene glycol (PEG) has been shown to render proteins nonimmunogenic and to greatly extend the length of time the protein remains in the blood and body fluids.[43] In particular, this process has been applied to asparaginase.

The use of L-asparaginase in the treatment of canine lymphosarcoma is discussed in Chapter 9. Briefly, the mechanism of action is a specific depletion of L-asparagine, resulting in the death of tumor cells that lack an endogenous synthetic capacity for L-asparagine. One of the major problems with asparaginase therapy is the immunogenicity of the enzyme. Production of anti-asparaginase antibodies results in an accelerated clearance of the enzyme that reduces the effectiveness of the therapy. Another limitation of asparaginase is its short half-life in the plasma, ranging from 2.5 hours in mice to 18 hours in humans. The PEG-asparaginase conjugate may resolve these two problems.

In a recent study, PEG-asparaginase, given as a single agent or in combination with other chemotherapeutic agents, was evaluated for its antitumor activity in 37 dogs with lymphosarcoma. This study showed that PEG-asparaginase had significant antitumor activity. When it was used as a single agent, 66% of the treated dogs showed response; with the addition of other chemotherapeutic agents, the response rate rose to 88%. Of 8 dogs that were considered chemotherapy failures (including native asparaginase), 4 showed response with PEG-asparaginase, suggesting that the PEG conjugate may be able to circumvent drug inactivation because of its reduced immunogenicity.[44]

Further investigation of the antitumor effects of PEG-asparaginase is needed, as is a comparison with native asparaginase with regard to efficacy, toxicity, and resistance. However, this ability of PEG conjugates to reduce immunogenicity and increase plasma half-life may play an important role in the use of similar agents in the treatment of cancer.

BONE MARROW TRANSPLANTATION

Bone marrow transplantation allows for high dosage cancer therapy that would be lethal without bone marrow replacement. In humans, this procedure has been used to treat leukemia patients. Although much experimental work has been done in animals, particularly in the dog, there have been few reports on the use of bone marrow transplantation in clinical veterinary oncology.

Autologous bone marrow transplantation has been used in conjunction with total body irradiation (TBI) in the treatment of dogs with malignant lymphoma. In one study, 34 of 57 dogs (60%) treated with combination chemotherapy (nitrogen mustard, oncovin, prednisone, L-asparaginase, and 6-mercaptopurine) achieved complete remission. Twelve of the dogs in remission had no further therapy and had a median disease-free survival of 73.5 days. Seventeen of the dogs in remission received 1100 rads TBI, which was followed by the infusion of fresh autologous bone marrow that had been aspirated from the dog immediately prior to the TBI. These dogs had a median disease-free survival of 206 days, which was significantly longer than the 73.5 days for the group that received chemotherapy alone. Two of the 17 dogs receiving bone marrow died of late transplant complications. This aspect of bone marrow transplantation needs further exploration. The findings of this study indicate that while dogs with malignant lymphoma are responsive to chemotherapy, the addition of TBI and rescue by infusion of the dog's own bone marrow markedly prolongs disease-free survival time.[45] Recent studies in the treatment of malignant lymphoma in dogs have given similar results. These studies investigated the effects of varying the dose of radiation, and it was found that increasing the dose led to greater toxicity and no measurable decrease in the relapse rate after transplantation.[46]

Currently, a study is underway in which bone marrow is being harvested from dogs with lymphosarcoma either before chemotherapy or when the cancer is in complete remission. The marrow is cryopreserved until the dog relapses, at which time TBI is performed, followed by infusion of the dog's preserved marrow. Engraftment by autologous cryopreserved bone marrow has been successful in normal, healthy dogs treated with TBI,[47] but there are not yet any results of the treatment of the dogs with lymphosarcoma. An indication of the effectiveness of this treatment may be available when this book is printed. If the treatment is successful, the approach has great potential as a salvage procedure when various types of cancer are treated with any therapy that is severely marrow suppressive. With the increasing capabilities of veterinary clinic facilities (*e.g.*, radiation therapy, nuclear medicine), bone marrow transplantation will soon play a significant role in cancer therapy for animals.

REFERENCES

1. De Clerq E: Suramin: A potent inhibitor of the reverse transcriptase of RNA tumour viruses. Cancer Lett 8:9–22, 1979
2. Cogan DC, Cotter SM, Kitchen LW: Effect of suramin on serum viral replication in feline leukemia virus-infected pet cats. Am J Vet Res 47:2230–2232, 1986
3. Yarchoan R, Klecker RW, Weinhold KJ, et al: Administration of 3'-azido-3'-deoxythymidine, an inhibitor of HTLVIII/LAV replication, to patients with AIDS or AIDS-related complex. Lancet March:575–580, 1985
4. Burroughs Wellcome Company: Announcing Retrovir[R] (zidovudine), the first effective treatment for certain AIDS and other serious HIV infections (drug brochure), 1987
5. Weinstein JN, Leserman LD: Liposomes as drug carriers in cancer chemotherapy. Pharmacol Ther 24:207–233, 1984
5a. MacEwen EG, Kurzman ID, Rosenthal RC, et al: Therapy of osteosarcoma in dogs with intravenous injection of liposome-encapsulated muramyl tripeptide. J Natl Cancer Inst (in press)
5b. MacEwen EG, Kurzman ID, Smith BW: Therapy of metastasis in canine osteosarcoma. In Lopez-Berestein G, Fidler IJ (eds): Liposomes in the Therapy of Infectious Diseases and Cancer, UCLA Symposium on Molecular and Cellular Biology, New Series, Vol. 89. New York, Alan R. Liss, pp. 117–124, 1989
6. Gabizon A, Meshorer A, Barenholz Y: Comparative long-term study of the toxicities of free and liposome-associated doxorubicin in mice after intravenous administration. J Natl Cancer Inst 77:459–469, 1986
7. Yatvin MB, Cree TC, Tegmo–Larsson IM, et al: Liposomes as drug carriers in cancer therapy: Hyperthermia and pH sensitivity as modalities for targeting. Strahlentherapie 160:732–740, 1984
8. Richardson RC: Targeted drug delivery. In Proceedings of the Groupe d'Etude en Oncologie: Diagnostic et Traitement des Tumeurs en Medicine Canine, pp. 22–26, 1986
9. Widder KJ, Morris RM, Poore GA, et al: Selective targeting of magnetic albumin microspheres containing low-dose doxorubicin: Total remission in Yoshida sarcoma-bearing rats. Eur J Cancer Clin Oncol 19:135–139, 1983
10. Sugibayashi K, Okumura M, Morimoto Y: Biomedical applications of magnetic fluids. III. Antitumor effect of magnetic albumin microsphere-encapsulated adriamycin on lung metastasis of AH7974 in rats. Biomaterials 3:181–186, 1982
11. Davis FM, Rao PN: Monoclonal antibodies in the diagnosis and treatment of cancer. In Sunkara PS (ed): Novel Approaches to Cancer Chemotherapy, pp. 23–92. Orlando, FL, Academic Press, 1984
12. Goodman DS: Vitamin S and retinoids in health and disease. N Engl J Med 310:1023–1031, 1984
13. Pawson BA, Ehrmann CW, Itri LM, et al: Retinoids at the threshold: Their biological significance and therapeutic potential. J Med Chem 25:1269–1277, 1982
14. Przybyszewska M, Szaniawska B, Janik P: Effect of 13-*cis*-retinoic acid on the spontaneous thymic

lymphoma development in AKR mice. Neoplasma 33:341–344, 1986

15. Evans AG, Madewell BR, Stannard AA: A trial of 13-*cis*-retinoic acid for treatment of squamous cell carcinoma and preneoplastic lesions of the head of cats. Am J Vet Res 46:2553–2557, 1985

16. Peck GL: Chemoprevention of cancer with retinoids. Gynecol Oncol 12:s331–s340, 1981

17. Eccles SA: Effects of retinoids on growth and dissemination of malignant tumors: Immunological considerations. Biochem Pharmacol 34:1599–1610, 1985

18. Watson RR, Moriguchi S: Cancer prevention by retinoids: Role of immunological modification. Nutr Res 5:663–675, 1985

19. Bollag W, Hartmann HR: Prevention and therapy of cancer with retinoids in animals and man. Cancer Surv 2:293–314, 1983

20. Prakash NJ, Schecter PJ, Mamont PS, et al: Inhibition of EMT6 tumor growth by interference with polyamine biosynthesis: Effects of alpha-difluoromethylornithine, an irreversible inhibitor of ornithine decarboxylase. Life Sci 26:181–194, 1980

21. Thompson HJ, Herbst FJ, Meeker LD, et al: Effect of D,L-alpha-difluoromethylornithine on murine mammary carcinogenesis. Carcinogenesis 5:1649–1651, 1984

22. Sunkara PS, Prakash NJ, Rosenberger AL, et al: Potentiation of antitumor and antimetastatic activities by alpha-difluoromethylornithine by interferon inducers. Cancer Res 44:2799–2802, 1984

23. Bartholeyns J: Treatment of metastatic Lewis lung carcinoma with DL-alpha-difluoromethylornithine. Eur J Cancer Clin Oncol 19:567–572, 1983

24. Sunkara PS, Prakash NJ: Inhibitors of polyamine biosynthesis as antitumor and antimetastatic agents. In Sunkara PS (ed): Novel Approaches to Cancer Chemotherapy. pp. 94–127. New York, Academic Press, 1984

25. Yarrington JT, Sprinkle DJ, Loudy DE, et al: Intestinal changes caused by DL-alpha-difluoromethylornithine (DFMO), an inhibitor or ornithine decarboxylase. Exp Mol Pathol 39:300–316, 1983

26. Abeloff MD, Slavid M, Luk G, et al: Phase I trial and pharmacokinetic studies of oral alpha-difluoromethyl-ornithine (DFMO). Proc Am Soc Clin Oncol 2:22, 1983

27. Sjoerdsma A, Schecter PJ: Chemotherapeutic implications of polyamine biosynthesis inhibition. Clin Pharmacol Ther 35:287–300, 1983

28. Silvestrini B, Hahn GM, Cioli V, et al: Effects of Lonidamine, alone or combined with hyperthermia in some experimental cell and tumor systems. Br J Cancer 47:221–231, 1983

29. Natali PG, Salsano F, Viroa M, et al: Inhibition of aerobic glycolysis in normal and neoplastic cells induced by Lonidamine. Oncology 41(suppl 1):7–14, 1984

30. Hahn GM: Potential for therapy of drugs and hyperthermia. Cancer Res 39:2264–2268, 1979

31. Kim JH, Kim SH, Alfieri A, et al: Lonidamine: A hyperthermic sensitizer of HeLa cells in culture and of the Meth-A tumor in vivo. Oncology 41(suppl 1):30–35, 1984

32. Gargus JL, Congleton GF: Antitumor bioassay—mice compound AF/T 1800, project 2101–100. Final report. Vol 2, Ref No 2206. Lonidamine IND. Hazelton Lab America, Madison, WI, 1981

33. Evans WK, Mullis SB: Phase II evaluation of Lonidamine in patients with advanced malignancy. Oncology 41(suppl 1):69–77, 1984

34. Tura S, Cavo M, Gobbi M, et al: Lonidamine in the treatment of chronic lymphocytic leukemia. Oncology 41(suppl 1):90–93, 1984

35. Kim JH, Alfieri A, Kim SH, et al: Radiosensitization of Meth-A fibrosarcoma in mice by Lonidamine. Oncology 41(suppl 1):36–38, 1984

36. Caputo A: Concluding remarks, Lonidamine. Proc 2nd Intl Symp, Vancouver, 1982. Oncology 41(suppl 1):121–123, 1984

37. Nambata T, Terada N, Mizutani T, et al: Characteristics of C3H/He mouse embryo cell lines established by culture with or without benzaldehyde. Gan No Rinsho 73:592–599, 1982

38. Kochi M, Takeuchi S, Mizutani T, et al: Antitumor activity of benzaldehyde. Cancer Treat Rep 64:21–23, 1980

39. Watanuki M, Sakaguchi K: Selective inhibition by benzaldehyde of the uptake of nucleosides and sugar into simian virus 40-transformed cells. Cancer Res 40:2574–2579, 1980

40. Marz R, Wohlhueter RM, Plagemann PGW: Relationship between thymidine transport and phosphorylation in Novikoff rat hepatoma cells as analyzed by a rapid sampling technique. J Supramol Struct 6:433–440, 1977

41. Plagemann PGW, Marz R, Wohlhueter RM: Uridine transport in Novikoff rat hepatoma cells and other cell types and its relationship to uridine phosphorylation and phosphorlysis. J Cell Physiol 97:49–72, 1978

42. MacEwen EG: Anti-tumor evaluation of benzaldehyde in the dog and cat. Am J Vet Res 47:451–452, 1986

43. Abuchowski A, van Es T, Palczuk NC, et al:

Alterations of immunological properties of bovine serum albumin by covalent attachment of polyethylene glycol. J Biol Chem 252:3578–3581, 1977

44. MacEwen EG, Rosenthal R, Matus R, et al: An evaluation of asparaginase:polyethylene glycol against canine lymphosarcoma. Cancer 59:2011–2015, 1987

45. Weiden PL, Storb R, Deeg HJ, et al: Prolonged disease-free survival in dogs with lymphoma after total-body irradiation and autologous marrow transplantation consolidation of combination-chemotherapy-induced remissions. Blood 54:1039–1049, 1979

46. Applebaum FR, Deeg HJ, Storb R, et al: Marrow transplant studies in dogs with malignant lymphoma. Tranplantation 39:499–504, 1985

47. Rosenthal RC: Autologous bone marrow transplantation for lymphoma. Proc ACVIM 6:397–399, 1988

16

TUMORS OF THE SKIN AND SUBCUTANEOUS TISSUES

Steven J. Susaneck
Stephen J. Withrow

INCIDENCE AND RISK FACTORS

Tumors of the skin and subcutaneous tissue are the most common tumors affecting dogs, accounting for 30% of all canine neoplasms. They are the second most common tumor in cats, accounting for 15% to 20% of feline tumors.[1] The incidence rate for benign and malignant neoplasms in the dog is reported to be 728 per 100,000 dogs at risk per year.[2] Tumors derived from mesenchymal tissues comprise about 55% of canine skin tumors, while 45% are of epithelial origin.[2-4] The most common mesenchymal tumors in the dog are histiocytomas, lipomas, and mast cell tumors.[2] In the cat the most common mesenchymal tumors are fibrosarcomas and mast cell tumors.[1] The most common epithelial tumors in the dogs are sebaceous gland tumors and papillomas, while the most common epithelial tumors in cats are basal cell tumors and squamous cell carcinomas.[1-3] Twenty percent of primary tumors of the skin and subcutaneous tissues of dogs are malignant, whereas in the cat 65% are malignant.[1-3]

The median ages for dogs and cats with skin tumors are 10.5 years and 12 years respectively.[2-4] There is no significant difference in the incidence by sex when all canine skin tumors are considered together.[5] Certain tumors, such as perianal adenomas, have a higher incidence in males, while other tumors may be overrepresented in females. Breeds with the highest incidence of skin tumors include bassett hound, boxer, bull mastiff, Scottish terrier, and weimaraner.[5,6] Canine breeds with the lowest incidence of skin tumors are Brittany spaniel, Chihuahua, Pekingese, Pomeranian and poodle.[5] Skin tumors show no breed predilection in cats.[7-9]

Specific etiologies have been proven for only a few tumors in the dog and cat. Several contributing factors in development of skin tumors include viruses,[10] solar and ionizing radiation,[11,12] hormones, as well as genetic and immunological influences. Tumors have also been associated with thermal injuries.[13]

Squamous papillomas (warts) in the young dog are of viral origin.[14] In the cat, the feline leukemia virus (FeLV) is associated with cutaneous lymphosarcoma.[15] Multiple fibrosarcomas occurring in young cats have been associated with the FeLV as well as the feline sarcoma virus (see Chapters 18 and 29). A viral etiology has been proposed for the canine mastocytoma, histiocytoma, and transmissible venereal tumor, but definite proof is lacking.

Ultraviolet irradiation from sunlight has been associated with squamous cell carcinomas in both the dog and the cat.[11,12]

PATHOLOGIC CLASSIFICATION

The heterogeneity of cutaneous structures that can be involved in a neoplastic process complicates the issue of classification. Generally, skin tumors are classified histologically according to the tissue of origin (epithelial, mesenchymal, melanotic, or round cell) and individual cell of origin if sufficient differentiation is present. They are further classified as to the degree of malignancy based on histological characteristics. In some cases, there is not a clear differentiation between malignant and benign skin tumors. Clinically, skin tumors are further classified according to the TNM (tumor-node-metastasis) system (see Appendix B), which allows the tumor to be described in exacting detail with regard to its clinical presentation. Finally, the location is a part of the classification of skin tumors. Some tumors behave differently when located in different areas of the body. An example of the difference in behavior due to location is the canine oral melanoma (usually malignant) as opposed to the canine cutaneous melanoma (usually benign). In addition, biologic behavior may vary for the same type of tumor in the dog as opposed to the cat.

HISTORY AND CLINICAL SIGNS

The history of an animal with a cutaneous tumor is variable. Commonly an owner discovers a growth while examining or grooming the pet. Benign tumors are more likely to have a history of slow growth from weeks to years. It is not unusual for benign epithelial tumors to be presented for ulceration due to self-trauma or secondary inflammation. Most benign tumors are well circumscribed, nonpainful, and freely moveable, and they incite a minimal inflammatory response. Malignant tumors are often rapidly growing, fixed to underlying structures, and ulcerated, and they often have ill-defined margins. Invasion into lymphatics and regional lymphatics is sometimes seen.

DIAGNOSTIC TECHNIQUES AND WORK-UP

One of the most important techniques used in the diagnosis and management of skin tumors is a thorough physical examination. Every tumor should be examined with respect to size, location, consistency, and presence or absence of fixation to underlying tissue and of ulceration of the overlying skin. In addition, a thorough examination of draining lymph nodes is important. Although the physical appearance, location, and growth pattern of a tumor may give the examiner a high degree of suspicion as to the type of tumor, it is imperative that some type of cytological or histopathological diagnosis be attained to properly plan therapy. The two most common diagnostic procedures for skin tumors are cytology and histopathology.

Aspiration cytology is a very important screening tool to differentiate neoplastic from inflammatory lesions (see Chapter 6). All cutaneous tumors should be evaluated by fine-needle aspiration cytology to aid in the planning of therapy. Several tumors such as round cell tumors and melanocytic tumors lend themselves well to cytological diagnosis. Cytology often allows one to differentiate between epithelial and connective tissue tumors, but special training is necessary to further subclassify these tumors. Cytologic examination of enlarged regional lymph nodes should be performed prior to surgery. Ulcerated or inflamed tumors may cause reactive lymphadenopathy without metastasis.

Histological examination of a suspected or known tumor is extremely important in planning therapy and determining prognosis. Histologic examination of a specimen will allow the pathologist to determine the degree of a malignancy and invasion, as well as whether surgical excision was adequate. The type of biopsy procedure is determined by size and location of the tumor. A small tumor in an easily accessible location should be treated by excisional biopsy and submission of the entire specimen for histologic examination. When dealing with large tumors or tumors in locations that don't allow easy excision, such as an extremity, an incisional biopsy should be performed to allow optimal therapeutic planning (see Chapter 7).

TREATMENT AND PROGNOSIS OF SPECIFIC TUMOR TYPES

Because skin tumors are often treated before the specific tumor type is known, the general principles of treatment will be discussed collectively. The specific form of therapy is determined by the nature of the primary disease, local and distant metastasis, and the anticipated behavior of the tumor. When disease is localized, the size and location will be important in determining the appropriate therapy.

Standard blade excision remains the treatment of choice for the majority of skin tumors. Standard surgical technique is employed with emphasis on wide surgical borders. When attempting to completely excise a tumor, it is better to leave an open wound if necessary, rather than to leave tumor. A major advantage of surgical excision of skin tumors is that completeness of surgery can be determined histologically. In the case of very large tumors, cytoreductive surgery may be employed for palliation or to facilitate other forms of therapy. The leading cause of failure for surgical excision is inadequate surgical margins. When dealing with large malignant tumors on extremities, amputation should be considered.

Cryosurgery may be very helpful in the treatment of skin tumors but is not essential (see Chapter 12). The main advantages are speed, avoidance of general anesthesia, and low cost. Indications for cryosurgery are small or multiple tumors in older animals, where anesthesia is a concern.

Radiation therapy may be used as either a primary or adjunctive form of therapy for residual tumor control. In some cases, radiation may be combined with hyperthermia to increase tumor control (see Chapters 10 and 13).

Chemotherapy, both systemic and topical, has been used in the treatment of skin tumors. To date, with the exception of cutaneous lymphsarcoma and mast cell tumors, very little is known about the efficacy of chemotherapy in the treatment of skin tumors.

TUMORLIKE LESIONS

Several types of tumorlike cutaneous and subcutaneous masses are encountered in veterinary medicine. These lesions are nonneoplastic but in some instances may mimic neoplastic lesions. The most common nonneoplastic lesions involving the skin of dogs and cats are cutaneous cysts. Cutaneous cysts are common in dogs and uncommon in cats. The most common of the epidermal cysts are epidermoid cysts, dermoid cysts, and follicular cysts.

Epidermoid cysts (epidermoid, epithelial inclusion cyst) are round to oval, firm to fluctuant, smooth, well-circumscribed lesions. They may be found anywhere in the body and may be solitary or multiple. These masses contain a gray to white-brown, cheesy material with bits of hair shafts and are usually covered by intact epithelium (Fig. 16-1). These cysts may become ulcerated or inflamed if the cystic contents are extruded into the adjacent tissues. The treatment of choice is surgery or cryosurgery. An alternate therapy is to lance and drain the cyst, peel out the lining, and cauterize with silver nitrate.

Dermoid cysts are similar to epidermoid cysts but are more complex in structure. They appear to be congenital or hereditary lesions. They may be single or multiple. Breeds which appear to be predisposed are boxers, Kerry blue terriers, and Rhodesian Ridgebacks.[16,17] Dermoid cysts of Rhodesian Ridgebacks and their crosses appear to be inherited. They are found on the dorsal midline, neck, and sacrum. In some cases the lesion may extend deep into the dog's back to the level of the spine. The treatment is surgery.

Follicular cysts are keratinous cysts derived from epithelium of the outer root sheath; they result from retention of follicular or glandular products due to obliteration of follicular orifices.

EPITHELIAL TUMORS

PAPILLOMAS

Papillomas include cutaneous papillomatosis, warts, verrucae, and squamous cell papillomas. They are common skin tumors in the dog but relatively rare in the cat. Two types of papillomas are recognized in the dog. In the young dog,

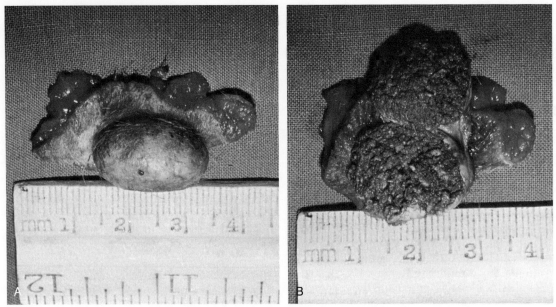

Figure 16-1. *(A)* Excised epidermoid cyst. Note hairless, circumscribed, dome-shaped appearance. *(B)* Typical appearance of brown, greasy, and granular material inside the cyst pictured in A.

papillomas are often multiple in nature and are most common on the head, eyelids, feet, and mouth (Fig. 16-2). These tumors are associated with a DNA virus that is species specific. Viral papillomatosis has been reported in the bovine, equine, and human species as well as in the dog.[10,14] Most virally induced papillomas in the young dog will undergo spontaneous regression.

The second type of papilloma is often seen in the older dog. These tumors are usually solitary but may be multiple and most commonly are located on the head, feet, eyelids, and genitalia.

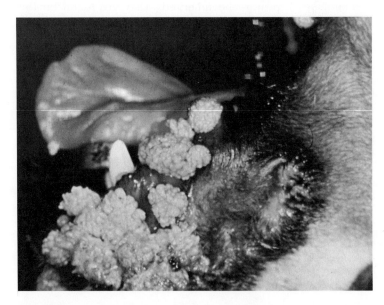

Figure 16-2. Multiple papillomas on the lip and gum of a young dog. These papillomas spontaneously regressed within 3 weeks.

Papillomas in the older dog are not associated with a viral etiology.

Papillomas appear as cauliflower-like growths with a finely fissured surface. They may be sessile or pedunculated and when traumatized will often bleed. Papillomas are usually benign, but malignant transformation into squamous cell carcinomas has been reported.[18] The treatment for solitary papillomas is surgery or cryosurgery, and the prognosis is excellent.

SQUAMOUS CELL CARCINOMAS (EPIDERMOID CARCINOMAS)

Squamous cell carcinoma (SCC) is a common tumor involving the skin in both the dog and the cat. Squamous cell carcinomas are usually found in unpigmented or lightly pigmented skin. The most common cutaneous locations for SCC in the dog are the toes, scrotum, nose, legs, and anus. The most common cutaneous locations for SCC in the cat are the nose, eyelids, lips, and pinnae. Tumors have also been reported affecting nonpigmented or lightly pigmented skin of the flank and abdomen in dalmation, beagle, whippet, and white English bull terrier dogs (Fig. 16-3).[13,19]

Squamous cell carcinoma may present as either a proliferative or erosive lesion. Proliferative lesions may vary from a red firm plaque to a cauliflowerlike lesion that often ulcerates. The erosive lesion, which is most common in the cat, initially starts as a shallow crusting lesion that may develop into a deep ulcer. SCC's arising from the digits often present as a chronic paronychia or osteomyelitis unresponsive to antibiotic treatment (Fig. 16-4). Multiple SCC involving the digits have been reported in large breeds with black skin and hair coat.[20]

The behavior and treatment of SCC is dependent on location. Tumors on the lips, nose and ears may start out as inflammatory lesions with an erythematous scaly appearance that later progress to erosive lesions. Generally squamous cell carcinomas involving the facial skin of felines are locally invasive but late to metastasize. The degree of local invasion can be quite severe. Tumors involving the nail beds of dogs are locally invasive, often invading the underlying bone. Lymph node metastasis and spread to other bones and lung is common. Tumors involving the skin of the flank and ventral abdomen are usually locally invasive with a low metastatic rate.[19]

The initial treatment of choice for periocular SCC in the cat is surgery or cryosurgery. For larger nonresectable or deeply invasive tumors, radiation therapy may be used. For tumors involving the ear, resection of the pinnae is indicated. Treatment of nasal planum tumors will be covered elsewhere (see Chapter 20). Subungual SCC is best treated by excision of

Figure 16-3. Typical appearance of a red, raised and ulcerated squamous cell carcinoma on the prepuce of a 5-year-old dalmation. Suture (arrow) denotes area of incisional biopsy. Surgical removal resulted in control for over two years, at which time a second lesion developed on the opposite flank.

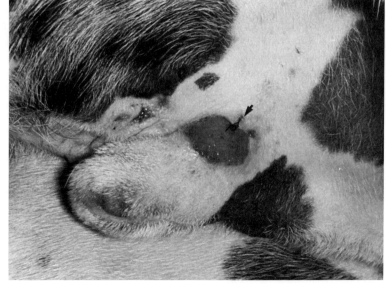

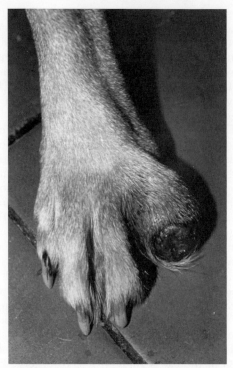

Figure 16-4. Squamous cell carcinoma of the digit. Extensive bone destruction was evident radiographically. The toe was amputated, and the dog died of metastatic disease to lung and lymph node 5 months later.

the affected digit. In some cases of extensive invasion and lymph node metastasis, amputation of the affected leg should be employed. Cisplatin has been used successfully to treat metastatic squamous cell carcinomas in a few cases.[21,21a] Squamous cell carcinomas involving the flank should be treated with wide surgical excision.

The prognosis of squamous cell carcinoma is dependent on location and the clinical stage at the time of diagnosis. The prognosis for SCC involving the ear, nose, and eyelid is good when the tumor is diagnosed early and complete surgical excision is possible. When lesions are more advanced and bone involvement is present the prognosis is guarded. Protecting susceptible cats from sunlight may aid in the prevention of initial or recurrent tumors. The prognosis for subungual tumors is guarded; local recurrence or metastasis is found in about one-third of the cases.[13]

BASAL CELL TUMORS

Basal cell tumors include basal cell epithelioma, basal cell carcinoma, and basiloid tumor. They are occasionally referred to inappropriately as basal cell carcinomas, probably in a carryover from human pathology. Since the tumor in domestic animals is almost always benign the preferred nomenclature is basal cell tumor. These tumors are common, representing 3% to 12% of all skin tumors in dogs and 15% to 18% of those in cats. They are generally found in middle-age dogs (6 to 9 years) and slightly older cats (9 to 10 years). There is no breed predilection in cats, whereas in dogs cocker spaniels and poodles have an increased incidence. Basal cell tumors are usually solitary, well-circumscribed, firm, hairless, dome-shaped, elevated masses from 0.5 to 10 cm in diameter (Fig. 16-5). Most basal cell tumors are freely movable masses firmly fixed to the overlying skin but rarely invading underlying fascia. They are most commonly located on the head, neck, and shoulders (Fig. 16-6). Feline basal cell tumors may be heavily pigmented or cystic and on occasion may ulcerate. There is no site predilection in the cat. Most basal cell tumors are benign, grow slowly, and may be present for months prior to diagnosis. The treatment of choice for basal cell tumors is surgical removal. In animals where anesthesia is a concern, cryosurgery is an alternative. The prognosis for basal cell tumors is good.

SEBACEOUS GLAND TUMORS

Sebaceous gland tumors represent a complex array of growths that can be divided into four groups based on histologic appearance. These are nodular hyperplasia, sebaceous adenoma, sebaceous epithelioma, and sebaceous adenocarcinoma. Sebaceous gland tumors are among the most common skin tumors in the dog, accounting for 6% to 35% of all skin tumors. Sebaceous gland tumors are rare in the cat. Modified sebaceous glands that may give rise to neoplastic growths are found in a variety of locations. Modified sebaceous glands of the eyelids form the meibomian glands. Perianal glands are also modified sebaceous glands and are a common location for tumor development in dogs. The ear contains modified sebaceous glands that give rise to ceruminous gland tumors.

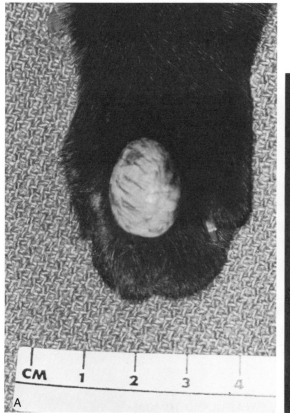
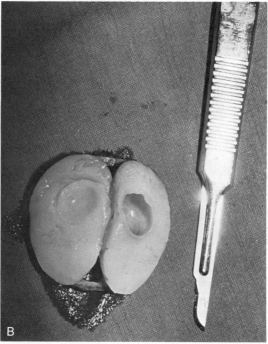

Figure 16-5. *(A)* Firm, circumscribed hairless basal cell tumor on the foot of a cat. *(B)* Cross-section of benign basal cell tumor seen in A. Note cystic center and well-defined margins.

Nodular sebaceous hyperplasia is a lesion arising from sebaceous glands that is characterized histologically by the accumulation of almost mature sebaceous glands. These tumorlike lesions, which often occur as multiple growths, are common in older dogs. Sebaceous gland adenomas are most common in older dogs and have been described most often in cocker spaniels, poodles, and breeds of dogs with kinky hair (Fig. 16-7).

Sebaceous gland tumors may involve the skin anywhere on the body; they are particularly frequent on the legs, neck, head, and anus.[21b] Sebaceous adenomas may be solitary or multiple and range in size from 0.5 to 3 cm in diameter. They are usually discrete, hairless, dome-shaped, or pedunculated, multilobulated masses. Ulceration due to trauma is common.

Sebaceous adenocarcinoma is an uncommon tumor in both the dog and the cat. Sebaceous gland adenocarcinomas are usually locally invasive and are characterized by ulceration and inflammation of the surrounding tissue.[21c] Although recurrence is common with sebaceous carcinomas, metastasis is rare (Fig. 16-8). Aggressive surgical resection is indicated for sebaceous adenocarcinomas. The treatment for benign sebaceous tumors is surgery or cryosurgery.

Ceruminous gland tumors are usually small, pedunculated, commonly melanotic single or multiple nodules in the external ear canal (Fig. 16-9). Cats with ceruminous gland tumors often present with a foul-smelling seropurulent discharge (otitits externa) that suggests an inflammatory lesion. Careful examination of the ear canal under anesthesia is often needed to reveal the tumor. The majority of ceruminous gland tumors are histologically malignant. Local lymph nodes should be carefully palpated and chest

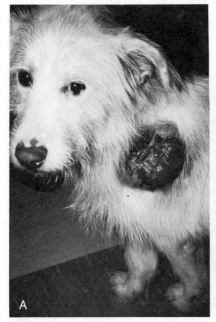
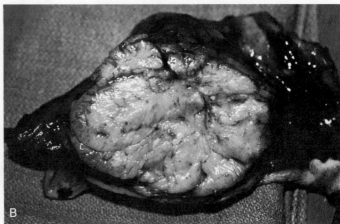

Figure 16-6. *(A)* Large basal cell tumor that had been slowly growing for two years. In spite of large size, fixation to underlying tissue and ulceration, surgery was curative. *(B)* Cross-section of basal cell tumor seen in A.

radiographs taken prior to surgery. The treatment of choice for ceruminous gland tumors is wide surgical excision. In some cases total ear canal resection is needed to remove the tumor. Because of the difficulty in completely removing ceruminous gland tumors (short of ear ablation), recurrences are common.

SWEAT GLAND TUMORS

Sweat gland tumors are the least common of the epithelial skin tumors in the dog and cat, accounting for less than 4% of all skin tumors in the dog. Most sweat gland tumors involve apocrine glands. Sweat gland tumors usually occur

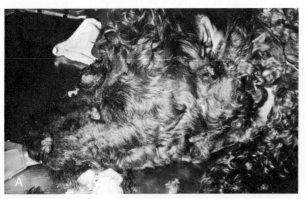
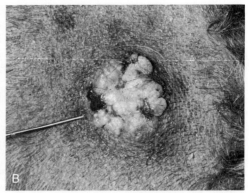

Figure 16-7. *(A)* Multiple sebaceous gland adenomas on the head of an aged poodle. *(B)* Close-up view of sebaceous adenoma prior to cryosurgery (thermocouple in place). Note roughened surface that is often greasy to the touch.

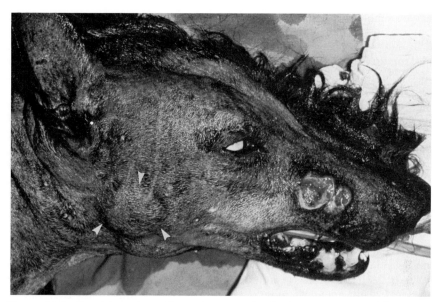

Figure 16-8. Scottish terrier with a sebaceous gland adenocarcinoma of the upper lip with metastasis to regional lymph nodes (arrows).

in dogs more than 8 years old; there is no sex or breed predilection. Sweat gland tumors may be either adenomas or adenocarcinomas and are most common to the head, neck, back, and flank. They are usually solitary, slow growing, and well-circumscribed tumors that are 1–4 cm in diameter. They are generally firm and on cut surface are fibrous and may be white and homogeneous or may contain small cysts containing clear yellow fluid. Sweat gland adenocarcinomas may be indistinguishable grossly from adenomas. Some may present as firm, poorly circumscribed masses infiltrating the skin; they are often ulcerated and moist and sometimes hem-

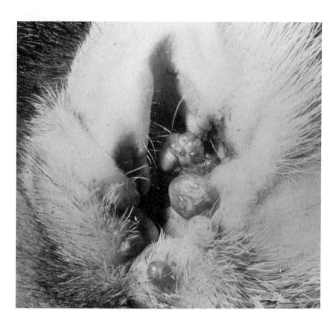

Figure 16-9. Multiple ceruminous gland tumors in ear canal of a cat. Complete ear canal ablation was necessary to attain local control. The cat was free of disease 18 months postoperatively.

orrhagic. Adenocarcinomas spread rapidly, are painful, and may give the impression of a cellulitis.

Sweat gland tumors in cats account for approximately 6% of feline skin tumors. They are most commonly located at the base of the ear, the dorsum of the head and neck, and the base of the tail. They are usually 1–2 cm in diameter and fixed to overlying skin; in some cases, they may be cystic. Roughly half the sweat gland tumors are histologically malignant. Malignant sweat gland tumors may metastasize rapidly to regional lymph nodes and the lungs.

Sweat gland tumors are treated with wide surgical excision. When surgical excision is not possible, or if surgery is incomplete, radiation therapy and combination chemotherapy using cyclophosphamide and doxorubicin may be used. Prognosis for sweat gland adenomas is good; the prognosis for sweat gland adenocarcinomas is guarded to poor.

INTRACUTANEOUS CORNIFYING EPITHELIOMAS (KERATOACANTHOMAS)

The canine intracutaneous cornifying epithelioma (ICE) is an epithelial proliferation arising from superficial epithelium between hair follicles, although it may appear to originate from adnexae.[21d] Canine intracutaneous cornifying epitheliomas present as two distinct clinical forms: (1) the solitary lesion, which may occur in any breed of dog, and (2) a multicentric form that usually occurs in arctic circle breeds (Norwegian elkhound and keeshond) (Fig. 16-10). Young male dogs seem to be at increased risk. The cause of ICE is unknown, but some evidence suggests genetic factors in the multicentric forms.

Most tumors are between 0.5 and 4.0 cm in diameter and have a pore opening to the surface. The pore usually contains a mass of keratin, which sometimes contains hair shafts. The tumors often contain a cheeselike material that can be manually expressed. Rupture of the tumor and extrusion of cystic contents to adjacent tissue may lead to a secondary inflammatory response. In some cases ICE may be located in the dermis and subcutaneous tissue without communication to the surface. Cytologically, these tumors are characterized by keratinous debris, clusters of squamous cells, and occasional cholesterol crystals. The treatment for solitary tumors is wide surgical removal. Multiple tumors may be treated with cryosurgery. Chemo-

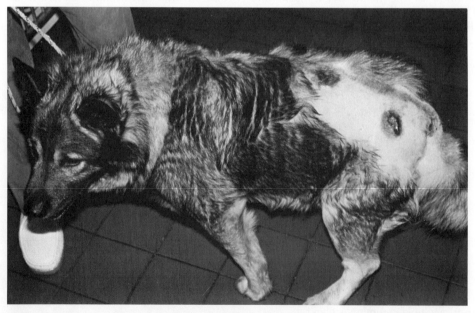

Figure 16-10. Intracutaneous cornifying epithelioma over the hip of a Norwegian elkhound. Surgical removal of this lesion was followed by development of two new lesions, in different sites, within 2 years.

therapy for multiple tumors has been suggested, but to date no clear efficacy has been demonstrated.[13]

TUMORS OF HAIR FOLLICLES
(HAIR MATRIX TUMORS)

Tumors of hair follicles in the dog account for about 5% of all skin tumors. Trichoepitheliomas and pilomatrixomas (necrotizing and calcifying epitheliomas) account for most of the hair follicle tumors. Hair follicle tumors are most common in dogs older than five years of age, and there is no sex predilection. Poodles and Kerry blue terriers are predisposed to develop pilomatrixomas.

Trichoepitheliomas are tumors derived from the follicular sheath. They account for 2% to 3% of canine skin tumors and 1.5% to 4% of feline skin tumors.[2] These tumors may show differentiation to either mature or incompletely developed hair follicles. Trichoepitheliomas may occur anywhere on the body but the most common location is on the back. Grossly, they are round to oval, well-circumscribed intradermal masses, 1–20 cm in diameter. The overlying skin may be atrophic, hairless, and often ulcerated from trauma. On cut section, small gray-white multiple foci are found separated by a thin connective tissue stroma. Trichoepitheliomas are rarely malignant and metastatic.

Pilomatrixomas are derived from hair matrix. They are firm, well-circumscribed, freely moveable masses. The skin overlying them is hairless and often ulcerated; on cut surface, it may be gritty due to mineral deposition. Tumors of hair follicles are generally benign, but malignant varieties have been reported. The treatment of choice is surgery, and the prognosis is excellent.

MESENCHYMAL TUMORS

Mesenchymal tumors are tumors derived from connective tissue. The most common mesenchymal tumors in the dog are fibrosarcomas, hemangiopericytomas, and lipomas. The most common mesenchymal tumors affecting the skin and subcutis of the cat include fibrosarcoma, malignant fibrous histiocytomas, and mast cell tumors (see Chapters 17, 18).

FIBROMAS AND FIBROSARCOMAS

Fibromas are benign tumors that arise from dermal or subcutaneous connective tissue. They are relatively infrequent in veterinary medicine. Fibromas do not show a breed or sex predilection. Grossly, they present as solitary, round to ovoid tumors that are firmly attached to the overlying epidermis. They are nonulcerated, sometimes hairless, and firm, and they range from 1 to 6 cm in diameter (Fig. 16-11). The treatment of choice is surgery, and the prognosis is excellent.

Fibrosarcomas are malignant tumors of fibroblasts. These tumors are common in cats and slightly less common in dogs. The clinical history and gross appearance of fibrosarcomas is quite variable, especially with respect to size. These tumors are poorly circumscribed and tend to infiltrate along tissue planes. Fibrosarcomas are locally very invasive and often recur after surgical removal. Metastasis occurs in about 10 percent of the cases and is usually hematogenous to the lungs.

The treatment of choice for fibrosarcomas is wide surgical excision. When an extremity is involved, amputation should be considered. Fibrosarcomas are relatively radioresistant and poorly responsive to chemotherapy. The prognosis is guarded to poor, and local recurrence is very common.

A syndrome of multicentric subcutaneous fibrosarcomas has been reported in young cats. These tumors are characterized by local invasiveness and rapid growth. They have been associated with the feline leukemia and sarcoma viruses.[22] No therapy is recommended for these cats (see Chapter 29).

HEMANGIOPERICYTOMAS

Hemangiopericytomas are thought to arise from pericytes, which are cells surrounding blood vessels that resemble smooth muscle cells. Hemangiopericytomas often resemble fibrosarcomas grossly and histologically. They occur most often in older dogs and are most common on the extremities (Fig. 16-12). On palpation these tumors may be firm and nodular with a rubbery consistency, or they may feel gelatinous and may mimic lipomas. They are slow growing but may ulcerate and become secondarily infected.

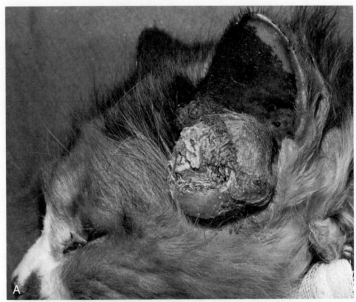

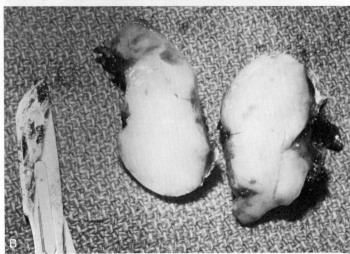

Figure 16-11. *(A)* Large peduncu-lated fibroma near ear canal of a 14-year-old cat. *(B)* Cross-section of fibroma seen in A. Note firm, tan to white homogeneous appearance on cross-section. Conservative removal of the mass resulted in local control 2 years postoperatively.

Although hemangiopericytomas may appear to be encapsulated, they are quite invasive locally.

Recurrence is common following conservative surgery. Metastasis occurs in about 5 percent of cases.[23] The treatment of choice is wide surgical excision. However, surgery combined with radiation therapy may reduce recurrence rates.[23a] In appendicular areas, where complete surgical excision is not possible, amputation should be considered.

HEMANGIOMAS AND HEMANGIOSARCOMAS

These tumors arise from the endothelium of capillaries. Hemangiomas and hemangiosarcomas can occur in the dermis or subcutis anywhere in the body. Both tumors are most common in older dogs and cats, although hemangiomas have been reported in younger dogs. A congenital hemangioma (hemartoma) has also been reported involving the skin. These tumors are more common in the dog than in the cat.

sions exist. When multiple organs are involved, chemotherapy should be considered. Combination chemotherapy using vincristine, doxorubicin, and cyclophosphamide has been suggested to be effective in treating hemangiosarcomas, but definitive proof of an increase in survival is still pending.[23b] The prognosis for hemangiomas is good while the prognosis for hemangiosarcomas is poor.

LIPOMAS AND LIPOSARCOMAS

Lipomas and liposarcomas[24-27] are benign and malignant tumors of fatty tissue. Lipomas are very common tumors of the subcutis in the dog but are rare in the cat. Lipomas are most common in older dogs, and females are affected three times more often than males.[28,29]

Lipomas may occur as individual tumors or may be multiple. They may occur anywhere on the body but are most common in the ventral regions of the abdomen and thorax. On rare occasions lipomas are reported within body cavities. Lipomas are very easily diagnosed by cytology. They are not premalignant and do not regress with weight loss. The treatment will vary with location and rate of growth. Slow growing or stable lipomas may not require any therapy. Most lipomas can be adequately treated by surgical excision (Fig. 16-13). The relative indications for removal include rapid growth (doubling in size in less than 1–2 months), cosmetic objectives of the owner, secondary infection, or interference with function of the animal. Intralesional injection of 10% calcium chloride has been used in the treatment of small solitary and multiple lipomas. Ten dogs with 18 lipomas were treated. At 6-month follow-up, four tumors had regressed completely and 14 were less than 50% of their original size.[30]

A variant of lipoma, termed infiltrating lipoma, has been described in the dog and cat.[31,32] This tumor, although histologically benign, is unencapsulated and infiltrates muscles, fasciae, joint capsules, and nerves. The invasive nature of this tumor makes surgical excision difficult short of amputation for appendicular locations.

MALIGNANT FIBROUS HISTIOCYTOMAS (EXTRASKELETAL GIANT CELL TUMORS)

These tumors have been reported most commonly in the cat. They are characterized by

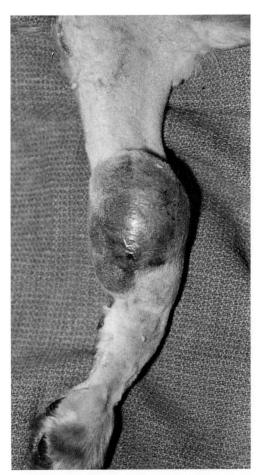

Figure 16-12. Large hemangiopericytoma on the foreleg of a dog. Complete surgical removal, short of amputation, is unlikely.

Hemangiomas are benign and well circumscribed, spherical to ovoid and generally small in size. Hemangiomas affect the dermis more frequently than the subcutis. Some tumors may resemble hematomas, and aspiration cytology may yield blood; however, hemangiosarcomas more commonly affect the subcutis and muscles. They are often poorly circumscribed, and invasion into adjacent tissue is usually present. Since cutaneous hemangiosarcomas may represent either primary or metastatic lesions, a thorough work-up is indicated when a hemangiosarcoma is suspected.

The treatment for solitary hemangiomas is surgical or cryosurgical removal. Treatment for hemangiosarcomas is surgery when isolated le-

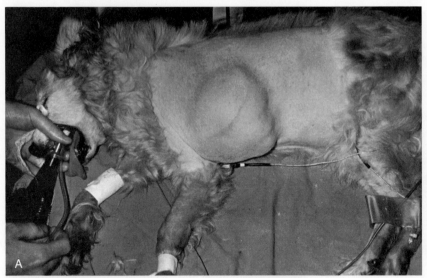

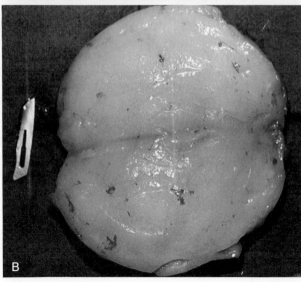

Figure 16-13. *(A)* Large lipoma on the chest and axilla of an older female dog. This mass took 3 years to reach this size. *(B)* Cross-section of a lipoma after surgical removal. Note soft and greasy appearance.

fibroblastlike cells, a degree of fibrogenesis, histiocytelike cells, and tumor giant cells. There is controversy as to the true nature of these tumors. In general they appear to be subcutaneous masses that are locally invasive and have a high rate of recurrence and a low metastatic rate. The treatment is wide surgical excision or amputation in the case of appendicular masses (see Chapter 18).

ROUND CELL TUMORS

All round cell tumors can involve the skin and subcutis. Cytologically these tumors are char-

acterized by discrete round cells. There are five different round cell tumors: histiocytoma, mast cell tumor, lymphosarcoma, transmissible venereal tumor (TVT), and plasmacytoma. Only the histiocytoma and plasmacytoma will be covered in this chapter.

HISTIOCYTOMAS

Canine cutaneous histiocytomas are common neoplasms that are unique in the dog. These tumors arise from the monocyte-macrophage cells in the skin. Histiocytomas account for between 10% and 20% of all skin tumors. They have a predilection for young dogs but may be seen in dogs of any age. Boxers and dachshunds are reported to be predisposed to histiocytomas, and there is no reported sex predisposition. Histiocytomas are very rare in species other than the dog. Only a few cases have been reported in the cat.[33]

Histiocytomas usually occur as a solitary, fast growing, nonpainful, dome-shaped, hairless intradermal lesion with a shiny and alopecic or ulcerated surface (Fig. 16-14). Tumors range from 0.5 to 4.0 cm in diameter, with the majority being 1 to 2 cm. Although most tumors are solitary, multiple histiocytomas have been reported.

Histiocytoma can usually be easily diagnosed by fine-needle aspiration cytology. These tumors consist of pleomorphic cells resembling monocytes. Nuclei of histiocytoma cells are variable in size and shape. The mitotic index may be quite high, and the cytoplasm is variable in

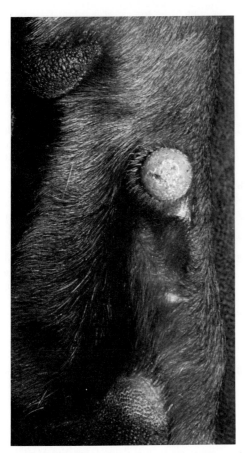

Figure 16-14. Typical appearance of a solitary histiocytoma on the foreleg of a young dog. Note hairless, circular, "button-like" appearance.

amount and stains pale blue. Histiocytomas may have a large lymphocytic, plasmacytic, or neutrophilic infiltrate. The differential diagnosis should include TVT, mast cell tumor, and cutaneous lymphosarcoma. Although rapid growth and high mitotic index are suggestive of a malignant tumor, these are benign tumors that may regress spontaneously. The treatment of choice for histiocytomas is surgery or cryosurgery, and the prognosis is excellent.

PLASMACYTOMA

Solitary cutaneous plasmacytomas have been reported independent of generalized myeloma.[34,34a] Plasmacytomas are usually solitary and have a predilection for the feet, lips, and ear canal. Most affected dogs are middle to old age dogs, and there is no sex predilection. In spite of a rapid rate of growth plasmacytomas can generally be controlled with conservative surgery. Local recurrence is rare and metastasis has not been reported.

LYMPHANGIOMA

Lymphangioma is a rare benign, usually cutaneous, tumor characterized by proliferating lymph vessels. Clinical signs are usually associated with drainage of lymph through the skin or an associated cystic mass.[35] Treatment involves surgical excision; however, recurrences can be seen. For recurrent tumors, radiation can be considered.[36]

MELANOCYTIC TUMORS

Tumors of melanocytes and melanoblasts are relatively common skin tumors in the dog, accounting for about 6% of all canine skin tumors. Melanocytic tumors are most common in older dogs (average age 9 years) with darkly pigmented skin. Males seem to be at greater risk than females. Melanomas are usually solitary and may occur anywhere on the body. The biological behavior of melanomas is influenced by the histologic appearance and the location of the tumor. Benign melanomas are well-circumscribed, dome-shaped, heavily pigmented nodules 0.5–2.0 cm in diameter (Fig. 16-15). Malignant melanomas are usually larger than benign tumors and are frequently ulcerated. The degree of melanin pigmentation may vary from amelanotic to highly pigmented. Melanomas arising

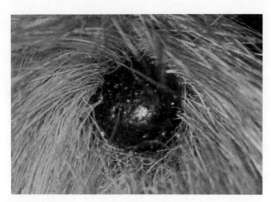

Figure 16-15. Typical picture of a raised cutaneous melanoma. The vast majority of melanomas occurring on haired skin are benign. This mass was biopsied and treated with cryosurgery.

from the digits and mucocutaneous junctions (except eyelids) have a higher rate of malignancy than those arising from skin elsewhere. Metastasis of malignant melanomas from the digits and mucocutaneous junctions is common; it usually occurs in the lymph node first and then the lungs. The treatment of choice is wide surgical excision. Chemotherapy and radiation have yielded poor results.

REFERENCES

1. Carpenter JL, Andrews LK, Holzworth J. Tumors and tumor like lesions. In Hosworth J (ed): Diseases of the Cat. Medicine and Surgery, pp. 406–596. Philadelphia, W.B. Saunders, 1987

2. Priester WA: Skin tumors in domestic animals. Data from 12 United States and Canadian colleges for veterinary medicine. J Natl Cancer Inst 50:457–466, 1973

3. Priester WA, Mantel N: Occurrence of tumors in domestic animals. Data from 12 United States and Canadian colleges of veterinary medicine. J Natl Cancer Inst 47:1333–1344, 1971

4. Dorn CR, Taylor DD, Frey EL, et al: Survey of animal neoplasms in Alameda and Costa counties in Calif. II. Cancer morbidity in dogs and cats from Alamedia county. J Natl Cancer Inst 40:307–318, 1968

5. Conroy JD: Canine skin tumors. J Am Anim Hosp Assoc 19:91–114, 1983

6. Howard EB, Nielson SW: Neoplasia of the boxer dog. Am J Vet Res 26:1121–1131, 1965

7. Cotchin E: Skin tumors of cats. Res Vet Sci 2:353–361, 1961

8. Engle GG, Brodey RS: A retrospective study of 395 feline neoplasms. J Am Anim Hosp Assoc 5:21–31, 1968

9. Dorn CR: Epidemiology of canine and feline tumors. J Am Anim Hosp Assoc 12:307–312, 1976

10. Allison AC: Viruses inducing skin tumors in animals. In Rook AJ, Walton CS (eds): Comparative Physiology and Pathology of the Skin, pp. 665–684. Oxford, Blackwell Scientific Publications, 1965

11. Dorn CR, Taylor D, Schneider R: Sunlight exposure and the risk of developing cutaneous and oral squamous cell carcinoma in white cats. J Natl Cancer Inst 46:1073–1078, 1971

12. Madewell BR, Conroy JD, Hodgkins EM: Sunlight skin cancer association in the dog. A report of 3 cases. J Cutan Pathol 8:434–443, 1981

13. Madewell BR, Theilen GH: Tumors and tumor-like conditions of epithelial origin. In Thielen GH, Madewell BR (eds): Veterinary Cancer Medicine, pp. 240–325. Philadelphia, Lea & Febiger, 1987

14. Watach AM, Hanson LE, Meyer RC: Canine papilloma. The structural characterization of oral papilloma virus. J Natl Cancer Inst 43:453–458, 1969

15. Dallman MJ, Noxon JO, Stogsdell P: Feline lymphosarcoma with cutaneous and muscle lesions. J Am Vet Med Assoc 181:161–168, 1982

16. Hofmeyer CFB: Dermoid sinus and the Ridgeback dog. J Small Anim Pract 4:5–8, 1963

17. Kral F, Schwartzman RM: Veterinary and comparative dermatology. Philadelphia, J.B. Lippincott, 1964

18. Watrach AM, Small E, Case MT: Canine papillomas: Progression of an oral papilloma to a carcinoma. J Natl Cancer Inst 45:915–920, 1970

19. Hargis AM, Thomassen RW, Phemister RD: Chronic dermatosis and cutaneous squamous cell carcinoma in the beagle dog. Vet Pathol 14:218–228, 1977

20. Madewell BR, Pool RR, Theilen GH, Brewer WG: Multiple subungual squamous cell carcinoma in five dogs. J Am Vet Med Assoc 180:732–734, 1982

21. Himsel CA, Richardson RC, Craig JA: Cisplatin chemotherapy for metastatic squamous cell carcinoma in two dogs. J Am Vet Med Assoc 189:1575–1578, 1986

21a. Knapp DW, Richardson RC, Bonney PL et al: Cisplatin therapy in 41 dogs with malignant tumors. J Vet Int Med 2:41–46, 1988

21b. Strafuss AC: Sebaceous gland adenomas in dogs. J Am Vet Med Assoc 169:640–642, 1976

21c. Strafuss AC: Sebaceous gland carcinoma in dogs. J Am Vet Med Assoc 169:325–326, 1976

21d. Stannard AA, Pulley LT: Intracutaneous cornifying epithelioma (keratoacanthoma) in the dog: A retrospective study of 25 cases. J Am Vet Med Assoc 167:385–388, 1975

22. Theilen GH, Madewell BR, Gardner MB: Hemopoietic neoplasms, sarcomas and related conditions. In Theilen GH, Madewell BR (eds): Veterinary Cancer Medicine, pp. 345–470. Philadelphia, Lea & Febiger, 1987

23. Postorino NC, Berg RJ, Powers BE, McChesney AE, Taylor RA, Withrow SJ: Prognostic variables for canine hemangiopericytoma: 50 cases (1979–1984). J Am Anim Hosp Assoc 24:501–509, 1988

23a. Evans SM: Canine hemangiopericytoma. Vet Rad 28:13–16, 1987

23b. Helfand SC: Chemotherapy for nonresectable and metastatic soft tissue tumors. Proceedings of the 10th Annual Kalkan Symposium, pp. 133–142, 1986

24. Garvin CH, Frey DC: Liposarcoma in a dog. J Am Vet Med Assoc 140:1073–1075, 1962

25. Jabara AG: Three cases of liposarcomas in dogs. J Comp Pathol 74:188–191 1964

26. Strafuss AC, Bozarth AJ: Liposarcoma in dogs. J Am Anim Hosp Assoc 9:183–187, 1973

27. Stephens LC, et al: Virus associated liposarcoma in malignant lymphoma in a kitten. J Am Vet Med Assoc 183:123–125, 1983

28. Strafuss AC, et al: Lipomas in dogs. J Am Anim Hosp Assoc 9:555–561, 1973

29. Theilen GH, Madewell BR: Veterinary Cancer Medicine, pp. 160–161. Philadelphia, Lea & Febiger, 1979

30. Albers GW, Theilen GH: Calcium chloride for the treatment of subcutaneous lipomas in dogs. J Am Vet Med Assoc 186:492–494 1985

31. Kramek BA, Spackman CJA, Hayden DW: Infiltrative lipoma in three dogs. J Am Vet Med Assoc 186:81–82, 1985

32. Esplin DG: Infiltrating lipoma in a cat. Feline Pract 14:24–25, 1984

33. Macy DW, Reynolds HA: The incidence, characteristics and clinical management of skin tumors in cats. J Am Anim Hosp Assoc 17:1026–1034, 1981

34. Lucke VM: Primary cutaneous plasmacytomas in the dog and cat. J Sm Anim Pract 28:49–55, 1987

34a. Rakich PM, Lattimer KS, Weiss R, et al: Mucocutaneous plasmacytomas in dogs: 75 cases (1980–1987). J Am Vet Med Assoc 194:803–810, 1989

35. Stambaugh JE, Harvey CE, Goldschmidt MH: Lymphangioma in four dogs. J Am Vet Med Assoc 173:759–761, 1978

36. Turrel JM, Lowenstine LJ, Cowgill CD: Response to radiation therapy of recurrent lymphangioma in a dog. J Am Vet Med Assoc 193:1432–1434, 1988

17

MAST CELL TUMORS

Dennis W. Macy
E. Gregory MacEwen

INCIDENCE AND RISK FACTORS

The neoplastic proliferation of mast cells is often referred to as mast cell tumor, histiocytic mastocytoma, or mast cell sarcoma, and systemic involvement as mastocytosis.[1-3] These are common tumors in the dog and represent 7% to 21% of all canine skin tumors and 11% to 27% of all malignant canine skin tumors.[4-6] In the cat, mast cell tumors represent 15% of all tumors.[7-8] No sex predilection has been found in the dog, but in the cat the ratio of male to female is 2:1.[9] Mast cell tumors have been reported in animals under a year of age but are most commonly encountered in middle-aged dogs and cats with mean ages of 8.5 years and 8.2 years respectively.[9-11] Risk factors for development of mast cell tumors include heredity, previous inflammation, and possibly viral infections. In dogs, mast cell tumors have been reported in essentially all breeds; however boxers, Boston terriers and other breeds of bulldog descendents are at higher risk for the development of this neoplasm.[12] The higher prevalence of this tumor in boxers, however, does not necessarily equate with higher mortality. Boxers accounted for 46% of the dogs in one mast cell tumor series; however, 45% of the tumors were of the well-differentiated type, while only 25% of the mast cell tumors in other breeds were of this favorable histology.[13] A similar relationship exists in the cat. Although 21% of the reported cutaneous mast cell tumors in one large series occurred in the Siamese breed, the tumor's histology and behavior differed significantly from mast cell tumors in other breeds of cats.[14] Siamese in the study developed mast cell tumors with morphologic features more characteristic of histiocytic mast cells. The tumors were seen in cats under 4 years of age and, although they were often multiple, usually underwent spontaneous regression in this breed. These observations in variation in biologic behavior based on breed suggests that a hereditary risk component exists within a species and may represent a modification in species susceptibility to this tumor.

Mast cell tumors have been reported to arise from sites of chronic inflammation in the dog and may be produced in mice by topical application of irritants.[11,15] However, a history of local inflammation is usually lacking in most feline and canine cases. In the dog, several studies have suggested the possibility of viral etiology in the development of mast cell tumors.[16,17] Mast cell tumors have been transmitted to susceptible laboratory dogs using tumor cell tissues or cell-free extracts.[16,17] Despite these findings, there is no epidemiologic evidence to suggest horizontal transmission if a virus is involved in the production of this tumor. Mast cell tumors in cats have not been associated with the feline leukemia virus.[18]

PATHOLOGY AND NATURAL BEHAVIOR

Mast cell tumors most frequently arise from the dermis and subcutaneous tissues in the dog and from the dermis, spleen, liver, and visceral lymphatics in the cat.[5,8] The incidence of mast cell tumors in specific tissue does not correlate with the normal concentration of mast cells in these tissues. For example, large numbers of mast cells are normally found in the lung and gastrointestinal tract but these sites exhibit low prevalence rates for the development of this tumor in dogs, cats, and human beings.[5,8,19]

Well-differentiated mast cells contain cytoplasmic granules. These granules become larger as the cell matures and contain a number of bioactive constituents, including histamine and heparin, which stain metachromatically with toluidine blue. Histiocytelike mast cells in cats have equivocal cytoplasmic granularity after staining with toluidine blue but are easily demonstrated an electron microscopy.[14] There is an inverse relationship between histamine and heparin content and mast cell differentiation. Differentiated mast cells contain 25 times more heparin than undifferentiated mast cells, and anaplastic or immature mast cells contain more histamine and less heparin.[16,20]

There is a wide variation in the histologic pattern seen in mast cell tumors. Several investigators applied a histologic grading system to canine mast cell tumors based on the degree of differentiation (Table 17-1). In all these studies, the tumors have been separated into anaplastic, intermediate and well differentiated groups.[11,13,21] In two studies, Grade I was assigned to the undifferentiated group, Grade II to the intermediate or differentiated group, and Grade III to the mature or well-differentiated group. The most recent study used a more universal system with a higher grade (Grade III) representing the most undifferentiated or anaplastic group of tumors (Table 17-2).[21] For the sake of clarity, groups should be simply referred to as undifferentiated, differentiated, and well-differen-

Table 17-1. Histologic Classification of Mast Cell Tumors

GRADE	BOSTOCK[13] GRADING	PATNAIK[21] GRADING	MICROSCOPIC DESCRIPTION
Anaplastic, immature, undifferentiated	1	3	Highly cellular, undifferentiated plasmic boundaries, irregular size and shape of nuclei; frequent mitotic figures; low number cytoplasmic granules.
Intermediate, differentiated	2	2	Cells closely packed with indistinct cytoplasmic boundaries; nucleus-to-cytoplasm ratio lower than that of anaplastic; mitotic figures infrequent; more granules than anaplastic.
Well-differentiated, mature	3	1	Clearly defined cytoplasmic boundaries with regular, spherical, or ovoid nuclei, mitotic figures rare; cytoplasmic granules large, deep staining, and plentiful.

Table 17-2.   Distribution of Mast Cell Tumors by Histologic Grade

INVESTIGATOR	NO. OF DOGS	UNDIFFER-ENTIATED (%)	INTER-MEDIATELY DIFFEREN-TIATED (%)	WELL-DIFFEREN-TIATED (%)
Hottendorf[11]	300	19	27	54
Bostock[13]	108	36	28	36
Patnaik[21]	83	36	43	20

tiated. The results of these studies indicate that histologic grading is helpful in predicting biologic behavior.

A pathologic grading system for feline mast cell tumors has also been reported.[22] Two histologic categories of mast cell tumors were described—the diffuse form (invasive) and the compact form. In the 65 cases studied, 29 of 65 (45%) were determined to be of the compact type and 55% to be of the diffuse (invasive) type. A follow-up study of 32 of these cases indicated the following findings: 12 of the 17 (70%) diffuse forms recurred or metastasized, while only 5 of the 15 (33%) compact forms demonstrated malignant behavior. Thus, the compact type was considered the more benign of the two forms.

Another system has been described for the cat[14] in which two distinct subclassifications of mast cell tumors appear to exist and to correlate with biologic behavior. The first is the mast cell type of mastocytoma. This type is present in the dermis and has a limited number of eosinophils

and plasma cells infiltrating the tumor. These mast cell tumors have strong metachromatic staining characteristics when stained with toluidine blue and usually occur in cats over 4 years of age. If solitary, they rarely recur following surgery; however anaplastic variants of this form are likely to recur or metastasize, as has been observed in the dog. A second more benign form of the disease occurs exclusively in young Siamese cats under 4 years of age. Lesions are multiple and have a subcutaneous location. They contain numerous eosinophils and plasma cells and have a weak orthochromatic staining characteristic. These tumors have been considered benign and will frequently regress within a 2-year period without therapy.

Mast cell tumors have been associated with gastrointestinal ulceration. In one study, 83% of necropsy dogs with mast cell tumors had gastrointestinal ulceration in the gastric fundus, pylorus or anterior segment of the duodenum (Fig. 17-1). In 15% of the cases, the ulcers had perforated the intestinal tract.[23] The mechanism of the gastrointestinal ulceration is thought to be related to the increased blood concentration of histamine released from the neoplastic mast cells.[23a] Elevated blood concentrations of histamine stimulates H_2 receptors, causing parietal cells to increase acid production, and increased gastric motility. Heparin tends to block the effects of histamine, but this is present in much lower concentrations in undifferentiated malig-

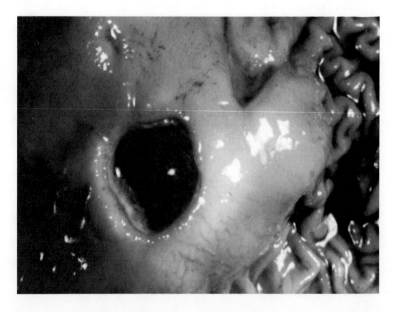

Figure 17-1. Perforated ulcer in the pylorus of a dog with an extensive mast cell tumor.

nant mast cells than in well differentiated mast cells. In addition to the increase in gastric acid production and gastric motility, histamine damages the vascular endothelium of arterioles and venules, causing the release of fibrolysin. It has been hypothesized that histamine may damage the gastric submucosal vasculature by causing small venule and capillary dilation, increasing endothelial permeability, and leading to intravascular thrombosis and ischemic necrosis of the mucosa. The pathogenesis of gastrointestinal ulceration associated with mast cell tumors appears to be related to the combination of vascular damage, increased gastric acid secretion, and hypermotility.

Delayed wound healing at the site of removal of mast cell tumors has been attributed to local effects of proteolytic enzymes and vasoactive amines released by the tumor. Recent studies in mice suggest that histamine released from mast cell tumors binds to H_1 and H_2 receptors of macrophages, resulting in the release of a fibroblastic suppressor factor that decreases normal fibroplasia and delays wound healing.[24] Both H_1 and H_2 blockers theoretically might be helpful in preventing wound dehiscence at sites of removal of mast cell tumors.

HISTORY AND CLINICAL SIGNS

Mast cell tumors may exist in cutaneous or extracutaneous locations. The most common sites in the dog for mast cell tumors are the skin of the trunk and perineal region (50%) and the skin of the extremities (40%). The remaining 10% arise from cutaneous sites of the head and neck. Mast cell tumors are reported to arise in multiple cutaneous locations in 11% of cases.[5,25] Although mast cell tumors can have marked extremes in physical characteristics, the cutaneous form generally has one of two separate appearances. The most common cutaneous form is a mass 1 to 10 cm in diameter. Most frequently the lesions are less than 3 cm in diameter, well circumscribed, raised, and firm to the touch. The surface may be erythematous or ulcerated and occasionally has a history of pruritus. The second cutaneous form of the disease is less common and is characteristically observed as a soft, poorly circumscribed raised lesion that is usually haired and lacks ulceration and erythe-

matous changes. This form may be mistaken as a lipoma on clinical examination. Some mast cell tumors have characteristics of both presentations.

Occasionally mechanical manipulation during examination of this tumor results in degranulation of mast cells, which results in erythema and wheal formation. This phenomenon has been observed in both dogs and cats and is referred to as "Darier's sign."[26] Regardless of the presentation, the largest dimension of the tumor is usually parallel to the skin surface. Although mast cell tumors may feel like discrete masses, microscopically most extend well beyond the palpable borders. Studies have determined that the size itself is not an indicator of malignancy.[13] Mast cell tumors vary in their growth rate and time from the first appearance to presentation to the veterinarian. Those mast cell tumors with the longest clinical history prior to presentation carry a better prognosis, presumably reflecting a slower growth rate.[13] Extracutaneous mast cell tumors without skin involvement are considered uncommon. The most common noncutaneous sites of involvement are the liver, spleen, or kidney. Other locations reported for extracutaneous involvement of mast cell tumors include the larynx, bone, gastrointestinal tract (including oral cavity), and trachebronchial lymph nodes.[27-29] Mast cell leukemia (mastocytosis) occurs rarely in the dog; when it is seen, malignant mast cells may be found in most tissues of the body as well as the peripheral blood.[30]

In the cat, there is less consensus on the tumor distribution. The older literature tends to suggest that 50% of the tumors arise from the viscera and 50% from the skin.[31] More recent studies suggest a higher percentage of cases are associated with primary cutaneous lesions. In the cat with primary cutaneous lesions, 40–60% are reported to be located on the head and neck.[31a] Seventy-five percent are considered to be solitary, and the remaining 25% have a multiple distribution.[14,18,22]

In cats, mast cell tumors can also arise in the intestines. The small intestine is most commonly involved and metastasis to regional lymph nodes is common. These cats present with vomiting, diarrhea, weight loss and anorexia. Cats with splenic involvement present with massive splenomegaly, vomiting, anorexia and an abdominal effusion may be present.

DIAGNOSTIC TECHNIQUES
AND WORK-UP

Diagnosis of mast cell tumors often can be made by examination of a fine-needle aspiration (Fig. 17-2), but excisional biopsy has been used traditionally for histologic grading. Cytologic grading may be as accurate as histologic grading because grading is dependent on cellular morphology and not architecture.[11,13,21] However, the value of histologic evaluation of the cut borders of the excised specimen (margins) makes excisional biopsies desirable.

The diagnostic work-up of mast cell tumors usually includes a number of procedures. In order for the clinician to be provided with the optimum treatment plan, several tests should be performed in addition to excisional biopsy or aspiration cytology of the primary lesion. These include a complete blood cell count (CBC), serum chemistry profile, and urinalysis. A CBC is valuable in assessing animals with mast cell tumors because those animal patients with systemic mastocytosis occasionally have peripheral eosinophilia and basophilia in addition to circulating mast cells.[30] Mastocytemia is a more common clinical phenomenon in the cat than in the dog.[31] The CBC may also give evidence of gastrointestinal bleeding or gastrointestinal perforation. Anemia has been reported in association with hypersplenism in visceral mast cell tumors in the cat.[32]

Buffy coat smears of blood samples may be examined microscopically for the presence of mast cells, but bone marrow smears appear to be more sensitive and are not associated with as many false positives. Recent studies have demonstrated that normal dogs have less than 1 mast cell per 1000 cells in the bone marrow. Investigators in human and veterinary oncology suggest mast cells in greater concentrations than 10/1000 cells are abnormal.[33] One series of cases found that 3 of 30 dogs with cutaneous mast cells had bone marrow involvement.[34] As a general rule, large tumors or visceral involvement are more commonly associated with mastocytemia. A clinical staging system has been proposed (Table 17-3) to help to further define the extent of tumor.

Any animal with mast cell tumor(s) should be carefully examined for lymphadenopathy in areas draining the primary tumor. Enlarged lymph nodes should be examined for the presence of mast cells as evidence of tumor spread. The presence of numerous mast cells and eosinophils in the regional lymph nodes indicates that the mast cell tumor is no longer localized and that therapy should be more aggressive than surgical excision alone.

Radiographic examinations are seldom useful in evaluation of dogs with mast cell tumors. However, abdominal radiographs may be useful in evaluating feline patients because of the high incidence of splenic involvement in cats with mast cell tumors. Primary mast cell tumors have been reported to arise from the bronchial tree, usually the peribronchial lymph nodes, but this location is extremely rare. Metastasis of mast cell tumors from cutaneous locations to pulmonary parenchyma does not usually occur except in animals with mastocytosis where the radiographic pattern is considered diffuse.[30] In cases of mast cell tumors that involve the hind limbs or the perineal or preputial area, abdominal

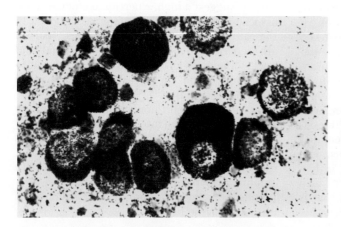

Figure 17-2. Fine-needle aspirate of an ulcerated skin lesion in a dog. A mast cell tumor can be recognized by the presence of individual round cells with round to oval nuclei that are obscured by an abundance of fine basophilic cytoplasmic granules. Numerous mast cell granules are present in the background. (Wright stain, 1000×); see Chapter 6 for further description.

**Table 17-3.   Clinical Staging System
for Mast Cell Tumors**

Stage I: One tumor confined to the dermis without
            regional lymph node involvement
                a. Without systemic signs
                b. With systemic signs
Stage II: One tumor confined to the dermis, with
            regional lymph node involvement
                a. Without systemic signs
                b. With systemic signs
Stage III: Multiple dermal tumors; large infiltrating
            tumors with or without regional lymph node
            involvement
                a. Without systemic signs
                b. With systemic signs
Stage IV: Any tumor with distant metastasis or
            recurrence with metastasis

radiographs may be helpful in detecting metastatic lymphadenopathy in the iliac and sublumbar lymph nodes.

Occult blood tests for gastrointestinal bleeding may be useful in evaluating patients with mast cell disease. In some cases, feces may contain small amounts of blood that are insufficient to produce melena. A positive occult blood test indicates GI hemorrhage, and if blood loss due to gastrointestinal parasites can be ruled out, bleeding due to intestinal neoplasia or gastric or duodenal ulceration must be considered. Most patients with positive occult blood in the feces will have large tumor volumes or CBC changes compatable with gastrointestinal blood loss.[26]

TREATMENT

Treatment of canine mast cell tumors consists of wide surgical excision, cryosurgery, chemotherapy, or radiation therapy, either individually or in various combinations. The therapeutic approach for mast cell tumors is based on the clinical stage and histologic grade of the tumor. Summary of the recommended treatments in the dog as they relate to clinical stage or histologic grade is given in Fig. 17-3.

Aggressive or high-grade mast cell tumor is treated by wide surgical excision, at least 3 cm of normal looking skin and subcutaneous tissue around the tumor should be removed when possible. The 3-cm recommendation is a guideline and might not be feasible when the tumor is located on the head or lower limbs or in the inguinal region. All excised tumor should be examined histologically for the completeness of excision. Histologic evidence of extension of the tumor beyond the surgical borders should prompt either a second, wider excision or radiation therapy of the tumor bed. If margins are not free of tumor and additional surgery or radiation is not possible, corticosteroids should be administered. With conservative surgery, more than 50% of mast cell tumors recur at the surgical site. In cats with localized cutaneous mast cell tumors, aggressive surgical excision may yield very good results. In one report of 14 cats with mast cell tumors, none of the tumors recurred or metastasized after excision.[31a]

Cats with splenic mast cell tumors benefit from splenectomy. Survival times of 2 months to 30 months have been reported following splenectomy, even in patients with evidence of systemic mastocytosis (Table 17-4).[35-37] Cryosurgery and hyperthermia have been useful in the treatment of mast cell tumors, especially in cases of multiple skin tumors.[38] In cases of mast cell tumors treated with cryosurgery and hyperthermia, hypotensive shock can result from large amounts of histamine being released from the treated tumors.[39] It is recommended that animal patients treated with either cryosurgery or hyperthermia be pretreated with H_1 and H_2 receptor antagonists such as Benadryl* and Tagamet† to protect against this complication. The tendency for local hemorrhage is frequently encountered during surgical excision or biopsy. Coagulation defects are thought to be associated with the heparin released from mast cell tumors.[40] Although abnormal coagulograms are found in a minority of canine patients, prolonged coagulation times are most consistently observed when they are measured on blood samples taken in or around the mast cell tumor. Protamine sulfate‡ has recently been recommended for use in dogs when prolonged local hemorrhage has been observed during surgery or postoperatively.§

Chemotherapy has been advocated for disseminated mastocytosis, and glucocorticoids are recommended most frequently. Oral prednisone and intralesional triamcinolone are widely used as palliative treatments for mast cell tumors in

* Parke Davis, Morris Plains, NJ.
† Smith, Kline & French Laboratories, Carolina, PR.
‡ Upjohn, Kalamazoo, MI.
§ Robinson G: Personal communication. Henry Bergh Hospital, New York City, 1986.

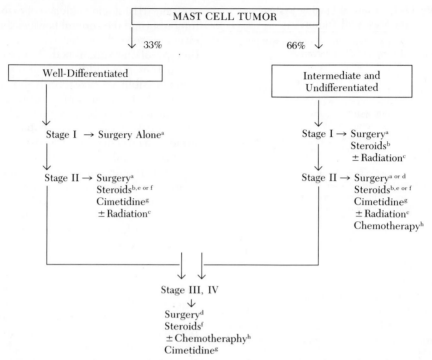

Figure 17-3. Suggested treatment of canine mast cell tumors based on clinical stage and histopathologic grade.

a. Surgery—excision of the tumor with a minimum of 2–3 cm between palpable tumor and incision line; such excision should include regional lymph node if cytologically positive or in close proximity.
b. Prednisone—2 mg/kg orally daily × 7 days, 1 mg/kg orally × 7 days, then 0.5 mg/kg orally × 14 days, then stop or proceed to f.
c. Radiation—4000 rads divided into 10 fractions to be administered every other day for 10 treatments. Generally used if inoperable and confined to regional areas.
d. Cytoreductive surgery—removal of as many tumors as possible.
e. Intralesional steroids—0.5–1.0 mg triamcinolone per centimeter of tumor administered every 2 weeks.
f. Prednisone—0.5–1.0 mg/kg orally daily.
g. Cimetidine—4 mg/kg, orally , four times daily.
h. Chemotherapy—vincristine 0.5–0.7 mg/m² IV every 2 weeks or vinblastine 2.0 mg/m² IV every 2 weeks

the dog. Although unproven, the use of glucocorticoids in combination with other anticancer drugs is reported superior to therapy with corticosteroids alone.[3,39] The only drug other than corticosteroids that has been demonstrated to have activity against mast cell tumors is L-asparaginase.[41] There is some evidence of efficacy of the vinca alkaloids, both vincristine and vinblastine; however published reports are not available. It is suggested that corticosteroids be used as the mainstay of cytotoxic therapy for canine and feline mast cell tumors and that once

resistance develops, other cytotoxic agents be used sequentially.

Glucocorticoid therapy frequently results in partial or occasionally complete remissions in canine mast cell tumors. However, cats appear to be less responsive to glucocorticoid treatment. The exact mechanism by which glucocorticoids exert their cytotoxic effects on mast cell tumors is unknown although it may be similar to the effects of glucocorticoids on lymphocytes. The susceptibility of mast cell tumors might depend on the presence of intracytoplasmic glucocorti-

Table 17-4.   Mastocytosis in the Cat Treated by Splenectomy

		BREED	SEX	AGE	POSTOP SURVIVAL (MONTHS)	CAUSE OF DEATH	NEOPLASTIC INVOLVEMENT
Case	1	DSH	F/S	16	15	Unknown	Spleen
	2	DLH	M/C	9	12*		Spleen, liver, cutaneous
	3	DSH	F/S	9	14	Heart (unrelated)	Spleen
	4	DSH	M/C	16	24*		Small intestine
	5	DSH	M/C	12	8	Unknown	Spleen
	6	DSH	F/S	12	34	Unknown	Spleen
	7	DSH	F/S	9	25	Duodenal ulcers, disseminated mastocytosis	Spleen
	8	DSH	F/S	7	28*		Spleen
	9	Maine	M/C	12	11*		Spleen
	10	DSH	M/C	4	2*		Spleen
	11	DSH	M/C	13	30	Toxic nephropathy	Spleen

* Still alive

coid receptor sites. Glucocorticoid receptor sites have recently been found in the cytoplasm of canine mast cell tumors.† Although sex steroid receptors for progesterone and estrogen have been recently described in dogs with canine mast cell tumors, the role of sex steroids in the treatment of canine mast cell tumors has yet to be fully investigated.[42] The type and route of administration (systemic vs. intralesional) of glucocorticoids appears to be unimportant. Fewer Cushingoid side-effects have been seen with short-acting glucocorticoids, such as prednisone or prednisolone, when used in the dog than intralesional triamcinolone. The usual dosage of prednisone is 0.5 to 1.0 mg/kg orally administered once daily and that of triamcinolone is 1 mg for every centimeter of diameter of tumor intralesionally, administered every 2 weeks.[26] Remission times are usually 10 to 20 weeks.[43] Dogs that are tumor free after 6 months, however, have a low incidence of recurrence; therapy is usually discontinued at this time. Tumor resistance may be caused by the emergence of mast cells with fewer or ineffective glucocorticoid receptors. Survival data based on histologic grade correlated with various chemotherapeutic regimens have not been reported.

Ancillary drug therapy is important with canine mast cells. Animals with mastocytosis or evidence of gastrointestinal bleeding or large volume mast cell disease should receive H_2 antagonists.[45] Cimetidine (Tagamet) reduces gastric acid production by competitive inhibition of the action of histamine on H_2 receptors of the gastric parietal cells. Ranitidine‡ is a newer H_2 antagonist that requires less frequent administration. The objective of the therapy is to prevent gastrointestinal ulceration associated with elevated levels of histamine and to treat ulcers already present. Some new evidence indicates that cimetidine may also alter the immune response to this tumor as well as activate certain alkylating agents.[44] Dogs and cats with evidence of gastrointestinal ulceration and bleeding might also benefit from sucralfate** therapy.[45] Because sucralfate interferes with absorption of cimetidine, these two drugs should be given at least 2 hours apart. The usual dosage of sucralfate is 1 g given orally. H_1 antagonists such as Benadryl may be used along with cimetidine prior to and following surgical removal of canine mast cell tumors to help prevent the negative effects of local histamine release on the fibroplasia phase of wound healing. H_1 antagonists may also be used with cryosurgery or hyperthermia therapy.[45] Another recommended ancillary medication is an antiserotonin agent (cyproheptadine). The use of this drug is controversial because serotonin has only been identified in rat and mouse mast cells and definitive studies in the dog and cat are lacking. The use of drugs that stabilize mast cells (sodium chromoglyco-

† Macy DW: Unpublished data. Colorado State University, 1986.

‡ Zantac, Glasgow, Inc., Fort Lauderdale, FL.
** Karafate, Marion Labs, Inc., Kansas City, MO.

late) has been described in the treatment of human patients with mastocytosis but not in animals.

Radiotherapy has been used alone or in combination with other treatment modalities. Most reports indicate remission rates of 48% to 77%, although responses were not evaluated relative to known prognostic variables and many patients were treated postsurgically instead of with measurable disease. Doses of 3000 to 4000 rads were used in these studies.[46-48] Radiation therapy is usually fractionated and delivered over a period of 3 to 4 weeks. The use of radiotherapy is somewhat expensive and is confined to referral centers. Mast cell tumors in regional lymph nodes and bone marrow appear to be more resistant to the effects of radiotherapy than those confined to the skin.[49,50]

PROGNOSIS

The natural behavior of mast cell tumors suggests that the prognosis of this tumor is dependent on the species, breed, histologic grade, tumor location, clinical stage, and growth rate, although this conclusion is not universally accepted. In general, cutaneous mast cell tumors carry a more guarded prognosis in the dog than in the cat, horse, or man. Mast cell tumors in the boxer dog are usually of a lower histologic grade than those in other breeds. Mast cell tumors in Siamese cats are also usually of the less malignant histiocytic type. Histologic grade has been shown to correlate with survival following surgical excision by at least two investigators.[13,21] (Table 17-5). The higher the histologic grade (more undifferentiated tumor), the poorer the prognosis. This criteria has not had universal acceptance, however, probably owing to the precise nature of histologic grading as well as to tumor heterogeneity. Canine mast cell tumors that remain localized with a slow growth pattern for long periods of time (perhaps months or years) are usually benign. Bostock[13] reported that dogs that had mast cell tumors for 28 weeks or longer before surgical removal had a favorable prognosis. Eighty-three percent of these dogs survived 30 weeks or longer after surgery. Of the dogs that had mast cell tumors for less than 28 weeks prior to surgical removal, only 25% survived 30 weeks. Similar studies have not been done in the cat. Location also may be an important prognostic indicator. Several investigators indicate that mast cell tumors located in the perineal, preputial, or inguinal areas as well as mucocutaneous junctions are more likely to recur or metastasize than those located in other parts of the body. In the dog, high-grade mast cell tumors usually extend beyond the palpable borders and are found in regional lymph nodes up to 76% of the time. Other organs frequently infiltrated by mast cell tumors in the dog include spleen, skin, liver, kidney, bone marrow, and heart. In summary for dogs, tumors located in the caudal half of the dog and those histologically classified undifferentiated, or Grade III, and with short clinical histories are more likely to metastasize internally and develop systemic mastocytosis.

In the cat, metastasis is less frequently observed.[31a] In one study 34 cats were treated with surgery alone.[22] Forty-one percent (14 cats) had no recurrence or metastases, 24% (8 cats) had local recurrence or developed mast cell tumors elsewhere in the skin with an average time to recurrence of 7 months (age 1–24 mos), 18% (6 cats) developed splenic involvement, and 17% (6 cats) developed regional or distant metastases.[22] As for dog mast cell tumors, metastasis occurs more frequently in the anaplastic types with high mitotic indices. The number of cutaneous lesions in cats does not necessarily indicate malignancy or the likelihood of visceral metastasis. Clinical staging and the extension of microscopic tumor masses beyond what might be detected clinically also play an important role in the failure of universal acceptance of the histologic grading system. In the cat, in addition to the histologic grading system described for the dog, the histiocytic mast cell variant tends to carry a better prognosis than the traditional mast cell tumor.

Table 17-5. Survival Times of Dogs Based on Histologic Grade

	NO. OF DOGS	% ALIVE	MONTHS POST-SURGERY
Bostock[13]			
Well-differentiated	39	77	6
Differentiated	30	45	6
Undifferentiated	45	13	6
Patnaik et al.[21]			
Well-differentiated	30	83	15
Differentiated	36	44	15
Undifferentiated	17	6	15

COMPARATIVE ASPECTS

Mast cell disease in man is rare. In humans, as in pet animals, there is a wide variation in the disease spectrum. Diseases characterized by mast cell infiltration of the skin and other organs include urticaria pigmentosa, mastocytosis, telangiectasia, macularis eruptiva persistans, diffuse mastocytosis, and systemic mastocytosis. The clinical appearance, symptomatology, and prognosis vary among clinical types. As in domestic animals, there appears to be a heritable factor that influences the disease in man. In man the disease usually occurs in young children (2–3 years of age) and has a better prognosis if it develops before puberty than in adult years. About 50% of the cases of mast cell disease spontaneously resolve at the time of puberty. In addition to cutaneous lesions, about one-third of the patients demonstrate clinical signs associated with the release of vasoactive compounds, including pruritus and flushing. These clinical signs have been associated with degranulation of mast cells and may be precipitated by exercise, heat, mechanical manipulation, spicy food, alcohol, and drugs such as codeine, morphine, and aspirin and may result in gastrointestinal ulceration, as seen in our domestic animals. Bone lesions, which have not been reported in the dog or cat, are reported in mastocytosis in people. The recommended treatment of isolated mastocytomas is surgical excision. Treatment of other forms of mastocytosis is symptomatic and not cytotoxic. Most therapies are directed at avoidance of stimuli that may result in degranulation. Sodium chromoglycolate, phototherapy, long-wave ultraviolet light, and antihistamines (including H_1 and H_2 blockers) are the mainstay of drug therapy.

REFERENCES

1. Smith HA, Jones TC: Veterinary Pathology, 3rd ed, pp. 269–274. Philadelphia, Lea & Febiger, 1966
2. Moulton JE: Tumors in Domestic Animals, pp. 31–32. Berkeley: University of California Press, 1978
3. Theilen GH, Madewell BR: Veterinary Cancer Medicine, pp. 178–183. Philadelphia, Lea & Febiger, 1979
4. Dorn ER, Taylor D, Schneider R, et al: Survey of animal neoplasms in Alameda and Contra Costa counties, California. II. Cancer morbidity in dogs and cats from Alameda County. J Natl Cancer Inst 40:307–318, 1968
5. Cohen D, Reif SS, Brodey RS, et al: Epidemiological analysis of the most prevalent sites and types of canine neoplasia observed in a veterinary hospital. Cancer Res 34:2859–2868, 1974
6. Priester WA: Skin tumors in domestic animals. Data from 21 US and Canadian colleges of veterinary medicine. J Natl Cancer Inst 50:457–466, 1973
7. Nielson SW: Spontaneous hematopoietic neoplasms in the domestic cat. NCI Monogr 32:73–94, 1969
8. Macy DW, Reynolds HA: The incidence, characteristic, and clinical management of skin tumors of cats. J Am Anim Hosp Assoc 17:1026–1034, 1981
9. Garner FM, Lingeman CH: Mast cell neoplasms of the domestic cat. Vet Pathol 7:517–530, 1970
10. Orkin M, Schwartzman RM: A comparative study of canine and human dermatology: Cutaneous tumors—The Mast cell and human mastocytoma. J Comp Dermatol 32:451–466, 1959
11. Hottendorf GH, Nielson SW: Survey of 300 extirpated canine mastocytomas. Zentralbl Veterinarmed [A] 14:272–281, 1967
12. Peters JA: Canine mastocytoma excess risk as related to ancestry. J Natl Cancer Inst 42:435–443, 1969
13. Bostock DC: The prognosis following surgical removal of mastocytomas in dogs. J Small Anim Pract 14:27–40, 1973
14. Wilcock BP, Yager JA, Zink MC: The morphology and behavior of feline cutaneous mastocytomas. Vet Pathol 23:320–324, 1986
15. Dunn TB, Patter H: A transplantable mast cell neoplasm in the mouse. J Natl Cancer Inst 18:587–601, 1957
16. Lombard LS, Moloney JB: Experimental transmission of mast cell sarcoma in dogs. Fed Proc 18:490–495, 1959
17. Nielson SW, Cole CR: Homologous transplantation of canine neoplasms. Am J Vet Res 27:663–672, 1961
18. Conter AW, Langloss VM: Long-term survival of two cats with mastocytosis. J Am Vet Med Assoc 172:160–161, 1978
19. Marquart DL, Wasserman SL: Mast cells in allergic disease and mastocytosis. West J Med 137:195–222, 1982
20. Oliver J, Bloom F, Mangieri C: On the origin of heparin: An examination of the heparin content and specific cytoplasmic particles of

neoplastic mast cells. J Exp Med 86:107–116, 1947

21. Patnaik AK, Ehler WN, MacEwen EG: Canine cutaneous mast cell tumor: Morphologic grading and survival time in 83 dogs. Vet Pathol 21:469–474, 1984

22. Holzinger EA: Feline cutaneous mastocytomas. Cornell Vet 63:87–93, 1973

23. Howard EB, Sawa TR, Nielsen SW, et al: Mastocytoma and gastroduodenal ulceration. Vet Pathol 6:146–158, 1969

23a. Fox LE, Rosenthal RC, Twedt DC et al: Plasma histamine and gastrin concentration in 17 dogs with mast cell tumors. J Vet Int Med 1989 (in press)

24. Kenyon AJ, Ramos L, Michaels EB: Histamine-induced suppressor macrophage inhibits fibroblast growth and wound healing. Am J Vet Res 44:2164–2166, 1983

25. Brodey RS: Canine and feline neoplasia. Adv Vet Sci Comp Med 14:309–354, 1970

26. Tams TR, Macy DW: Canine mast cell tumors. Compend Contin Ed 3(10):869–877, 1981

27. Stannard AA, Pulley LT: Tumors of the skin and soft tissues. In Moulton JE (ed): Tumors in Domestic Animals, pp. 16–74. Berkeley, University of California Press, 1978

28. Patnaik AK, MacEwen EG, Black AP, et al: Extracutaneous mast-cell tumor in the dog. Vet Pathol, 19:608–615, 1982

29. Patnaik AK, Twedt DC, Manetta SM: Intestinal mast cell tumor in a dog. J Small Anim Pract 21:207–212, 1980

30. Davis AP, Hayden DW, Klausner TS, et al: Noncutaneous systemic mastocytosis and mast cell leukemia in a dog: Case report and literature review. J Am Anim Hosp Assoc 17:361–368, 1981

31. Nielson SW, Howard EB, Wolke RF: Feline mastocytosis. In Clark WJ, Howard EB, Hackett PL (eds): Myeloproliferative Disorders of Animals and Man, pp. 359–370. Oak Ridge, TN, US Atomic Energy Commission, 1970

31a. Buerger RG, Scott DW: Cutaneous mast cell neoplasia in cats: 14 cases (1975–1985). J Am Vet Med Assoc 190:1440–1444, 1987

32. Madewell BR, Gunn C, Gribble DH: Mast cell phagocytosis of red blood cells in a cat. Vet Pathol 20:638–640, 1983

33. O'Keefe DA, Couto C, et al: Systemic mastocytosis in the dog. J Vet Int Med 1:75–80, 1987

34. Fowler EH, Wilson GP, Roenish WJ, et al: Mast cell leukemia in three dogs. J Am Vet Med Assoc 149:281–285, 1966

35. Guerre R, Millet P, Groulade P: Systemic mastocytosis in a cat: Remission after splenectomy. J Small Anim Pract 20:769–772, 1979

36. Liska WD, MacEwen EG, Zaki FA, et al: Feline systemic mastocytosis: A review and results of splenectomy in seven cases. J Am Anim Hosp Assoc 15:589–597, 1979

37. MacEwen EG, Mooney S, Brown NO, et al: Management of feline neoplasms. In Holzworth J (ed): Diseases of the Cat, pp. 597–618. Philadelphia, W.B. Saunders, 1987

38. Borthwick R: Cryosurgery in veterinary practice: A preliminary report. Vet Rec 86:683–685, 1970

39. Hess P: Canine mast cell tumors. Vet Clin North Am (Small Anim Pract) 42(1):133–143, 1977

40. Hottendorf GH, Nielson SW, Kenyon AJ: Canine mastocytoma. I. Blood coagulation in dogs with mastocytoma. Vet Pathol 2:129–141, 1965

41. Hardy W, Old LJ: L-Asparaginase in the treatment of neoplastic diseases of the dog, cat and cow. In Grundman E, Oettgen HF (eds): Experimental and Clinical Effects of L-Asparginase, pp. 131–136. New York, Springer Verlag, 1970

42. Elling H, Ungemach FR: Sexual hormone receptors in canine mast cell tumour cytosol. J Comp Pathol 92:629–630, 1982

43. Calvert CA: Canine viral and transmissible neoplasm. In Greene CE (ed): Clinical Microbiology and Infectious Diseases of the Dog and Cat, pp. 469–545. Philadelphia, W.B. Saunders, 1984

44. Dorr RT, Soble MV, Albert DS: Interaction of cimitidine but not ranitidine with cylophosphamide in mice. Cancer Res 46:1795–1799, 1986

45. Macy DW: Canine and feline mast cell tumors: Biologic behavior, diagnosis and therapy. Sem Vet Med Surg 1:72–83, 1986

46. Gillette EL: Veterinary radiotherapy. J Am Vet Med Assoc 157:1707–1712, 1976

47. Gillette EL: Radiation therapy of canine and feline tumors. J Am Anim Hosp Assoc 12:359–562, 1976

48. McClelland RB: The treatment of mastocytomas in dogs. Cornell Vet 54:517–519, 1964

49. Kitamura Y, Yokoyama M, Sonoda T, et al: Different radiosensitivities of mast-cell precursors in bone marrow and skin of mice. Radiat Res 93:147–156, 1983

50. Turrel JM, Kitchell BE, Miller LM et al: Prognostic factors for radiation treatment of mast cell tumor in 85 dogs. J Am Vet Med Assoc 193:936–940, 1988

18

SOFT TISSUE SARCOMAS

E. Gregory MacEwen
Stephen J. Withrow

INCIDENCE AND RISK FACTORS

Soft tissue sarcomas are malignant neoplasms arising from tissues derived from the primitive mesenchyme. They are relatively rare, constituting about 1% of all malignant tumors. The annual incidence rates of soft tissue sarcomas in dogs and cats are much greater than the rate in humans, and the canine rate is approximately twice that of the cat. Fibrosarcoma, hemangiosarcoma, and hemangiopericytoma are major types of soft tissue sarcoma in the dog, and the annual incidence of soft tissue sarcomas in the dog is about 35 per 100,000 dogs at risk.[1] In the cat the annual incidence is about 17 per 100,000 cats at risk.[1]

Little is known about the epidemiologic or etiologic factors of importance in animals with soft tissue sarcomas. There is no proven genetic predisposition to the development of soft tissue sarcomas. In cats, a viral cause has clearly been demonstrated; feline multicentric fibrosarcomas have been associated with the feline sarcoma virus (FeSV) (see section on oncogenic viruses in Chapter 29). FeSV induces multiple fibrosarcoma of young cats (3 years or younger), whereas the more common solitary fibrosarcomas that are not associated with FeSV develop in cats with a mean age of 10 years. In the dog, soft tissue sarcomas tend to be reported in the larger breeds, including the St. Bernard, basset hound, German shepherd, golden retriever, English setter, Great Dane, and pointer. In dogs sarcomas have been associated with radiation, trauma, and parasites (see Chapter 2).

PATHOLOGY AND NATURAL BEHAVIOR

The term "soft tissue sarcoma" refers to a large variety of malignant tumors arising in the soft tissues that are grouped together because of similarities in pathologic appearance, clinical presentation, and behavior. In general, sarcomas arise largely, though not exclusively, from mesodermal structures and largely, though not exclusively, from connective tissue cells. Some

167

sarcomas arise from ectodermal structures and some from epithelium. Table 18-1 depicts the cell derivation of soft tissue tumors. Hemangiosarcomas, oral sarcomas, and feline virus-induced sarcomas are covered separately in other chapters.

Soft tissue sarcomas tend to have several important common features with regard to their biologic behavior:

1. They may arise from any anatomical site in the body.
2. They tend to have poorly defined margins and infiltrate through and along fascial planes.
3. Local recurrence after conservative surgical resection is common.
4. They tend to metastasize through hematogenous methods. Regional lymph node metastasis in unusual (except for synovial cell sarcoma).

Many of the soft tissues can undergo malignant transformation into a sarcoma. Because of the large number of different soft tissues, a variety of histologically distinct types have been identified. Each of these tissues can also give rise to benign tumors, which can also have a somewhat aggressive behavior and become locally invasive. It is important to distinguish these locally invasive but nonmetastasizing tumors from those that are truly benign and those that are truly malignant. Many times the overall course of disease and prognosis may be based not only on the histologic type of tumor, but also on the histopathologic grade of the malignancy.

Some sarcomas are difficult to categorize correctly as to the specific tissue of origin. Highly undifferentiated tumors may be designated simply as soft tissue sarcomas, without any further classification.

FIBROMA/FIBROSARCOMA

A fibroma is a benign tumor of fibrocytes; it originates in dermal collagen in which it forms a nodule covered with epidermis. Fibromas occur as single or multiple tumors and usually involve the subcutaneous tissue. They are usually very firm and well circumscribed. Fibromas are characterized by fibroblasts and collagen fibers.

Most fibrosarcomas arise from the skin, subcutaneous tissue, or palate, and represent malignant or transformed fibrocytes. The tumor tissue is very cellular, with closely packed spindle-shaped fibroblasts showing many mitotic figures. The fibrosarcoma is a malignant tumor with a tendency to grow to quite a large size, to invade deeper structures such as tendons, fascia, and muscles, and to produce ulceration of the epidermis.

HEMANGIOPERICYTOMA

A malignant tumor of the subcutis, the hemangiopericytoma is considered to originate in ad-

Table 18-1. Cell of Origin, Tumor Types, and Metastatic Potential of Common Soft Tissue Neoplasms

CELL OF ORIGIN	BENIGN	MALIGNANT*	METASTATIC POTENTIAL†	RELATED CHAPTER
Fibrocyte	Fibroma	Fibrosarcoma	+/++	19
Fibrocyte/histiocyte	—	Fibrous histiocytoma	+	
Myxomatous tissue	Myxoma	Myxosarcoma	+/++	
Pericyte of blood vessel	Hemangiopericytoma	Hemangiopericytoma	+	
Endothelial cells of blood vessels and lymphatic vessels	Hemangioma	Hemangiosarcoma	+++	30
	Lymphangioma	Lymphangiosarcoma	+	
Adipose	Lipoma	Liposarcoma	++	
Nerve	Neurofibroma	Neurofibrosarcoma	+	27
	Schwannoma	Malignant schwannoma	+	
Smooth muscle‡	Leiomyoma	Leiomyosarcoma	+	19, 23
Osteocyte	Osteoma	Osteosarcoma	+++	21
Chondrocyte	Chondroma	Chondrosarcoma	+/++	21
Synovial cell		Synovial cell sarcoma	++	21
Skeletal muscle	Rhabdomyoma	Rhabdomyosarcoma	++	21

* Some neoplasms are so primitive and anaplastic that they can only be classified as undifferentiated sarcoma or undifferentiated spindle cell sarcomas.
† +, low; ++, moderate; +++, high.
‡ Probably of blood vessel smooth muscle as opposed to the more common gastrointestinal or reproductive tract neoplasms.

ventitial pericytes of small blood vessels. It occurs as a nodular, lobulated, and poorly defined tumor. It may appear to be clinically encapsulated, but the capsule is really compressed tumor cells as opposed to benign encapsulation. Most adhere to deeper tissues and infiltrate underlying fascia and muscle. These tumors are considered malignant with a high likelihood of local recurrence after conservative treatment. The metastatic rate for hemangiopericytoma is less than 10%. They tend to grow slowly and can range in size from 0.5 cm to over 10–12 cm in diameter. In some cases, they can easily be confused with lipomas.

The tumor occurs most commonly on the extremities or around the perineal region. The histologic criteria for making a diagnosis of hemangiopericytoma include typical whorling—the arrangement of plump spindle cells in a circular pattern around open or collapsed vessels.

NEUROFIBROMA/NEUROFIBROSARCOMA

Neurofibromas and neurofibrosarcomas are tumors originating in endo- and perineural connective tissue. They are malignant tumors of neurosheath origin and have been referred to as neurogenic sarcomas, malignant schwannomas, and malignant neurolemmomas. These tumors can occur anywhere in the body. Close association with the nerve may be necessary in order to differentiate a neurofibrosarcoma from a fibrosarcoma or hemangiopericytoma.

Neurofibromas may cause nodular enlargement and resulting compression of nerves. They may involve the brachial or lumbosacral plexi and result in paralysis and pain (see Chapter 27).

LIPOMA/LIPOSARCOMA

The lipoma is a frequent tumor of dogs and less common in cats; it is usually well circumscribed and ovoid, consisting of mature fat cells. It appears most commonly in older female dogs. The ventral regions of the abdomen and thorax and sternal regions are most commonly affected. They are not premalignant (see Chapter 16).

Liposarcomas are rare malignant lesions of adipose tissue. They tend to be aggressive and locally invasive, and they may metastasize to lungs, liver, and bone.[2] They tend to occur in subcutaneous tissue of the ventral aspects of the body.[3] Mitoses are frequent as is infiltration into veins, lymphatics, and underlying muscle and fascia. On palpation, these tumors tend to have a very firm texture and be poorly defined.

Infiltrative lipomas are invasive and nonencapsulated masses that may be difficult to remove (see Chapter 16).

HEMANGIOMA/HEMANGIOSARCOMA

The hemangioma is a frequent, benign tumor of the dermis in dogs and less commonly in cats. It consists of blood-filled spaces lined by young endothelial cells. It can frequently occur in younger dogs and is usually small (0.5–2 cm in diameter) and well circumscribed.

The hemangiosarcoma (also called malignant endothelioma) is the malignant counterpart of the hemangioma and is characterized by great cellularity, many mitoses, and small-size neoplastic blood vessels. The tumor often involves the spleen, but it may occur anywhere. (See Chapter 30 for a discussion of hemangiosarcoma.)

LYMPHANGIOMA/LYMPHANGIOSARCOMA

Lymphangiomas appear as soft or firm masses usually involving the skin. Lymphangiomas arise from lymphatic endothelial cells and are extremely rare in the skin of both dogs and cats. They are usually soft and may appear invasive. Lymphangiosarcomas usually arise from the subcutaneous tissues, but they can occur in sites such as liver, pericardium, and nasopharynx. They tend to have a low metastatic potential.

RHABDOMYOSARCOMA

Rhabdomyosarcomas are malignant tumors derived from striated muscle cells. They consist of large, pleomorphic, elongated tumor cells, so-called strap cells, which may show cross striation in their eosinophilic cytoplasm. These tumors tend to be locally invasive and can metastasize to lungs, liver, spleen, kidneys, and adrenal gland. They tend to be diffuse, infiltrative, and poorly circumscribed. Some rhabdomyosarcomas can also be termed "botryoid"—they have a polypoid or grapelike appearance. Botryoid rhabdomyosarcomas have usually been reported in the bladder of large young dogs. (See Chapter 26.)

SYNOVIAL SARCOMA

Synovial sarcomas are malignant neoplasms thought to arise from tendosynovial tissue in either joints, bursa, or tendon sheaths and are considered rare in dogs and even rarer in cats. The synovial sarcomas tend to invade tendons, muscles, and bone and to originate from periarticular tissue rather than the synovium of joints, tendons, or bursa. They commonly recur following conservative surgical excision. Even after amputation, stump recurrences may be observed. Extensive bone destruction has been reported, and metastasis will occur in up to 50% of cases. (See Chapter 21.)

LEIOMYOMA/LEIOMYOSARCOMA

Leiomyomas (fibroleiomyoma, polyps) and leiomyosarcomas are tumors that arise from smooth muscle. They are found as firm, white, lobulated masses in any part of the gastrointestinal tract from esophagus to rectum. They also are found to originate in the spleen and genitourinary tract. Benign lesions are usually small, localized, and encapsulated with cells resembling normal smooth muscle. Many leiomyomas occur within the gastrointestinal tract and have been associated with chronic blood loss. Tumors affecting the vagina or vulva are usually pedunculated and often protrude from the vulva (see Chapter 23).

Leiomyosarcomas commonly arise in the retroperitoneal space, the spleen, or the gastrointestinal tract. They tend to be highly aggressive and can metastasize widely.

MALIGNANT FIBROUS HISTIOCYTOMA (MFH)

Malignant fibrous histiocytomas are uncommon tumors characterized as primitive, pleomorphic sarcoma cells with partial fibroblastic and histiocytic differentiation. They are usually firm, invasive tumors arising in the subcutis and rarely metastasize. In cats MFH have also been called giant cell tumors of soft tissue. They seem to behave the same in the cat and the dog; they are invasive, frequently recur, and have low metastatic potential.[4]

HISTORY AND CLINICAL SIGNS

Soft tissue sarcomas most often present as soft tissue masses. Because these lesions arise in compressible soft tissues and are often far from vital organs, the tumors may be quite large before any appreciable clinical signs occur. Sarcomas may present as soft subcutaneous masses such as a hemangiopericytoma or lipoma, or they may be more firm and invasive into surrounding tissues, such as a fibrosarcoma. There is marked variability in the physical features of soft tissue sarcomas, but they are generally firm and adherent (fixed) to skin, muscle, or bone.

Leiomyosarcomas are seen most commonly in the digestive and urogenital tracts. In the gastrointestinal tract the clinical signs are usually obstructive in nature and perforations may occur. Smooth muscle sarcomas of the bladder present with signs of hematuria and dysuria.

DIAGNOSTIC TECHNIQUES AND WORK-UP

Soft tissue sarcomas should be suspected in all animals with soft tissue masses. Aspiration or needle biopsy usually does not play a major role in the diagnosis of primary soft tissue sarcoma. Although fine-needle aspiration is very useful in the diagnosis of lipomas, tumor cells from sarcomas are difficult to exfoliate, and inadequate specimens are often obtained from a fine-needle aspiration. Incisional biopsy is the most accurate way to obtain a definitive diagnosis. The incisional biopsy should be performed through a carefully placed incision so as not to compromise subsequent radical excision of the lesion or interfere with radiotherapy. Care should be taken to obtain excellent hemostasis. Hematomas resulting from biopsy of soft tissue sarcomas lead to spread of tumor far beyond the site of natural tumor invasion—that is, along the path of the hematoma.

Other diagnostic tests that are important include radiographic evaluation of the primary tumor and of the thoracic cavity to rule out distant metastasis. In some cases sarcomas may invade bone. Dystrophic calcification is a feature of some anaplastic sarcomas and is also a characteristic of extraskeletal osteosarcomas.

Although regional lymph node metastasis is not a common feature associated with sarcomas, the regional lymph node should be carefully examined. An investigation of the node should include palpation to assess size, mobility, and texture; if the node is enlarged, it should be further evaluated by fine needle cytology or needle biopsy. The important sites to evaluate for metastasis include lungs, liver, and bones.

A CBC and chemistry profile should be performed on all animals going to surgery with a suspected sarcoma. Hypoglycemia has been identified in dogs with large intra-abdominal sarcomas.[5] If splenic involvement is suspected, then particular attention should be directed to possible anemia and thrombocytopenia.

TREATMENT

SURGERY

Soft tissue sarcomas grow in the path of least resistance and push surrounding tissue before them. This surrounding tissue forms a pseudocapsule (not a true capsule) and always contains invasive prongs of malignant tissue. For this reason shelling (marginal resection) out of a soft tissue sarcoma is rarely curative. In fact, excision through the pseudocapsule often spreads the tumor into surrounding tissue planes and can greatly complicate further surgical treatment or radiation therapy.

Radical surgical excision remains the most effective treatment to control local disease. Surgical excision should be as aggressive as possible, removing as much of the surrounding normal fascial planes and tissue compartments as possible. Overlying skin and subcutaneous tissue should also be removed. Pathologic evaluation of margins should be performed and reexcision immediately undertaken if the first excision was incomplete. Common surgical mistakes include "shelling out" or removal of the tumor in pieces. Both procedures result in seeding of the surgical field (see Chapter 8). The application of these principles requires, of course, that the tumor be located in an area in which acceptably wide margins of normal tissue can be removed (at least 2- to 3-cm margins). Any areas of fixation (including bone and fascia) should be excised en bloc with the mass (Fig. 18-1). Any marginal area of concern to the surgeon should be tagged with fine suture or submitted as a separate specimen for histologic analysis. When the tumors occur in locations such as the extremities or whenever clear margins cannot be obtained without an unacceptable functional impairment, amputation may be the best approach. The level of amputation recommended is often the proximal attachment of involved muscles or one joint

above the lesion. In most cases it is best to do a disarticulation of the limb at the attachment to the body.

CHEMOTHERAPY

The use of chemotherapy has shown very promising results in humans, but few studies have evaluated the effectiveness of chemotherapy in dogs and cats.[6-9] Chemotherapeutic drugs used to treat sarcomas include doxorubicin, cyclophosphamide, dacarbazine (DTIC), and vincristine. The reader is referred to Chapter 9 for the specific dosages of the various chemotherapeutic agents. One combination that we and others have found somewhat effective is doxorubicin and cyclophosphamide with or without the addition of vincristine.[7] This combination is particularly effective in treating fibrosarcomas, undifferentiated sarcomas, myxosarcomas, and synovial sarcomas. We have also found this approach effective in cats with various sarcomas. In a study of 13 cats with nonresectable soft tissue sarcomas,[6] treatment consisted of combination chemotherapy (cyclophosphamide, vincristine, and methotrexate); 8 cats (61%) had a measurable reduction in tumor volume. No complete responses were noted. It appears that a doxorubicin-based combination would be the optimal approach. In certain sarcomas a 50% response rate can be anticipated, and the duration of response can vary between a matter of a few weeks to as long as 8 to 12 months.[7,9]

RADIATION

Soft tissue sarcomas are generally thought to be resistant to conventional doses of irradiation (40 to 48 Gy).[10,11] Although higher doses have higher control rates, the chances of normal tissue complications also increases. These tumors do not rapidly regress after radiation, and "control" may be defined as a slowly regressing or stable-sized mass. Combinations of chemotherapy or hyperthermia with irradiation are showing promise for improved control over irradiation alone.[12,13]

Radiation may also be used preoperatively to "shrink" an inoperable tumor or "sterilize" the peripheral extensions of the tumor to make curative surgery possible. Postoperative irradiation may be used if surgical removal is incomplete and further surgery is not feasible.

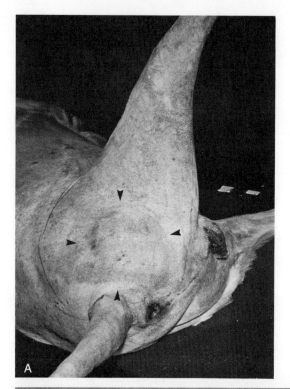

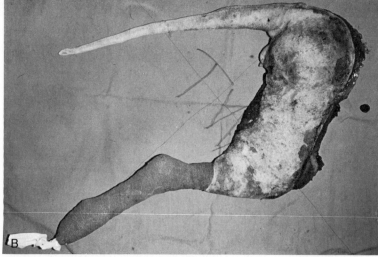

Figure 18-1. *(A)* 15-year-old dog with a large fibrosarcoma (arrows) over the tuber ischii with fixation to ischium and tail. Tumor also extended to area of greater trochanter. *(B)* Tumor fixation and location mandated removal of the tail, ischium, acetabulum, and leg to achieve tumor-free margins. Function and cosmetics were excellent, and patient remains free of disease 2 years later.

TREATMENT OF SELECTED TUMORS

Lipoma/Liposarcoma

Surgical excision is the treatment of choice for a lipoma. Infiltrative lipomas require more aggressive surgery because the potential for recurrence is high. Liposarcomas require extensive surgery and respond poorly to chemotherapy and radiation therapy.

Fibroma/Fibrosarcoma

For fibrosarcomas wide local excision is of paramount importance because the tumors infiltrate along fascial planes well beyond their apparent gross margin. Radiation therapy has generally been unsuccessful; however, a preliminary report suggests that radiation and local hyperthermia may have benefit in small localized fibrosarcomas.[12] Postoperative chemotherapy using doxorubicin and cyclophosphamide has been beneficial in retarding recurrence after surgery. In our experience, approximately 25% to 35% of the nonresectable or recurrent fibrosarcomas treated with combination chemotherapy (adriamycin-cyclophosphamide) have at least a partial (>50%) response. This therapy is still considered palliative.

Hemangiopericytoma

Wide aggressive surgery is the treatment of choice for hemangiopericytomas. Because these tumors are locally invasive, the recurrence rate with surgery is from 7.5% to 56%.[14–21] Tumors with a high mitotic index are more likely to recur. Complete regressions have been reported after a combined therapy of hyperthermia and irradiation.[13] In addition, partial regression has been reported after using doxorubicin.[18]

PROGNOSIS

The prognosis for canine soft tissue sarcoma depends on the histologic type, degree of cellular differentiation, number of mitotic figures, location and success of a complete surgical excision. The metastatic potential of the various sarcomas is summarized in Table 18-1.

FIBROSARCOMA

As a general rule, approximately 10% to 30% of fibrosarcomas metastasize after a complete surgical removal. In one study only 5% had not recurred in a 2-year period after radiation therapy.[10] Another study found a 50% recurrence rate in 1 year with combined hyperthermia and radiation therapy.[12]

HEMANGIOPERICYTOMA

Hemangiopericytomas are one of the most common soft tissue sarcomas, and limb locations are most common. A recent review of 34 canine hemangiopericytoma cases treated principally by aggressive surgery revealed that local control can be achieved in 90% of cases at 2 years postoperatively (Fig. 18-2).[14] Other reported recurrence rates, often with short-term follow-up, range from 25% to 60%.[15–17,21] Size, site, and histologic grade were not prognostic.[14] Tumors excised within 2 months of being detected did better than those with longer histories.

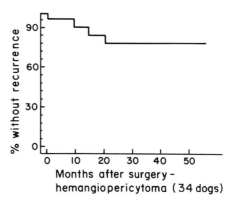

Figure 18-2. Probability of recurrence after aggressive surgical removal of hemangiopericytoma in 34 dogs.[14]

Recurrent tumors were harder to control than those previously untreated, reinforcing the need to perform the first surgery aggressively and early in the course of the disease. Multiple surgeries are sometimes necessary; the mean time to recurrence is 16 months.[14] Recurrence times tend to get shorter with multiple surgeries, and metastatic potential may increase.

Adjuvant radiation therapy after incomplete surgical removal has yielded an approximate 40% control rate at 2 years.[14,19] Control rates (no increase in size) for radiation alone, without surgical debulking, are approximately 50% at 1 year and 20% at 2 years.[22] The tumor control dose for 50% controlled patients at one year (TCD_{50}) was 45.3 Gy in 10 fractions over 3 weeks (Fig. 18-3).[22] Normal tissue complications at higher dosages can be significant and the optimal dose, dose per fraction, and number of fractions to control sarcomas are yet to be determined.[23]

LIPOSARCOMA

Therapy is with aggressive surgical resection. Overall, liposarcomas have a very high local recurrence rate. Metastasis can also occur.

FELINE SOFT TISSUE SARCOMA

The cat is generally similar to the dog in terms of types and behavior of soft tissue sarcoma seen. Two exceptions are the rarity of feline hemangiopericytoma and the presence of a virally induced multicentric fibrosarcoma in young cats.

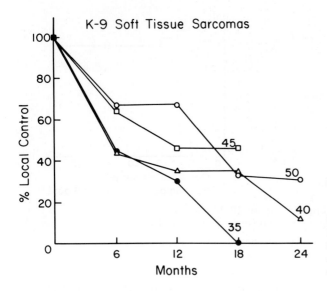

Figure 18-3. Probability of local control of various canine soft tissue sarcomas as a reflection of dose. A clear-cut dose response can be seen at 1 year. Patients were treated with radiation only[22] (eg, 45 = 45Gy = 4500 rads).

Fibrosarcoma (nonvirally induced) accounts for over 50% of feline soft tissue sarcomas in most published reports. Over half of all fibrosarcomas occur on the limb, making complete excision difficult short of amputation.[9,24]

As in the dog, wide resection is mandatory. Without always defining the aggressiveness of surgical removal, one report revealed a 2-year survival of over 50%,[24] and another report revealed only a 40% 9-month survival.[25] The latter reported that histologic grade and tumor location were prognostic variables.[25] Tumors of the pinna and flank did not recur, while 70% of tumors located on the head, back, and leg recurred. Low-grade tumors had a median survival of 128 weeks, while high-grade tumors had a median survival of 16 weeks. Most cats were euthanatized due to local recurrence; only 11% of the tumors metastasized.[25]

Limited attempts at treatment with radiation, chemotherapy, or immunotherapy have not significantly improved local control or survival to date.[9]

CANINE CARDIAC TUMORS

Primary cardiac tumors are rare. Those that have been reported include hemangiosarcoma, fibrosarcoma, mixed-cell sarcoma, hemangioma, fibroma, rhabdomyoma, neurofibroma, and mesothelioma.[26–31]

Clinical signs associated with primary cardiac tumors depend on tumor location, size, degree of infiltration, and metastatic potential.[27] Intraluminal tumors can cause cavity obliteration, or venous and valvular obstruction. Tumors involving the myocardium will induce arrhythmias, electrocardiographic changes, and myocardial failure. Pericardial tumors may cause pericardial and pleural effusion.

Diagnosis is based on thoracic radiography, two-dimensional echocardiography,[26–27] electrocardiography and pericardial fluid analysis.[32] Surgical exploration or endomyocardial biopsy will be necessary to obtain a histopathologic diagnosis in most cases.

Treatment will depend on the location, degree of infiltration and histopathologic tumor type. Surgery and chemotherapy has been used to treat cardiac hemangiosarcoma (see chapter 30).

COMPARATIVE ASPECTS[33]

In general, soft tissue sarcomas have a similar pathologic appearance, clinical presentation, and behavior in humans and animals. A specific difference is the higher incidence at an early age in people as opposed to animals (except, rhabdomyosarcomas are seen in young dogs). Most sarcomas recognized in humans are recognized in animals, although the specific incidences may vary markedly. The more common histologic types in humans, in order, are fibrosarcoma, liposarcoma, rhabdomyosarcoma, unclassified, malignant fibrous histiocytoma, synovial sarcoma, leiomyosarcoma, and neurofibro-sarcoma.

As in animals, the most common site appears to be the limbs (58%) followed by the trunk (30%) and the head and neck (12%). Metastasis would appear to be more common in human soft tissue sarcoma then in dogs. This is partially explained by the higher numbers of hemangiopericytomas, which have a low metastatic rate, seen in the dog.

Well-defined prognostic variables in humans include histologic grade, necrosis, site, size, lymph node involvement, and aggressiveness of surgery.

Standard treatment is with aggressive surgical resection, but radiation and chemotherapy (often doxorubicin combinations) used before or after resection may allow effective limb-sparing treatment in a significant number of patients.

Overall 5-year survival rates are 40% to 50%. Permanent local control with the first treatment is most likely to produce long-term survival.

REFERENCES

1. Dorn ER: Epidemiology of canine and feline tumors. J Am Amin Hosp Assoc 12:307–312, 1976

2. Doster AR, Tomlinson MJ, Mahaffey EA, et al: Canine liposarcoma. Vet Pathol 28:87–88, 1986

3. Strafuss AC, Bozarth AJ: Liposarcoma in dogs. J Am Anim Hosp Assoc 9:183–187, 1973

4. Allen SW, Duncan JR: Malignant fibrous histiocytoma in a cat. J Am Vet Med Assoc 192:90–91, 1988

5. Leifer CE, Peterson ME, Matus RE et al: Hypoglycemia associated with nonislet cell tumors in 13 dogs. J Am Vet Med Assoc 186:53–55, 1985

6. Brown NO, Hayes AA, Mooney S, et al: Combined modality therapy in the treatment of solid tumors in cats. J Am Anim Hosp Assoc 16:719–722, 1980

7. Helphan SC: Chemotherapy for nonresectable and metastatic soft tissue tumors. Proceedings Kal Kan Symp, Columbus, OH, 1986

8. White RAS: Clinical diagnosis and management of soft tissue sarcomas. In Gorman NT (ed): Oncology: Contemporary Tissues in Small Animal Practice, pp. 243–270. New York, Churchill-Livingstone, 1986

9. MacEwen EG, Mooney S, Brown NO, Hayes AA: Management of feline tumors. In Holzworth J (ed): Diseases of the Cat, pp. 597–606. Philadelphia, W.B. Saunders, 1987

10. Hilmas DE, Gillette EL: Radiotherapy of spontaneous fibrous connective-tissue sarcomas in animals. J Natl Cancer Inst 56:365–368, 1976

11. Banks WC, Morris E: Results of radiation treatment of naturally occurring animal tumors. J Am Vet Med Assoc 166:1063–1064, 1975

12. Brewer WG, Turrel JM: Radiotherapy and hyperthermia in the treatment of fibrosarcomas in the dog. J Am Vet Med Assoc 181:146–150, 1982

13. Richardson RC, Anderson VL, Voorhees WD, et al: Irradiation-hyperthermia in canine hemangiopericytomas: Large-animal model for therapeutic response. J Natl Cancer Inst 73:1187–1194, 1984

14. Postorino NC, Berg RJ, Powers BE, et al: Prognostic variables for canine hemangiopericytoma: 50 cases (1979–1984). J Am Anim Hosp Assoc 24:501–509, 1988

15. Mills JHL, Nielson SW: Canine hemangiopericytomas: A survey of 200 tumors. J Small Anim Pract 8:599, 1967

16. Mulligan RM: Hemangiopericytoma in the dog. Am J Pathol 31:773, 1955

17. Yost DH, Jones TC: Hemangiopericytoma in the dog. Am J Vet Res 19:159, 1958

18. Richardson RC: Solid Tumors. Vet Clin North Am 15:557–568, 1985

19. Evans SM: Canine hemangiopericytoma: A retrospective analysis of response to surgery and orthovoltage radiation. Vet Radiol 28:13–16, 1987

20. Fossum TW, Couto CG, DeHoff WD et al: Treatment of hemangiopericytoma in a dog using surgical excision, radiation, and a thoracic pedicle graft. J Am Vet Med Assoc 193:1440–1442, 1988

21. Graves GM, Bjorling DE, Mahaffey E: Canine hemangiopericytoma: 23 cases (1967–1984). J Am Vet Med Assoc 192:99–102, 1988

22. McChesney SL, Withrow SJ, Gillette EL, et al: Radiotherapy of canine soft tissue sarcomas. J Am Vet Med Assoc 194:60–63, 1989

23. McChesney SL, Gillette EL, Dewhirst MW: Influence of WR 2721 on radiation response of canine soft tissue sarcomas. Int J Radiat Oncol Biol Phys 12:1957–1963, 1986

24. Brown NO, Patnaik AK, Mooney S, et al: Soft tissue sarcomas in the cat. J Am Vet Med Assoc 173:744–749, 1978

25. Bostock DE, Dye MT: Prognosis after surgical excision of fibrosarcomas in cats. J Am Vet Med Assoc 175:727–728, 1979

26. Atkins CE, Badertscher RR, Greenlee P et al: Diagnosis of an intracardiac fibrosarcoma using two dimensional echocardiography. J Am Anim Hosp 20:131–137, 1984

27. Vicini DS, Didier PJ, Ogilvie GK: Cardiac fibrosarcoma in a dog. J Am Vet Med Assoc 189:1486–1488, 1986

28. Luginbull H, Detweiler DK: Cardiovascular lesions in dogs. Ann NY Acad Sci 127:517–540, 1965

29. Jubb KVF, Kennedy PC, Palmer N: Pathology of domestic animals, 3rd ed, Vol 3 pp. 32–35. New York, Academic Press Inc., 1985

30. Lombard CW, Goldschmidt MH: Primary fibroma in the right atrium of a dog. J Small Anim Pract 21:439–448, 1980

31. Harbison ML, Godleshi JJ: Malignant mesothelioma in urban dogs. Vet Pathol 20:531–540, 1983

32. Sisson D, Thomas WP, Ruehl WW et al: Diagnostic value of pericardial fluid analysis in the dog. J Am Vet Med Assoc 184:51–55, 1984

33. Rosenberg SA, Suit HD, et al: Sarcomas of the soft tissue and bone. In DeVita VT (ed): Cancer: Principles and Practice of Oncology, pp. 1037–1093. Philadelphia, J.B. Lippincott, 1982

19

TUMORS OF THE GASTROINTESTINAL SYSTEM

The Oral Cavity

Stephen J. Withrow

INCIDENCE AND RISK FACTORS

Collectively, oral cancer accounts for 6% of canine cancer and is the fourth most common cancer overall.[1] In the cat, it accounts for 3% of all cancers. Tumors of unusual sites, types, or behavior will be covered at the end of this chapter: tonsillar squamous cell carcinoma, tongue tumors, viral papillomatosis, canine eosinophilic granuloma complex, epulis, inductive fibroameloblastoma, nasopharyngeal polyp, eosinophilic granuloma in cats, and undifferentiated malignancy of young dogs. A general summary of the common oral tumors is found in Table 19-1.

PATHOLOGY AND NATURAL BEHAVIOR

The oral cavity is a very common site for a wide variety of malignant and benign cancers. Although most cancers are fairly straightforward histologically, some have confusing nomenclature or extenuating circumstances that warrant discussion.

Oral fibrosarcoma often looks surprisingly benign histologically, and even with large biopsy samples the pathologist is forced to read out fibroma or low-grade fibrosarcoma. If the cancer in question is rapidly growing, recurrent, or invading bone, however, the clinician should consider treatment as for malignant cancer. Fibrosarcoma is locally very invasive but metastasizes in less than 20% of cases (usually to the lungs).

Malignant melanoma can present a confusing histopathologic picture if the tumor or the biopsy section does not contain melanin. A histopathologic diagnosis of undifferentiated sarcoma should be looked upon with suspicion for possible underlying melanoma. Melanoma has a strong predilection to metastasize to regional lymph nodes and then lung. Metastasis to lung only or to other sites is not uncommon.

177

Table 19-1. Summary of Common Oral Cancers of the Dog and Cat

	CANINE				FELINE	
	Sq. cell carcinoma* (SCC)	Fibrosarcoma (FS)	Melanoma (MM)	Dental	Sq. cell carcinoma (SCC)	Fibrosarcoma (FS)
FREQUENCY (%)	20–30%	10–20%	30–40%	5%	70%	20%
AGE (YR)	10	7	12	9	10	10
SEX PREDILECTION	Equal	M > F	M > F	F > M	None	None
PATIENT SIZE	Larger	Larger	Smaller	None		
SITE PREDILECTION	Rostral mandible	Palate	Buccal mucosa	Rostral mandible	Mandible or maxillary bone; tongue	Gingiva
REGIONAL LYMPH NODE METASTASIS	Rare (except tonsil and tongue)	Rare	Common	Never	Occasional	Rare
DISTANT METASTASIS	Rare (except tonsil and tongue)	Occasional	Common	Never	Rare, but few live long enough to see metastasis	Occasional
GROSS APPEARANCE	Red, cauliflower, raised, ulcerated	Flat, firm, ulcerated	2/3 pigmented, ulcerated	Like SCC	Proliferative in pharynx; minimal visible disease in oral cavity	Firm
BONE INVOLVEMENT†	Variable	Common	Variable	Always	Common	Common
RADIATION RESPONSE	Good	Poor	Poor?	Excellent	Poor	Poor
SURGERY RESPONSE	Good rostral Fair caudal	Poor to fair (esp. large lesions)	Fair to good	Excellent	Poor	Fair to good
PROGNOSIS	Good rostral Poor caudal	Poor to fair	Poor to fair	Excellent	Very poor	Fair
USUAL CAUSE OF DEATH	Distant disease	Local disease	Distant disease	Rarely tumor related	Local disease	Local disease
COMMENTS	Behavior varies dramatically from front (good) to back (poor) of oral cavity	Often looks benign histologically but very invasive biologically	Presence or absence of pigment is not prognostic	May be confused with SCC histologically	Many tumors of mandible and maxilla have little or no visible oral disease but severe deep invasion of bone	

* Nontonsillar

† Varies with site, if adherent to bone, must consider bone involved.

Squamous cell carcinoma is usually a straight-forward histologic diagnosis. It is the most common feline oral malignancy. Severe and extensive involvement of bone is common in the cat. The metastatic rate in cats is somewhat unknown because the local disease is rarely controlled enough to permit observation of the long-term metastatic potential. Metastasis in the dog is very site dependent; the rostral oral cavity has a low metastatic rate, and the caudal tongue and tonsil have high metastatic potential. Metastasis is to lymph node and lung.

The terminology for the epulides and dental tumors has been recently revised by some authors.[2] The "traditional" epulides are similar to gingival hyperplasia in appearance and are usually confined to one or two sites at the gum margin. They are slow growing, firm, and generally covered by intact epithelium. Most are firmly attached, and some are pedunculated. These are classified as fibrous epulides or ossifying epulides, depending on the presence or absence of bone. A third class recently has been termed acanthomatous epulides instead of adamantinomas, as previously described. Some pathologists use the terms interchangeably. These are much more locally invasive and virtually always invade bone. They do not metastasize.

HISTORY AND CLINICAL SIGNS

Most patients present with a mass in the mouth noticed by the owner. Cancer in the caudal pharynx, however, is rarely seen by the owner; the patient presents with increased salivation, weight loss, halitosis, bloody discharge, dysphagia, or occasionally cervical lymphadenopathy. Loose teeth, in a patient with generally good dentition, should alert the clinician to possible underlying neoplastic bone lysis (especially in the cat).[3]

DIAGNOSTIC TECHNIQUES AND WORK-UP

The diagnostic evaluation of oral cancer is critical owing to the wide range of cancer behavior and therapeutic options available. If the cancer is suspected of being malignant, thoracic radiographs can be performed prior to biopsy. The most likely cancers to have positive chest radiographs at the time of diagnosis are melanoma and squamous cell carcinoma of the caudal oral and pharyngeal area. Most animals will require a short general anesthesia for careful palpation, regional radiographs, and a biopsy.

Animals with cancers that are adherent to bone, other than simple epulides, should be regionally radiographed under anesthesia (Fig. 19-1). When 40% or more of the cortex is destroyed, lysis may be observed. However, apparently normal radiographs do not rule out bone invasion. This evaluation will assist in determining the clinical stage of cancer and the extent of resection when surgery is indicated.

Regional lymph nodes (mandibular and retropharyngeal) should be carefully palpated for enlargement or asymmetry. When abnormal (or even just palpable), they should be aspirated with a fine needle. This is especially important for melanoma and caudally situated squamous cell carcinoma.

The last step, under the same anesthesia, is a large incisional biopsy. Oral cancers are commonly infected, inflamed, or necrotic, and it is important to obtain a large specimen. Electrocautery may distort the specimen and should only be used for hemostasis after blade incision. Large samples of healthy tissue at the edge and center of the lesion increase the diagnostic yield. The biopsy site should be in such a position as to be easily included in a possible resection. For small lesions (epulides, papillomas, or labial mucosa melanomas), curative intent resection (excisional biopsy) may be undertaken at the time of initial evaluation. For more extensive disease, waiting for biopsy results to accurately plan treatment is encouraged.

Cytologic preparations of oral cancers may not be rewarding because necrosis and inflammation commonly accompanies these conditions.

THERAPY

Surgery, cryosurgery, and irradiation are the principal therapies used for tumors in the mouth. When feasible, surgical excision is the most economical, fastest, and most curative treatment. Radical surgeries, such as mandibulectomy and partial maxillectomy, are well tolerated by the patient. They are indicated for lesions that have extensively invaded bone, are not believed responsive to radiation, or are too large for cryosurgery (Tables 19-2 and 19-3).[4-8a] Margins of at least 2 cm are necessary for malignant cancers such as squamous cell carcinoma, ma-

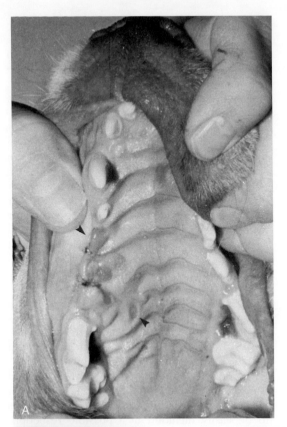

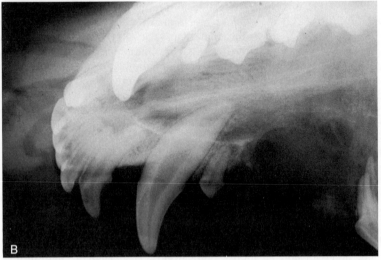

Figure 19-1 *(A)* Fibrosarcoma of the lateral hard palate in a 3-year-old male vizsla. Tumor is firm, flat, and relatively non-aggressive in appearance. *(B)* Lateral oblique radiograph of dog in A. Note marked destruction of maxilla and loss of teeth. This dog was treated with a partial maxillectomy and remains free of cancer at 3 years postoperatively.

lignant melanoma, and fibrosarcoma in the dog. Squamous cell carcinoma in the cat should have wider margins yet, owing to its high local recurrence rate.

Cryosurgery may be indicated for lesions less than 1 inch in diameter and fixed or minimally invasive into bone (see Chapter 12). Larger lesions should generally be surgically resected.

Table 19-2.   Various Mandibulectomies

MANDIBULECTOMY PROCEDURE	AREA REMOVED	INDICATIONS	COMMENTS
Unilateral rostral		Lesions confined to rostral hemi-mandible; not crossing midline	Most common tumor types are squamous cell carcinoma and adamantinoma, which don't require removal of entire affected bone; tongue lags to resected side
Bilateral rostral		Bilateral rostral lesions crossing the symphysis	Tongue will be "too long" and some cheilitis of chin skin will occur; has been performed as far back as PM4 but preferably at PM1 or PM2
Vertical ramus		Low-grade boney or cartilaginous lesions confined to vertical ramus	These tumors are variously called chondroma rodens or multilobular osteoma; TM joint may be removed—cosmetics and function excellent
Complete unilateral		High-grade tumors with extensive involvement of horizontal ramus or invasion into medullary canal of ramus	Usually reserved for aggressive tumors; function and cosmetics good
Segmental		Low-grade midhorizontal ramus cancer, preferably not into medullary cavity	Poor choice for highly malignant cancer in medullary cavity because growth along mandibular artery, vein, and nerve is common

More extensive lesions in bone often result in a fracture (mandible) or oronasal fistula (maxilla) if aggressively frozen. Cancer of soft tissue only should be surgically excised rather than treated with cryosurgery.

Hyperthermia offers no advantage over cryosurgery or surgery if it is used alone. In fact, bone penetration is less reproducible with heat as opposed to cold treatment. Hyperthermia at moderate temperatures (42–43°C) may, however, be used as an effective adjunct to irradiation (see Chapters 10 and 13).

Radiation therapy is used in three general settings:

1. When the tumor is known to be responsive to radiation—acanthomatous epulis (adamantinoma)[9,10] or squamous cell carcinoma[11,12]

Table 19-3.   Various Maxillectomies

MAXILLECTOMY PROCEDURE	AREA REMOVED	INDICATIONS	COMMENTS
Unilateral rostral		Lesions confined to hard palate on one side	One-layer closure
Bilateral rostral		Bilateral lesions of rostral hard palate	Usually requires double-layer closure of overlapping or opposing lip
Lateral		Laterally placed midmaxillary lesions	Single-layer closure if small defect, two-layer if large
Bilateral		Bilateral palatine lesions	High rate of closure dehiscence because lip flap rarely reaches side to side; may result in permanent oronasal fistula

2. When a cancer of any histology is inoperable
3. To "clean up" remaining cancer when there is known postoperative residual disease

Local and regional disease control is the goal of treatment. No known effective chemotherapeutic agents exist for cancers likely to metastasize (malignant melanoma, squamous cell carcinoma, or fibrosarcoma) (see Chapter 9). Slight short term response was noted for 5 dogs with oral squamous cell carcinoma treated with cisplatin.[12a] Combinations of doxorubicin and cyclophosphamide have also yielded some responses in cats.[12b] Adjuvant immunotherapy with Bacille Calmette Guérin (BCG) or levamisole has failed to improve survivals in malignant melanoma in the dog. A slight improvement in survival was demonstrated for patients with advanced local malignant melanoma treated with surgery and *Corynebacterium parvum* as opposed to surgery alone.[13]

PROGNOSIS

The prognosis for acanthomatous epulis/adamantinoma is excellent with surgery or irradiation. Recurrence rates for these tumors after aggressive resection are less than 5%.[4,6] Radiation therapy controls in excess of 90% of these tumors.[9] A syndrome in which a malignant cancer develops in the irradiated site may occur in up to 20% of patients.[9,14] The tumor may be of epithelial or mesenchymal origin and usually takes several years to develop.

The outlook for squamous cell carcinoma varies widely according to site and species. Canine cancers in the rostral mouth are curable with surgery[4] or irradiation,[12,12c,12d] while those of tonsil or base of tongue are highly metastatic and likely to recur locally or regionally.[11,15] Local control of feline squamous cell carcinoma is very poor with either surgery or radiation therapy;[7,16,17] 1-year survivals rarely exceed 10%. In a series of 52 cats with oral squamous cell carcinoma treated with various combinations of surgery, radiation, chemotherapy and hyperthermia, the median survival was 2.0 months, with only 2 cats living longer than 1 year.[17a]

Overall, approximately 25% of dogs with oral malignant melanomas survive 1 year or more.[13,18] The only known variables that have prognostic significance are size (< 2 cm diameter is a better prognosis) and ability of first treatment to afford local control.[13,18,19] Dogs with tumors < 2 cm in diameter have a median survival of 511 days, as opposed to dogs with lymph node involvement or tumors greater than 2 cm in diameter, whose median survival is 164 days (Fig. 19-2).[13] Recurrent malignant melanoma does worse than disease that is locally controlled with the first attempt.[18] Age, breed, sex, degree of pigmentation, microscopic appearance, and anatomic site are not prognostic.[18]

Local control of fibrosarcoma is more of a problem than metastasis. The best 1-year survivals with almost any treatment are no better than 25% to 40%.[4–8] Fibrosarcomas are generally considered radiation resistant.[20,21] Mean survival after radiation of 17 dogs was only 7 months.[22] Radiation combined with regional hyperthermia improved local control rates to 50% as measured at 1 year in a series of 10 cases.[23]

Eighty-one dogs with mandibular tumors and 61 dogs with maxillary tumors were treated with either mandibulectomy or maxillectomy. The cumulative proportion surviving at 1 and 2 years following mandibulectomy was 45% and 35%. For dogs treated with maxillectomy the 1 and 2

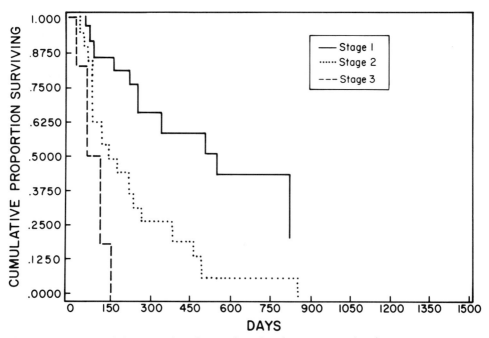

Figure 19-2. Survival duration of 89 dogs with oral melanoma treated with surgery or surgery and *Corynebacterium parvum*. Stage 1 is tumor diameter less than 2 cm; Stage 2 is tumor diameter between 2 and 4 cm. Both Stages 1 and 2 have negative lymph nodes. Stage 3 is tumor diameter greater than 4 cm or any size tumor with positive lymph nodes. Stage 1 was associated with a significant increase in survival time (p = 0.024).[13]

year survival was 47% and 24% respectively. Improved survival was demonstrated when tumor free margins were achieved. Benign tumors survived better than malignant tumors but a statistically significant difference between the various malignant types was not demonstrated. Most dogs that died or were euthanized were because of local recurrence.[23a]

SELECTED SITES OR CANCEROUS CONDITIONS IN THE ORAL CAVITY

Tonsillar Squamous Cell Carcinoma

This cancer is 10 times more common in animals living in urban as opposed to rural areas, implying an etiologic association with environmental pollutants.[24] Most primary tonsillar cancer is squamous cell carcinoma. Lymphosarcoma can affect the tonsils but is usually accompanied by regional or generalized lymphadenopathy. Other cancer, especially malignant melanoma, may metastasize to tonsil as well. Cervical lymphadenopathy, ipsi- or contralateral, is a common presenting sign, even with very small primary cancers. Fine-needle aspirates of these lymph nodes or excisional biopsy of the tonsil will confirm the diagnosis. Thoracic radiographs will be positive in a large percentage of cases. This disease is considered metastatic at diagnosis in over 90% of patients. Simple tonsillectomy is almost never curative but probably should be done bilaterally owing to the high percentage of bilateral disease.[25] Cervical lymphadenectomy, especially for large and fixed nodes, is rarely curative and should be considered diagnostic only. Regional radiation (pharynx and cervical lymph nodes) is capable of controlling local disease in over 75% of the cases; however, survival remains poor, with only 10% of affected animals alive at 1 year.[11] The cause of death is local disease early and systemic disease (usually lung metastasis) later. To date, no known effective chemotherapeutic agents exist for canine or feline squamous cell carcinoma, although bleomycin has been used with very limited success.[26] Recent reports suggest some beneficial effects with cisplatin against tonsillar squamous cell carcinoma with or without concomitant radiation therapy. In spite of some partial and complete responses, the one year survival was less than 10%.[12a,26a]

Tongue[15]

Cancer confined to the tongue is rare. White dogs appear to be at higher risk for squamous cell carcinoma, even though lack of pigment would not seem to be as much a problem as it is in other, more exposed areas of the body (nose, eyelids, and ears). The most common cancer of the canine tongue is squamous cell carcinoma (~50%) followed by granular cell myoblastoma, melanoma, mast cell, fibrosarcoma, and a wide variety of histologic types. Feline tongue tumors are usually squamous cell carcinomas, and most are located on the ventral surface near the frenulum. Presenting signs are similar to other oral cancers and mass lesions. Ulceration may be seen (especially with squamous cell carcinoma).

With the animal under general anesthesia, the tongue may be biopsied with a wedge incision and closed with horizontal mattress sutures. Hemorrhage may be profuse before suturing. Regional lymph nodes should be aspirated for staging purposes if they are palpable. Treatment is generally surgery; irradiation is reserved for inoperable cancer or cancer metastatic to lymph nodes. Partial glossectomy can be performed for the rostral half (mobile tongue) or longitudinal half of the tongue. Eating and drinking may be slightly impaired, but good hydration and nutrition can be maintained postoperatively. Up to 50% removal will compromise grooming in cats and may result in poor hair coat hygiene.

The prognosis for tongue tumors varies according to site and type of cancer. Cancer in the rostral (mobile) tongue has a better prognosis for any of the following reasons:

1. It may be detected earlier because the owner can see the lesion.
2. The caudal tongue may have richer lymphatic and vascular channels to allow metastasis.
3. Rostral lesions are easier to excise with wide margins.

Even so, the 1-year survival with surgery or radiation for squamous cell carcinoma of the tongue is rarely over 25%. Metastasis to regional lymph nodes and to other sites is common.

Granular cell myoblastoma is a curable cancer. These cancers may look large and invasive, but they are almost always removable (Fig. 19-3).

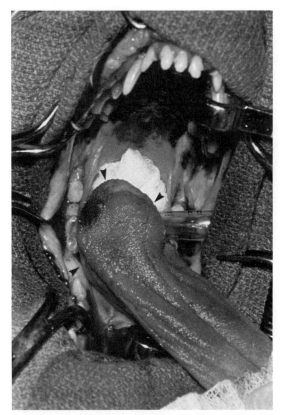

Figure 19-3. This large granular cell myoblastoma was easily removed surgically. The patient had a recurrence 2 years postoperatively, which was again removed, and the dog is free of disease 3 years after the last surgery.

Permanent local control rates exceed 80%. They may recur, but repeated surgeries are usually possible. This cancer is rarely metastatic. Local control in four of six tongue melanomas was obtained by surgery, and the metastatic rate was less than 50% in this small series.[15] The behavior of other tongue cancers is generally unknown because these conditions are rare.

Viral Papillomatosis[27]

This condition is transmitted by a viral agent (papilloma virus) from dog to dog. Affected animals are generally young. The lesions appear wartlike and are generally multiple in the oral cavity, pharynx, tongue, or lips. A biopsy can be performed if necessary, but visual examination is usually diagnostic (Fig. 16-2). Most patients never suffer any significant side-effects of

this disease, though an occasional dog has such marked involvement as to require surgical debulking in order to permit swallowing. Although uncommon, papillomas of the oral mucosa have been observed to progress to squamous cell carcinoma.[27a] The majority of patients undergo a spontaneous regression of disease within 4 to 8 weeks which resists a subsequent viral challenge. For recalcitrant cases, a wide variety of treatments have been tried: crushing of lesions *in situ* to "release" antigen, autogenous vaccines, and chemotherapy.[28] These methods are seldom required, and the prognosis without them is excellent.

Canine Oral Eosinophilic Granuloma[29,30]

This disease affects young dogs (1–7 years) and may be heritable in the Siberian husky. It is histologically similar to the feline disease, with eosinophils and granulomatous inflammation predominating. The granulomas typically occur on the lateral and ventral aspects of the tongue. They are raised and frequently ulcerated, and they may mimic more malignant cancers in appearance. Treatment with corticosteroids or conservative surgical excision is generally curative, although spontaneous regression may occur. Recurrences are uncommon.

Epulis

Benign, gingivally located proliferations of tissue in the dog are termed epulides; they may be fibromatous or ossifying.[2] They are usually firm, 1 to 4 cm in diameter, and variably fixed to the bone at the gum line (Fig. 19-4). Mild ulceration may occur, but most epulides are covered by epithelium. Epulides rarely invade bone, and treatment is conservative blade excision.[30a] The rare recurrent lesion may require more aggressive destruction of the base with electrocautery or cryosurgery. These tumors are rare in the cat.

Inductive Fibroameloblastoma[31,32]

This rare odontogenic tumor primarily affects young cats (6 months to 2 years) and has a predilection for the region of the upper canine teeth and maxilla. Radiographically the tumor site shows variable degrees of bone destruction and expansion of the maxillary bones (Fig. 19-5). Tooth deformity is common. Smaller lesions are treated with surgical debulking and cry-

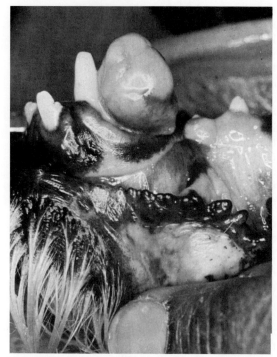

Figure 19-4. Typical appearance of a fibromatous epulis on the gum line of an 8-year-old dog. The mass is firmly adherent to underlying bone but non-invasive on radiographs. Conservative removal was curative.

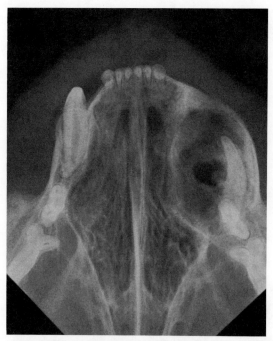

Figure 19-5. Radiograph of 1-year-old cat with a large inductive fibroameloblastoma of entire lateral maxilla. Note displacement of teeth and expansile nature of bone distortion. This patient was treated with radiation therapy and is in clinical remission 3 years after treatment.

osurgery or premaxillectomy. Larger lesions respond to radiation. Local treatment needs to be aggressive, but control rates are good and metastasis has not been reported.

Nasopharyngeal Polyp in Cats

This disease tends to affect young cats; most are less than 2 years old. No definitive breed or sex predilection is known.[33] Clinical signs include sneezing, swallowing problems, rhinitis, and difficulty in breathing. Firm, fleshy masses can be seen or palpated in the caudal pharynx or above the soft palate (Fig. 19-6). Occasionally, masses can be visualized in the external ear canal.[34] Skull radiographs may reveal fluid or tissue in the tympanic bullae.[35] Most lesions originate in the bullae or eustachian tube and grow toward the pharynx to become a pedunculated mass. Treatment through the oral cavity is by traction and ligation of as much of the stalk as possible; however, recurrences may occur when that is the only treatment. If radiographs

reveal tissue in the bullae, a combined oral removal and bullae osteotomy may be required to effect a cure. The disease is probably not truly neoplastic but rather primarily or secondarily inflammatory.

Eosinophilic Granuloma in the Cat[36,37,37a]

This condition is also known as rodent ulcer, indolent ulcer, or most commonly eosinophilic granuloma. It occurs more commonly in females, and the average age is 5 years. The etiology is unknown.

Any oral site is at risk, but the disease is most common on the upper lip near the midline (Fig. 19-7). The history is usually that of a slowly progressive (months to years) erosion of the lip. Biopsies are often necessary to differentiate the condition from true cancers.

Various treatments are proposed, including prednisone at 1–2 mg/kg BID × 30 days orally or IM methyl prednisolone acetate* at 20 mg/

* Depo-Medrol, Upjohn, Kalamazoo, MI

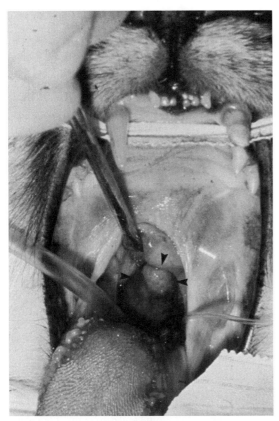

Figure 19-6. Nasopharyngeal polyp can be visualized as soft palate is pulled forward. This lesion is attached to a stalk emanating from the eustachian tube.

cat SQ every 2 weeks; megestrol acetate[†]; hypoallergenic diets; radiation; surgery or cryosurgery; and immunotherapy.[37a] The prognosis for complete and permanent recovery is only fair, although in rare cases, spontaneous regression may occur.

Undifferentiated Malignancy of Young Dogs[38]

This condition is seen in dogs under 2 years of age (range, 6–22 months). Most patients are large breeds, and there is no sex predilection. The disease is manifest by a rapidly growing mass in the area of the hard palate, upper molar teeth, or maxilla and orbit. Biopsies reveal an undifferentiated malignancy of undetermined histogenesis. Most patients present with lymph node metastasis, and at necropsy five of six had metastasis beyond the head and neck. No effective treatment has been proposed, although conceptually, chemotherapy would be necessary. Most patients are euthanatized within 30 days of diagnosis because tumor growth is progressive and uncontrolled.

Papillary Squamous Cell Carcinoma in Young Dogs[38a]

This disease is seen in dogs less than six months old and affects the maxilla or the mandible. A proliferative mass with bone lysis is common.

† Ovaban, Schering, Kenilworth, NJ

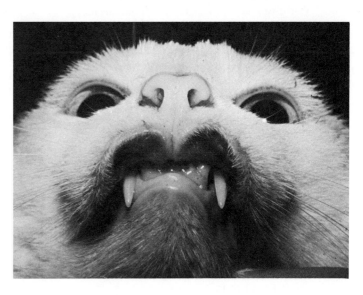

Figure 19-7. Typical erosive eosinophilic granuloma on the upper lip of a female cat.

Debulking surgery combined with radiation appears to be curative.

Neuroendocrine (Merkel) Cell Tumors[38b]

This tumor may occur in the skin or oral cavity of the dog. It is a round cell tumor that has only recently been recognized as a separate histologic and clinical entity. Based on four treated oral cases the prognosis with surgical removal would appear to be excellent.

COMPARATIVE ASPECTS[39]

The vast majority of oral cavity cancer in humans is squamous cell carcinoma. It is associated with alcohol and tobacco use and usually occurs in patients older than 45 years.

Treatment is generally surgery, radiation, or both. Chemotherapy has a limited role for local disease but has shown promise, often in combination with radiation, for advanced cancer.

Prognosis is strongly correlated to histologic grade, stage, and site. The pharynx and caudal tongue have worse prognoses than the rostral tongue and oral cavity.

REFERENCES

1. Hoyt RF, Withrow SJ: Oral malignancy in the dog. J Am Anim Hosp Assoc 20:83–92, 1984
2. Dubielzig RR: Proliferative dental and gingival diseases of dogs and cats. J Am Anim Hosp Assoc 18:577–584, 1982
3. Madewell BR, Ackerman N, Sesline DH: Invasive carcinoma radiographically mimicking primary bone cancer in the mandibles of two cats. J Am Vet Radiol Soc 27:213–215, 1976
4. Withrow SJ, Holmberg DL: Mandibulectomy in the treatment of oral cancer. J Am Anim Hosp Assoc 19:273–286, 1983
5. Withrow SJ, Nelson AW, Manley PA, Biggs DR: Premaxillectomy in the dog. J Am Anim Hosp Assoc 21:49–55, 1985
6. White RAS, Gorman NT, Watkins SB, Brearley MJ: The surgical management of bone-involved oral tumours in the dog. J Small Anim Pract 26:693–708, 1985
7. Bradley RL, MacEwen EG, Loar AS: Mandibular resection for removal of oral tumors in 30 dogs and 6 cats. J Am Vet Med Assoc 184:460–463, 1984
8. Salisbury SK, Richardson DC, Lantz GC: Partial maxillectomy and premaxillectomy in the treatment of oral neoplasia in the dog and cat. Vet Surg 15:16–26, 1986
8a. Penwick RC, Nunamaker DM: Rostral mandibulectomy: A treatment for oral neoplasia in the dog and cat. J Am An Hosp Assoc 23:19–25, 1987
9. Thrall DE: Orthovoltage radiotherapy of acanthomatous epulides in 39 dogs. J Am Vet Med Assoc 184:826–829, 1984
10. Langham RF, Mostosky UV, Schirmer RG: X-ray therapy of selected odontogenic neoplasms in the dog. J Am Vet Med Assoc 170:820–822, 1977
11. MacMillan R, Withrow SJ, Gillette EL: Surgery and regional irradiation for treatment of canine tonsillar squamous cell carcinoma: Retrospective review of eight cases. J Am Anim Hosp Assoc 18:311–314, 1982
12. Gillette EL: Radiation therapy of canine and feline tumors. J Am Anim Hosp Assoc 12:359–362, 1976
12a. Shapiro W, Kitchell BE, Fossum TW: Cisplatin for treatment of transitional cell and squamous cell carcinomas in dogs. J Am Vet Med Assoc 193:1530–1533, 1988
12b. Mauldin GN, Matus RE, Patnaik AK et al: Efficacy and toxicity of doxorubicin and cyclophosphamide used in the treatment of selected malignant tumors in 23 cats. J Vet Int Med 2:60–65, 1988
12c. Gillette EL, McChesney SL, Dewhirst MW: Response of canine oral carcinomas to heat and radiation. Int J Rad Oncol Biol Phys 13:1861–1867, 1987
12d. Evans SM, Shofer E: Canine oral nontonsillar squamous cell carcinoma: Prognostic factors for recurrence and survival following orthovoltage radiation therapy. Vet Radiol 29:133–137, 1988
13. MacEwen EG, Patnaik AK, Harvey HJ, et al: Canine oral melanoma: Comparison of surgery versus surgery plus *Corynebacterium parvum*. Cancer Invest 4:397–402, 1986
14. Thrall DE, Goldschmidt MH, Biery DN: Malignant tumor formation at the site of previously irradiated acanthomatous epulides in four dogs. J Am Vet Med Assoc 178:127–132, 1981
15. Beck ER, Withrow SJ, McChesney AE, et al: Canine tongue tumors: a retrospective review of 57 cases. J Am Anim Hosp Assoc 22:525–532, 1986
16. Bostock DE: The prognosis in cats bearing squamous cell carcinoma. J Small Anim Pract 13:119–125, 1972
17. Cotter SM: Oral pharyngeal neoplasms in the cat. J Am Anim Hosp Assoc 17:917–920, 1981
17a. Postorino NC, Turrel JM, Withrow SJ: Feline oral squamous cell carcinoma: A retrospective

study of 52 cats. Vet Cancer Soc Newsletter 12:6, 1988

18. Harvey HJ, MacEwen GE, Braun D, et al: Prognostic criteria for dogs with oral melanoma. J Am Vet Med Assoc 178:580–582, 1981

19. Dewhirst MW, Sim DA, Forsyth K, et al: Local control and distant metastases in primary canine malignant melanomas treated with hyperthermia and/or radiotherapy. Int J Hyperthermia 1:219–234, 1985

20. Hilmas DE, Gillette EL: Radiotherapy of spontaneous fibrous connective-tissue sarcomas in animals. J Natl Cancer Inst 56:365–368, 1976

21. Creasty WA, Phil D, Thrall DE: Pharmacokinetic and anti-tumor studies with the radiosensitizer misonidazole in dogs with spontaneous fibrosarcomas. Am J Vet Res 43:1015–1018, 1982

22. Thrall DE: Orthovoltage radiotherapy of oral fibrosarcomas in dogs. J Am Vet Med Assoc 159–162, 1981

23. Brewer WG, Turrel JM: Radiotherapy and hyperthermia in the treatment of fibrosarcomas in the dog. J Am Vet Med Assoc 181:146–150, 1982

23a. Schwarz PD, Withrow SJ: Mandibular and maxillary resection as a treatment of oral cancer: Long term followup and survival. The 8th Annual Conf, Vet Cancer Soc, Estes Park, Colo., 8:6, 1988

24. Reif JS, Cohen D: The environmental distribution of canine respiratory tract neoplasms. Arch Environ Health 22:136–140, 1971

25. Todoroff RJ, Brodey RS: Oral and pharyngeal neoplasia in the dog: A retrospective survey of 361 cases. J Am Vet Med Assoc 175:567–571, 1979

26. Buhles WC, Theilan GH: Preliminary evaluation of bleomycin in feline and canine squamous cell carcinomas. Am J Vet Res 34:289–291, 1973

26a. Brooks MB, Matus RE, Leifer CE et al: Chemotherapy versus chemotherapy plus radiotherapy in the treatment of tonsillar squamous cell carcinoma in the dog. J Vet Int Med 2:206–211, 1988

27. Norris AM, Withrow SJ, Dubielzig RR: Oropharyngeal neoplasms. In Harvey CE (ed): Oral Disease in the Dog and Cat. Veterinary Dentistry, pp. 123–139. Philadelphia, W.B. Saunders, 1985

27a. Watrach AM, Small E, Case MT: Canine papilloma: Progression of oral papilloma to carcinoma. J Nat Cancer Inst 45:915–920, 1970

28. Calvert CA: Canine viral and transmissible neoplasias. In Greene CE (ed): Clinical Microbiology and Infectious Diseases of the Dog and Cat, pp. 461–478. Philadelphia, W.B. Saunders, 1984

29. Potter KA, Tucker RD, Carpenter JL: Oral eosinophilic granuloma of Siberian huskies. J Am Anim Hosp Assoc 16:595–600, 1980

30. Madewell BR, Stannard AA, Pulley LT, et al: Oral eosinophilic granuloma in Siberian husky dogs. J Am Vet Med Assoc 177:701–703, 1980

30a. Bjorling DE, Chambers JN, Mahaffey EA: Surgical treatment of epulides in dogs: 25 cases (1974–1984). J Am Vet Med Assoc 190:1315–1318, 1987

31. Dubielzig RR, Adams WM, Brodey RS: Inductive fibroameloblastoma: An unusual dental tumor of young cats. J Am Vet Med Assoc 174:720–722, 1979

32. Hawkins CD, Jones BR: Adamantinoma in a cat. Aust Vet J 59:54–55, 1982

33. Bradley RL, Noone KE, Saunders GK, et al: Nasopharyngeal and middle ear polypoid masses in five cats. Vet Surg 14:141–144, 1985

34. Harvey CE, Goldschmidt MH: Inflammatory polypoid growths in the ear canal of cats. J Small Anim Pract 19:669–677, 1978

35. Parker NR, Binnington AG: Nasopharyngeal polyps in cats: Three case reports and a review of the literature. J Am Anim Hosp Assoc 21:473–478, 1985

36. Scott DW: Chapter 11. Disorders of Unknown or Multiple Origin. J Am Anim Hosp Assoc 16:406–411, 1980

37. McClelland RB: X-ray therapy in labial and cutaneous granulomas in cats. J Am Vet Med Assoc 125:469–470, 1954

37a. MacEwen EG, Hess PN: Evaluation of effect of immunomodulation of the feline eosinophilic granuloma complex. J Am An Hosp Assoc 23:519–526, 1987

38. Patnaik AK, Lieberman PH, Erlandson RA, et al: A clinicopathologic and ultrastructural study of undifferentiated malignant tumors of the oral cavity in dogs. Vet Pathol 23:170–175, 1986

38a. Ogilvie GK, Sundberg JP, O'Banion MK et al: Papillary squamous cell carcinoma in three young dogs. J Am Vet Med Assoc 192:933–936, 1988

38b. Whiteley LO, Leininger JR: Neuroendocrine (Merkel) cell tumors of the canine oral cavity. Vet Path 24:570–572, 1987

39. Million RR, Cassisi NJ, Wittes RE: Cancer in the head and neck. In DeVita VT et al (ed): Cancer: Principles and Practice of Oncology, pp. 301–386. Philadelphia, J.B. Lippincott, 1982

Salivary Glands

Stephen J. Withrow

INCIDENCE AND RISK FACTORS

Primary salivary gland cancer is very rare in the dog and cat. Most cases are reported in older patients (10 to 12 years) and no breed or sex predilection has been determined.[1]

PATHOLOGY

The vast majority of salivary cancers are adenocarcinomas. They can arise from major (parotid, mandibular, sublingual, zygomatic) or minor glands. The parotid gland is most commonly affected. The tumors are locally very invasive, and metastasis to regional lymph nodes is common. Distant metastasis has been reported but may be slow to develop.

HISTORY AND CLINICAL SIGNS

Symptoms are nonspecific and generally include a unilateral, firm, painless swelling of the upper neck (mandibular and sublingual), base of the ear (parotid), upper lip or maxilla (zygomatic), or mucous membrane of lip (accessory or minor salivary tissue).

Major differential diagnoses are mucoceles, abscesses, or lymphosarcoma.

DIAGNOSTIC TECHNIQUES AND WORK-UP

Fine-needle aspiration cytology of masses in these locations should help differentiate mucoceles and abscesses from cancer. Regional radiographs will usually be normal but may reveal periosteal reaction on adjacent bones or displacement of surrounding structures. Needle core or wedge biopsies will usually be necessary to make a definitive diagnosis.

THERAPY

When possible, aggressive surgical removal should be performed. Unfortunately, most lesions are invasive and widely extensive throughout the region, which contains numerous vital structures.

Radiation therapy resulted in good local control and prolonged survival in three reported cases.[2] Chemotherapy for salivary gland adenocarcinoma has been largely unreported.

PROGNOSIS

The prognosis for salivary gland cancer is generally unknown. Clinical experience on a limited number of cases would indicate that aggressive local resection (usually histologically incomplete) followed by adjuvant radiation can attain permanent local control and long-term survival.[2]

COMPARATIVE ASPECTS[3]

Salivary gland tumors are more common in older humans than in animals and account for 4% of head and neck neoplasms. The parotid gland is most commonly affected. A wide array of benign and malignant neoplasms are recognized. Treatment is with surgical excision, and radiation is used for inoperable disease or after incomplete removal. Five-year survival usually exceeds 75% but is dependent on clinical stage at treatment and histologic type.

REFERENCES

1. Koestner A, Buerger L: Primary neoplasms of the salivary glands in animals compared to similar tumors in man. Pathol Vet 2:201–226, 1965
2. Evans SM, Thrall DE: Postoperative orthovoltage radiation therapy of parotid salivary gland adenocarcinoma in three dogs. J Am Vet Med Assoc 182:993–994, 1983
3. Million RR, Cassisi NJ, Wittes RE: Cancer in the head and neck. In DeVita VT (ed): Cancer: Principles and Practice of Oncology, pp. 301–395. Philadelphia, J.B. Lippincott, 1982

Esophageal Cancer

Stephen J. Withrow

INCIDENCE AND RISK FACTORS

Cancer of the esophagus is rare; it accounts for less than 0.5% of all cancer in the dog and cat.[1] Sarcomas secondary to *Spirocerca lupi* infestation have been reported in areas of Africa and the southeastern United States[2] (see Chapter 2). No cause is known for the more common carcinomas. Most animals affected are older, and no sex or breed predilection is evident.

PATHOLOGY AND NATURAL BEHAVIOR

The more commonly reported histologic types include squamous cell carcinoma, leiomyosarcoma, fibrosarcoma, and osteosarcoma. Rarely, benign neoplasms such as leiomyoma may be encountered.[1a] Paraesophageal tumors such as thymic, heart base, or thyroid may also invade the esophagus.[1] In cats, squamous cell carcinomas are usually seen in females and are located in the middle third of the esophagus just caudal to the thoracic inlet.[3,4]

Most esophageal cancers are locally invasive, and metastasis is to draining lymph nodes, hematogenously or by direct extension.

HISTORY AND SIGNS

Signs other than those of general debilitation and weight loss include pain on swallowing, dysphagia, and regurgitation of undigested food. Pneumonia secondary to aspiration may also be noted. Hypertrophic osteopathy has been reported, especially with *Spirocerca lupi*-induced sarcomas.[2]

DIAGNOSTIC TECHNIQUES AND WORK-UP

It is generally evident from the history that the patient is suffering from a partial or complete upper gastrointestinal obstruction. Plain radiographs may reveal retention of gas within the esophageal lumen, a mass, or esophageal dilation proximal to the cancer. A positive contrast esophagram with or without fluoroscopy generally reveals a stricture or mass lesion in the lumen.[1] Esophagoscopy allows visualization of the lesion, which is frequently ulcerated. Several biopsies should be taken because necrosis and inflammation are often prominent. The risk of esophageal perforation during the biopsy is generally minimal.

Open surgical biopsy via thoracotomy, abdominal exploratory, or cervical exploration is another option to obtain tissue for a diagnosis. *Spirocerca lupi* ova may be detected in the feces.

THERAPY

Therapy for malignant cancer of the esophagus is difficult at best because the disease in most cases is advanced.[5] Intrathoracic resections are further complicated by poor exposure, lengthy resections, tension on the anastomosis, and "normal" healing problems of the thoracic esophagus. For lesions in the caudal esophagus or cardia, gastric advancement through the diaphragm can be attempted.

Chemotherapy has rarely been attempted. Radiation therapy for the cervical esophagus can be attempted but is of limited value for the intrathoracic esophagus because large volumes of normal tissues, such as lung and heart, tolerate it poorly.

PROGNOSIS

Except for the rare, benign lesion or lymphosarcoma, the prognosis is very poor for cure or palliation.

COMPARATIVE ASPECTS[6]

Esophageal cancer (principally squamous cell carcinoma) is rare in humans, yet accounts for 7000 deaths per year in the United States. Marked geographic variance in worldwide incidence implies numerous environmental influences, including tobacco, alcohol, highly seasoned foods, and nitrosamines.

Most esophageal cancers have extensive local tumor growth and lymph node involvement, precluding curative treatment. Combinations or single use of surgery, radiation, and chemotherapy have resulted in 5-year survivals of less than 20% for the more common advanced disease. A variety of palliative bypass procedures for inoperable disease are also performed (esophagogastrostomy, intraluminal intubation, dilation, and gastrostomy).

REFERENCES

1. Ridgeway RL, Suter PF: Clinical and radiographic signs in primary and metastatic esophageal neoplasms of the dog. J Am Vet Med Assoc 174:700–704, 1979
1a. Hartzband LE: What is your diagnosis? Esophageal leiomyoma. J Am Vet Med Assoc 193:369–370, 1988

2. Bailey WS: *Spirocerca lupi:* A continuing inquiry. J Parasitol 58:3–22, 1972
3. Carpenter JL, Andrews LN, Holzworth J: Tumor and tumor-like lesion. In Holzworth J (ed): Diseases of the Cat, p. 492. Philadelphia, W.B. Saunders, 1987
4. Cotchin E: Neoplasms in cats. Proc R Soc Med 45:671, 1952
5. McCaw D, Pratt M, Walshaw R: Squamous cell carcinoma of the esophagus in a dog. J Am Anim Hosp Assoc 16:561–563, 1980
6. Rosenberg JC, Schwade JG, Vaitkevicius VK: Cancer of the esophagus. In DeVita VT (ed): Cancer: Principles and Practice of Oncology, pp. 499–533. Philadelphia, J.B. Lippincott, 1982

Exocrine Pancreas

Stephen J. Withrow

INCIDENCE AND RISK FACTORS

Exocrine cancer of the pancreas is very rare (< 0.5%) in the dog and even more uncommon in the cat.[1] Older female dogs have been described as being at higher risk.[2,3]

PATHOLOGY AND NATURAL BEHAVIOR

Almost all cancers of the pancreas are epithelial and most are adenocarcinomas of ductular or acinar origin. Nodular hyperplasia is a common asymptomatic finding in older dogs or cats. In the vast majority of cases, malignant cancer has metastasized to regional or distant sites before a diagnosis can be made.

HISTORY AND CLINICAL SIGNS

The history and clinical signs of pancreatic cancer are vague and nonspecific. Weight loss, anorexia, vomiting, abdominal distention, icterus (with common bile duct obstruction), and depression are common symptoms. Alternatively, patients may present with symptoms of metastatic disease. Abdominal effusions can develop because of tumor implants on the peritoneum or compression of the postcava.

DIAGNOSTIC TECHNIQUES AND WORK-UP

Most hematologic and biochemical evaluations are nonspecific; they may include mild anemia, neutrophilia, and bilirubinemia (if the common bile duct is occluded).[1] Elevations of serum amylase and lipase are inconsistent. In extreme cases, signs of pancreatic insufficiency may be exhibited.[4] Positive-contrast upper gastrointestinal radiographs may reveal slowed gastric emptying and occasionally compression or invasion of the duodenum.

Ascites may be a clinical sign and, when present, may reveal malignant cells on cytologic examination. Most tumors are not palpable through the abdominal wall.

Ultrasonography should be a useful diagnostic tool, but few reports exist to document its efficacy. Most diagnoses are made at exploratory laparotomy.

THERAPY

Most nonislet cell carcinomas of the pancreas are metastatic (regional lymph nodes and liver) or locally very invasive at the time of diagnosis. If the liver, peritoneal cavity, or draining lymph nodes are positive for tumor, heroic surgery should generally not be performed. Complete pancreatectomy or pancreaticoduodenectomy (Whipple's procedure) has been described in humans but carries a high operative mortality without significant cure rates.[5] Palliative gastrointestinal bypass (gastrojejunostomy) is a short-term option if bowel obstruction is imminent. Radiation and chemotherapy have shown limited value in humans and animals.

PROGNOSIS

The outlook for this disease in animals is very poor because of its critical location and advanced stage at diagnosis. One-year survival after diagnosis, regardless of treatment, has not been reported.[1]

COMPARATIVE ASPECTS[6]

Pancreatic exocrine carcinoma affects over 20,000 humans per year in the United States. In most patients disease has progressed beyond the pancreas at the time of initial diagnosis. Seventy-five percent of the cancers are located in the head of the pancreas, and the remainder in the body and tail. Direct extension to duodenum, bile duct, and stomach, as well as common metastasis to lymph node and liver, make treatment difficult.

When possible, pancreaticoduodenectomy (Whipple procedure) or complete pancreatectomy is the treatment of choice. However, operative mortality ranges from 5% to 30%. Palliative bypass of the biliary tree and duodenum is commonly performed for inoperative lesions.

Traditional external beam radiation therapy is generally palliative rather than curative. Intraoperative and interstitial radiation are being explored as means for delivering high dosages to the tumor while sparing normal radiosensitive structures. Chemotherapy alone or in combination with radiation or surgery has demonstrated some improvement in survival. Overall 5-year survival for all patients remains less than 5%.

REFERENCES

1. Davenport D: Pancreatic carcinoma in twenty dogs and five cats. Proceedings 5th Annual Vet Cancer Soc Meeting, W. Lafayette, Ind., 1985
2. Kircher CH, Nielson SW: Tumours of the pancreas. Bull WHO 53:195–202, 1976
3. Anderson NV, Johnson KH: Pancreatic carcinoma in the dog. J Am Vet Med Assoc 150:286–295, 1967
4. Bright JM: Pancreatic adenocarcinoma in a dog with a maldigestion syndrome. J Am Vet Med Assoc 187:420–421, 1985
5. Cobb LF, Merrell RC: Total pancreatectomy in dogs. J Surg Res 37:235–240, 1984
6. MacDonald JS, Gunderson LL, Cohn I: Cancer of the pancreas. In DeVita VT (ed): Cancer: Principles and Practice of Oncology, pp. 563–889. Philadelphia, J.B. Lippincott, 1982

Gastric Cancer

Stephen J. Withrow

INCIDENCE AND RISK FACTORS

Gastric cancer is more common than esophageal cancer but still accounts for less than 1% of all malignancies. No definitive etiology is known, although long-term administration of nitrosamines may induce carcinomas in dogs.[1] The average age of affected carcinoma patients is 8 years, with a 2.5:1 ratio of males to females. No clear-cut breed predilection has been identi-

fied.[2,3] Leiomyomas tend to occur in very old dogs (average age 15 years).[4]

PATHOLOGY AND NATURAL BEHAVIOR

Adenocarcinoma accounts for 60% to 70% of cancers of the canine stomach. It is often schirrous (firm and white serosally) and has been termed linitis plastica (leather bottle) because of its firm and nondistensible texture. Lesions can be diffusely infiltrative and expansile (often with a central crater and ulceration), or they may look more polypoid.[5] Other reported canine malignancies include leiomyosarcoma, lymphosarcoma, and fibrosarcoma. Leiomyosarcoma is less metastatic. Adenocarcinoma frequently spreads to regional lymph nodes (50% to 60% at necropsy) or to the liver and lung.[3,5,6] Adenocarcinomas have been described as diffuse or interstitial, but little clinical significance can be associated with these variants.[3] Benign lesions are generally leiomyomas, hypertrophic gastropathy, or adenomas.[7–11] Feline gastric adenocarcinoma is rare, and the stomach is the least commonly affected gastrointestinal site in the cat.[12,13] Lymphosarcoma is the most common gastric tumor in the cat and may be solitary or one component of systemic involvement. Most cats with gastric lymphosarcoma test negatively for feline leukemia virus.

HISTORY AND CLINICAL SIGNS

The most common history is one of progressive vomiting (the vomit is often tinged with blood or "coffee grounds"), anorexia, and weight loss. The weight loss may be a result of poor digestion, loss of protein and blood from an ulcer, or generalized cachexia. Duration of symptoms is from weeks to many months.

DIAGNOSTIC TECHNIQUES AND WORK-UP

Laboratory and noncontrast radiographs are generally not diagnostic. A microcytic hypochromic anemia is common. Occult blood in the feces may be detected. Liver enzymes may be elevated owing to hepatic metastasis or obstruction of the common bile duct. Thoracic radiographs are only rarely positive for metastasis.

Positive or double contrast gastric radiographs may reveal a mass lesion extending into the lumen (Fig. 19-8). Ulceration is also a common finding. Delayed gastric emptying, poor motility, or delayed adherence of contrast material

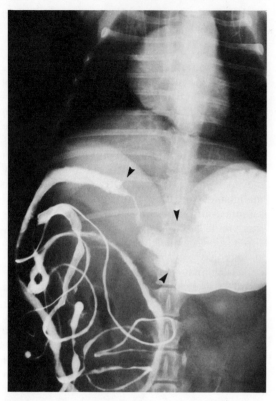

Figure 19-8. Ventrodorsal view of a dog with gastric cancer. Note filling defect and partial outflow obstruction of gastric antrum and pylorus.

to an ulcerated tumor may also be detected. Fluoroscopy may aid in determining motility alterations. Malignancies tend to be sessile, and adenocarcinoma tends to occur most commonly on the lesser curvature and gastric antrum (Fig. 19-9). Benign lesions may be pedunculated or well circumscribed.

Gastroscopy with a flexible endoscope generally reveals larger lesions that can be biopsied. Several samples should be taken because most gastric tumors have superficial necrosis, inflammation, and ulceration. In some patients, the lesions are submucosal only, making endoscopic biopsy difficult. False negative biopsies through the gastroscope may occur, however. Open surgical biopsy is the most definitive method of diagnosis.

THERAPY

Except for lymphosarcoma, surgery is the most common form of treatment for gastric cancer.

As with esophageal cancer, curative resection is complicated by advanced disease in a difficult operative area (lesser curvature, antrum, and pylorus) with a frequently debilitated patient. At the time of surgery, a careful evaluation of liver and regional lymph nodes should be made to stage the cancer adequately. Lymph node metastasis can be quite varied, and all abdominal lymph nodes should be examined. If the cancer is felt to be localized to the stomach at laparotomy, a curative resection may be attempted. If possible, wide partial gastrectomy or antrectomy followed by a gastroduodenostomy (Billroth I) should be performed because increased morbidity is associated with more extensive surgery, such as complete gastrectomy and gastrojejunostomy (Billroth II).[14] Lesions requiring biliary bypass and very extensive surgery (complete gastrectomy) are generally too advanced to make these procedures worthwhile in terms of survival. For obstructive lesions thought inoperable for cure, or metastatic, it is possible to perform a palliative gastrojejunostomy to allow passage of food into the intestine, although this procedure is associated with significant postoperative morbidity.[14a]

Radiation therapy is rarely used because surrounding normal tissue (liver and intestine) poorly tolerates it. Nonresectable lymphosarcoma may be dramatically reduced with lower doses of irradiation than are required for other tumors. No effective chemotherapy is known for adenocarcinoma.

Lymphosarcoma may be excised if it is localized, or it responds to conventional chemotherapy[15] (see Chapter 29). The need for postoperative chemotherapy after "complete" resection of lymphosarcoma is unknown. If a careful search of other body sites fails to reveal cancer and if the margins of resection are free of tumor, chemotherapy may not be necessary.

PROGNOSIS

The prognosis for most malignant gastric cancer is poor. Even if surgery can be performed, most patients are dead within 6 months as a result of recurrent or metastatic cancer.[16–19] Few adenocarcinoma patients are operable for cure, and the short-term morbidity with radical resection can be high. Palliation via bypass can be achieved for 1 to 6 months. Animals with benign lesions can be cured with complete surgical excision.

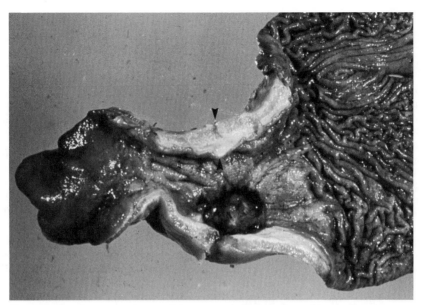

Figure 19-9. Gross specimen of the stomach from a dog with gastric adenocarcinoma. Note large ulcer and fibrous thickening of stomach wall in area of gastric antrum (arrow). This patient had metastasis to regional lymph nodes and liver.

COMPARATIVE ASPECTS

Gastric cancer is the sixth most common cause of cancer death in humans. Adenocarcinoma comprises over 90% of all malignant gastric cancers. Multiple socioeconomic, geographic, and environmental factors are associated with risk of tumor development.

Most lesions are firm, ulcerative, and located in the antrum or lower third of the stomach, as in the dog. Most are detected late in the course of disease and have direct tumor extension to surrounding organs, lymph node metastasis, or systemic metastasis.

Treatment is surgical resection when possible or less effective radiation and chemotherapy. Five-year survival for all patients is less than 10%; for those deemed operatively to have "localized" disease it is 30%.

REFERENCES

1. Sasajima K, Kawachi T, Sano T, et al: Esophageal and gastric cancers with metastasis induced in dogs by N-ethyl-N'-nitro-N nitrosoguanidine. J Natl Cancer Inst 58:1789–1794, 1977

2. Sautter JH, Hanlon GF: Gastric neoplasms in the dog: A report of 20 cases. J Am Vet Med Assoc 166:691–696, 1975

3. Patnaik AK, Hurvitz AI, Johnson GF: Canine gastric adenocarcinoma. Vet Pathol 15:600-607, 1978

4. Patnaik AK, Hurvitz AI, Johnson GF: Canine gastrointestinal neoplasms. Vet Pathol 14:547–555, 1977

5. Murray M, Robinson PB, McKeating FJ, et al: Primary gastric neoplasia in the dog: A clinico-pathological study. Vet Rec 91:474–479, 1972

6. Lingeman CH, Garner FM, Taylor DON: Spontaneous gastric adenocarcinomas of dogs: A review. J Natl Cancer Inst 47:137–149, 1971

7. Walter MC, Goldschmidt MH, Stone EA, et al: Chronic hypertrophic pyloric gastropathy as a cause of pyloric obstruction in the dog. J Am Vet Med Assoc 186:157–161, 1985

8. Kipnis RM: Focal cystic hypertrophic gastropathy in a dog. J Am Vet Med Assoc 173:182–184, 1978

9. Happe RP, Van Der Gaag W, Wolvekamp THC, Van Toorenburg J: Multiple polyps of the gastric mucosa in two dogs. J Small Anim Pract 18:179–189, 1977

10. Culbertson R, Branam JE, Rosenblatt LS:

Esophageal/gastric leiomyoma in the laboratory beagle. J Am Vet Med Assoc 183:1168–1172, 1983

11. Hayden DW, Nielsen SW: Canine alimentary neoplasia. Zbl Vet Med A20:1–22, 1973

12. Brodey RS: Alimentary tract neoplasms in the cat: A clinicopathologic survey of 46 cases. Am J Vet Res 27:74–80, 1966

13. Turk MAM, Gallina AM, Russell TS: Nonhematopoietic gastrointestinal neoplasia in cats: A retrospective study of 44 cases. Vet Pathol 18:614–620, 1981

14. Beaumont PR: Anastomotic jejunal ulcer secondary to gastrojejunostomy in a dog. J Am Anim Hosp Assoc 17:133–237, 1981

14a. Suka FA, Withrow SJ, Nelson AW et al: Billroth II gastrojejunostomy in dogs: Stapling technique and postoperative complications. Vet Surg 17:211–219, 1988

15. MacEwen EG, Mooney S, Brown NO, et al: Management of feline neoplasms. In Holzworth J (ed): Diseases of the Cat, Vol 1, pp. 597–606. Philadelphia, W.B. Saunders, 1987

16. Olivieri M, Gosselin Y, Sauvageau R: Gastric adenocarcinoma in a dog: Six-and-one-half month survival following partial gastrectomy and gastroduodenostomy. J Am Anim Hosp Assoc 20:78–82, 1984

17. Elliott GS, Stoffregen DA, Richardson DC, et al: Surgical, medical, and nutritional management of gastric adenocarcinoma in a dog. J Am Vet Med Assoc 185:98–101, 1984

18. Walter MC, Matthiesen DT, Stone EA: Pylorectomy and gastroduodenostomy in the dog: technique and clinical results in 28 cases. J Am Vet Med Assoc 187:909–914, 1985

19. McDonald AE: Primary gastric carcinoma of the dog: review and case report. Vet Surg 3:70–73, 1978

20. MacDonald JS, Gunderson LL, Cohen I: Cancer of the stomach. In DeVita VT (ed): Cancer: Principles and Practice of Oncology, pp. 534–562. Philadelphia, J.B. Lippincott, 1982

Hepatic Tumors

Nancy C. Postorino

INCIDENCE AND RISK

Primary hepatic tumors are rare. They account for 0.6% to 1.3% of all canine neoplasms,[1,2] and only a few feline cases have been reported.[3–7]

Most malignant hepatic tumors occur in older animals at an average age of 10 years.[1] No breeds appear to be at increased risk of developing primary liver tumors. The etiology is unknown, but experimental exposure to certain carcinogens, especially aflatoxins, pyrollizidine alkaloids, and diethylnitrosamine has been shown to induce primary hepatic tumors.[8,9] Metastatic tumors are more common than primary neoplasms in the liver because of the dual afferent blood supply of the hepatic artery and portal vein.[10]

PATHOLOGY AND NATURAL BEHAVIOR

Five neoplasms of epithelial origin affect the hepatobiliary system of domestic animals. These include hepatocellular carcinoma, bile duct carcinoma, hepatocellular adenoma, bile duct adenoma, and hepatoblastoma.[1,11] Carcinoid tumors of neuroectodermal origin also arise from the hepatobiliary system.[12] In the dog, bile duct adenomas are not clinically significant and hepatoblastomas have not been documented. Therefore, hepatocellular carcinoma, bile duct carcinoma, hepatocellular adenoma, and carcinoid tumors are the clinically significant tumor types that will be discussed in this section. Hepatocellular carcinomas are the most common malignant tumor of the canine and feline liver.[1] Males appear to be at increased risk for developing these tumors.[1,2] Grossly, hepatocellular carcinoma may be massive, nodular, or diffuse.[1] The massive form is the most common and consists of a large mass affecting a single liver lobe with smaller metastatic masses often scattered throughout other lobes of the liver. The left liver lobes are more often affected by massive hepatocellular carcinomas.[1] The nodular form of the disease consists of multiple discrete nodules of variable size within several lobes. In the diffuse form of hepatocellular carcinoma, large areas of the liver are infiltrated by nonencapsulated neoplastic tissue. The metastatic rate of these tumors is high and somewhat dependent on subtype; 100% of the diffuse, 93% of the nodular, and 36.6% of the massive type demonstrate metastasis at the time of diagnosis.[1] The most common metastatic sites are the hepatic lymph nodes, lung, and peritoneum.[1,12]

Bile duct carcinomas are the second most common primary hepatobiliary tumor of dogs.[12] Bile duct carcinomas occur more frequently in female dogs.[1] Three sites give rise to these tumors: intrahepatic bile ducts, extrahepatic bile ducts, and the gallbladder.[2,14] In dogs, intrahepatic bile ducts are the most common site of origin.[12] As with hepatocellular carcinoma, the disease has three gross forms: massive, nodular, and diffuse.[12] Bile duct carcinomas are highly metastatic tumors; the reported rate of metastasis is 87.5%.[2,12] The most common sites of metastasis are the hepatic lymph nodes, lung, and peritoneum.[14] The nodular and diffuse forms can sometimes be difficult to differentiate from nodular hyperplasia, cirrhosis, or chronic active hepatitis. The highly metastatic nature of this tumor helps differentiate it clinically from these other diseases.[12]

Hepatocellular adenomas are benign tumors that are more common than their malignant counterpart. They are usually single masses but can occur as multiple tumors and often are pedunculated. They can be difficult to differentiate histologically from nodular hyperplasia. However, compression of the surrounding hepatic parenchyma is characteristic of adenomas.

Carcinoid tumors arise from neuroectodermal tissue or the amine precursor uptake and decarboxylation (APUD) cells of the biliary epithelium. They are rare, accounting for less than 15% of all hepatic tumors.[15] They require specific silver stains to identify their characteristic intracytoplasmic granules.[12,15] Grossly they are diffuse, micronodular, or nodular tumors that affect all lobes of the liver.[15] Hemorrhage, necrosis, and calcification occur throughout these tumors. Because of their APUD origin, they may be capable of secreting vasoactive peptides and amines, but this has not been documented in the dog.[15] A metastatic rate of 90% is reported,[15] most commonly to the hepatic lymph nodes and peritoneum.[15]

The cat may develop primary liver tumors as well, although the incidence is rare. Benign and malignant tumors of hepatocellular origin occur, but hepatic adenomas are very rare. Carcinomas may be nodular, massive, or diffuse. Metastases at the time of diagnosis are found in 28% of cats with liver carcinomas. Tumors of the intrahepatic bile ducts are more common. Bile duct adenocarcinoma is the most frequently reported feline liver tumor. Females are more commonly affected; the incidence is reported to be 11 females to 3 males. Once again, the signs are nonspecific, and 78% of the tumors will have

metastasized to the lungs, lymph nodes, and intestinal serosa by the time of diagnosis.[3] Intrahepatic bile duct adenocarcinomas have been associated with liver fluke infestations.[3,4] Bile duct adenomas are also seen, being the third most common primary tumor type affecting the feline liver.[3] Other tumor types are rare; they include tumors of the extrahepatic bile ducts and the gallbladder.[3]

Myelolipomas are tumorlike nodules composed of mature adipose tissue and bone marrow elements, most commonly found in the adrenal glands, tissues of the paravertebral, intrathoracic, retroperitoneal, and presacral regions and the mesentery of man. They have been reported in both wild and domestic cats.[5–7]

Metastatic liver tumors are more common than primary ones in both the dog and the cat. Metastasis from any site may occur, but the most common primary tumors are gastrointestinal tumors, hemangiosarcomas, pancreatic tumors, and mammary adenocarcinomas. The history and clinical presentation will often mimic primary hepatic tumors.[2]

HISTORY AND CLINICAL SIGNS

Animals with hepatic tumors usually present with variable histories of vague, nonspecific clinical signs, such as anorexia, weight loss, vomiting, and polydipsia.[2,9] Most gallbladder tumors do not show clinical signs until the gallbladder is occluded. Occasionally, an animal may show signs of central nervous system disease due to hepatoencephalopathy or hypoglycemia secondary to the tumor.

Physical examination may reveal a palpable cranial abdominal mass as well as abdominal distention from ascites or hemoperitoneum.[9] Pale mucous membranes are a common finding, but it is quite rare for the animal to be clinically icteric.[1,12]

DIAGNOSIS AND WORK-UP

The most consistent laboratory abnormalities are increased serum alkaline phosphatase (ALP) secondary to cholestasis and increased serum alanine aminotransferase (SALT) and serum aspartate aminotransferase (SAST) caused by hepatocellular necrosis or increased enzyme production by neoplastic tissues.[2,13] In humans, the ratio of SAST to SALT is suggestive of histologic type. Hepatocellular carcinomas are associated with a ratio of greater than 1:1, and bile duct carcinomas usually give ratios of less than 1:1. In one series of canine patients, a ratio of less than 1:1 was associated with hepatocellular or bile duct carcinoma, and a ratio of greater than 1:1 was associated with sarcomas or carcinoid tumors.[1] It is rare for the serum bilirubin or sulfobromophthalein (BSP) retention to be elevated. Serum protein levels are usually within normal limits, although one study showed elevations in globulin levels along with decreases in albumin levels.[2] These changes may be explained by alterations in hepatic synthesis and degradation as well as possible increased antigenic stimulation resulting in increased globulin production. Serum bile acid levels will be elevated with hepatic neoplasia, but this is not definitive for tumors.[16] A nonregenerative anemia is a common finding due to anemia of chronic disease. However, regenerative anemia can occur if the tumor actively bleeds into the peritoneum.[1,9]

Hypoglycemia is another reported abnormality that can be attributed to the tumor's increased use of glucose or production of hormones with insulinlike activity.[2] The liver's decreased production of clotting factors can cause coagulation abnormalities. The most consistent clotting abnormalities associated with hepatic neoplasia are shortened thrombin clotting time, decreased Factor VIII:C levels, and increased Factor VIII:Ag levels.[17] A coagulogram should be performed in all cases prior to biopsy or any surgical procedure.

Abdominocentesis should be performed in animals presented with ascites. In some cases, neoplastic cells can be identified in the fluid, especially when peritoneal metastases are present. Other diagnostic tests include abdominal radiography to help localize the abdominal mass to the liver. Abdominal ultrasound may be used to characterize the internal structure of the tumor, to confirm the organ of origin, to aid in defining the extent of the disease, and possibly to identify previously undetected metastases.[10,18] Thoracic radiographs should be performed on patients with suspect hepatic tumors to identify pulmonary metastases.

Despite all these noninvasive techniques, neoplastic tissue must be obtained to arrive at a definitive diagnosis of hepatic tumor. Tissues may be obtained via percutaneous biopsy, laparoscopy, or laparotomy. Laparotomy is the most definitive method and has the advantage of being both diagnostic and in some cases therapeutic as well. Percutaneous liver biopsy or laparoscopic biopsy is considered when the disease is diffuse and surgical treatment is considered unlikely.

TREATMENT

Surgical excision is the treatment of choice for hepatic tumors (Fig. 19-10).[19] Because they are insidious, many tumors are nonresectable by the time of presentation. Up to 75% of the liver may be resected without significant clinical dysfunction.[9] Hepatic regeneration occurs rapidly and is usually complete within 6 to 8 weeks. There are no controlled studies in veterinary medicine to support the use of chemotherapy for nonresectable hepatic tumors or as an adjuvant treatment. Remissions are reported for humans with hepatic tumors,[13,19] but the overall response rates and survival times are less than encouraging. Hepatic dearterialization has been described in the dog[20] and may be a palliative treatment for unresectable primary hepatic tumors.

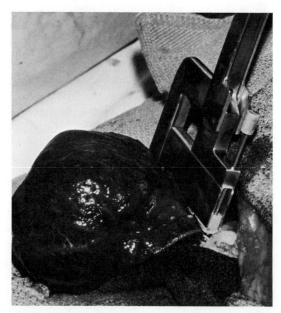

Figure 19-10. Dog with hepatic adenoma at surgery. Mass was removed with staples, and dog is alive and free of disease at 18 months.

PROGNOSIS

The prognosis for benign hepatic tumors following excision is good; survival times greater than 2 years have been reported.[9] Malignant hepatic tumors carry a poor prognosis, even when resection is possible and no visible metastases are noted at surgery. Survival times of less than 80 days following surgery are reported for most malignant hepatic cancer.[9] The size of the tumor is not a reliable indicator of prognosis because many large, solitary, well-encapsulated tumors can be successfully removed.[9] It appears that the degree of invasiveness and resectability, as well as the presence of metastases, are the most reliable indicators of survival.[9]

The prognosis for cats with primary liver tumors is poor because most of the tumors have metastasized by the time of diagnosis.[3] The prognosis following surgical excision of myelolipomas is good; most animals are free of the disease more than 1 year after treatment.[5]

COMPARATIVE ASPECTS

Primary tumors of the hepatobiliary system are rare and highly lethal tumors in man. Gallbladder carcinoma is the most common tumor type followed by hepatocellular carcinoma and cholangiocarcinoma. Two-thirds of hepatocellular carcinomas are the nodular form, 30% are massive, and 5% are diffuse. An encapsulated form also occurs in 4% of the cases and is less aggressive than other forms of the disease. Adenocarcinomas represent 85% of all the tumors that occur in the gallbladder and bile duct.[21]

The etiology of hepatobiliary tumors is unknown, but an increased frequency has been associated with preexisting liver disease, especially cirrhosis, hepatitis B infections, steroid and hormone therapy, cholelithiasis, liver fluke infestations, and ulcerative colitis.[21]

As in other animals, clinical signs are nonspecific; abdominal pain, jaundice, weight loss, and an acute onset of ascites are common. Unfortunately, the similarity of symptoms of benign and malignant disease often confuses the diagnosis. Surgery is the treatment of choice, but because the symptoms are vague, the disease is often advanced beyond the limits of excision at the time of diagnosis. Radiation therapy can be effective, though the liver tolerates only a limited dosage of radiation. Chemotherapy is used for advanced neoplasms. Mitomycin-C has shown the best results, and responses have been reported with combinations of doxorubicin, bleomycin, and 5-fluorouracil. Hepatic artery infusion is useful for delivering chemotherapy directly to the tumor.[21]

Prognosis is poor. Patients treated with resection have a 5-year survival rate of less than 20%, and in advanced, unresectable tumors, the 5-year survival rate is zero.[21]

REFERENCES

1. Patnaik AK, Hurvitz AI, Lieberman PH: Canine hepatic neoplasms: A clinicopathologic study. Vet Pathol 17:553–564, 1980

2. Strombeck DR: Clinicopathologic features of primary and metastatic neoplastic disease of the liver in dogs. J Am Vet Med Assoc 173:267–269, 1978

3. Carpenter JL, Andrews LK, Holzworth J: Tumors and tumor-like lesions. In Holzworth J (ed): Diseases of the Cat, pp. 500–505. Philadelphia, W.B. Saunders, 1987

4. Feldman BF, Strafuss AC, Gabbert N: Bile duct carcinoma in the cat: Three case reports. Fel Pract, pp. 33–39, Jan, 1976

5. Gourley IM, Popp JA, Park RD: Myelolipomas of the liver in a domestic cat. J Am Vet Med Assoc 158:2053–2057, 1974

6. Ikede BO, Downey RS: Multiple hepatic myelolipomas in a cat. Can Vet J 13:160–163, 1972

7. Lombard LS, Fortna HM, et al: Myelolipomas of the liver in captive wild felidae. Vet Pathol 5:127–134, 1968

8. Hirao K et al: Primary neoplasms in dog liver induced by diethylnitrosamine. Cancer Res 34:1870–1882, 1974

9. Liska W: Canine hepatomas and hepatocellular carcinomas. Resident seminar presented at The Animal Medical Center, New York, NY, April 9, 1975

10. Nyland TG, Park RD: Hepatic ultrasonography in the dog. Vet Radiol 24:74–84, 1983

11. Strombeck DR: Hepatic neoplasms. In (ed): Small Animal Gastroenterology. Santa Barbara, Stonegate Publishing, 1979

12. Patnaik AK, Hurvitz AI, et al: Canine bile duct carcinoma. Vet Pathol 18:439–444, 1981

13. Al-Sarraf M, Kithier K, Vaitkevivius VK: Primary liver cancer: A review of clinical features, blood groups, serum enzymes, therapy and survival of 65 cases. Cancer 33:574–582, 1974

14. Strafuss AC: Bile duct carcinoma in dogs. J Am Vet Med Assoc 169:429, 1976

15. Patnaik AK, Lieberman PH, et al: Canine hepatic carcinoids. Vet Pathol 18:445–453, 1981

16. Center SA, Baldwin BH, et al: Bile acid concentrations in the diagnosis of hepatobiliary disease in the dog. J Am Vet Med Assoc 187:935–940, 1985

17. Badylak SF, Dodds WJ, Van Vleet JF: Plasma coagulation factor abnormalities in dogs with naturally occurring hepatic disease. Am J Vet Res 44:2336–2340, 1983

18. Feeney DA, Johnston GR, Hardy RM: Two-dimensional gray-scale ultrasonography for assessment of hepatic and splenic neoplasia in the dog and cat. J Am Vet Med Assoc 184:68–81, 1984

19. Evans AE, Land VJ, et al: Combination chemotherapy (vincristine, adriamycin, cyclophosphamide, and 5-fluorouracil) in the treatment of children with malignant hepatoma. Cancer 50:821–826, 1982

20. Gunn C, Gourley IM, Koblick PD: Hepatic dearterialization in the dog. Am J Vet Res 47:170–175, 1986

21. MacDonald JS, Gunderson LL, Adson MA: Cancer of the hepatobiliary system. In DeVita VT (ed): Cancer: Principles and Practice of Oncology, pp. 590–615. Philadelphia, J.B. Lippincott, 1982

Tumors of the Intestinal Tract

Rodney C. Straw

INCIDENCE AND RISK FACTORS

Tumors of the intestine are uncommon in domestic animals; they represent less than 1% of all malignancies. Intestinal tumors occur most commonly in the rectum or colon of dogs and the small intestine of cats. No definitive etiologic factors for development of intestinal neoplasia are known for the dog or the cat.

Adenocarcinoma is the most common intestinal tumor in the dog,[1] and leiomyosarcoma is the most common sarcoma.[2] Adenomatous polyps are reported to be the most common tumor in the canine rectum.[3] In the feline intestinal tract, lymphosarcoma is reported most frequently,[4-7] then adenocarcinoma and mast cell

tumor.[8] Other tumors affecting the intestinal tract include fibrosarcoma,[9,10] undifferentiated sarcoma,[1] carcinoids,[11-15] leiomyomas,[1,3] plasmacytoma,[3,3a] and neurolemmoma.[16] A ganglioneuroma and a neoplasm of globule leukocytes have been reported in cats.[17,18]

Carcinoma of the intestine occurs in older animals. The mean age of affected dogs is 9 years (range, 1 to 14 years) and 10 years for cats (range, 2 to 17 years). One study of nonlymphoid intestinal neoplasia reported that male dogs outnumbered females (21:11) and that female cats were affected more often than males cats (9:5),[1] although others have reported no sex predisposition for feline nonlymphoid gastrointestinal neoplasia.[19,20]

Siamese cats are reported to have a higher frequency of small intestinal adenocarcinoma than other breeds.[1,19-21] In one report 70% of cats with small intestinal adenocarcinoma were Siamese; however, cats with adenocarcinoma of the cecum, colon, and rectum were more commonly domestic cats.[8] Boxers,[22] collies,[8] and German shepherds[8] may be predisposed to development of intestinal cancer, although in a recent series none of the canine breeds were overrepresented.[1]

Leiomyosarcomas of the intestines of dogs were diagnosed in less than 0.2% of 10,270 canine necropsies reviewed.[16] They occur most commonly in the cecum and jejunum, and the mean and median age of affected dogs is 11 and 10.5 years.[1,2,16] One report indicated that younger dogs may be affected with small intestinal leiomyosarcoma.[23] There is no apparent breed predilection, and females may be more commonly affected than males.[16]

Lymphosarcoma occurs predominantly in middle-aged dogs, and there is conflicting data in the literature regarding a possible sex predilection. In one study of 144 canine lymphosarcoma cases, 6.9% were alimentary in origin.[24] Lymphosarcoma of the feline intestine is often part of a multicentric disease.[19] In a study of 76 cases of feline alimentary lymphoma which excluded cats with multicentric disease, there appeared to be no breed or sex predilection.[25] The mean age of affected cats was 10.6 years (range, 4 to 17 years) and the small intestine was the most common site (41/76) with the jejunum and ileum most frequently affected.[25] These tumors are thought to arise from B-lymphocytes in the lamina propria.[8,26] In one study, 41 cats with intestinal lymphosarcoma were tested for the presence of feline leukemia virus, and 4.9% were positive[25] (see Chapter 29).

Mast cell tumors are more common in the feline than the canine intestine. The mean age for cats with mast cell tumors of the intestine is 13 years (range, 7 to 21 years). All reported cases, in a series of 28, occurred in domestic short- or longhairs, and there was no sex predilection.[8] A primary mast cell tumor in the ileocecal region has been described in a dog.[27]

Intestinal carcinoids occur rarely and affect older dogs. No sex or breed predisposition has been determined. In dogs, carcinoids are mainly located in the duodenum, colon, and rectum.[22] Six cases of intestinal carcinoids, and one case of adenocarcinoid have been reported in dogs.[13-15] Intestinal carcinoids have been reported in the cat; most feline carcinoids develop in the stomach or small intestine.[11]

PATHOLOGY AND NATURAL BEHAVIOR

Intestinal neoplasms in dogs and cats are usually malignant. Of nonlymphoid intestinal neoplasms in 32 dogs and 14 cats, 88% of the canine tumors and all of the feline tumors were malignant.[1] Half of the canine rectal tumors showed transition from benign polypoid lesions to adenocarcinomas in one study.[13] Some polypoidlike lesions are malignant, and those greater than 1.0 cm in diameter generally have a more anaplastic appearance, may recur after excision,

and may progress to become invasive adenocarcinoma.[22]

Adenocarcinoma of the canine and feline intestine is usually in an advanced stage at the time of diagnosis. Extension of the neoplasm beyond the bowel wall was found in 86% of dogs at necropsy;[1] lymph nodes, liver, lungs, and adjoining sections of the gastrointestinal wall were the most common sites of metastasis.[13] Results of a study of small intestinal adenocarcinoma in 32 cats indicated that 71% had gross or histologic evidence of metastatic disease at the time of diagnosis.[20] In cats, the most common metastatic sites are abdominal serosa, followed by lymph nodes, lung, and liver.[19] Regional lymph node metastasis was identified in 5 of 11 cats with gastrointestinal carcinoma.[20a]

Adenocarcinoma has been described as annular when the lumen is constricted 360° by tumor (Fig. 19-11), or as intraluminal when there is neoplastic growth into the lumen as well as infiltration into the wall.[13] One histologic classification divides canine adenocarcinoma into four groups that may overlap: acinar, solid, mucinous, and papillary.[22] Acinar adenocarcinoma may be either annular or intraluminal. Papillary forms are usually intraluminal, and mucinous adenocarcinomas are annular in the small intestine but intraluminal in the rectum.[13]

Tumors involving large bowel may grow slowly and spread predominantly horizontally with few distant metastases; this is often the case with papillary adenocarcinoma.[13,22] Acinar, solid, and mucinous adenocarcinoma tend to show more

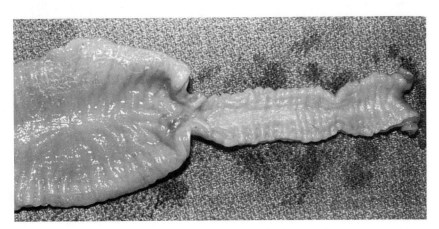

Figure 19-11. Gross specimen of annular intestinal adenocarcinoma removed from the cat in Fig. 19-15. This patient survived 18 months and succumbed to lymph node and omental metastasis.

vertical growth and to extend into bowel wall, serosa, and other organs. There is one case report of a signet ring carcinoma of the colon with secondary meningeal carcinomatosis.[22a]

The clinical and gross appearance of feline intestinal adenocarcinoma is similar to that in dogs.[22] In cats, the tumors have been reported to be located most frequently in the jejunum; the second most frequent location is the ileum and least frequent the ileocecal region.[20] Similar morphologic types are described, and osteochondroid metaplasia is a frequent feature of adenocarcinoma in the cat.[19,22]

Leiomyosarcomas of the canine intestine are locally invasive, malignant smooth muscle neoplasms that are slow to metastasize, although extension to regional lymph nodes has been reported.[2] Dogs with these tumors can be asymptomatic, and the diagnosis may be an incidental finding at necropsy or exploratory surgery (Fig. 19-12). Some animals are presented because of melena and may have anemia.

Animals with the alimentary form of lymphoma may have focal or diffuse neoplastic infiltrates of the bowel wall (Fig. 19-13) which may also involve the mesenteric lymph nodes, liver, and spleen.

Carcinoids can be expansile and infiltrative, and larger neoplasms are usually more malignant and likely to metastasize, especially to the liver.[13,22] Feline intestinal mast cell tumors metastasize to the mesenteric lymph nodes most commonly; other metastatic sites include the liver, the spleen, and rarely, the lungs.[22]

HISTORY AND SIGNS

The most common finding in animals with intestinal neoplasia is weight loss of several days to over 6 months' duration.[1,19] The tumor may cause ulceration of the intestinal mucosa and resultant hemorrhage. Intestinal obstruction or abscessation may also occur. Septic peritonitis was associated with a duodenal leiomyosarcoma in a dog.[23] Vomiting, anorexia, and depression are also commonly found. Less common signs include constipation, icterus, diarrhea, ascites, melena, and dehydration. Tenesmus, hematochezia, dyschezia, and occasionally intermittent anal eversion may be seen in dogs with colorectal neoplasia.[3,13,21,28,29] Signs of obstructive bowel disease may be present or a malabsorption syndrome may occur, especially with diffuse lymphosarcoma. Tumor infiltrates may occasionally obstruct lymphatics and lead to steatorrhea due to lymphangiectasia. Carcinoids of the small bowel are usually slow growing. The clinical signs may be related to the primary tumor—that is, nonspecific pain and intermittent obstruction with associated vomiting. Bleeding is unusual. Although not documented in dogs, carcinoid tumors may be associated with clinical features dependent on hormones or amines produced by the tumor. The most common clinical signs are chronic diarrhea and weight loss. Serotonin (5-HT) is commonly associated with carcinoids in humans.

DIAGNOSTIC TECHNIQUES AND WORK-UP

An abdominal mass, dilated intestinal loops, thickened bowel or intra-abdominal lymphadenopathy may be detected on careful abdominal palpation. Adenomatous polyps or carcinoids may evert through the anus. Most rectal cancer can be detected on digital palpation as firm annular rings. In a study of canine colorectal adenocarcinoma, 63% (49/78) of the dogs had masses that were palpable on rectal exam.[29]

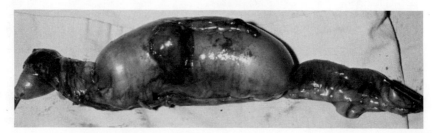

Figure 19-12. Gross specimen of the small intestinal leiomyosarcoma removed from the dog in Fig. 19-14. This patient is alive and free of disease more than 2 years postoperatively.

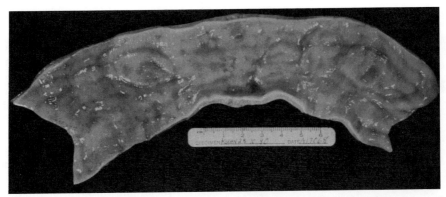

Figure 19-13. Gross specimen of bowel from a cat with diffuse alimentary form of lymphosarcoma.

Hematologic and biochemical profiles are often normal although anemia or hypoproteinemia may be present owing to bleeding into the intestine.

Pulmonary metastases are rarely detected on thoracic radiography. Plain abdominal radiographs may reveal a mass, enlarged lymph nodes, or signs of intestinal obstruction. Positive-contrast upper gastrointestinal studies may delineate an intramural (Fig. 19-14) or annular (Fig. 19-15) lesion, and diffuse intestinal neoplasia may appear as ragged filling defects along the bowel wall. Barium enemas may help establish the extent of colorectal tumors (Fig. 19-16) and double-contrast studies may define small lesions.[29a] Colonoscopy and proctoscopic examination can be a valuable diagnostic aid in the identification and biopsy of lesions of the colon and rectum, and because adenocarcinoma can be diffuse or have multiple lesions, endoscopy is recommended for staging and planning treatment.[29,30] A definitive diagnosis of intestinal neoplasia can only be made on histologic examination of biopsy material.

THERAPY

The most common treatment for intestinal neoplasia is surgical resection. Margins of at least 4 to 8 cm should be strived for. Suspicious lesions (especially in the liver and regional lymph nodes) should be biopsied during abdominal procedures. Careful attention to surgical technique in anastomosis is important owing to the

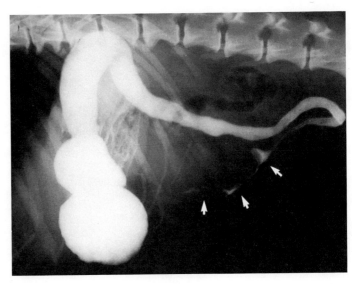

Figure 19-14. Lateral projection of an upper gastrointestinal contrast study of a dog with intestinal leiomyosarcoma. Note the intramural filling defect in the small intestine (arrows).

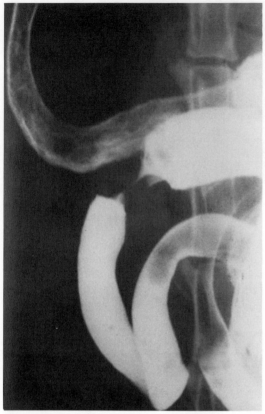

Figure 19-15. Ventrodorsal projection of an upper gastrointestinal contrast study of a cat with annular intestinal adenocarcinoma. Note typical "apple core" like lesion.

frequent debilitated state of the patient and potential for poor healing.

Tumors of the small intestine, cecum, and colon are treated by means of a midline abdominal approach. Tumors of the rectum (especially adenocarcinoma) pose special problems for the surgeon (Fig. 19-17). About one-half of dogs with midrectal adenocarcinoma (a site where >50% of these tumors occur) have luminal obstruction requiring resection to alleviate signs.[29] Various techniques, such as end-to-end anastomosis (usually requiring a pelvic osteotomy for access), rectal pull-through, or the dorsal rectal approach have been described.[31,32] However, the short length of mesorectum, the location of the affected segment within the bony pelvis, and the problems associated with surgery of the large intestine cause significant morbidity (infection, incontinence, dehiscence, and stricture) and mortality when wide removals are undertaken. Considering the morbidity, mortality (3 out of 4 in one report[29]), and poor tumor control achieved for large invasive rectal tumors, it is questionable whether surgery should be undertaken in some cases. Local excision and cryosurgery for adenocarcinoma of the colon have significantly extended the life of dogs compared with other methods of surgical treatment; however, 82% (9/11) treated with cryosurgery suffered complications (rectal prolapse, stricture, perineal hernia, and recurrence).[29] Electrosurgery or laser surgery may be considered where

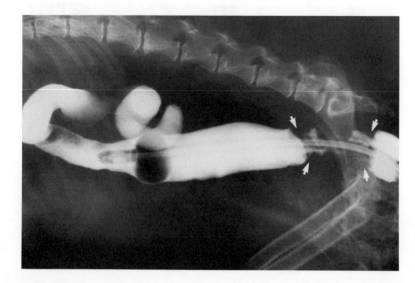

Figure 19-16. Positive-contrast barium enema in a dog showing a prepelvic and intrapelvic rectal adenocarcinoma (arrows).

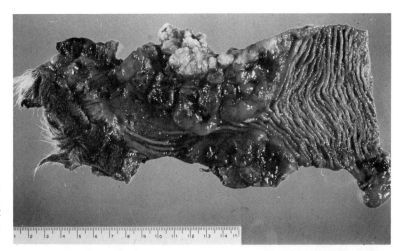

Figure 19-17. Gross specimen of rectal adenocarcinoma from a dog. Tumor usually occurs at pelvic brim, making resection difficult.

rectal adenocarcinoma is not annular and is in a distal location where it can be completely prolapsed.

Rectal polyps may be pedunculated or have a sessile base (Figs. 19-18 and 19-19). Most polyps are within 2 cm of the anus. They may be multiple but usually appear singularly. They are treated by surgical excision, electrosurgery, or cryosurgery. Masses that are not accessible by digital exteriorization require rectal pro-

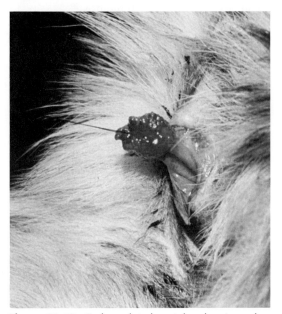

Figure 19-18. Pedunculated rectal polyp in a dog. This mass was biopsied and frozen and has not recurred in more than 2 years.

lapse.[33] With epidural anesthesia, which provides excellent muscle relaxation, gentle traction applied to four stay sutures placed equidistantly around the rectum in the mucosal folds allows exposure of the lesion. Polyps with sessile bases are best managed with cryosurgery or electrosurgery.[33] Once the mass is exposed, its stalk is transfixed with a ligature and the mass is removed. The base is then frozen with a cryoprobe.

Surgery is indicated in obstructive intestinal lymphosarcoma or where bowel perforation has occurred. Biopsies and cytologic evaluation of impression smears of adjacent intestine, lymph nodes, spleen, and liver should be performed to clinically stage the disease. Chemotherapy protocols for lymphosarcoma can be employed as adjuvant therapy or as the major form of therapy in diffuse disease (see Chapter 29). Diffuse canine alimentary lymphosarcoma does not respond as well to chemotherapy as multicentric disease, but solitary or nodular gastrointestinal lymphosarcoma responds better to chemotherapy. In a study of 23 cats with alimentary lymphosarcoma treated with L-asparaginase, vincristine, cyclophosphamide, methotrexate and prednisone, the mean survival time was 25.3 weeks.[25] The method of diagnosis (lesional biopsy or resection of a solitary tumor) did not affect survival time. In this report, four cats received prednisone alone; their mean survival was 7.3 weeks.

High-dosage radiotherapy has been reported as a treatment for adenocarcinomas of the distal half of the rectum and anal canal.[34] The rectum was prolapsed with stay sutures, and doses of

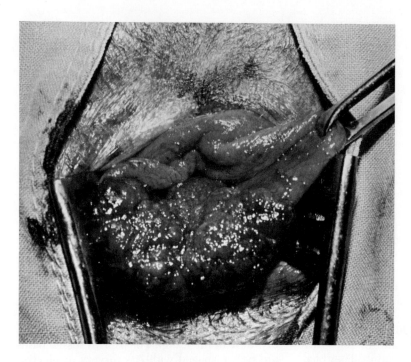

Figure 19-19. Canine adenomatous polyp with a sessile base.

between 15 and 25 Gy were delivered from an orthovoltage x-ray teletherapy unit with the beam restricted by a cone. The cone diameter was 1 cm greater than the diameter of grossly visible tumor. In early or small recurrent lesions in six dogs ($T_1N_0M_0$ and $T_2N_0M_0$), the treatment was technically feasible and safe; toxicity was limited to occasional, transient tenesmus. Three dogs had no evidence of disease at 5, 6, and 31 months, and 3 others had local recurrence at 1, 6, and 7 months. High-dosage radiotherapy may represent a suitable alternative to surgery for selected cases.

Adjuvant chemotherapy for intestinal adenocarcinoma and leiomyosarcoma has been recommended,[35] but the efficacy of such treatment has not been reported in the dog and cat.

PROGNOSIS

Twenty-three dogs with colonic or rectal intestinal adenocarcinoma treated only with fecal softeners had a mean survival time of 15 months.[29] Clinical signs of metastasis were not observed in any of the 78 dogs with colorectal adenocarcinoma in the same study. In another study, dogs with surgically managed malignant epithelial tumors had a mean survival time of 6.9 months; local recurrence was the reason for euthanasia in every case.[30] Dogs with single, pedunculated, polypoid adenocarcinoma lesions had a mean survival time of 32 months; those with nodular or cobblestonelike lesions had a mean survival time of 1.6 months.[29]

Dogs with colonic or rectal intestinal adenocarcinoma are usually euthanized because of failure to control dyschezia and hematochezia. The surgeon must consider control of these clinical signs an important goal. A prognosis is based on the ability to achieve this goal. The form and severity of disease are also prognostic indicators.

In one report, 23 cats with small intestinal adenocarcinoma were treated with intestinal resection and end-to-end anastomosis. Eleven cats either died or were euthanatized within 2 weeks of surgery. Twelve cats survived an average of 15 months following surgery (range 1.5 to 50 months). Five of these cats were staged with extension to mesenteric lymph nodes, two had disease confined to the bowel, and five were not staged. Five cats died with known or suspected recurrence, five died of unknown causes, one was euthanatized for an unrelated cause, and one was alive at 50 months after surgery. The five cats with known lymph node metastasis had a mean survival time of 12 months.[20] The median survival time of 10 cats with gastrointestinal adenocarcinoma treated surgically was 2.5 months (range 0 to 24 mos.) However, in this report, those cases that died of non-tumor causes were not censored from the survival statistics.[20a]

An excellent prognosis can be expected with completely excised polyps; however, recurrence is possible, especially with large or sessile lesions. Malignant transformation is also possible.[30]

Diffuse intestinal lymphoma carries a poor prognosis; solitary nodular lymphoma does better. Insufficient data are available to adequately evaluate the prognosis for patients with intestinal carcinoids; however, surgical resection is recommended where possible. One report suggested a favorable prognosis after complete surgical resection of canine intestinal leiomyosarcoma.[2] In this study, 3 of 5 dogs treated with surgical resection were alive a minimum of 12 months following resection with no evidence of recurrence or metastasis. Two dogs developed metastasis, 3 months and 12 months postexcision, and 1 dog died 1 month postexcision with no evidence of metastasis or local recurrence. In a report of dogs with small intestinal carcinomas, 4 were treated with surgical excision and 3 of these survived 6 months or longer.[29a]

COMPARATIVE ASPECTS

Small intestinal neoplasms are rare in humans; they account for about 1% of all gastrointestinal malignancies.[36] Colorectal cancer, however, is one of the most common internal malignancies in the United States; there are approximately 140,000 cases per year.[37,38] No factors have been definitely implicated in the etiology of small intestinal or colorectal neoplasia, although it appears likely to be related to carcinogens within the bowel lumen. A low-fat, high-fiber diet, as well as selenium and calcium, may be protective. It has been speculated that local factors in the small intestine (alkaline pH, rapid transit, less abrasive contents than colon, high level of benzopyrene hydroxylase in small bowel mucosa, high concentration of IgA, and relative absence of bacteria) may function to prevent the development of cancer or to clear or deactivate potential carcinogens. Some bowel diseases have a high predilection for colorectal cancer; these include familial polyposis syndromes and chronic ulcerative colitis. A family history of colorectal

cancer increases the risk of developing colon cancer 3-fold. Although there is some debate as to the origin of colorectal cancer, there is good evidence for a transition of adenomatous polyps to carcinoma. It is not known how often colorectal cancer arises in previously benign polyps, but it seems that the longer polyps are allowed to grow and the larger they become, the greater the likelihood that cancer will develop from them. Different types of polyps have different potentials for malignant transformation. Villous polyps have 10 times the malignant potential, and intermediate type 6 to 7 times the malignant potential, that adenomatous polyps have.[37]

Treatment is surgical resection of bowel and adjacent mesentry. Radiation therapy may minimize local recurrence, and there is intense interest currently in the use of intraoperative radiation as an adjuvant to surgery. Chemotherapy has limited value in advanced colorectal cancer and has minimal benefit as an adjuvant to surgery.

Many prognostic variables affect the survival of people with colorectal cancer (clinical and anatomic features that can be determined from history, physical examination, radiologic examination, endoscopic examination, and pathologic variables determined from a study of the resected specimen); however, the survival rates after "curative resection" largely depend on tumor stage. With negative lymph nodes and tumor contained within the bowel wall, 5-year survival is 86%, but for patients with positive lymph nodes and disease seen grossly through the wall, 5-year survival is 22%.

REFERENCES

1. Birchard SJ, Couto CG, Johnson S: Nonlymphoid intestinal neoplasia in 32 dogs and 14 cats. J Am Anim Hosp Assoc 22:533–537, 1986
2. Bruecker KA, Withrow SJ: Intestinal leiomyosarcomas in six dogs. J Am Anim Hosp Assoc 24:281–284, 1987
3. Holt PE, Lucke VM: Rectal neoplasia in the dog: A clinicopathological review of 31 cases. Vet Rec 116:400–405, 1985
3a. MacEwen EG, Patnaik AK, Johnson GF et al: Extramedullary plasmacytoma of the gastrointestinal tract in two dogs. J Am Vet Med Assoc 184:1396–1398, 1984
4. Brodey RS: Alimentary tract neoplasms in the cat: A clinicopathologic survey of 46 cases. Am J Vet Res 27:74–80, 1966

5. Cotchin E: Some tumors of dogs and cats of comparative veterinary and human interest. Vet Rec 71:1040–1050, 1959

6. Engle GG, Brodey RS: A retrospective study of 395 feline neoplasms. J Am Anim Hosp Assoc 5:21–31, 1969

7. Head KW: Tumors of the lower alimentary tract. Bull WHO 53:167–186, 1976

8. Carpenter JL, Andrews LK, Holzworth J: Tumors and tumor-like lesions. In Holzworth J (ed): Diseases of the Cat Medicine and Surgery, pp. 406–596. Philadelphia, W.B. Saunders, 1987

9. Howard DR, Schirmer RG, Ulrey VM, Michel RL: Adenocarcinoma in the ileum of a young dog. J Am Vet Med Assoc 162:956–958, 1973

10. Brodey RS, Cohen D: An epizootiological and clinicopathological study of 95 cases of gastrointestinal neoplasms in the dog. Proceedings of the 101st Annual Meeting, Am Vet Med Assoc, pp. 167–179. Chicago, Am Vet Med Assoc, 1964

11. Carakostas MC, Kennedy GA, Kittleson MD, Cook JE: Malignant foregut carcinoid in a domestic cat. Vet Pathol 16:607–609, 1979

12. Sykes GP, Cooper BJ: Canine intestinal carcinoids. Vet Pathol 19:120–131, 1982

13. Patnaik AK, Hurvitz AI, Johnson GF: Canine intestinal adenocarcinoma and carcinoid. Vet Pathol 17:149–163, 1980

14. Patnaik AK, Leiberman PH: Canine goblet-cell carcinoid. Vet Pathol 18:410–413, 1981

15. Giles RC, Hildebrandt PK, Montgomery CA: Carcinoid tumor in the small intestine of a dog. Vet Pathol 11:340–349, 1974

16. Patnaik AK, Hurvitz AI, Johnson GF: Canine gastrointestinal neoplasms. Vet Pathol 14:547–555, 1977

17. Patnaik AK, Lieberman PH, Johnson GF: Intestinal ganglioneuroma in a kitten: A case report and review of the literature. J Small Anim Pract 19:735–742, 1978

18. Finn JP, Schwartz LW: A neoplasm of globule leukocytes in the intestine of a cat. J Comp Pathol 82:323–328, 1972

19. Turk MAM, Gallina AM, Russel TS: Nonhematopoietic gastrointestinal neoplasia in cats: A retrospective study of 44 cases. Vet Pathol 18:614–620, 1981

20. Kosovsky JE, Matthiesen DT, Patnaik AK: Small intestinal adenocarcinoma in cats: 32 cases (1978–1985). J Am Vet Med Assoc 192:233–2235, 1988

20a. Cribb AE: Feline gastrointestinal adenocarcinoma: A review and retrospective study. Can Vet J 29:709–711, 1988

21. Patnaik AK, Liu SK, Johnson GF: Feline intestinal adenocarcinoma: A clinicopathologic study of 22 cases. Vet Pathol 13:1–10, 1976

22. Barker IK, VanDreumel AA: The alimentary system. In Jubb KVF et al (eds): Pathology of Domestic Animals, 3rd ed, Vol 2, pp. 1–237. New York, Academic Press, 1985

22a. Strampley AR, Swayne DE, Prasse KW: Meningeal carcinomatosis secondary to a colonic signet-ring carcinoma in a dog. J Am An Hosp Assoc 23:655–658, 1987

23. Larahu LJ, Center SA, Flanders JA, Dietze AE, et al: Leiomyosarcoma in the duodenum of a dog. J Am Vet Med Assoc 183:1096–1097, 1983

24. Theilen GH, Madewell BR: Tumors of the digestive tract. In Theilen GH, Madewell BR (eds): Veterinary Cancer Medicine, 2nd ed, Philadelphia, Lea & Febiger, 1979

25. Fulton LM, Mooney S, Matus RE, Hayes AA, et al: Alimentary lymphosarcoma in 76 cats. J Am Vet Med Assoc, in press.

26. Hardy WD Jr: Hematopoietic tumors of cats. J Am Anim Hosp Assoc 17:921–940, 1981

27. Patnaik AK, Twedt DC, Marretta SM: Intestinal mast cell tumor in a dog. J Small Anim Pract 21:207–212, 1980

28. Seiler RJ: Colorectal polyps of the dog: A clinicopathologic study of 17 cases. J Am Vet Med Assoc 174:72–75, 1979

29. Church EM, Mehlhaff CJ, Patnaik AK: Colorectal adenocarcinoma in dogs: 78 cases (1973–1984). J Am Vet Med Assoc 191:727–730, 1987

29a. Gibbs C, Pearson H: Localized tumors of the canine small intestines: A report of 20 cases. J Sm Anim Prac 27:507–519, 1986

30. White RAS, Gorman NT: The clinical diagnosis and management of rectal and pararectal tumors in the dog. J Small Anim Pract 28:87–107, 1987

31. McKeown DB, Cockshutt JR, Partlow GD, Dekleer VS: Over-the-top approach to the caudal pelvic canal and rectum in the dog and cat. Vet Surg 13:181–184, 1984

32. Anderson GI, McKeown DB, Partlow GD, Percy DH: Rectal resection in the dog: A new surgical approach and the evaluation of its effect on fecal continence. Vet Surg 16:119–125, 1987

33. Seim HB: Diseases of the anus and rectum. In Kirk RW (ed): Current Veterinary Therapy, IX, pp. 901–921. Philadelphia, W.B. Saunders, 1986

34. Turrel JM, Theon AP: Single high-dose irradiation for seleted canine rectal carcinomas. Vet Radiol 27:141–145, 1986

35. Walshaw R: The small intestine. In Gourley IM, Vasseur PB (eds): General Small Animal Surgery, pp. 343–384. Philadelphia, J.B. Lippincott, 1985

36. Sindelar WF: Cancer of the small intestine. In DeVita VT et al (eds): Cancer: Principles and Practice of Oncology, pp. 616–642. Philadelphia, J.B. Lippincott, 1982

37. Sugarbaker PH, MacDonald JS, Gunderson LL: Colorectal cancer. In DeVita VT et al (eds): Cancer: Principles and Practice of Oncology, pp. 643–723. Philadelphia, J.B. Lippincott, 1982

38. Cohen AM, Kaufman SD, Kadish SP: Cancer of the colon and rectum. In Cady B (ed): Cancer Manual, 7 ed, pp. 212–221. Boston, American Cancer Society, Massachusetts Division, 1986

Perianal Tumors

Stephen J. Withrow

INCIDENCE AND RISK FACTORS

Perianal tumors are very common in the male and rare in the female dog. Perianal adenomas comprise over 80% of all perianal tumors and are the third most common tumor in the male dog.

Risk factors vary from male to female and from benign to malignant (Table 19-4). The older, sexually intact male is at high risk for perianal adenomas, implying an androgen dependency, whereas both castrated and intact

Table 19-4. Perianal Tumors

	MALE		FEMALE	
	Benign	Malignant	Benign	Malignant
CELL TYPE	Sebaceous	Sebaceous (very rare apocrine)	Sebaceous	Apocrine (anal sac)
TUMOR TYPE	Perianal adenoma	Perianal adenocarcinoma	Perianal adenoma	Anal sac adenocarcinoma
FREQUENCY	Common	Rare (10:1 benign)	Rare	Rare
HORMONAL FACTORS	Usually intact, testosterone dependent?	None	Ovariohysterectomized, *i.e.*, lack of estrogen*	Usually ovariohysterectomized but no proven hormone regulation
LOCATION AND APPEARANCE	Superficial hairless perineum; single, multiple, or diffuse; may be on prepuce or tailhead	Usually single, invasive, often ulcerated	Superficial and single	Subcutaneous at 4 or 8 o'clock, firm and fixed
PARANEOPLASTIC SYNDROMES	None	None (*very* rarely hypercalcemia)	None	Over 90% have hypercalcemia
METASTATIC PATTERN	None	First to regional nodes, then further, up to 50% of time, especially with multiple recurrence	None	Very common to regional lymph nodes and then further
SPECIAL WORK-UP	None; cytology may have difficulty telling benign from malignant	Caudal abdominal x-rays	None	Caudal abdominal x-rays; possible chest x-rays; calcium levels and renal function
TREATMENT	Castration, surgical or cryosurgical removal of tumors†	Wide excision and lymphadenectomy if involved; radiation or chemotherapy if inoperable; castration of little benefit	Surgery or cryosurgery†	Wide excision of primary, lymphadenectomy; consider radiation PO to primary and metastatic lymph node sites
PROGNOSIS	Excellent, less than 10% recurrence rate	Fair, recurrence is common but may take many months and several surgeries can be done	Excellent	Poor, less than 10% one year survival

* If multiple or large (malelike), consider testosterone secretion from adrenal (with or without Cushing's signs).
† Estrogens cause regression but carry risk of bone marrow suppression. Adenomas respond to radiation therapy, but surgery is cheaper, faster, and safer.

males develop perianal adenocarcinoma implying no hormonal dependency. Adenomas are more prevalent in the cocker spaniel, beagle, bulldog, and Samoyed than in other breeds.[1]

A high incidence of associated interstitial cell tumors has been reported for males with adenomas, suggesting testosterone production as a cause.[1] However, a true cause-and-effect relationship has not been demonstrated because interstitial cell tumors are common incidental findings in nontumor-bearing, older, intact males. Perianal adenomas in the female occur almost exclusively in ovariohysterectomized animals. Rarely, testosterone secretion from the adrenal glands (with or without signs of Cushing's disease) may stimulate perianal adenoma formation.[1a] Most older females with aprocrine gland (anal sac) adenocarcinoma are ovariohysterectomized, but a true hormonal dependence has not been shown because most older females have been ovariohysterectomized.

Perianal tumors are not commonly recognized in the cat because the cat has no glands analogous to the circumanal (perianal) glands in the dog.

PATHOLOGY AND NATURAL BEHAVIOR

Almost any tumor can occasionally affect the perianal region, including lymphosarcoma, squamous cell carcinoma, melanoma, and mast cell tumor; however, the most common are those of the sebaceous cells of the perineum. These have been called circumanal hepatoid cells because of their morphologic resemblance to liver cells. The histologic distinction between adenomas and adenocarcinomas may not always be clear, and clinically there may be an intermediate condition called invasive perianal adenoma which may look benign under the microscope yet be invasive in the patient.

The malignant anal sac (apocrine gland) adenocarcinoma is generally only seen in the female and is distinct from the male perianal sebaceous gland adenocarcinoma clinically and histologically. Both male and female forms of adenocarcinoma are locally invasive. Metastasis to regional lymph nodes is common in females at the time of presentation[2] and occurs later in the course of disease in males.[3]

HISTORY AND CLINICAL SIGNS

The history of benign lesions is that of a slow growing (months to years) mass or masses that are nonpainful and usually asymptomatic. These may be single, multiple, or diffuse (similar to generalized hyperplasia or hypertrophy of the perianal tissue) (Fig. 19-20). Most occur on the hairless skin area around the anus, although they may extend to haired regions and can develop on the prepuce, scrotum, or tailhead (stud tail or "caudal tail gland") (Fig. 19-21). Benign lesions may ulcerate and becomes infected but are rarely adherent or fixed to deeper structures. They are usually fairly well circumscribed, 0.5 to 3 cm in diameter, and elevated from the perineum.

The male perianal adenocarcinoma may look similar to an adenoma, but it tends to grow faster, be firmer, become ulcerated, adhere to deeper tissues (or the anal and rectal canals), recur following treatment, and generally be larger than an adenoma. Obstipation or dyschezia can be seen with larger masses. Castrated males with new or recurrent perianal tumors should raise the clinician's suspicion of malignant rather than benign disease because adenocarcinomas are not hormonally dependent.

Females (and *very* rarely males) with anal sac adenocarcinoma generally present for systemic signs of hypercalcemia (see paraneoplastic syndromes, Chapter 5) or occasionally obstruction at the anal canal.[4,5] Rarely, regional bone metastasis or direct extension of tumor from sublumbar (iliac) lymph nodes into the lumbar vertebrae with associated pain or fracture may be seen. An externally visible mass, as seen in the male, is rarely observed.

DIAGNOSTIC TECHNIQUES AND WORK-UP

In the male, a routine geriatric work-up prior to anesthesia is desirable. Thoracic radiographs to evaluate for lung metastasis are probably not cost effective unless they are indicated for other cardiopulmonary evaluation. Caudal abdominal radiographs to evaluate regional lymph node size are indicated if adenocarcinoma is suspected (castrated dog, recurrent disease, or physical characteristic of malignancy) (Fig. 19-22). A rectal exam may reveal palpable evidence of sublumbar lymphadenopathy. Fine-needle aspiration cytology, to differentiate benign from malignant tumors in the male, has been unrewarding in my experience.

The anal sac adenocarcinoma of the female requires careful evaluation for stage of disease and the systemic effects of hypercalcemia. Cau-

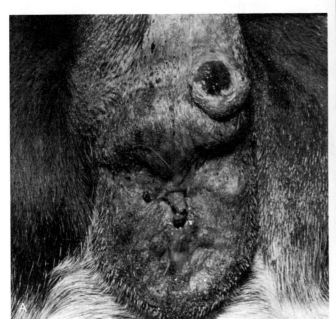
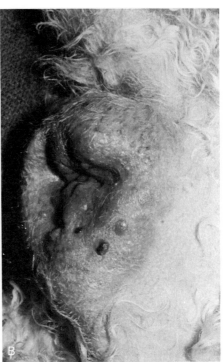

Figure 19-20. *(A)* Typical small and ulcerated perianal adenoma can be seen at 1 o'clock. Treatment with castration and cryosurgery was curative. *(B)* Diffuse 360° involvement of the perianal region with perianal adenoma. Aggressive resection or cryosurgery should not be performed but rather castration, followed by a waiting period of several months for partial regression, and then local treatment for residual disease.

dal abdominal radiographs are always indicated and, if positive, should be followed by thoracic radiographs. It is uncommon to discover pulmonary metastasis without obvious regional lymph node metastasis. A fine-needle aspirate is helpful in differentiating cancer from infection and usually demonstrates pleomorphic malignant cells. Most females with this cancer have an elevated serum calcium level.[2,5] This may result in significant renal damage, which will modify the prognosis and anesthetic risk. Depending on the level of hypercalcemia and renal function, aggressive saline diuresis and diuretic administration may be in order prior to surgery (see Chapter 5).

A careful rectal exam should be performed to detect possible lymphadenopathy and the clinical degree of fixation prior to surgery. These tumors in the female have characteristic clinical appearances and rarely require a biopsy before treatment. Males with clinical (fixed, large, ulcerated) or historical (previously castrated, recurrent) evidence of malignancy may require a wedge or punch biopsy to differentiate benign from malignant so that the desired extent of surgery can be determined.

THERAPY

Castration and tumor removal with surgery or cryosurgery is effective for the vast majority of adenomas.[6] For diffuse or large lesions situated on or in the anal sphincter, castration to allow reduction in tumor volume followed by an observation period of several months may permit safer and easier mass removal. This will only be effective for hormone-dependent benign lesions. Estrogens have been used in the past to reduce tumor volume, but they carry a significant risk of bone marrow suppression and should only be used when owners absolutely refuse castration or anesthesia. Rarely, estrogens are used to help reduce the size of a large tumor prior to surgery. In one study, 69% of irradiated adenomas regressed for at least 1 year.[7] The cost and added morbidity of radiation makes this treatment a

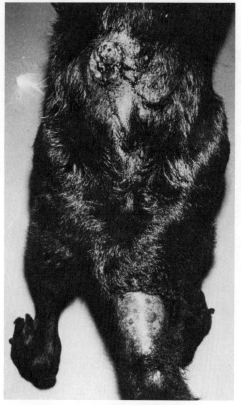

Figure 19-21. Dorsal view of a male dog with an ulcerated skin mass over the lumbar region and a thickened, hairless area over the tailhead. Both lesions were perianal adenoma.

last alternative for most clinicians. Adenomas in the female are managed by simple excision or cryosurgery.

Perianal adenocarcinomas in the male are more locally invasive than their benign counterparts and generally do not respond to castration. Aggressive surgical removal with adequate margins is indicated. Removal of one-half or more of the anal sphincter is possible with return of continence within a few weeks. Recurrent disease becomes more difficult to resect. Regional lymph node metastasis can be excised in over half the cases. Resectability cannot be reliably predicted preoperatively, and large volume is not a contraindication to caudal abdominal exploration and lymphadenectomy. Some nodes "shell out" readily, while others are very invasive. For inoperable local or regionally confined (lymph node) disease, radiation therapy may be effective in slowing the disease progression but is only rarely curative. Doxorubicin (± cyclophosphamide) or *cis*-platinum has resulted in some short-term partial remissions. Radiation or chemotherapy may convert a marginally operable tumor to an operable one.

Anal sac adenocarcinoma in the female is generally locally invasive and has spread to regional lymph nodes in virtually all cases regardless of radiographic findings. Treatment with surgery is done as in the malignant male disease with the exception of routine abdominal exploration and lymphadenectomy. Radiation

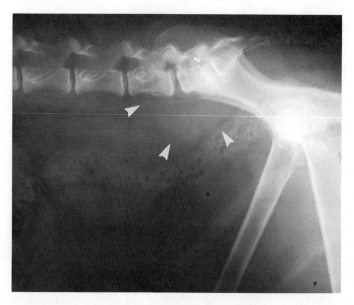

Figure 19-22. A lateral radiograph of the caudal abdomen in a male dog with perianal adenocarcinoma. Note metastatic involvement of sublumbar/iliac lymph nodes and displacement of large bowel.

and chemotherapy may be used as in the male. Removal of the tumor results in reversal of the hypercalcemia. Return of hypercalcemia post-operatively usually signals recurrence or metastasis.

PROGNOSIS

The prognosis for the various subsets of this disease location are widely divergent. For benign adenomas in the male, over 90% will be cured with castration and mass removal. Occasional recurrences are usually treated successfully but should be rebiopsied to rule out carcinoma.

Adenocarcinoma in the male is difficult to cure because local recurrence is common and may require numerous palliative resections over several years.[1] Unfortunately, most adenocarcinomas are not suspected or known until after a conservative resection. If the clinician is more sensitized to preoperatively diagnosing malignancy, more aggressive initial resection should improve survivals. The emergence of regional or distant metastasis may take many years in the male. In a series of 41 male dogs with perianal adenocarcinoma 15% had metastasis at presentation. Only stage of disease (T_2 No Mo or less) had an influence on survival. Tumors 5 cm or less in diameter had median survivals in excess of 2 years when surgically resected[8a] (Fig. 19-23).

Anal sac adenocarcinoma in the female carries the worst prognosis; very few patients are alive at 1 year. The cause of death is either renal failure secondary to hypercalcemia or local disease symptoms.[2,5,8] Most reports to date have concentrated on the pathophysiology of the disease rather than therapy. Aggressive resection with postoperative radiation has resulted in remissions longer than 1 year in a limited number of cases in my experience.

COMPARATIVE ASPECTS[9]

No similar hormone-dependent disease exists in humans. The most common cancer of the perianal skin is squamous cell carcinoma (epidermoid carcinoma). Chronic anal irritation (fissure, fistulas, and so forth) may precede tumor development.

REFERENCES

1. Wilson GP, Hayes HM: Castration for treatment of perianal gland neoplasms in the dog. J Am Vet Med Assoc 174:1301–1303, 1979

1a. Dow SW, Olson PN, Rosychuk RAW et al: Perianal adenomas and hypertestosteronemia in a spayed bitch with pituitary-dependent hyperadrenocorticism. J Am Vet Med Assoc 192:1439–1441, 1988

2. Meuten DJ, Cooper BJ, Capen CC, Chew DJ, Kociba GJ: Hypercalcemia associated with an adenocarcinoma derived from the apocrine glands of the anal sac. Vet Pathol 18:454–471, 1981

3. Nielsen SW, Aftosmis J: Canine perianal gland tumors. J Am Vet Med Assoc 144:127–135, 1964

4. Rubin S, Shivaprasad HL: Hypercalcemia associated with an anal sac adenocarcinoma in a castrated male dog. Comp Cont Educ 7:348–352, 1985

5. Hause WR, Stevenson S, Meuten DJ, Capen CC: Pseudohyperparathyroidism associated with

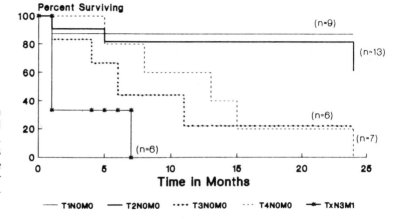

Figure 19-23. Survival duration in 41 male dogs with perianal adenocarcinoma based on stage. Note that dogs with small tumors (T_1 or T_2) without lymph node involvement will do well after aggressive removal of the primary.

adenocarcinomas of anal sac origin in four dogs. J Am Anim Hosp Assoc 17:373–379, 1981

6. Liska WD, Withrow SJ: Cryosurgical treatment of perianal gland adenomas in the dog. J Am Anim Hosp Assoc 14:457–463, 1978

7. Gillette EL: Veterinary radiotherapy. J Am Vet Med Assoc 157:1707–1712, 1970

8. Goldschmidt MH, Zoltowski C: Anal sac gland adenocarcinoma in the dog: 14 cases. J Small Anim Pract 22:119–128, 1981

8a. Vail DM, Withrow, SJ, Schwarz PD: Perianal adenocarcinoma in the canine male: A retrospective study of 41 cases. J Am Anim Hosp (in press)

9. Sugarbaker PH, Gunderson LL, MacDonald JS: Cancer of the anal region. In DeVita VT (ed): Cancer: Principles and Practice of Oncology, pp. 724–731. Philadelphia, J.B. Lippincott, 1982

20

TUMORS OF THE RESPIRATORY SYSTEM

Stephen J. Withrow

THE NASAL PLANUM

INCIDENCE AND RISK FACTORS

Cancer of the nasal planum is rare in the dog and fairly common in the cat. The development of squamous cell carcinoma (SCC) has been correlated with exposure to ultraviolet light and lack of protective pigment.[1] It is classically seen in older, lightly pigmented cats.

PATHOLOGY AND NATURAL BEHAVIOR

By far the most common cancer is squamous cell carcinoma. Depending on the timing of biopsy, this tumor may be reported as carcinoma *in situ*, superficial SCC, or deeply infiltrative SCC. It may be locally very invasive but only rarely metastasizes.

Other cancers reported in this site are lymphoma, fibrosarcoma, hemangioma, melanoma, mast cell tumor, fibroma, and eosinophilic granuloma. Immune-mediated disease may present as erosive or crusty lesions on the nose but is rarely proliferative and usually affects other sites.

HISTORY AND CLINICAL SIGNS

Invasive SCC is usually preceded by protracted disease (months to years) that progresses through the following stages (Fig. 20-1): crusting and erythema, superficial erosions and ulcers (carcinoma *in situ* or early SCC), and finally, deeply invasive and erosive lesions. Associated eyelid and ear pinna lesions may be seen if these sites lack pigment. Patients have often been treated with corticosteroids or topical ointments with little response.

DIAGNOSTIC TECHNIQUES AND WORK-UP

Erosive or proliferative lesions should have a deep wedge biopsy to determine the degree of invasion and histologic type of disease. These biopsies require a brief anesthetic owing to the sensitivity of the nasal planum. Hemorrhage can

215

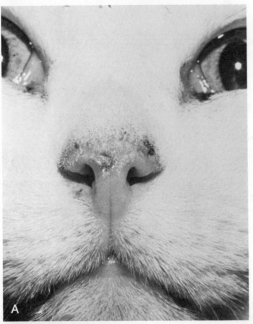

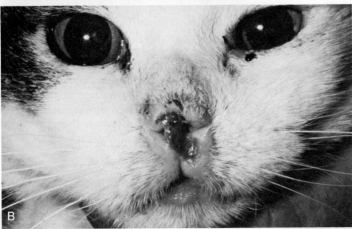

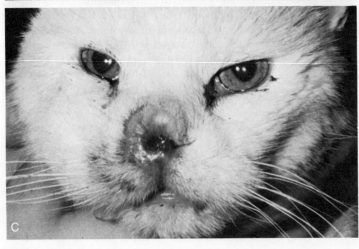

Figure 20-1. (A) Crusting and erythema of a white cat's nose which had been slowly progressing for 8 months. Six months later the lesion was confirmed by biopsy as carcinoma *in situ*. Treatment would be with cryosurgery or hyperthermia. (B) A cat with invasive squamous cell carcinoma that has caused some erosion of the nasal planum but is still confined to the nasal planum. Nosectomy was curative. (C) A cat with a 2-year history of progressive nasal ulceration and deformity. The nasal planum is markedly deformed and the surrounding skin up to the eyelids is swollen and infiltrated with squamous cell carcinoma. Even nosectomy would not be curative. Note concomitant eyelid lesions, which are carcinoma *in situ*. No treatment was offered.

be profuse and usually requires one or two sutures to appose the edges. Rarely, dilute epinephrine (1:10,000) can be injected locally or topically applied to arrest capillary oozing. Cytologic scrapings or superficial biopsies are of little value because they only reveal inflammation, which may accompany both cancer and noncancerous conditions. Lymph nodes are rarely involved except in very advanced disease, and thoracic radiographs are invariably negative for metastasis.

THERAPY

It may be possible to prevent or arrest the course of the preneoplastic disease by limiting exposure to the sun or by tattooing to add pigment protection. Topical sunscreens are readily licked off and rarely help. When inflammation and ulceration are present, it is very difficult to maintain the tattoo, which is rapidly removed by macrophages. Even under the best of circumstances, tattooing has to be repeated at yearly intervals. Attempts to increase epithelial differentiation with synthetic derivatives of vitamin A have been unsuccessful.[2]

SCC, and probably other neoplasms as well, falls into two general categories: (1) superficial, minimally invasive disease, and (2) deeply infiltrating disease. Superficial cancers can be managed effectively by almost any method, including cryosurgery, hyperthermia, or irradiation.[3] These methods are preferred over blade excision because of hemostatic and cosmetic considerations.

Deeply invasive cancer on the other hand is generally resistant to these treatments. In particular, radiation therapy, which would have the greatest chance of preserving the cosmetic appearance of the nose, has had poor local control rates for bigger and more invasive SCC in the dog and the cat.[4,5] Expectations for radiation with other tumor types would have to be extrapolated from radiation results achieved at more conventional sites.

Complete excision of invasive cancer of the nasal planum can be performed in the cat with an acceptable comestic result. With the cat under general anesthesia, the nasal planum is completely removed by means of a 360° skin incision, which also transects the underlying turbinates (Fig. 20-2). A single cutaneous purse-string suture of 3-0 nylon is used to pull the skin into an open circle (1 cm in diameter) around the airways. The site will crust and scab over. The scab is removed at suture removal (often requiring sedation), and healing of the skin with two patent "nostrils" is complete by 1 month. Functional and cosmetic results are good in the cat (Fig. 20-3) and fair in the dog. This probably is the treatment of choice for invasive lesions that have not extensively involved the lip or surrounding skin.[5a]

PROGNOSIS

The outlook for SCC is good for early, noninvasive disease. Later development of new sites of neoplasia on other areas of the planum is

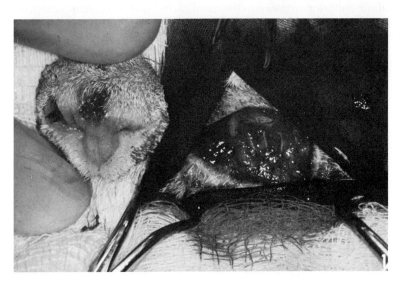

Figure 20-2. Operative view of resected nasal planum in a cat with invasive carcinoma that was confined to the nasal planum.

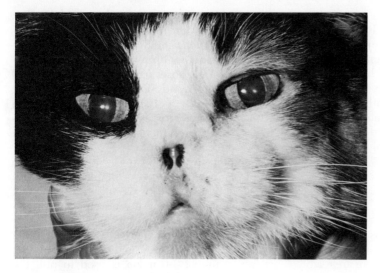

Figure 20-3. One year postoperative view of a cat after nosectomy for squamous cell carcinoma. Note well-healed skin around patent airways. This cat remains free of disease 28 months postoperatively.

common, however, because the underlying causes are not reversed. In later stages, the disease can be cured with aggressive surgery, but it is poorly responsive to most other treatments. In my experience, 7 of 10 cats with invasive SCC of the nasal planum treated with wide resection (nosectomy) were free of recurrent disease at 1 year.[5a] Since SCC rarely metastasizes from this site, even untreated animals with advanced cancer can live a long time, albeit with an ulcerated and deforming cancer.

COMPARATIVE ASPECTS[6]

Cancer of the human nasal skin and nasal vestibule (anterior entrance to the nasal cavity) may be induced by ultraviolet light as in the cat. Lack of protective pigment is also a contributing factor. Squamous cell carcinoma of the vestibule is treated with radiation (interstitial or external beam) or surgery. Surgery generally entails resection of nasal skin and cartilage and reconstruction with composite ear skin and cartilage, nasolabial flaps, or a prosthesis. Local control is generally good.

NASAL TUMORS

INCIDENCE AND RISK

Intranasal cancer comprises approximately 1% of all canine neoplasms.[7] It has been speculated, but unproven, that dolichocephalic breeds (those

with a long nose) or dogs living in urban environments with resultant nasal filtering of pollutants may be at higher risk.[8,9] The average age of patients is 10 years, and medium to large breeds may be more commonly affected. A slight male predilection has been reported.[8]

These tumors are less common in the cat.

PATHOLOGY AND NATURAL BEHAVIOR

Carcinomas (mainly adenocarcinoma, squamous cell carcinoma, and undifferentiated carcinoma) comprise nearly two-thirds of intranasal cancers.[10] Sarcomas (fibrosarcoma, chondrosarcoma, osteosarcoma, and undifferentiated sarcoma) comprise the bulk of the remaining cancers.[11] All of these malignancies are characterized by progressive local invasion. The metastatic rate is generally considered low.

Rarely, transmissible venereal cell cancer and polyps or fibromas are seen.[12] The cat has a higher percentage of lymphosarcoma (usually FeLV negative) than the dog.[13]

HISTORY AND CLINICAL SIGNS

Although many intranasal diseases have overlapping clinical signs, a strong presumption of cancer can be made for older animals with an intermittent and progressive history of initially unilateral epistaxis (Table 20-1). The average length of signs before diagnosis is 3 months.[7] If facial deformity, and to a lesser degree epiphora, are present, the diagnosis is almost always can-

Table 20-1. Nasal Tumors: Differential Diagnosis for Common Intranasal Diseases*

	CANCER	BACTERIAL, FUNGAL	FOREIGN BODY	BLEEDING DIATHESIS
Age	Older	Any	Younger? Indiscriminate sniffing?	Younger if heritable?
Type discharge	Bloody > seromucoid > purulent	Purulent (occasionally epistaxis)	Seromucoid and ultimately purulent	Bloody
Symmetry	Unilateral initially	Often bilateral	Unilateral	Unilateral
Epiphora	Common	Occasional	No	No
Facial deformity	Common	Rare (temporal atrophy and ulcerated rhinarium)	No	No
Onset	Insidious, intermittent, progressive	Insidious, intermittent, progressive	Acute	Acute
Duration of signs	Months	Months to years	?	?
CNS signs	Occasionally	Rare	No	No
Frequency	Rare/common	Common	Rare	Rare
Sneezing	Yes	Yes	Yes, peracute and severe initially	Yes

* "Allergic" rhinitis has been so poorly defined that it is not discussed here. Trauma has also been omitted because an injury severe enough to cause epistaxis is almost invariably obvious clinically.

cer. "Apparent" response to a variety of symptomatic treatments is commonly seen.

When dealing with a history predominantly of epistaxis, a careful search for evidence in support of systemic bleeding disorders should be made before performing a biopsy (travel history for Ehrlichia, abnormal bleeding from previous surgery, hematuria, and so forth).

DIAGNOSTIC TECHNIQUES AND WORK-UP

A definitive diagnosis requires a tissue biopsy even though radiographs and historical information can be highly suggestive. Before skull radiographs and biopsy are performed, it is important to rule out a systemic bleeding problem as carefully as possible. Attention to platelet count, clotting of venipuncture sites, presence of hematuria, retinal changes (hemorrhage or hyperviscosity), presence of petechial hemorrhages, and possibly a clotting time should determine if serious bleeding will occur subsequent to the biopsy.

Nasal radiographs are generally required to define the extent of disease, to provide a presumptive diagnosis, and to locate that area within the nose most likely to yield diagnostic material with a biopsy.[14] Standard radiographs include lateral, dorsal ventral, frontal sinus, and open-mouth oblique views. Probably the most rewarding views are an open-mouth VD oblique (to show caudal nasal cavity and cribriform plate) or the isolated nasal cavity exposure with the film placed in the mouth and exposed in the DV plane (Fig. 20-4). Asymmetrical destruction of turbinates or superimposition of a soft tissue mass over the turbinates, especially in the caudal half of the nose, are classic radiographic changes of cancer. Bone destruction or erosion is also common with cancer. Fluid in one or both frontal sinuses without bony erosion is usually secondary to outflow obstruction of the normal mucoid secretions and not neoplastic infiltration. Computed tomography would be an ideal diagnostic tool if it were more readily available, especially as it relates to cribriform plate and orbital invasion (Fig. 20-5).

While the patient is anesthetized for radiography, a tissue biopsy should be obtained. A transnostril core sample is usually easily procured for biopsy.[15] According to the location of the lesion on radiographs, either a punch biopsy needle or a large bore (3–5 mm) plastic cannula is passed up the nostril and directed to the tumor.[15] With either technique, it is important to avoid penetrating the cribriform plate. Biopsy instruments should be marked with tape (punch) or cut off (plastic core) so as to avoid penetrating farther than the distance from the tip of the nares to the medial canthus of the eye (Fig. 20-6). Tumors are usually strongly suspected when the tissue obtained is white or yellow rather than turbinate only. Mild hemorrhage is to be expected and will subside within a few minutes. If hemorrhage is severe, the unilateral carotid artery can be permanently ligated in the neck.

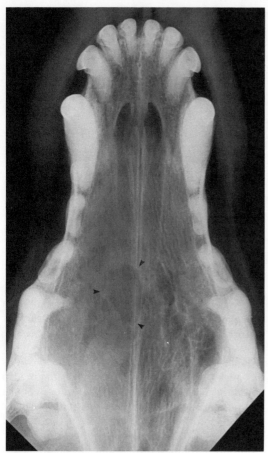

Figure 20-4. Dorsal ventral radiograph of the nasal cavity with film placed in the mouth. Note asymmetry. Bone lysis (small arrow) and loss of turbinate detail implies tumor in the caudal half of the nasal cavity.

Cats or small dogs may be biopsied with a curette passed up the nostril and into the tumor.

Attempts at nasal washing and fluid retrieval for cytologic examination have been generally unrewarding and are not recommended as the sole means of diagnosis.[7] Rhinoscopy is only rarely needed to facilitate tissue procurement.[16]

A lymph node aspirate is positive in 10% of cases (especially carcinomas), and thoracic radiographs are usually normal.

If any central nervous system signs exist, a sample of cerebrospinal fluid should be procured to help in determining the potential extension of disease to the dura or farther across the cribriform plate. Increased pressure, increased

protein, and an increased cell count suggest brain involvement.[17]

Culture and sensitivity testing for bacterial evaluation is seldom helpful in the therapy of primary bacterial rhinitis or rhinitis secondary to a tumor.

THERAPY

Therapy is directed principally at local disease control. Unfortunately, this disease usually presents in a relatively advanced stage in a critical location near the brain and eyes (Fig. 20-7). Bone invasion occurs early, and curative surgery is virtually impossible. Although surgical removal by rhinotomy has been recommended, its high rate of acute and chronic morbidity, without significant extension of life,[7,10] makes it rarely indicated unless other adjuvant therapies, such as radiation, are available.

Radiation therapy has the advantage of treating the entire nasal cavity, including any extension of cancer into the bone, where surgery cannot remove it. It is unclear whether surgical debulking before radiation is of benefit. Debulking is probably necessary when using orthovoltage radiation, but it may not be necessary with high-energy radiation, such as cobalt or megavoltage.[18,19] Doses of 40 to 48 Gy are usually delivered in 10 to 12 fractions over 3 to 4 weeks to the caudal three-fourths of the nasal cavity and frontal sinuses if indicated.[19] Either a single dorsal portal or bilateral opposed portals (preferred) are used. Although rhinitis as a result of surgery and radiation can be severe, it will usually subside within 1 or 2 months. Owners may be required to clean the nostrils several times a day, and rarely is the patient's nasal cavity completely normal. Ocular changes can be expected if both eyes receive irradiation to 40 Gy in 3 weeks. Keratoconjunctivitis sicca is very common and corneal ulcers and cataract formation often occur at doses over 40 Gy.[20]

Cats are usually treated with radiation therapy only, owing to their poor tolerance of rhinotomy and the marked radiosensitivity of their tumors, especially lymphoid ones.[13]

Unilateral or bilateral carotid artery ligation may palliate the symptoms of epistaxis for 3 months or longer without damage to the brain.[21]

Chemotherapy (systemic or intranasal drops), immunotherapy, and cryosurgery have not improved survival rates.[7,22]

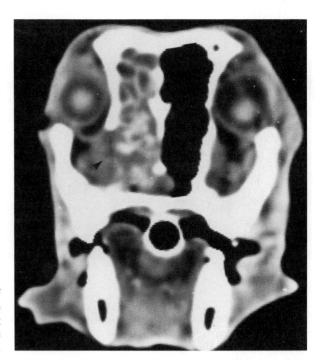

Figure 20-5. Computed tomographic image of a dog with nasal cancer taken in the transverse plane at the level of the orbit. Note involvement of the left side of the nasal cavity with invasion and destruction of the medial boney orbit (arrow).

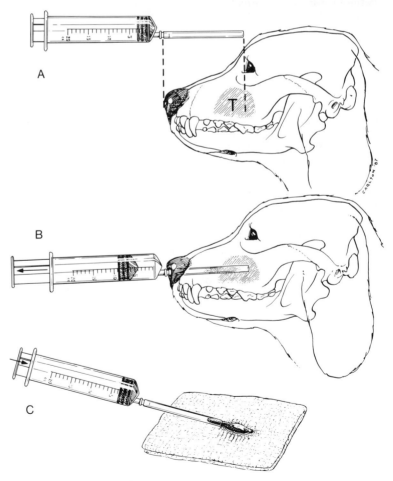

Figure 20-6. (A) Illustration of the dog skull showing caudally situated tumor (T). Plastic cannula for core aspirate has been shortened to extend no deeper than the medial canthus of the eye to avoid injury to the brain. (B) Cannula is introduced into nasal cavity through the nares. Slight resistance is usually felt as the tumor is entered. Negative pressure is applied as cannula is redirected in various angles. (C) Tissue and blood are expelled onto a gauze sponge, where blood is separated from tissue. Tissue is then submitted for histologic evaluation.[15]

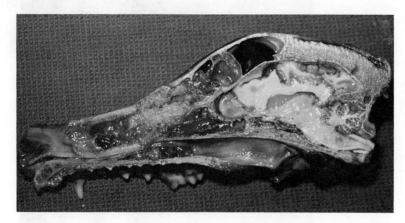

Figure 20-7. Cross-section of a dog's skull with atypical intranasal carcinoma. Note mid to caudal position of tumor in nasal cavity, erosion of dorsal nasal bones, dark mucous in frontal sinus secondary to obstruction, and close proximity of tumor to cribriform plate. Complete surgical resection is impossible.

PROGNOSIS

Overall, the prognosis for canine nasal tumors is poor. The mean survival for surgery, chemotherapy, immunotherapy, cryosurgery, or no treatment is 3 to 5 months.[7,22,23]

The only improvements in survival rate have been with radiation therapy, usually combined with surgical debulking. Mean survival in various reports ranges from 8 to 25 months.[19,23,24] One-year survivals range from 38% to 57%, and 2-year survivals range from 30% to 48%.[19,24] The prognosis for carcinomas is better than that for sarcomas, and adenocarcinomas respond better than squamous cell carcinoma or undifferentiated carcinoma (Fig. 20-8).[24]

It is difficult to analyze end results after radiation and surgical debulking because clinical symptoms resulting from treatment may be similar to those of the tumor before treatment.[19] Few dogs are truly cured if they are followed to autopsy. In a series of 19 autopsied patients treated at Colorado State University with radiation or radiation and surgery, 18 had evidence of local recurrence, 10 had lymph node metastasis, and 9 had metastasis beyond the head and neck (usually to the lung). Mean survival in this series of patients was 10 months. As improvements in local control and survival continue to progress, the metastatic potential of nasal malignancies in the dog will increase.

Far fewer cats have been treated, but survival, especially of those with lymphoid neoplasms, appears excellent. In a series of 6 cats (3 lymphosarcomas, 2 carcinomas, and 1 chondrosarcoma) treated with 40 Gy of radiation, the mean survival was 19 months; two patients were still alive at 12 and 14 months when this was written.

Clinical improvement of patients with lymphoid tumors is very fast, complete, and probably permanent.[13]

COMPARATIVE ASPECTS[25]

Cancer of the nasal cavity and paranasal sinuses is rare in humans. It generally affects persons over 40 years of age and is twice as common in men as in women. The most common cancer is squamous cell carcinoma. Etiologic factors for adenocarcinoma include work in occupations associated with wood dust, boot making, and the flooring industry.

The disease is variably invasive locally and reasonably late to metastasize. Surgery or irradiation are the standard treatments, depending on stage, site, and type of cancer. Five-year control rates vary from 50% to 75%.

LARYNX AND TRACHEA

INCIDENCE AND RISK FACTORS

Cancer in either the larynx or trachea is rare. Young animals with active osteochondral ossification sites are at higher risk for benign tracheal osteocartilaginous tumors that grow in synchrony with the rest of the musculoskeletal system.[26] Laryngeal oncocytomas also appear to occur in young mature dogs.[27,28]

PATHOLOGY AND NATURAL BEHAVIOR

Reported canine laryngeal tumors include oncocytoma (rhabdomyoma), osteosarcoma, chondrosarcoma, adenocarcinoma, melanoma, gran-

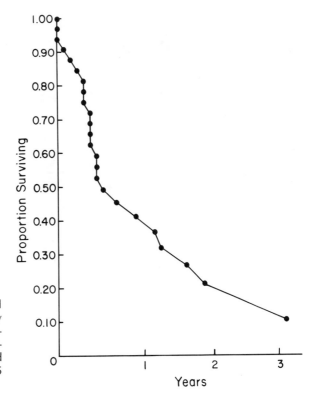

Figure 20-8. Survival curve of 33 dogs with nasal cancer treated with high-energy radiation therapy at Colorado State University. Most patients received 40 Gy in 10 fractions in 3 weeks. Twenty-eight tumors were carcinomas. Survivals should increase with the current use of 48 Gy in 15 fractions in 3 weeks.

ular cell myoblastoma, undifferentiated carcinoma, fibrosarcoma, mast cell tumor, and squamous cell carcinoma.[29–30b] Oncocytomas in the dog may attain a large size, are minimally invasive, and do not appear to metastasize.[27,28] Most other laryngeal tumors are locally very invasive with a significant metastatic potential. Feline laryngeal neoplasms are more commonly lymphosarcomas, although squamous cell carcinomas and adenocarcinomas have been reported.[30,31]

Reported tracheal cancer includes lymphosarcoma, chondrosarcoma, adenocarcinoma, and squamous cell carcinoma. Tracheal leiomyomas and polyps have also been reported.[32–34] Several reports of benign tracheal osteochondral tumors exist in the literature.[26,35] These lesions grow from the cartilaginous rings and are composed of cancellous bone capped by cartilage. They may reflect a malfunction of osteogenesis rather than true cancer and are benign.[35]

The larynx and trachea may be secondarily invaded by neoplasms such as lymphosarcoma and thyroid adenocarcinoma.

HISTORY AND CLINICAL SIGNS

Patients with laryngeal tumors usually present with a progressive change in voice or bark, exercise intolerance, dysphagia, or aspiration. Tracheal tumor patients usually present with coughing and exercise intolerance. Since osteochondral lesions of young dogs grow at the same rate as the rest of the skeleton, they cause the most pronounced symptoms during or after the skeletal growth spurt.

Laryngeal and tracheal tumors are generally not palpable externally.

DIAGNOSTIC TECHNIQUE AND WORK-UP

Laryngeal tumors can usually be biopsied under direct visualization. Regional radiographs may reveal the lesion but are rarely necessary.[29]

Tracheal tumors offer more of a diagnostic challenge but can be biopsied with the use of fiberoptic instruments or a rigid bronchoscope (Fig. 20-9). Alternately, open surgical biopsy, often coupled with excision, can be performed.

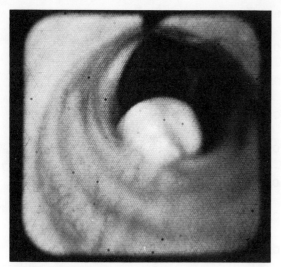

Figure 20-9. Fiberoptic view of tracheal osteochondroma in a 5-month-old dog.

Plain radiographs or a tracheogram may reveal a mass narrowing the lumen (Fig. 20-10).

THERAPY

Benign laryngeal cancers such as oncocytomas can be successfully removed with preservation of function.[27] Complete laryngectomy with a permanent tracheostomy is an option used in humans but has had limited use in veterinary medicine.[31, 36–38] Depending on suspected radioresponsiveness, invasive cancers can be treated with irradiation to better preserve laryngeal function. Radiation should control lymphosarcoma in the dog or cat larynx or trachea. Chemotherapy ($\pm$ surgery) may also be effective.[39]

Tracheal tumors, especially benign osteochondral tumors, should be treated with resection (Fig. 20-11). Full-thickness removal with end-to-end anastomosis can be easily performed on up to 3 or 4 rings. Experimentally, up to 50% of tracheal length has been removed with successful closure.[40]

Phototherapy with bronchoscopy has been successfully used in humans for small lesions (carcinoma *in situ* or early carcinoma), but these lesions are only rarely recognized in the dog.

PROGNOSIS

Benign lesions of the trachea or larynx carry a good prognosis if they can be surgically resected. Most dogs with resectable oncocytomas live more than a year and may be presumed cured.[27] Very limited information is available for malignancies because very few have been treated and reported.

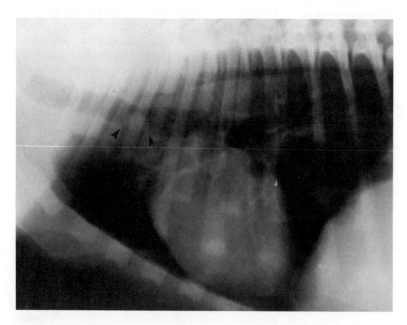

Figure 20-10. Lateral thoracic radiograph of dog in Fig. 20-9. Note intraluminal mass on floor of trachea (arrows).

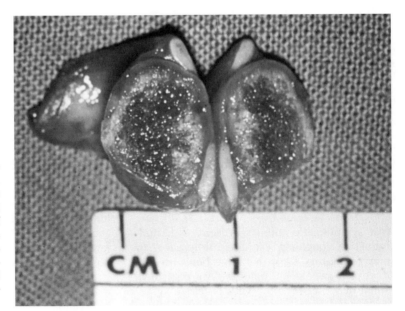

Figure 20-11. Resected tumor and associated tracheal cartilage rings of dog in Fig. 20-9 and 20-10. Tumor is bisected and has typical appearance of cancellous bone with a cartilaginous cap. The patient recovered uneventfully from surgery and survived for over 5 years, when it was lost to follow-up.

COMPARATIVE ASPECTS[41]

Laryngeal cancer is common in humans (2% of all cancers) and is related to smoking and alcohol consumption. Squamous cell carcinoma accounts for nearly all cancers. Earlier detection than in animals due to changes in voice make treatment more feasible.

The disease appears to progress through stages of development from dysplasia, to carcinoma *in situ*, to minimally invasive carcinoma, to invasive carcinoma. Sixty percent of patients with carcinoma present with local disease only, 30% with regional nodal metastasis, and 10% with distant metastasis. Treatment is surgery (partial or complete laryngectomy) or radiation. Local control and cure rates are good to excellent.

Tracheal cancer (independent of lung cancer) is very rare.

PRIMARY LUNG CANCER

INCIDENCE AND RISK FACTORS

Compared to humans, dogs very rarely develop primary lung cancer, which accounts for only 1% of all canine cancers diagnosed. It is even more uncommon in the cat. Attempts to cor-

relate urban living[42] and passive cigarette smoking with canine lung cancer have not as yet shown an association. However, dogs trained to smoke cigarettes (with or without concomitant asbestos instillation) through a tracheostomy develop lung cancer at a dramatically increased rate.[43,44] The average age at diagnosis is 10 years, and there is no apparent sex or breed predilection. Metastatic disease from nonlung cancer primaries is much more common than primary lung cancer in the dog and the cat.

PATHOLOGY AND NATURAL BEHAVIOR

Almost all cancers are carcinomas, the most common being adenocarcinoma.[45–47] Adenocarcinomas are further classified by location as bronchial, bronchoalveolar, or alveolar carcinoma. Carcinomas can be further graded as differentiated or undifferentiated, and undifferentiated ones have a higher incidence of metastasis.[45] Squamous cell carcinoma is less commonly reported. Benign tumors and primary sarcomas are rare.[45]

Metastasis can occur through lymphatics, through the airways, hematogenously or transpleurally. Over 50% of undifferentiated adenocarcinomas and over 90% of squamous cell carcinomas metastasize.[45]

Table 20-2.   Differential Diagnosis of Solid Lung Masses

	PRIMARY LUNG CANCER	METASTATIC LUNG CANCER	GRANULOMATOUS DISEASE
Age	Old	Old	Variable
Location	Especially caudal lobes, slight trend to right side	Any lobe (peripheral?)	Random (plant awn granulomas often caudal ventral)
Fever, leukocytosis	Rare	Rare	Occasional, more common acutely
Hilar lymphadenopathy on radiographs	Occasional	Rare	More common
Incidence	Rare	Common	Rare
Historical information	None	Known primary cancer	Travel? for fungal

HISTORY AND CLINICAL SIGNS

Most symptomatic animals present with non-productive coughing, exercise intolerance, or other respiratory signs that have been present for several weeks to months. An occasional animal may be presented with peracute symptoms secondary to hemothorax, pneumothorax, or malignant pleural effusion.[47a]

Paraneoplastic syndromes, common in humans, are rare (or unrecognized) in animals; the most common one is hypertrophic pulmonary osteopathy.[47,48] When present, the animal may be seen for lameness or swollen legs.

DIAGNOSTIC TECHNIQUES AND WORK-UP

Many diagnostic techniques are available but only rarely indicated. Once a thoracic radiograph demonstrates a solitary lung mass, the next step is generally surgical removal. Deciding which lung lesions are likely to be primary lung cancer and treatable with surgery is the clinical dilemma. However, a strong presumptive diagnosis can be made before surgery (Table 20-2).

Radiographs usually demonstrate a well-demarcated, spherical mass that is usually solitary. The caudal lung lobes are most commonly affected (Fig. 20-12). Multiple or miliary lesions are less commonly seen. Hilar lymphadenopathy is uncommonly seen on radiographs even though positive lymph nodes may be removed at surgery. Pleural effusion may also be detected.[49,49a]

Bronchoscopy for tissue or brush biopsy may be of diagnostic value for centrally located lesions that extend into the bronchus.[50] Transtracheal lavage is only rarely diagnostic. Transthoracic fine-needle aspirates can be quite rewarding for larger lesions located in a peripheral location, but it is common for these tumors to have a

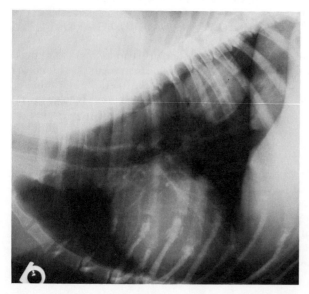

Figure 20-12. Lateral radiograph of 12-year-old dog with well-circumscribed mass in caudal lung lobe. This mass was surgically removed via lobectomy and diagnosed as adenocarcinoma. The patient died 26 months later of unrelated causes; autopsy revealed no evidence of cancer.

necrotic center, which may confuse interpretation.[51-53] However, bronchoscopy, tracheal lavage, and fine-needle aspirates are really not necessary before surgery for solitary lesions since the treatment (*i.e.*, lobectomy) is the same for all etiologies. Unless the owner desires an accurate diagnosis or prognosis before surgery, the diagnosis and treatment should be combined.

Pleural effusions, on the other hand, should be carefully assessed because malignancy in this case carries a very poor prognosis and may preclude surgical intervention.

THERAPY

Once a diagnosis of solitary lung mass in a patient who can tolerate anesthesia is made, thoracotomy is generally the next step. Regardless of etiology, surgical removal is the treatment of choice. At the very least, an accurate diagnosis and staging can be attained.

A standard intercostal incision over the 4th to 6th interspace generally allows complete lung lobe removal and hilar lymph node biopsy. Partial lobectomy can be accomplished for very peripherally located tumors, but a complete lobectomy is the rule. Careful palpation of other lobes may reveal further nodules for removal. The use of stapling equipment (TA-55 or -90)* has allowed quick and secure lobectomy to be performed in most patients but is not required (Fig. 20-13).[53,54]

Other methods of therapy such as radiation and chemotherapy have been largely untried. Normal lung tissue will generally not accept doses of irradiation required to kill cancer without serious consequences such as fibrosis. In a very limited series of cases, multidrug chemotherapy with vindesine ± *cis*-platinum may have shown some benefit.[53]

Malignant pleural effusions can be treated with systemic chemotherapy or intrapleural chemotherapy with such agents as thiotepa. Alternately, sclerosing agents such as tetracycline or talc have been used.[55,55a]

Metastatic lung cancer is treatable on rare occasions.[56-58] The criteria for surgery in a human patient with metastasis are relative; they include complete control of the primary cancer (the longer the better), absence of other known

metastatic sites, a "favorable histology" (this is not established in veterinary medicine but generally includes sarcomas), a slow doubling time (more than 40-day doubling of tumor diameter), and probably fewer than five lesions. Cases for removal of metastatic lung nodules in dogs and cats should be chosen carefully (Fig. 20-14).[59,59a]

PROGNOSIS

The best prognosis is seen in patients with solitary lesions of small diameter (< 2 in), negative lymph nodes, and no malignant pleural effusion and who were diagnosed without symptoms. In this group of patients, over 50% can be expected to live at least 1 year postoperatively. Of the malignant cancers, adenocarcinomas have a better prognosis than squamous cell carcinoma, which is often diffuse at diagnosis. One paper reported a mean survival of 8 months for three dogs with squamous cell carcinomas and of 19 months for eight with adenocarcinomas.[53] Canine patients with tumors located in the periphery of the lung or near the base of the lung had better survivals (mean of 18 months) than those with tumors involving the entire lobe (mean of 8 months). Similarly, small tumors (< 100 cc^3, 2-in diameter) had a mean survival of 20 months, whereas large tumors (> 100 cc^3) had a mean survival of 8 months. Patients with lymph node involvement have a decreased survival[59b] (Fig. 20-15).

The cat responds to surgical resection of lung tumors similarly to the dog in my experience, but very little information is published to substantiate this statement.

COMPARATIVE ASPECTS[60]

Primary lung cancer develops in over 100,000 people per year in the United States. It is the leading cause of cancer-related death in men over 35 years of age and the second leading cause in women. It is strongly associated with smoking.

Bronchial or bronchoalveolar carcinomas and bronchial mucinous gland carcinomas comprise over 90% of lung cancers. The most common histologic types, in order, are squamous cell carcinoma, adenocarcinoma, small cell carcinoma (oat cell), and large cell carcinoma.

Paraneoplastic syndromes, seen in over 50% of cases, are common and diverse.

* Autosuture, U.S. Surgical, Norwalk, CT.

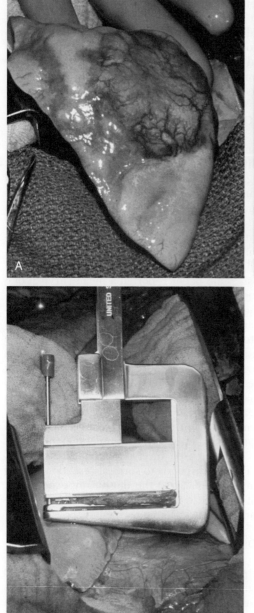

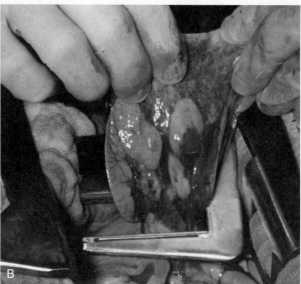

Figure 20-13. *(A)* Operative view of lung cancer from patient in Fig. 20-12. Note typical raised lesion with superficial neovascularization. *(B)* Lung lobe is lifted up and surgical staples placed at level of proximal main stem bronchus. *(C)* Stapler has been fired to release a double row of capital B-shaped stainless steel staples. Lung mass is then removed, and the instrument is released. The artery, vein, and bronchus are inspected for possible small leaks, which are sutured.

Surgical resection is the treatment of choice for most lesions. If resection for cure can be performed, up to 30% of patients with non-small-cell cancer may survive 5 years. Small cell carcinoma has historically carried the worst prognosis, but chemotherapy is becoming increasingly successful. Radiation is generally reserved for nonresectable tumors or for palliation.

MISCELLANEOUS CONDITIONS OF THE LUNG

Canine Lymphomatoid Granulomatosis[61]

In a series of 8 cases, canine lymphomatoid granulomatosis affected young to middle-aged dogs with no breed or sex predilection. The most consistent laboratory abnormalities were circulating basophilia (6) and leukocytosis (5).

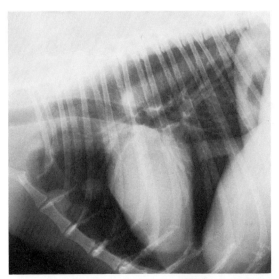

Figure 20-14. Lateral radiograph of a 10-year-old Irish setter who had undergone forelimb amputation for osteosarcoma 8 months previously. Note two spherical lesions in apical lung lobes. These lesions increased in diameter only 25% in 40 days, and they were surgically removed with a partial lobectomy. This patient did well for 8 more months, when a rib metastasis was noted. No further lung cancer was noted.

Radiographic changes include lung lobe consolidation or large pulmonary granulomas (7), and tracheobronchial lymph node enlargement (6) (Fig. 20-15). Definitive diagnosis was based on histologic examination of involved tissues (generally an open biopsy). Predominant findings were angiocentric and angiodestructive infiltration of the pulmonary parenchyma by large lymphoreticular and plasmacytoid cells, along with normal lymphocytes, eosinophils, and plasma cells. This infiltrate was characteristically centered around the small- to medium-sized arteries and veins.

Treatment consisted of immunosuppressive therapy and was attempted in 5 dogs. Drugs used included cyclophosphamide, vincristine, and prednisone. Three of the 5 treated dogs achieved a complete response as evidenced by both clinical and radiographic resolution of signs (Fig. 20-16). These three animals remained in complete remission at 7, 12, and 32 months from the time of diagnosis and initiation of therapy. One dog was euthanatized because of progression of signs following treatment with prednisone alone, and 1 dog who was treated with combination chemotherapy developed lym-

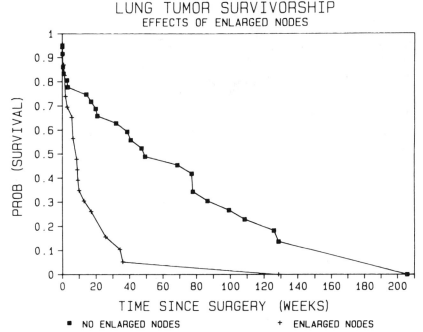

Figure 20-15. Survival curve of 76 dogs with and without enlarged lymph nodes secondary to pulmonary neoplasia. Normal size lymph nodes were associated with a significant survival improvement (p < 0.01)[59b]

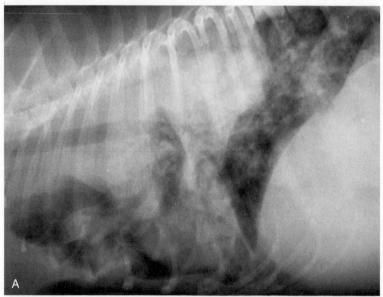

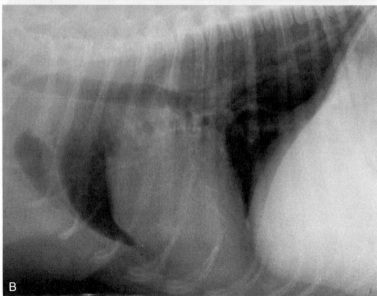

Figure 20-16. Lateral radiograph of a 3-year-old dog demonstrating a large perihilar mass with additional peripheral parenchymal lung pathology. *(B)* Lateral radiograph of dog in A 1 year after chemotherapy with cyclophosphamide, vincristine, and prednisone. Chemotherapy was given for 6 months, and the dog remains in remission 3 years later.

phoblastic leukemia 2 months after initiating therapy. Two dogs were euthanatized at the time of diagnosis, and the remaining dog was treated with surgical excision of a mass lesion located on the external nares (only case without lung disease).

The etiology of lymphomatoid granulomatosis remains unknown; it may represent a preneoplastic, immune-mediated, or allergic disease. The disease responds to combination chemotherapy and carries a good prognosis with ade-

quate treatment. Lymphomatoid granulomatosis must be recognized as a distinct disease entity with a much better prognosis than other more commonly diagnosed primary or metastatic diseases affecting the canine lung.

Malignant Histiocytosis in Bernese Mountain Dogs[62,63]

This recently described condition was reported in 10 male and 1 female Bernese Mountain dogs. Nine dogs were closely related, suggesting a genetic predisposition. Most patients were middle-aged (range 4 to 10 years, mean 7 years). Respiratory signs were the most common complaint, although weight loss, lethargy, and anorexia were also noted. Three patients were presented for neurologic abnormalities. Most patients had radiographic evidence of a large pulmonary nodule (> 5 cm in diameter), and smaller nodules were visible as well. Clinically or at necropsy all patients had metastasis beyond the lung tissue. The most common sites of metastasis were lymph node, liver, kidney, and central nervous system (two brain, three epidural space). Treatment was rarely attempted in this series, but it is obvious that surgical resection is limited to diagnostics and that some form of systemic chemotherapy is indicated. Combination chemotherapy using doxorubicin, cyclophosphamide and vincristine has been used in a few cases with significant responses (> 75% regression) for as long as 6 months.[†]

REFERENCES

1. Hargis AM: A review of solar-induced lesions in domestic animals. Comp Cont Educ 3:287–294, 1981

2. Evans AG, Madewell BR, Stannard AA: A trial of 13-*cis*-retinoic acid for treatment of squamous cell carcinoma and preneoplastic lesions of the head in cats. Am J Vet Res 46:2553–2557, 1985

3. Grier RL, Brewer WG, Theilen GH: Hyperthermic treatment of superficial tumors in cats and dogs. J Am Vet Med Assoc 177:227–233, 1980

4. Carlisle CH, Gould S: Response of squamous cell carcinoma of the nose of the cat to treatment with x-rays. Vet Radiol 23:186–192, 1982

5. Thrall DE, Adams WM: Radiotherapy of squamous cell carcinomas of the canine nasal plane. Vet Radiol 23:193–195, 1982

5a. Withrow SJ, Straw RC: Resection of the nasal planum in nine cats and five dogs. J Am Anim Hosp Assoc in press, 1989

6. Levene MB, Harley HA, Goldwyn RM: Cancers of the skin. In DeVita VT, et al (eds): Cancer: Principles and Practice of Oncology, pp. 1094–1123. Philadelphia, J.B. Lippincott, 1982

7. MacEwen EG, Withrow SJ, Patnaik AK: Nasal tumors in the dog: Retrospective evaluation of diagnosis, prognosis, and treatment. J Am Vet Med Assoc 170:45–48, 1977

8. Stunzi H, Hauser B: Tumours of the nasal cavity. Bull WHO 53:257–263, 1976

9. Reif JS, Cohen D: The environmental distribution of canine respiratory tract neoplasms. Arch Environ Health 22:136–140, 1971

10. Madewell BR, Priester WA, Gillette EL, et al: Neoplasms of the nasal passages and paranasal sinuses in domesticated animals as reported by 13 veterinary colleges. Am J Vet Res 37:851–856, 1976

11. Patnaik AK, Lieberman PH, Erlandson RA, et al: Canine sinonasal skeletal neoplasms: Chondrosarcomas and osteosarcomas. Vet Pathol 21:475–482, 1984

12. Weir EC, Pond MJ, Duncan JR, et al: Extragenital occurrence of transmissible venereal tumor in the dog: literature review and case reports. J Am Anim Hosp Assoc 14:532–536, 1978

13. Straw RC, Withrow SJ, Gillette EL, et al: Use of radiotherapy for the treatment of intranasal tumors in cats: Six cases (1980–1985). J Am Vet Med Assoc 189:927–929, 1986

14. Gibbs C, Lane JG, Denny HR: Radiological features of intra-nasal lesions in the dog: A review of 100 cases. J Small Anim Pract 20:515–535, 1979

15. Withrow SJ, Susaneck SJ, Macy- DW, et al: Aspiration and punch biopsy techniques for nasal tumors. J Am Anim Hosp Assoc 21:551–554, 1985

16. Rudd RG, Richardson DC: A diagnostic and therapeutic approach to nasal disease in dogs. Comp Cont Educ 7:103–112, 1985

17. Bailey CS, Higgins RJ: Characteristics of cisternal cerebrospinal fluid associated with primary brain tumors in the dog: A retrospective study. J Am Vet Med Assoc 188:414–417, 1986

18. Feeney DA, Johnston GR, Williamson JF, et al: Orthovoltage radiation of normal canine nasal passages: Assessment of depth dose. Am J Vet Res 44:1593–1596, 1983

19. Thrall DE, Harvey CE: Radiotherapy of malignant nasal tumors in 21 dogs. J Am Vet Med Assoc 183:663–666, 1983

20. Roberts SM, Lavach JD, Severin GA, et al: Ophthalmic complications following megavoltage irradiation of the nasal and paranasal cavities in dogs. J Am Vet Med Assoc 190:43–47, 1987

21. Clendenin MA, Conrad MC: Collateral vessel development after chronic bilateral common carotid artery occlusion in the dog. Am J Vet Res 40:1244, 1979

[†] MacEwen EG, personal communication, 1989

22. Withrow SJ: Cryosurgical therapy for nasal tumors in the dog. J Am Anim Hosp Assoc 18:585–589, 1982

23. Norris AM: Intranasal neoplasms in the dog. J Am Anim Hosp Assoc 15:231–236, 1979

24. Adams WM, Withrow SJ, Walshaw R, et al: Radiotherapy of malignant nasal tumors of 67 dogs. J Am Vet Med Assoc 191:311–315, 1987

25. Million RR, Cassisi NJ, Wittes RE: Cancer in the head and neck. In DeVita VT, et al (eds): Cancer: Principles and Practice of Oncology, pp. 301–395. Philadelphia, J.B. Lippincott, 1982

26. Withrow SJ, Holmberg DL, Doige CE, Rosychuk RAW: Treatment of a tracheal osteochondroma with an overlapping end-to-end tracheal anastomosis. J Am Anim Hosp Assoc 14(4):469–473, 1978

27. Meuten DJ, Calderwood-Mays MB, Dillman RC, Cooper BJ, et al: Canine laryngeal rhabdomyoma. Vet Pathol 22:533–539, 1985

28. Pass DA, Huxtable CR, Cooper BJ, Watson ADJ, Thompson R: Canine laryngeal oncocytomas. Vet Pathol 17:672–677, 1980

29. Wheeldon EB, Suter PF, Jenkins T: Neoplasia of the larynx in the dog. J Am Vet Med Assoc 180:642–647, 1982

30. Saik JE, Toll SL, Diters RW, Goldschmidt MH: Canine and feline laryngeal neoplasia: A 10 year survey. J Am Anim Hosp Assoc 22:359–365, 1986

30a. Flanders JA, Castleman W, Carberry CA et al: Laryngeal chondrosarcoma in a dog. J Am Vet Med Assoc 190:68–70, 1987

30b. Turk MA, Johnson GC, Gallina AM et al: Canine granular cell tumor (myoblastoma): A report of four cases and a review of the literature. J Sm Anim Prac 24:637–645, 1983

31. Vasseur PB: Laryngeal adenocarcinoma in a cat. J Am Anim Hosp Assoc 17:639–641, 1981

32. Bryan RD, Frame RW, Kier AB: Tracheal leiomyoma in a dog. J Am Vet Med Assoc 178:1069–1070, 1981

33. Black AP, Liu S, Randolph JF: Primary tracheal leiomyoma in a dog. J Am Vet Med Assoc 179:905–907, 1981

34. Hendricks JC, O'Brien JA: Tracheal collapse in two cats. J Am Vet Med Assoc 187(4):418–419, 1985

35. Carb A, Halliwell WH: Osteochondral dysplasias of the canine trachea. J Am Anim Hosp Assoc 17:193–199, 1981

36. Nelson AW, Wykes PM: Upper respiratory system. In Slatter DH (ed): Textbook of Small Animal Surgery, pp. 950–990. Philadelphia, W.B. Saunders, 1985

37. Harvey CE: Speaking out. J Am Anim Hosp Assoc 22:568, 1986

38. Crowe DT, Goodwin MA, Greene CE: Total laryngectomy for laryngeal mast cell tumor in a dog. J Am Anim Hosp Assoc 22:809–816, 1986

39. Schneider PR, Smith CW, Feller DL: Histiocytic lymphosarcoma of the trachea in a cat. J Am Anim Hosp Assoc 15:485–487, 1979

40. Nelson AW: Lower respiratory system. In Slatter DH (ed): Textbook of Small Animal Surgery, pp. 950–990. Philadelphia, W.B. Saunders, 1985

41. Million RR, Cassisi NJ, Wittes RE: Cancer in the head and neck. In DeVita VT et al (eds): Cancer: Principles and Practice of Oncology, pp. 348–358. Philadelphia, J.B. Lippincott, 1982

42. Reif JS, Cohen D: The environmental distribution of canine respiratory tract neoplasms. Arch Environ Health 22:136–140, 1971

43. Auerbach O, Hammond EC, Kirman D, et al: Pulmonary neoplasms. Arch Environ Health 21:754–768, 1970

44. Humphrey EW, Ewing SL, Wrigley JV, et al: The production of malignant tumors of the lung and pleura in dogs from intratracheal asbestos instillation and cigarette smoking. Cancer 47:1994–1999, 1981

45. Moulton JE, von Tscharner C, Schneider R: Classification of lung carcinomas in the dog and cat. Vet Pathol 18:513–528, 1981

46. Koblik PD: Radiographic appearance of primary lung tumors in cats. Vet Radiol 27:66–73, 1986

47. Brodey RS, Craig PH: Primary pulmonary neoplasms in the dog: A review of 29 cases. J Am Vet Med Assoc 147:1628–1643, 1965

47a. Dallman MJ, Martin RA, Roth L: Pneumothorax as the primary problem in 2 cases of bronchoalveolar carcinoma in the dog. J Am An Hosp Assoc 24:710–714, 1988

48. Sorjonen DC, Braund KG, Hoff EJ: Paraplegia and subclinical neuromyopathy associated with a primary lung tumor in a dog. J Am Vet Med Assoc 180:1209–1211, 1982

49. Biery DN: Differentiation of lung diseases of inflammatory or neoplastic origin from lung diseases in heart failure. Vet Clin North Am 4:711–721, 1974

49a. Barr FJ, Gibbs C, Brown PJ: The radiographic features of primary lung tumors in the dog: A review of thirty-six cases. J Sm Anim Pract 27:493–505, 1986

50. Venker–van Haagen AJ, Vroom MW, Heijn A, et al: Bronchoscopy in small animal clinics:

an analysis of the results of 228 bronchoscopies. J Am Anim Hosp Assoc 21:521–526, 1985

51. Berquist TH, Bailey PB, Cortese DA, et al: Transthoracic needle biopsy. Accuracy and complications in relation to location and type of lesion. Mayo Clin Proc 55:475-481, 1980

52. Roudebush P, Green RA, Digilio KM: Percutaneous fine-needle aspiration biopsy of the lung in disseminated pulmonary disease. J Am Anim Hosp Assoc 17:109–116, 1981

53. Mehlhaff CJ, Leifer CE, Patnaik AK, et al: Surgical treatment of primary pulmonary neoplasia in 15 dogs. J Am Anim Hosp Assoc 20:799–803, 1984

54. LaRue SM, Withrow SJ, Wykes PM: Lung resection using surgical staples in dogs and cats. Vet Surg 16:238–240, 1987

55. Laing EJ, Norris AM: Pleurodesis as a treatment for pleural effusion in the dog. J Am Anim Hosp Assoc 2:193–196, 1986

55a. Shapiro W, Turrel J: Management of pleural effusion secondary to metastatic adenocarcinoma in a dog. J Am Vet Med Assoc 192:530–532, 1988

56. Spanos PK, Payne WS, Ivins JC, et al: Pulmonary resection for metastatic osteogenic sarcoma. J Bone Jt Surg 58A:624–628, 1976

57. Huth JF, Holmes EC, Vernon SE: Pulmonary resection for metastatic sarcoma. Am J Surg 140:9–16, 1980

58. Roth JA, Putnam JB, Wesley MN, et al: Differing determinants of prognosis following resection of pulmonary metastases from osteogenic and soft tissue sarcoma patients. Cancer 55:1361–1366, 1985

59. Hause WR: Treatment of musculoskeletal tumors of the dog and cat, selected cases. Proc 4th An Kal Kan Symp, Columbus, Ohio, pp. 45-52. 1980

59a. Withrow SJ, Straw RC, Richter SC et al: Pulmonary metastasectomy for canine osteosarcoma. The 8th Annual Conf, Vet Cancer Soc, Estes Park, Colo, 8:2, 1988

59b. Ogilvie GK, Weigel RM, Haschek WM et al: Prognostic factors for tumor remission and survival in dogs after surgery for primary lung tumors: 76 cases (1975–1985). J Am Vet Med Assoc, in press, 1989

60. Minna JD, Higgins GA, Glatstein EJ: Cancer of the lung. In DeVita VT et al (eds): Cancer: Principles and Practice of Oncology, pp. 396–474. Philadelphia, J.B. Lippincott, 1982

61. Postorino NC, Wheeler SL, Park RD, et al: Canine pulmonary lymphomatoid granulomatosis: 8 cases (1981–1986). J Vet Int Med, 3:15–19, 1989

62. Rosin A, Moore P, Dubielzig R: Malignant histiocytosis in Bernese mountain dogs. J Am Vet Med Assoc 188:1041–1045, 1986

63. Moore PF: Systemic histiocytosis in Bernese mountain dogs. Vet Path 21:554–557, 1984

21

TUMORS OF THE SKELETAL SYSTEM

Susan Margaret LaRue
Stephen J. Withrow

OSTEOSARCOMA IN DOGS

INCIDENCE AND RISK FACTORS

Eighty percent of primary bone tumors in dogs are osteosarcomas, which represent 2% to 7% of all canine malignancies.[1,2] Osteosarcoma is estimated to occur in more than 6000 dogs in this country per year, and that figure may be increasing with the growing popularity of large and giant breeds. It is primarily a disease of middle-aged to older animals; the median age is 7 years.[3,4] However, osteosarcoma has been reported in dogs as young as 6 months, and an early prevalence peak occurs at 18–24 months.[5] Osteosarcoma is most likely to occur in large and giant breeds.[3,6] Fewer than 5% of cases reported have occurred in dogs weighing less than 25 pounds, and the tumor appears to be more size than breed related.[3,6] Males are more frequently affected than females, except in St. Bernards, where the female is most often affected.[3]

The etiology of canine osteosarcoma is not known. The occurrence of osteosarcoma in littermates and the ability to induce the disease in fetal puppies injected with osteosarcoma cells has led to speculation of a viral etiology.[7,8] However, no progress has been made in isolating a virus. The tendency of osteosarcoma to occur in major weight-bearing bones and late closing physes, plus the propensity in large and giant dogs, may point to multiple minor trauma as an inciting factor. The resulting increase in cell turnover may result in increased mutagenesis in these sites. Osteosarcomas have also been associated with metallic implants used for fracture repair, chronic osteomyelitis, and fractures in which no internal repair was used.[9–13] In these instances a diaphyseal location is much more common than in dogs with spontaneously occurring osteosarcoma.[14] Ionizing radiation has been shown to produce osteosarcoma in beagles exposed to radon, plutonium, and strontium. Osteosarcomas have also been associated with bone infarcts.[15,16] The cause of the infarcts, a condition quite unusual in bone, is unknown, but apparently not associated with embolic tumor shower. Osteosarcomas associated with bone infarcts often occur in smaller breeds.

PATHOLOGY AND NATURAL BEHAVIOR

The term osteosarcoma is synonymous with osteogenic sarcoma, meaning bone-forming tumor. This describes the hallmark histologic finding, the appearance of tumor-produced osteoid. The sarcoma cells are plump, polygonal to spindle shaped, and the osteoid produced is variably mineralized. Generally canine osteosarcomas are invasive and cellular, with pleomorphic cells and often numerous mitotic figures, indicating an aggressive tumor. Canine osteosarcoma can vary in the type and quantity of matrix produced and pattern of cell arrangement; it is subclassified as osteoblastic, chondroblastic, fibroblastic, and telangiectatic (vascular). These patterns may vary from tumor to tumor or even within the same tumor. Hence, small biopsy samples may be misdiagnosed as chondrosarcoma, fibrosarcoma, or hemangiosarcoma. It is therefore important to obtain follow-up histologic analysis of the entire tumor following therapy.

More than 75% of osteosarcomas occur in long bones, and the remainder occur in the axial skeleton.[3] The metaphyseal region is most frequently affected. The tumor is twice as likely to occur in the front limb than the rear, and the distal radius and proximal humerus are the two most common locations.[17] Tumors in the elbow region are uncommon. In the rear limbs, tumors are evenly distributed between the distal femur, distal tibia, and proximal tibia; the proximal femur is a slightly less common site.[3] The skull (maxilla and mandible) and the ribs, at the costochondral junction, are major sites for osteosarcoma of the axial skeleton, but vertebral bodies and pelvis also may be affected.[3] Multicentric osteosarcoma occurs, but represents less than 10% of total cases.[18] Osteosarcoma is a highly metastatic tumor; 90% of affected animals not receiving chemotherapy will develop metastasis, generally to the lungs, within 1 year of amputation or control of the primary tumor.[3,19]

HISTORY AND CLINICAL SIGNS

Dogs with osteosarcoma generally present with a lameness associated with a mild traumatic episode. This history can often lead to misdi-agnosis of a strain or sprain. The pain is likely due to microfractures provoked by osteolysis or to pressure on the periosteum and surrounding tissues. The lameness worsens and swelling becomes apparent. Less frequently dogs present with pathologic fractures or with diffuse edema of the distal extremity due to lymphatic or venous blockage by a tumor located in the proximal extremity. Dogs with tumors arising from flat bones present with local swelling, and in tumors affecting the ribs, respiratory compromise may result. Tumors in the nasal cavity result in nasal obstruction and facial deformity. Tumors involving the vertebral spine may result in neurologic dysfunction.

DIAGNOSTIC TECHNIQUES AND WORK-UP

Radiographic analysis should include at least two views of the suspected site. Radiographic changes include a mixed appearance of osteolysis and bony proliferation, though either change may dominate (Fig. 21-1). Early in the course of the tumor, osteolysis can be punctate and focal. However, by the time of diagnosis there is generally significant cortical disruption and extension of the tumor into adjacent soft tissues. The osteolysis may predispose the bone to pathologic fracture. Bone proliferation includes both normal periosteal reaction and tumor osteoid production. The appearance of tumor osteoid ranges from focal areas of increased density to a generalized increase in density. Late in the course of the disease the tumor may take on a sunburst appearance as tumor osteoid radiates perpendicularly from the tumor. The transitional zone from tumor to normal bone is often poorly defined. Periosteal reaction is not specific to the tumor, but rather a response to injury of the bone.

Subperiosteal new bone formation blends with normal-appearing reactive bone beyond the periphery of the tumor, causing a triangular formation of new bone known as Codman's triangle. When seen Codman's triangle is a harbinger of an aggressive malignant lesion that has invaded soft tissue. This sign does not necessarily persist through the course of the disease, as tumor expansion can eliminate it. In most cases, the tumor does not invade or cross the articular cartilage, but may cross joints by extension along the joint capsule. It may, however, invade the adjacent bone of a two-bone system, although

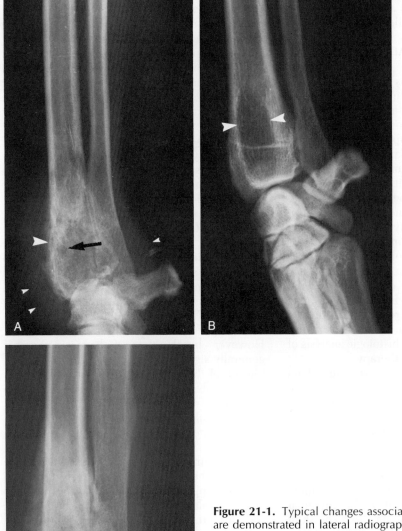

Figure 21-1. Typical changes associated with primary bone tumors are demonstrated in lateral radiographs of distal radii in three dogs with histologically confirmed osteosarcoma. *(A)* Note areas of punctate lysis (black arrow) and cortical destruction (large white arrowhead) as well as areas of increased bone density. Soft tissue swelling is evident both cranially and caudally (small white arrowheads). *(B)* Radiographic changes seen here are primarily lytic. The lysis (white arrowheads) is confined to the medullary cavity and has not yet caused cortical destruction. *(C)* Radiographic changes are predominantly proliferative in this example. Regions of periosteal proliferation (large white arrowhead) as well as areas that may represent tumor osteoid production (small white arrowheads) are observed. Regions of punctate osteolysis (black arrow) are also detected.

irritation from the tumor can cause periosteal reaction to occur in the second bone.

In addition to osteosarcoma, other conditions that must be considered when a dog presents with a lytic and proliferative bony condition are other primary bone tumors, such as chondrosarcoma and fibrosarcoma; round cell tumors, such as plasma cell myeloma and lymphoma, which can originate in bone; metastatic spread from other primary tumor sites; and bacterial or fungal osteomyelitis. Other primary bone tumors are discussed later in this chapter. Round cell tumors of bone are unusual; their radiographic appearance is generally lytic.[20] Histologic evaluation is generally necessary to diagnose these tumors. Metastatic spread to bone can occur with almost any primary malignant tumor. Dogs presenting with bony lesions should always be carefully evaluated for other tumor sources. Dogs with bacterial osteomyelitis usually have a history of penetrating trauma (including open fractures or orthopedic surgery) and persistent draining tracts. Dogs with fungal infection of bone have generally traveled into fungal endemic regions, and a travel history should always be part of the history. Fungal infections occur through respiratory and hematogenous routes. With coccidioidomycosis, the respiratory phase has often resolved by the time the osteomyelitis occurs, and although thoracic radiographs are indicated, the most common finding on these dogs is occasional enlargement of the hilar lymph nodes. In contrast, the respiratory phase of blastomycosis is generally still active at the time of boney involvement. Thoracic radiographs may reveal diffuse miliary nodular interstitial pneumonia. These pulmonary changes are distinct and generally not confused with metastatic disease. Animals with blastomycosis are often debilitated, and the disease is usually widely disseminated. Diagnosis can sometimes be made by the detection of spores on cytologic evaluation of regional lymph nodes. Fungal lesions can occur anywhere in bone, but the metaphyseal region is most common, due to superior blood supply. Multiple lesions can occur and do not rule out osteosarcoma, which can be multifocal. Animals of any age can contract fungal infections, but young or immunologically suppressed dogs are most susceptible.[21]

Although a presumptive diagnosis of osteosarcoma can be based on compatible signalment, history, and radiographic changes, definitive diagnosis requires biopsy and histologic evaluation. Bone biopsy can be performed quickly and accurately with an 8- or 11-gauge Jamshidi* type biopsy needle (Fig. 21-2).[22] In bone, the center of the neoplastic lesion is most likely to yield a diagnostic sample.[23] This is because bone surrounding almost any insult, including trauma, infection, and neoplasia, can become reactive. Samples containing only reactive bone are at best recognized as inadequate and at worst misdiagnosed as benign lesions. Therefore the lesion should be measured on the radiograph with reference to a nearby landmark, generally the adjacent joint. At the time of biopsy the radiographs should be in view, and a sterile ruler available. At least two biopsy samples should be obtained, one running through the center of the lesion, and one starting at the center and angling toward the periphery of the tumor. It is important that discernible cores of bone and medullary or extramedullary tissue be obtained. In extremely lytic tumors it may be necessary to sample at the periphery of the tumor in order to obtain an acceptable core of tissue.[22] Bone biopsies must be obtained with sterile techniques. Any appropriate general anesthetic regime may be used. In some instances, particularly with an extremely lytic lesion, heavy sedation and local anesthesia may be adequate for restraint.

If osteosarcoma is diagnosed, a thorough search should be made for any apparent spread of the disease. Physical examination should include palpation of lymph nodes, all extremities, the spine, and the abdominal cavity. Lymph node metastasis is rare, but fine-needle aspiration of enlarged regional lymph nodes should be performed. Thoracic radiographs should be taken during inspiration, and should include a ventrodorsal view and lateral radiographs taken on both sides. Metastatic osteosarcoma in the lungs is usually not seen until the nodules are bigger than 6–8 mm. The nodules are round and are usually found in the periphery of the lungs. It is most common to find clusters of nodules, but single nodules are occasionally detected. Radio-

* Jamshidi bone marrow needle, American Pharmaseal Co., Valencia, CA. Bone marrow biopsy needle, Sherwood Medical Co., St. Louis, MO.

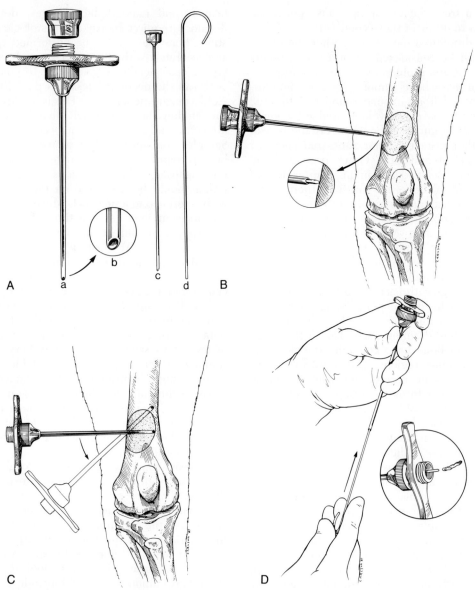

Figure 21-2. *(A)* The Jamshidi type biopsy needle: cannula and screw-on cap (a), tapered point (inset b), pointed stylet to advance cannula through soft tissue (c), and probe to expel specimen from cannula (d). *(B)* With the stylet locked in place, the cannula is advanced through soft tissue until bone is reached. Inset: close-up of portion of bone with stylet up to cortex. *(C)* The stylet removed and the bone cortex penetrated with the cannula. The cannula is withdrawn and the procedure is repeated with redirection of the needle. *(D)* The probe is then inserted into the tip of the cannula and the specimen expelled through the cannula base (insert).[22]

graphically detectable lung metastases are found at the time of initial presentation in fewer than 5% of dogs with osteosarcoma.[18] A radiographic

bone survey, including lateral radiographs of all bones, reveals additional neoplasia in up to 10% of cases.[18] Nuclear bone scans may also be employed to detect multiple sites of bone involvement. Although these radiographic studies are low yield, the importance of recognizing apparent metastatic disease in determining appropriate therapeutic alternatives warrants the procedures. Additionally, a complete blood count, serum biochemical panel, and urinalysis should be performed to help assess the dog's overall physical condition.

THERAPY AND PROGNOSIS

Successful treatment of osteosarcoma includes local tumor control as well as the treatment of systemic tumor spread. Historically, a number of methods of treatment have been attempted with dismal results. Radiation therapy for local tumor control was unsuccessful.[24,25] Cryotherapy combined with surgical debulking also failed to control local tumor and was fraught with complications.[26] En bloc surgical resection is generally impossible without removing neurovascular structures vital for limb function, and marginal resections alone do not provide tumor control. Amputation alone generally provides good primary tumor control; however, long-term survival is poor owing to metastatic spread.[27] Various chemotherapeutic and immunologic agents were used adjuvantly with amputation in attempts to improve long-term survival. BCG vaccine, high dosages of methotrexate with leucovorin rescue, doxorubicin, RA233 (mopidamole), and combinations of drugs have had no positive effect on survival.[28–34,34a] A recently completed study using liposome encapsulated muramylpeptides (MTP) combined with surgical amputation showed evidence of reduced metastasis and prolonged survival when compared to dogs treated with surgery alone.[34b,34c]

Early attempts at limb sparing, using a combination of surgical debulking, chemotherapy, and radiation therapy or local hyperthermia and radiation therapy were also unsuccessful.[35–37] However, more recent adjuvant chemotherapeutic regimes and limb-sparing procedures have encouraging results and should be considered as treatment alternatives, particularly when the animal is free of apparent tumor spread.

Amputation alone is aimed at achieving local tumor control. It is very important that the tumor be removed en bloc. The extent of the tumor should be estimated from radiographic and physical exam findings before surgery is planned. Forequarter amputation (including the scapula) is advocated for tumors anywhere on a front limb. Large tumors of the proximal humerus may necessitate removal of the pectoral muscles. Amputation at the level of the proximal one third of the femur may be adequate for tumors below the stifle, while hip disarticulation is necessary for tumors of the distal femur. Osteosarcoma of the proximal femur may require resection of the acetabulum (subtotal hemipelvectomy) en bloc with the femur to ensure complete removal.

Local tumor control is good following amputation, but 90% of dogs develop metastatic disease, generally to the lungs, within 1 year of amputation and the mean survival is only 3 to 6 months. Despite the poor long-term survival, amputation for osteosarcoma provides a number of advantages. The quality of life of these animals is generally excellent.[38] Recovery from surgery and adaptation to the loss of limb is quick. The animal's attitude and mobility often improves owing to relief of pain. Thoracic radiographs may be evaluated every 3 months. The metastatic pattern for dogs not receiving adjuvant therapy is generally that of diffuse nodularity in all lung lobes. If solitary or slow-growing nodules appear, the dog may be a candidate for thoracotomy and metastatectomy (see Chapter 20).

Amputation combined with certain chemotherapeutic agents may enhance survival. In one study, 19 dogs received adjuvant chemotherapy two weeks following amputation.[38a] Doxorubicin (30 mg/m^2 IV) was administered on day one and cisplatin (60 mg/m^2 IV) was administered on day 21. The treatment cycle was repeated twice. Survival was compared with 19 dogs who underwent amputation only. The median survival of the 19 dogs treated with amputation and chemotherapy was 300 days, which was significantly longer than the median survival of 175 days in dogs treated with surgery alone.

Similar survival times were obtained when a cisplatin was administered at 40–50 mg/m^2 for 2 to 6 treatments at 28-day intervals,[38b] or at 70 mg/m^2 for two treatments 21 days apart (personal communication, RC Straw, Colorado State University, 1989) (Fig. 21-3).

The optimal dose of cisplatin, the number of doses, and the timing of administration has not been determined. The role of doxorubicin as an adjuvant drug is not certain.[34a,39] Current recommendations include intravenous administra-

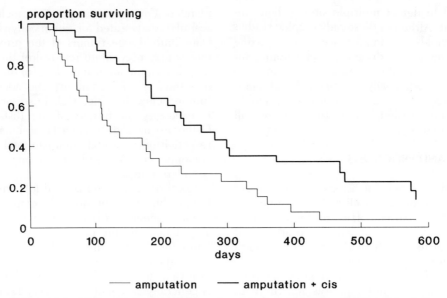

Figure 21-3. Kaplan Meier probability of survival of 35 dogs receiving amputation only and 32 dogs who received amputation and two intravenous doses of cisplatin at 70 mg/m². This difference in survival is statistically significant (p = 0.007) (Straw RC, Withrow SJ, Richter SL et al: Colorado State University, 1989)

tion of cisplatin at 60–70 mg/m², started as soon after surgery as the status of the patient permits. It should be repeated at 21 day intervals for at least two treatments, and preferably 3 to 6 treatments.

Limb-sparing procedures in dogs are relatively new and are available at a limited number of referral centers.[39a] The goals of limb sparing are to obtain local tumor control, provide a pain-free and functional limb, and enhance long-term survival. The procedures usually involve chemotherapy or radiation followed by surgical excision of the tumor and replacement of the bone with an allograft. A prospective pilot limb-sparing study at Colorado State University involving 20 dogs used various doses and routes of delivery (intravenous, intra-arterial) of *cis*-platinum.[40] Additionally, some dogs received conventional fractionated radiotherapy. After chemotherapy or chemotherapy and radiation, the tumors were resected and replaced with a cortical allograft (Fig. 21-4). Local tumor control was obtained in 69% of the cases. Limb function was good to excellent in 75% of the dogs; dogs with forelimb-sparing procedures had improved limb usage. One-year survival was 55%, and 2-year survival

was 35%. In spite of improved survival most patients ultimately died of metastatic osteosarcoma. Optimal dosages and methods of drug administration have yet to be determined.

Osteosarcomas of the axial skeleton may be aggressively excised; however, local control is difficult to achieve, and long-term survival is poor. In a series of dogs with primary bone tumors of the ribs, few dogs survived more than 4 months after diagnosis.[41] Combined modality therapy may offer the best prognosis.

A dog with apparent tumor spread at the time of diagnosis has a dismal prognosis. If the dog's general health has not deteriorated and the limb is adversely affecting the quality of life, amputation can be considered. Treatment with intravenous *cis*-platinum at 70 mg/m² may delay the progression of the disease.*

Useful prognostic indicators have not been found for canine osteosarcoma. One article positively correlated tumor diameter, volume, and extension into soft tissues with the presence of metastasis.[5] However, in dogs with no apparent

* Straw RC: Personal Communication, 1989

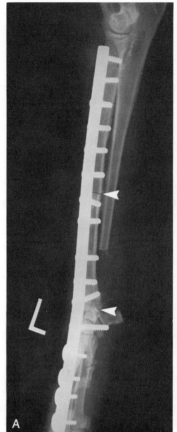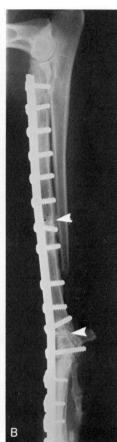

Figure 21-4. *(A)* Postoperative radiograph of a limb-sparing procedure to remove an osteosarcoma of the distal radius in a 10-year-old female golden retriever. Arrowheads depict the proximal and distal aspects of the cortical allograft. The distal ulna was removed and not replaced. Dog also received two doses of cisplatin. *(B)* Radiographic appearance of the same limb 3 months after surgery. Note healing of both the proximal and distal osteosynthesis sites. This dog was still alive with excellent limb function 24 months following surgery.

metastatic spread, no parameters have been identified by which to predict the development of metastasis following treatment.

COMPARATIVE ASPECTS

Osteosarcoma in dogs closely resembles osteosarcoma in humans.[3,42] Histologically the diseases are virtually indistinguishable, and osteosarcomas in both human and dog are likely to be a high histologic grade. The tumor rapidly metastasizes in both species. Following amputation without chemotherapy, metastasis occurs within 2 years in 80% of humans and within 1 year in 90% of dogs affected. Tumors in both species appear to be radioresistant and show responsiveness to *cis*-platinum. The disease tends to affect large males more commonly in both species, and the lesions are likely to occur in the metaphyseal region of weight-bearing bones.

The two major differences are the age of affected individuals and prevalence. Osteosarcoma in humans is generally a disease of adolescents, and it is a rare tumor, affecting only 800–1000 people per year in this country. The striking similarities, combined with the abundance of canine cases each year, make osteosarcoma in dogs an excellent model for study of osteosarcoma in man.

PAROSTEAL OSTEOSARCOMA

Parosteal osteosarcoma, also called juxtacortical or surface osteosarcoma, differs from intra-osseous osteosarcoma in its radiographic and histologic appearance as well as its biologic behavior. Histologically, the tumor is composed of well-differentiated regions of cartilage, fibrous tissue, and reactive bone. Some areas may appear more typical of intra-osseous osteosarcoma, with sarcomatous cells and tumor-produced osteoid. However, some areas of the tumor are difficult to differentiate histologically from reactive bone. Radiographically the tumor has a homogenous matrix. It generally arises from a thick pedicle and grows proximally and distally, outgrowing the base of the origin. The tumor does not cause gross destruction of the cortex, and does not invade the medullary cavity. Diagnosis must be based on both the histologic and radiographic findings.

Animals with parosteal osteosarcoma present with signs similar to those seen in animals with intra-osseous osteosarcoma; however, the signs may have been in evidence for an extended time.

Parosteal osteosarcomas behave less aggressively than intra-osseous ones, and with complete excision local control can be obtained. The tumor can metastasize, but it is thought the long-term survival is much better than with intra-osseous osteosarcoma.[43,44]

Therapy should be directed at obtaining local tumor control. Aggressive *en bloc* resection may be performed. On the extremities, a bone saw or osteotome may be used to remove the tumor and the adjacent cortical bone. If it is deemed necessary to remove full cortical thickness, then an allogenous or autogenous cortical graft may be used in conjunction with a bone plate for structural support. *En bloc* resections of parosteal osteosarcoma of the zygomatic arch have been successfully performed.[44]

Following resection, the margins of the tumor should be carefully examined for tumor infiltration. If infiltrated margins are present, the use of adjuvant chemotherapy, radiation therapy, or complete limb amputation should be considered.

OTHER PRIMARY BONE TUMORS OF DOGS

Primary bone tumors other than osteosarcoma are reported to represent roughly 20% of canine bone malignancies. Recent data imply that biopsy samples without accompanying evaluation of the remainder of the tumor specimen following treatment or euthanasia may result in misdiagnosis of some osteosarcomas as chondrosarcoma, fibrosarcoma, undifferentiated sarcoma, or hemangiosarcoma.[22] Thus the true incidence of these tumors is in question. The limited number of nonosteosarcoma cases makes it difficult to study the biologic behavior of these tumors; however trends for incidence and prognoses are available. It is important that true cases of nonosteosarcomatous bone tumors be recognized and given appropriate prognosis and therapy.

CHONDROSARCOMA

Chondrosarcoma is the second most common primary bone tumor, representing up to 10% of canine bone malignancies.[45,46] Chondrosarcoma occurs most often in large breeds, but giant breeds are less commonly affected. Chondrosarcoma can occur at almost any age, but peak occurrence is middle age. Flat bones are most commonly affected, with the nasal turbinates, ribs, maxilla, and pelvis the most common sites.

Histologically, chondrosarcomas are characterized by the production of neoplastic chondroid and mucinous intracellular matrix. Plump nuclei, sometimes in pairs, lie within lacunae in the tumor matrix. Mitotic figures may be scant or numerous, but when seen they are helpful in suggesting chondrosarcoma over chondromas. Undifferentiated regions may be present, and the cartilage may undergo ossification by a process similar to endochondral ossification, but malignant cells do not make new tumor osteoid.

The radiographic appearance is difficult to distinguish from osteosarcoma or other bone tumors (Fig. 21-5). Histologic evaluation is necessary for definitive diagnosis, but small biopsy samples must be interpreted with caution.

Dogs with chondrosarcoma of the ribs generally present with a firm swelling at the costochondral junction. Chondrosarcomas of the pelvis are usually quite large by the time of presentation and can often be detected by internal or external palpation. Chondrosarcomas of the ribs have been successfully excised with rib and chest wall resection techniques.[41] Similarly, amputation provides local control of chondrosarcomas of the extremity. Hemipelvectomy is generally necessary to control pelvic chondrosarcoma. True chondrosarcomas appear less likely to metastasize to the lung or other organs than osteosarcomas are; however, data on survival following treatment is limited. One paper

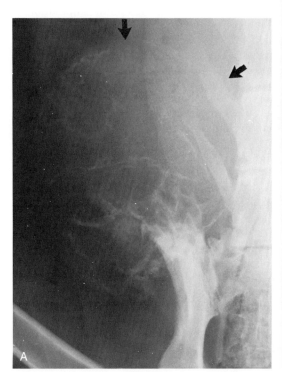
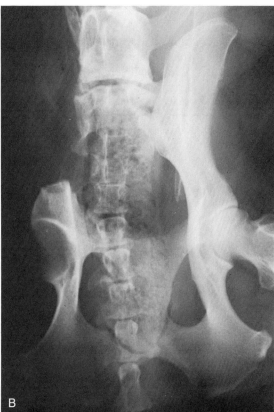

Figure 21-5. *(A)* The radiographic appearance of this ileal chondrosarcoma in a 6-year-old Labrador retriever is lytic and productive. The arrows depict the extent of the tumor. *(B)* Radiographic appearance following subtotal hemipelvectomy and partial sacrectomy. This dog is alive and free of disease 26 months following surgery.

suggested that the metastatic rate for skeletal chondrosarcoma in dogs is approximately 17%.[46a] Recommended therapy is aggressive surgery to obtain local tumor control (Fig. 21-5). Response of chondrosarcomas to radiation and chemotherapy is poor.

HEMANGIOSARCOMA

Hemangiosarcoma is thought to represent 2% to 3% of primary bone tumors.[46] It is primarily a disease of middle-aged dogs (mean age, 6.2 years),[47] but it can occur at almost any age. Males are affected more often than females (1.6:1). Primary bone hemangiosarcoma can occur in dogs of any size. Breeds commonly affected include the Great Dane, boxer, and German shepherd.[47]

The axial skeleton is more frequently affected than the appendicular skeleton (57%:43%), and the ribs and proximal humeri are the most frequently involved sites.

Hemangiosarcoma is a highly metastatic tumor. Virtually 100% of affected dogs will develop metastatic disease within 1 year of primary tumor diagnosis. Hemangiosarcoma can metastasize to the lungs, liver, kidney, adrenals, heart, omentum, peritoneum, or bone. Dogs with osseous hemangiosarcoma may present with tumors at other locations, making it difficult to ascertain the primary site.

Hemangiosarcoma is defined as a malignancy of vascular endothelial cells or their precursors. Histologically the disease is characterized by the formation of ill-defined, irregular vascular channels. Cords and clumps of spindle-shaped cells with large, pleomorphic nuclei align along strands of collagen and form small vascular spaces. Invasion of bone by the tumor and osteolysis due to numerous osteoclasts are apparent. Fingerlike extensions invade adjacent soft tissue structures. Unfortunately, the histologic changes are similar to those observed in telangiectatic osteosarcoma, and a conclusive diagnosis based on a small sample can be misleading.

History and presenting signs are the same as seen in osteosarcoma. Osteolysis is the dominant radiographic change, although the radiographic appearance cannot be conclusively distinguished from osteosarcoma (Fig. 21-6). When performing the bone biopsy, special care should be taken to obtain adequate tissue samples. Hemangiosarcomas often have vascular spaces and hemorrhage, which render samples nondiagnostic. It may be necessary to biopsy at the periphery of the tumor in order to obtain distinct cores of tissue.

If hemangiosarcoma is diagnosed, an aggressive search should be made for any apparent spread of the disease. In addition to the work-up suggested for osteosarcoma, an ultrasound evaluation of the heart should be performed to locate any evidence of right atrial involvement. If no apparent spread is found, amputation of the involved extremity may improve the quality of life until the animal succumbs from metastatic disease. Lesions involving the axial skeleton are generally not controlled by surgery. No chemotherapeutic regimes are known to enhance survival, although recent work suggests some activity with the use of vincristine, doxorubicin, and cyclophosphamide.[39]

FIBROSARCOMA

Osseous fibrosarcoma occurs in older dogs and affects the axial skeleton more commonly than the appendicular skeleton.[48] Histologically, the disease is characterized by well to poorly differentiated spindle-shaped tumor cells producing collagen in variable amounts. The surrounding bone is invaded, giving rise to lysis. Reactive bone can be seen at the tumor margins, but no tumor-produced osteoid is evident. Information on the biologic behavior of the tumor is limited, but it is believed that fibrosarcomas are less likely to metastasize than other primary bone tumors.

Radiographically, fibrosarcoma cannot be distinguished from other primary bone tumors. Diagnosis is dependent on the biopsy and subsequent histologic evaluation of the tumor. Amputation is the therapy of choice. No evidence exists to support the use of chemotherapy following amputation.

SYNOVIAL CELL SARCOMA

Incidence and Risk Factors

Synovial cell sarcomas are rarely reported tumors in dogs. Synovioma, synovial sarcoendothelioma, and malignant synovioma are terms that have been used to describe the tumor; however, synovial cell sarcoma is the preferred name. The tumor tends to occur in large, but not giant breeds, and males are more commonly affected than females.[49,50] It is primarily a disease of middle-aged to older animals with a mean age of 8 years and a range of 2–14 years.

Pathology and Natural Behavior

Synovial sarcomas are mesenchymally derived, and the histologic appearance mimics that of

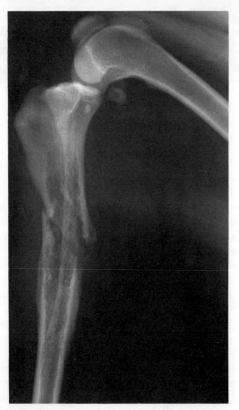

Figure 21-6. Lateral radiograph of the tibia of a 9-year-old Shetland sheepdog. Note extreme lysis and pathologic fracture. The histologic diagnosis was hemangiosarcoma.

synovial tissues. However, the tumor is not thought to originate in the synovial lining cells. Rather, it is believed to originate from nonspecific connective tissue outside of the synovial membrane.[51]

Histologically, the tumor is composed of two cell types. The synovial component is composed of cells that may vary in appearance from plump to elongated. The cytoplasm stains deeply, and the nucleus is eccentric. The cells may be grouped in packets or cords, or it may be diffusely intermingled with the fibrosarcomatous cells. The fibrosarcomatous cells have a spindle shape and may produce collagen or reticulum fibers. These cells stain poorly and have indistinct borders. The fibrosarcomatous cell type tends to predominate, resulting often in a misdiagnosis of nondifferentiated sarcoma or fibrosarcoma.

Synovial sarcomas are found in the extremities and are most commonly associated with major joints. Although grossly they appear circumscribed, they are locally invasive and thus may be difficult to control with surgical resection. Metastasis is reported to occur in up to 31% of cases and may involve the lungs or regional lymph nodes. Stump recurrences following amputation have been observed, even when the original tumor was far distal to the surgical site. Whether these recurrences are due to skip lesions or local nodal involvement is not known.

History and Clinical Signs

Dogs with synovial cell sarcomas generally present with lameness that may or may not be accompanied by a soft tissue mass. The progression of the tumor may vary from slow and insidious to rapid and may be accompanied by bony destruction. The degree of lameness may be associated with the amount of bony lysis. Radiographic evidence of a soft tissue mass is generally present and may be the only radiographically detectable abnormality (Fig. 21-7). When bony lysis is present, it usually involves both bones of the joint. The lysis may be permeated or poorly demarcated, and periosteal reaction may be present.

Diagnosis must be confirmed by histologic evaluation. The biopsy specimens should include tissues from both the bone and the soft tissue mass. Bone biopsy can be easily obtained with the Jamshidi biopsy technique previously described. A small wedge biopsy should be obtained from the soft tissue mass. Entering the joint is not necessary. Cytologic evaluation of regional lymph nodes should be obtained when possible. Thoracic radiographs should also be done.

Therapy and Prognosis

Amputation is currently the therapy of choice for synovial sarcomas. Forequarter amputation is advised for tumors of the front limb. A proximal femoral amputation is currently advocated for tumors of or below the tibial tarsal joint. A coxofemoral disarticulating amputation should be performed for most stifle tumors. Excision of the tumor alone may result in local recurrence. Chemotherapy alone, using doxorubicin and cyclophosphamide, has been reported in a dog that underwent tumor remission and was alive 36 months following therapy.[52]

In humans with synovial sarcomas, the tumor bed is routinely irradiated following surgical excision.[53] Local control is good if only microscopic amounts of tumor remain in the field. Although this method has not been explored extensively in veterinary medicine, it may be worthy consideration if amputation is not a viable alternative.

GIANT CELL TUMORS

Giant cell tumors of bone are rare in dogs. They occur most commonly in long bones, and no age, breed, sex, or size factors have been identified. Radiographically, the appearance is similar to that of other bone tumors. Multinucleated giant cells are common in many bone tumors; thus histologic diagnosis is dependent on more than the presence of giant cells. The tumor is characterized by two populations of malignant cells: stromal cells and multinucleated giant cells. The giant cells contain from 2 to 30 centrally aggregated nuclei. They are generally well differentiated, with minimal pleomorphism or mitotic figures. The natural behavior of the tumor is not known in dogs. There have been reports of long-term survival following surgical excision.[54] Treatment should focus on establishing local control of the tumor, and amputation is the preferred surgery when the lesions involve the long bones.

MALIGNANT MESENCHYMOMA

Malignant mesenchymoma is an unusual tumor in dogs. It is characterized histologically by a

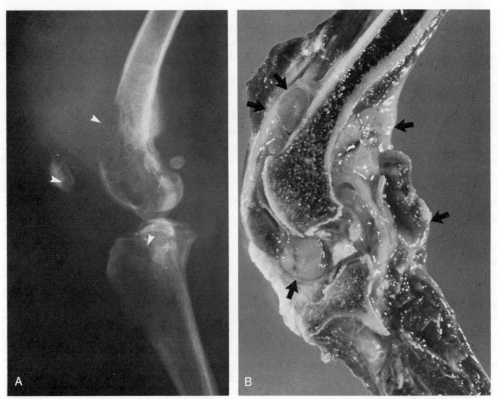

Figure 21-7. *(A)* Lateral radiograph of the stifle joint of a 9-year-old poodle demonstrates lytic involvement of the femur, tibia, and patella (white arrowheads). The patella is pushed cranially due to tumor proliferation. The histologic diagnosis was synovial cell sarcoma. *(B)* In this gross specimen of the patient seen in A the extent of soft tissue involvement can be appreciated (arrows depict tumor).

mixture of two or more mesenchymal derivatives not commonly associated (*e.g.*, fibrosarcoma, hemangiosarcoma, chondrosarcoma, osteosarcoma, and so forth). No breed or sex predilections are known. Radiographic characteristics include both lytic and proliferative changes, with multiple cystic compartments. The biologic behavior of this tumor in dogs is not well characterized, although locally the tumor is quite invasive. Amputation is probably the best method of obtaining local tumor control.

BENIGN BONE TUMORS AND NONTUMOROUS BONE LESIONS

OSTEOMAS

Osteomas are dense, well-circumscribed lesions of bone that are generally firmly attached to normal bone. Radiographically they appear sclerotic (Fig. 21-8). Their density makes it difficult to obtain biopsy specimens. The use of a Michele trephine is often necessary to obtain an adequate core of tissue. Histologically the lesion is difficult to distinguish from reactive bone. Thus the diagnosis must be based on radiographic, clinical, and histologic findings. Treatment is not generally warranted unless the osteoma interferes with function or is cosmetically unacceptable to the owner. Surgical excision is the treatment of choice. An osteotome may be necessary to separate the osteoma from adjacent bone.

MULTILOBULAR OSTEOMA

Multilobular osteoma is a term used for chondroma rodens and osteochondroma of the skull; it is synonymous with canine aponeurotic fi-

treated dogs, 7 had local recurrence with a median time to local recurrence of 14 months. Seven dogs also developed metastasis to lung with a median time to metastasis of 14 months as well. Overall median survival was 21 months.[55a] Without intervention, local growth of the tumor continues, and pressure on vital structures in the area can lead to the demise of the animal. Radiographically, the tumors are characterized by an amorphous pattern of radiodensity. The tumor often has a granular appearance (Fig. 21-9). The margins of the lesion are generally well defined.

Surgical resection is the treatment of choice, and it can be curative. Incomplete removal may result in tumor regrowth.[55a] The effectiveness of primary or adjuvant radiation or chemotherapy is unknown although minimal response was noted for either treatment in a small series of dogs.[55a]

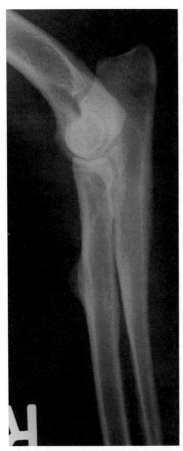

Figure 21-8. Lateral radiograph of the proximal radius of a 2-year-old male Irish setter. The histologic diagnosis was osteoma.

broma. Multilobular osteomas are hypothesized to arise from a focal area of perturbed periosteal activity.[55]

Although uncommon, multilobular osteoma is the most frequently seen tumor of the canine skull. The tumor generally occurs in middle-aged to older dogs (mean age, 7 years) but has been reported in dogs as young as 13 months.

Multilobular osteoma generally affects dogs of medium and large breeds. Occurrence in giant breeds is unusual. Multilobular osteoma most commonly involves the parietal crest, the tempero-occipital region, and the base of the zygomatic process. Although the tumor was not originally thought to be highly metastatic, a review of 16 cases that includes extensive follow-up periods revealed that up to 50% of these tumors may eventually metastasize.[55a] Of twelve

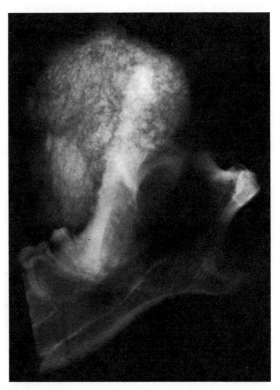

Figure 21-9. Radiograph of a multilobular osteoma (chondroma rodens) on the surgically excised mandible of a 9-year-old large, mixed breed dog. The tumor is granular in appearance, and the margins are well defined. The dog was alive and free of disease 24 months following surgical excision.

MULTIPLE CARTILAGINOUS EXOSTOSES (OSTEOCHONDROMATOSIS)

Multiple cartilaginous exostoses is a developmental condition of growing dogs. Because diagnosis is often incidental, the incidence of the disease may be underestimated. No breed or sex predilection is apparent; however evidence supports a hereditary basis.[56,57]

The condition is characterized by polyostotic osteochondroma formation. These cartilage-capped bony growths protrude from the surface of bone (Fig. 21-10). The lesions can occur on any bone formed by endochondral ossification, but the vertebra, ribs, and long bones are most commonly affected. The nodule may continue to grow until skeletal maturity is reached, when the nodule usually persists unchanged. These lesions can, however, transform to malignancies (usually osteosarcoma or chondrosarcoma) later in life.[58] The likelihood of malignant transformation increases with increasing numbers of lesions. The histologic appearance of the benign lesion is characterized by a cartilaginous cap giving rise to a stalk of trabecular bone by means of orderly endochondral ossification. The cortical surfaces of the bony stalk and adjacent bone are confluent.[58a]

Dogs generally present with a bony swelling that may be painful. While the nodule grows, it gives the appearance of moving closer to the diaphysis of the bone. Pain and lameness are due to pressure on soft tissues in the region and mechanical interference by the nodule with normal soft tissue movements associated with ambulation.

Radiographs of the lesion show a sessile or pedunculated bony mass. A presumptive diag-nosis can be based on radiographic findings, clinical signs, and signalment. If histologic confirmation is necessary, it is important to obtain tissue from both the cap and the stalk.

Treatment is dependent on the severity of signs. If signs do not abate at skeletal maturation, surgical excision of the nodule may be necessary. The owner should be informed of the hereditary aspects of the disease, and use of the dog for breeding should be discouraged. Additionally the owner should be apprised of the possibility of malignant transformation and instructed to seek immediate counsel if the appearance of the nodule changes.

BONE CYSTS

Bone cysts are uncommon in dogs. Bone cysts are classified as simple, subchondral, or aneurysmal. Simple bone cysts may be either mono- or polyostotic and occur in the metaphyseal region. They have been reported in both large and small dogs, and appear most commonly in dogs under 1 year of age. Histologic examination reveals cavities lined with fibrous connective tissue. Multinucleate giant cells may be abundant. Dogs generally present with a lameness due to microfractures in the bone or fluid distension impinging on soft tissue structures. Radiographic evaluation reveals a well-circumscribed lytic lesion in the metaphyseal region (Fig. 21-11). The cyst may appear compartmentalized, and thinning of the surrounding cortical bone may be apparent.

Subchondral bone cysts differ from simple bone cysts only in location. Subchondral bone cysts, also known as juxtacortical bone cysts, are

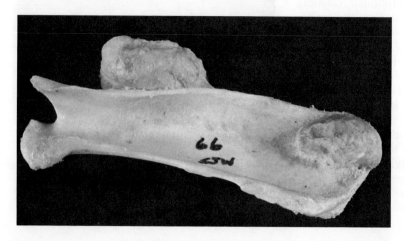

Figure 21-10. Gross appearance of two multiple cartilagenous exostoses on the scapula of a dog.

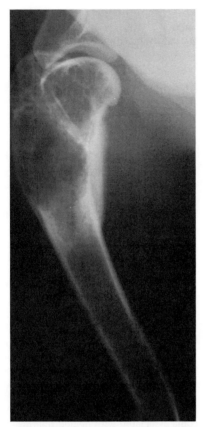

Figure 21-11. Lateral radiograph of a metaphyseal bone cyst in a 2-year-old bearded collie. Compartmentalization and thinning of the surrounding cortical bone is apparent.

located between the growth plate and the articular cartilage.

If pain from simple or subchondral bone cysts persists, therapy is indicated. If possible, therapy should be delayed until the adjacent growth plate is closed. The cyst should be surgically curetted and an effort made to remove the tissue lining. Bone chips or cancellous graft may be packed into the defect. The growth plate and joint should not be entered.

Aneurysmal bone cysts are proposed to be formed by aneurysmic vessels in the region. Aneurysmal bone cysts may be more aggressive in appearance and behavior. The soft tissue component may become large, and severe erosion of the surrounding bone may occur. Histologic evaluation reveals blood-filled cavities lined by proliferative fibrous tissue with active fibroblasts, hemosiderin-laden macrophages, and some multinucleated cells.

Destruction of the bone occurs without surgical intervention. Surgical curettage and packing of the defected with cancellous bone graft or bone chips has been recommended for this condition.

METASTATIC TUMORS OF BONE

Metastatic spread to bone can occur with almost any malignancy. Metastatic lesions have been reported in a variety of locations, although the most common site may be the lumbar vertebrae and pelvis owing to the common occurrence of urogenital malignancies (prostate, bladder, urethra, and mammary)[59] that may drain to these sites. Because metastatic bone tumors often cannot be distinguished radiographically from primary bone tumors, they must be considered whenever a dog presents with a lytic and proliferative bony lesion or lesions. Bone scintigraphy is a useful technique for detection of osseous metastasis in small animals.[59a]

BONE TUMORS IN CATS

Bone tumors occur rarely in cats. This section will discuss bone lesions in cats that represent a clinical entity distinct from those seen in dogs.

FELINE OSTEOSARCOMA

Osteosarcoma is the most common bone tumor affecting cats.[60] Osteosarcoma is generally seen in older female domestic short-hair cats, and the lesions tend to occur in the hind limbs.[60-62] Osteosarcoma is reported less often in the front limbs and flat bones, with the skull and pelvis as the predominant flat bone locations. Clinical signs generally include pain in the extremity and localized swelling. Presentation with pathologic fracture is not uncommon. Osteosarcoma in cats has also been reported at the sites of previous long bone fractures.

Histologic evaluation of feline osteosarcoma shows changes similar to those observed in dogs.

Radiographic changes typical for osteosarcoma in cats include osteolysis and bony proliferation, although the primarily lytic tumors are more common.[61] Complete cortical destruction with extension into soft tissue structures can occur.

Parosteal osteosarcoma is also recognized in the cat. This form of osteosarcoma progresses slowly. Radiographically it is defined by a dense, homogenous proliferation of bone that is adjacent to the outer bone cortex. Invasion of the cortex does not occur until late in the course of the disease. Histologically the tumor is well differentiated.

Although histologic and radiographic similarities exist between osteosarcoma in the dog and cat, they represent distinct clinical entities, and information about the dog should not be extrapolated to the cat because the biologic behavior of the tumors differ. Pulmonary metastasis is much less common in the cat. In one study involving cats undergoing amputation for osteosarcoma of the appendicular skeleton the median survival was greater than 48 months.[61] Amputation of the affected extremity is therefore the recommended therapy. Ambulation following amputation in cats is usually excellent.

Osteosarcomas of the axial skeleton are more difficult to treat, owing to the inability to achieve local tumor control with surgery alone. Treatment of these tumors should include an aggressive surgical attempt to excise the entire tumor. Combining surgery with chemotherapy or radiation therapy to enhance local tumor control may be warranted, but at this time there are no established protocols.

FELINE OSTEOCHONDROMATOSIS

Feline osteochondromatosis (multiple cartilaginous exostoses) is primarily a disease of young adult cats. Unlike osteochondromatosis in dogs, the disease in cats does not manifest until after skeletal maturity. No apparent breed or sex predilections exist, and a hereditary influence has not been established. Histologically and radiographically the disease resembles that of the dog. The disease in cats, however, is progressive. Growth of the nodules is continuous, and malignant transformation may occur. The disease is associated with and perhaps induced by the feline leukemia virus.[63] The prognosis for cats affected with this disease is grave.[63]

REFERENCES

1. Dorn CR, Taylor DON, Schneider R, Hibbard HH: Survey of animal neoplasms in Alameda and Contra Costa Counties, California. II. Cancer morbidity in dogs and cats from Alameda County. J Natl Cancer Inst 40:307–318, 1968

2. Priester WA, editor. The occurrence of tumors in domestic animals. NCI Monogr No. 54. November 1980.

3. Brodey RS, Riser WH: Canine osteosarcoma: A clinicopathologic study of 194 cases. Clin Orthop 62:54–64, 1969

4. Phillips L, Hager D, Parker R, Yanik D: Osteosarcoma with a pathologic fracture in a six-month-old dog. Vet Radiol 27:18–19, 1986

5. Misdorp W, Hart AAM: Some prognostic and epidemiologic factors in canine osteosarcoma. J Natl Cancer Inst 62:537–545, 1979

6. Tjalma RA: Canine bone sarcoma: Estimation of relative risk as a function of body size. J Natl Cancer Inst 36:1137–1150, 1966

7. Bech-Nielsen S, Haskins ME, Reif JS, Brodey RS, Patterson DF, Spielman R: Frequency of osteosarcoma among first-degree relatives of St. Bernard dogs. J Natl Cancer Inst 60:349–353, 1978

8. Owen LN: Transplantation of canine osteosarcoma. Eur J Cancer 5:615–620, 1969

9. Rosin A, Rowland GN: Undifferentiated sarcoma in a dog following chronic irritation by a metallic foreign body and concurrent infection. J Am Anim Hosp Assoc 17:593–598, 1981

10. Bennett D, Campbell JR, Brown P: Osteosarcoma associated with healed fractures. J Small Anim Pract 20:13–18, 1979

11. Stevenson S, Holm RB, Pohler OEM, Fetter AW, Olmstead ML, Wind AP: Fracture-associated sarcoma in the dog. J Am Vet Med Assoc 180:1189, 1982

12. Sinibaldi K, Rosen H, Liu S-K, DeAngelis M: Tumors associated with metallic implants in animals. Clin Orthop 118:257–266, 1976

13. Knecht CD, Priester WA: Osteosarcoma in dogs: A study of previous trauma, fracture and fracture fixation. J Am Anim Hosp Assoc 14:82–84, 1978

14. Dougherty TF, Stove BJ, Lee JH, et al: Growth dynamics of beagle osteosarcomas. Growth 35:119–125, 1971

15. Dubielzig RR, Biery DN, Brodey RS: Bone sarcomas associated with multifocal medullary bone infarction in dogs. J Am Vet Med Assoc 179:64–68, 1981

16. Prior C, Watrous BJ, Penfold D: Radial diaphyseal osteosarcoma with associated bone infarctions in a dog. J Am Anim Hosp Assoc 22:43–48, 1986

17. Knecht CD, Priester WA: Musculoskeletal tumors in dogs. J Am Vet Med Assoc 172:72–74, 1978

18. LaRue SM, Withrow SJ, Wrigley RH: Radiographic bone surveys in the evaluation of primary bone tumors in dogs. J Am Vet Med Assoc 188:514–516, 1986

19. Brodey RS: Surgical treatment of canine osteosarcoma. J Am Vet Med Assoc 147:729–735, 1965

20. Osborne CA, Perman V, Sautter JH, Stevens JB, Hanlon GF: Multiple myeloma in the dog. J Am Vet Med Assoc 153:1300–1319, 1968

21. Maddy KT: Coccidioidomycosis in animals. Vet Med 54:233–242, 1959

22. Powers BE, LaRue SM, Withrow SJ, Straw RC, Richter SL: Jamshidi needle biopsy for diagnosis of bone lesions in small animals. J Am Vet Med Assoc 193:205–210, 1988

23. Wykes SJ, Withrow SJ, Powers BE, Park RD: Closed biopsy for diagnosis of long bone tumors accuracy and results. J Am Anim Hosp Assoc 21:489–494, 1985

24. Banks WC, Morris E: Results of radiation treatment of naturally occurring animal tumors. J Am Vet Med Assoc 166:1063–1066, 1975

25. Silver IA: Use of radiotherapy for the treatment of malignant neoplasms. J Small Anim Pract 13:351–358, 1972

26. Withrow SJ: Application of cryosurgery to primary malignant bone tumors in dogs (Phase I Study). J Am Anim Hosp Assoc 16:493–496, 1980

27. Brodey RS, Abt DA: Results of surgical treatment in 65 dogs with osteosarcoma. J Am Vet Med Assoc 168:1032–1035, 1976

28. Owen LN, Bostock DE, Lavelle RB: Studies on therapy of osteosarcoma in dogs using BCG vaccine. J Am Vet Radiol 18:27–29, 1977

29. Owen LN, Bostock DE: Clinical management of neoplasia. 2. Chemotherapy and immunotherapy. J Small Anim Pract 19:223–288, 1978

30. Cotter SM, Parker LM: High-dose methotrexate and leucovorin rescue in dogs with osteogenic sarcoma. Am J Vet Res 39:1943–1945, 1978

31. Meyer JA, Dueland RT, MacEwen EG, Macy DW, Hoefle WD, Richardson RC, Alexander JW, Trotter E, Hause WR: Canine osteogenic sarcoma treated with amputation and MER, adverse effects of splenectomy on survival. Cancer 49:1613–1616, 1982

32. Hamilton HB, LaRue SM, Withrow SJ: The effect of RA233 on metastasis in naturally occurring canine osteosarcomas. Am J Vet Res 48:1380–1382, 1987

33. Weiden PL, Deeg HF, Graham TC, Storb R: Canine osteosarcoma failure of intravenous or intralesional BCG as adjuvant immunotherapy. Cancer Immunol Immunother 11:69–72, 1981

34. Henness AM, Theilen GH, Park RD, Buhles WC: Combination therapy for canine osteosarcoma. J Am Vet Med Assoc 179:1076–1081, 1977

34a. Madewell BR, Leighton RL: Amputation and doxorubicin for treatment of canine and feline osteosarcoma. Europ J Cancer 14:287–293, 1978

34b. MacEwen EG, Kurzman IP, Smith BW et al: Therapy of osteosarcoma in dogs with intravenous injection of liposome encapsulated muramyltripeptide. J Nat Cancer Inst, in press, 1989

34c. Smith BW, MacEwen EG: Therapeutic considerations for the treatment of canine osteosarcoma of the extremities. Companion Anim Prac, Oct, 20–24, 1987

35. Lord PF, Kapp DS, Morrow D: Increased skeletal metastases of spontaneous canine osteosarcoma after fractionated systemic hyperthermia and local x-irradiation. Cancer Res 41:4331–4334, 1981

36. LaRue SM: Limb salvage for canine osteosarcoma using surgery, tourniquet induced hypoxia and radiation. Abstract, Vet. Ortho. Soc., Copper Mountain, February 1985

37. Theilen GH, Leighton R, Pool RR, Park RD: Treatment of canine osteosarcoma for limb preservation using osteotomy, adjuvant radiotherapy and chemotherapy (a case report). Vet Med Small Anim Clin February 179–183, 1977

38. Withrow SJ, Hirsch VM: Owner response to amputation of a pet's leg. Vet Med Small Clin March 332–334, 1979

38a. Mauldin GN, Matus RE, Withrow SJ et al: Canine osteosarcoma: Treatment by amputation vs. amputation and adjuvant chemotherapy using doxorubicin and cisplatin. J Vet Int Med 2:177–180, 1988

38b. Shapiro W, Fossum TW, Kitchell BE et al: The use of cisplatin for treatment of appendicular osteosarcoma in dogs. J Am Vet Med Assoc 192:507–511, 1988

39. Helfand SC: Chemotherapy for nonresectable and metastatic soft tissue tumors. Proceedings. KalKan Symposium, Columbus, Ohio. October 1986

39a. Vasseur P: Limb preservation in dogs with primary bone tumors. Vet Clin No Amer 17:889–903, 1987

40. LaRue SM, Withrow SJ, Power BE et al: Multidisciplinary limb sparing for canine osteosarcoma. J Am Vet Med Assoc, accepted, 1989

41. Feeney DA, Johnston GR, Grindem CB, Toombs JP, Caywood DD, Hanlon GF: Malignant neoplasia of canine ribs: Clinical, radiographic, and pathologic findings. J Am Vet Med Assoc 180:927–933, 1982

42. Brodey RS: The use of naturally occurring cancer in domestic animals for research into human cancer: General considerations and a review of canine skeletal osteosarcoma. Yale J Biol Med 52:345–361, 1979

43. Banks WC: Parosteal osteosarcoma in a dog and a cat. J Am Vet Med Assoc 158:1412–1415, 1971

44. Withrow SJ, Doige CE: En bloc resection of a juxtacortical and three intra-osseous osteosarcomas of the zygomatic arch in dogs. J Am Anim Hosp Assoc 16:867–872, 1980

45. Ling GV, Morgan JP, Pool RR: Primary bone tumors in the dog: A combined clinical, radiographic and histologic approach to early diagnosis. J Am Vet Med Assoc 165:55–67, 1974

46. Brodey RS, McGrath JT, Reynolds H: A clinical and radiological study of canine bone neoplasms. Part I. J Am Vet Med Assoc 134:53–71, 1959

46a. Brodey RS, Misdorp W, Riser W et al: Canine skeletal chondrosarcoma: A clinicopathologic study of 35 cases. J Am Vet Med Assoc 165:68–78, 1974

47. Bingel SA, Brodey RS, Allen HL, Riser WH: Haemangiosarcoma of bone in the dog. J Small Anim Pract 15:303–322, 1974

48. Liu S-K, Dorfman HD, Hurvitz AI, Patnaik AK: Primary and secondary bone tumours in the dog. J Small Anim Pract 18:313–326, 1977

49. Lipowitz AJ, Fetter AW, Walker MA: Synovial sarcoma of the dog. J Am Vet Med Assoc 174:76–81, 1979

50. Madewell BR, Pool RR: Neoplasms of joints and related structures. Vet Clin North Am 8:511–521, 1978

51. King ES: Tissue differentiation in malignant synovial tumours. J Bone Joint Surg 34B:97–115, 1952

52. Tilmant LL, Gorman NT, Ackerman N, Calderwood Mays MB, Parker R: Chemotherapy of synovial cell sarcoma in a dog. J Am Vet Med Assoc 188:530–532, 1986

53. Carson JH, Harwood AR, Cummings BJ, Fornasier V, Langer F, Quirt I: The place of radiotherapy in the treatment of synovial sarcoma. Int J Radiat Oncol Biol Phys 7:49–53, 1981

54. Crow SE, Hall AD, Walshaw R, Wortman JA: Giant cell tumor (osteoclastoma) in a dog. J Amer Anim Hosp Assoc 15:473–476, 1979

55. Pool RR: Tumors of bone and cartilage. In Moulton J, ed: Tumors of Domestic Animals, 2nd ed, pp. 89–149. Berkley, University of California Press, 1978

55a. Straw RC, LeCouter RA, Withrow SJ, et al: Multilobular osteochondrosarcoma of the canine skull: 16 cases (1978–1988). J Am Vet Med Assoc 1989, in press

56. Chester DK: Multiple cartilaginous exostoses in two generations of dogs. J Am Vet Med Assoc 159:895–897, 1971

57. Gee BR, Doige CE: Multiple cartilaginous exostoses in a litter of dogs. J Am Vet Med Assoc 156:53–59, 1970

58. Doige CE, Pharr JW, Withrow SJ: Chondrosarcoma arising in multiple cartilaginous exostoses in a dog. J Am Anim Hosp Assoc 14:605–611, 1978

58a. Doige CE: Multiple cartilaginous exostosis in dogs. Vet Path 24:276–278, 1987

59. Brodey RS, Reid CF, Sauer RM: Metastatic bone neoplasms in the dog. J Am Vet Med Assoc 148:29–43, 1966

59a. Lamb CR: Bone scintigraphy in small animals. J Am Vet Med Assoc 191:1616–1622, 1987

60. Quigley PJ, Leedale AH: Tumors involving bone in the domestic cat: A review of 58 cases. Vet Pathol 20:670–686, 1983

61. Bitetto WV, Patnaik AK, Schrader SC, Mooney SC: Osteosarcoma in cats: 22 cases (1974–1984). J Am Vet Med Assoc 190:91–93, 1987

62. Turrel JM, Pool RR: Primary bone tumors in the cat: A retrospective study of 15 cats and a literature review. Vet Radiol 23:152–166, 1982

63. Pool RR, Harris JM: Feline osteochondromatosis. Feline Pract 5:24, 1975

22

ENDOCRINE TUMORS

Steven L. Wheeler

Many common endocrine diseases occur as a result of neoplasia involving the endocrine system. In this chapter, emphasis is placed on the more common tumors of the endocrine system, including canine thyroid tumors, feline hyperthyroidism, hyperadrenocorticism, and insulin-producing islet cell tumors. Other less common endocrine tumors are also discussed.

CANINE THYROID TUMORS

INCIDENCE AND RISK FACTORS

Thyroid tumors are uncommon in the dog; the reported incidence rates are 1.2% to 3.75%,[1-5] and the tumors account for 10% to 15% of all head and neck neoplasias.[4] The average age of dogs with thyroid adenomas is about 10 years, with a range of 5 to 15 years.[1-4,7] The average age of dogs with thyroid carcinomas is similar (mean 9 years; range, 4 to 18 years).[1-4,6,7] Most studies do not reveal any sex predilection.[1-4,7] Among breeds, boxers are thought to be predisposed to adenomas, and beagles, boxer, and golden retrievers to have a higher prevalence of carcinomas.[1-4,7]

The incidence of thyroid tumors in dogs has been shown to vary according to geographical location; the tumors are more common in areas of endemic goiter secondary to iodine deficiency.[8] Laboratory rodents fed iodine-deficient diets have also shown an increased incidence of thyroid tumors.[9] However, even though goiter in both man and dogs has declined in the United States with the introduction of iodized salt, the incidence of thyroid tumors has not shown a parallel decrease.[10] There are also no experimental studies demonstrating an increased incidence of thyroid tumors in dogs placed on iodine-deficient diets. Finally, since the histologic changes seen with iodine deficiency can be similar to those seen with tumors,[11,12] the incidence of tumors in iodine-deficient areas may be overestimated.

PATHOLOGY AND NATURAL BEHAVIOR

Carcinomas represent the majority (63% to 87.5%) of thyroid neoplasias detected clinically.[1-4,7] Adenomas are detected clinically less than 50% of the time and are most often only found as incidental findings at necropsy.[2,3] Adenomas are usually well-encapsulated, freely movable, unilateral masses that may vary in size from microscopic to several centimeters in diameter and may be cystic or solid. Thyroid carcinomas can vary in size from microscopic to greater than 10 cm in diameter, but they usually have tumor volumes exceeding 100 cm^3 at the time of diagnosis.[5] About two-thirds of thyroid carcinomas are unilateral, and bilateral tumors usually represent more extensive disease.[7] Thyroid carcinomas may arise from ectopic mediastinal thyroid tissue and have been reported to occur at the heart base.[13,13a] Carcinomas may be encapsulated but commonly display invasive growth into the esophagus, trachea, larynx, cervical musculature, and blood vessels (Fig. 22-1). Hematogenous spread to the lung and lymphatic extension to cervical lymph nodes are the most common routes and sites of metastasis.[2,3,7] Carcinomas have also been described to metastasize to adrenal glands, kidneys, myocardium, liver, and brain.[7] Most carcinomas are of the follicular type but can be classified as compact, or papillary, carcinomas. Histologic classification among the various carcinomas has not been shown to be of prognostic significance in the dog. However, tumor volume has been shown to be directly related to metastatic behavior. In one study, only 14% of dogs with tumor volume less than 20 cm^3 had metastases, while 74% of dogs with tumor volumes between 21 and 100 cm^3, and 100% with tumors greater than 100 cm^3, had metastases.[7] Thyroid medullary carcinomas, arising from the calcitonin-producing C cells of the thyroid gland, are uncommon in dogs.[13b]

HISTORY AND CLINICAL SIGNS

Adenomas are not commonly detected clinically but, when seen, are usually presented for asymptomatic cervical masses.[2,7] The duration of clinical signs prior to presentation may be from a few weeks to many years. Adenomas usually palpate as small, freely movable, firm or cystic, nonpainful masses. Carcinomas are also usually presented for evaluation of a cervical mass.

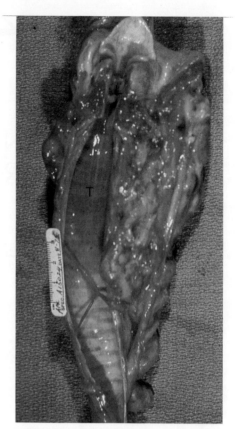

Figure 22-1. Thyroid carcinoma invading into larynx (L), trachea (T), and cervical blood vessels.

Dysphagia, dyspnea, and change in the dog's bark may also be noted.[1-3,6,7] Less frequently, regurgitation, precaval syndrome (Fig. 22-2), weight loss, and excessive hemorrhage secondary to disseminated intravascular coagulation are seen. The duration of signs prior to presentation is usually less than 3 months. Physical examination reveals a firm, nonpainful, movable (Fig. 22-3) or fixed neck mass (Fig. 22-4). Larger tumors may descend ventrally toward the thoracic inlet.

Rijnberk noted that approximately 20% of all canine thyroid tumors were hyperfunctional and resulted in a hyperthyroid state.[14] Clinical signs most commonly seen with hyperthyroidism were polydipsia, polyuria, and weight loss in spite of adequate caloric intake. Weakness, fatigue, restlessness, heat intolerance, and panting are reported less often. Physical examination may reveal muscle atrophy, prominent apex heart beat, and bounding pulses. However, other

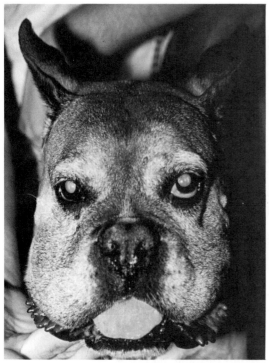

Figure 22-2. Precaval syndrome, resulting in pronounced facial edema, secondary to an invasive thyroid carcinoma in a boxer.

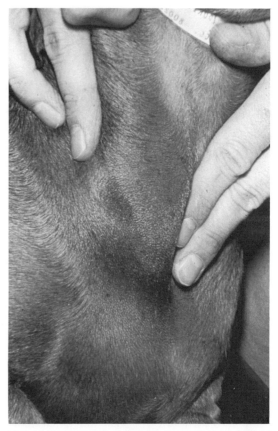

Figure 22-3. Freely movable ·noninvasive thyroid carcinoma in a dog. Surgical removal alone resulted in local and systemic control for more than 4 years.

investigators have reported a low incidence of hyperthyroidism, with most dogs being euthyroid, in fact, hypothyroidism was the only abnormality in thyroid function noted.[3] Hypothyroidism may occur secondary to tumor destruction of normal thyroid tissue with bilateral involvement. However, hypothyroidism has also been noted to occur with unilateral tumors and may occur secondary to the tumor's production of biologically inactive thyroid hormone, which inhibits pituitary thyrotropin (TSH) secretion and thereby results in atrophy of the normal thyroid tissue.[15]

DIAGNOSTIC TECHNIQUES AND WORK-UP

Differential diagnosis of cervical masses includes abscess, granuloma, salivary mucocele, metastatic tonsillar squamous cell carcinoma, lymphoma, carotid body tumors, and regional soft tissue sarcomas. Aspiration cytology should be performed to help rule out abscess, mucocele, and lymphoma. Thyroid carcinoma cells are often seen via aspiration cytology but may be obscured by hemodilution owing to the marked vascularity of these tumors. The feathered edge of the slide is the most likely area to see neoplastic cells. Histopathology is needed to establish a definitive diagnosis. Prior to obtaining a biopsy, thoracic and cervical radiographs should be made. Cervical radiographs are useful in identifying the location of the mass, proximal airway, and esophagus prior to performing a biopsy. In the majority of cases, adequate tissue for diagnosis may be obtained with a percutaneous needle biopsy, but open surgical biopsies may also be performed. Since these tumors are highly vascular, hemorrhage may be significant. Aspiration cytology should be performed on regional lymph nodes for staging purposes. Lymph node metastasis may develop in a cranial (most common) or caudal direction from the primary tumor.

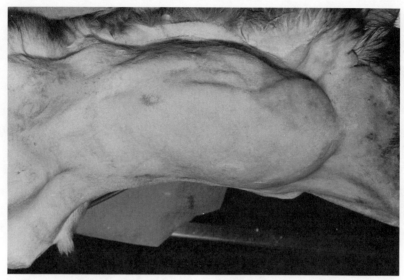

Figure 22-4. Large, fixed, invasive thyroid carcinoma in a dog. (Head is to the right.) Surgical removal should not be attempted on a tumor as extensive as this.

Nuclear scans using radioactive iodine isotopes (usually ^{123}I) or sodium pertechnetate (technetium [99]m) may occasionally be helpful in establishing the location and extent of the primary tumor and detecting lymph node and pulmonary metastases.[3,4,15] The functional status of the thyroid should be ascertained, preferably with the use of TSH stimulation testing, to detect underlying hypothyroid or hyperthyroid states. Thyroid storm (massive release of thyroid hormone into the circulation) has not been reported following TSH administration in dogs with thyroid tumors.

THERAPY

Complete surgical excision is the treatment of choice for adenomas and should be curative. For noninvasive (*i.e.*, freely movable) carcinomas, complete surgical excision is also the treatment of choice (Fig. 22-5). Tumors should be approached by a ventral midline incision, and vital structures such as the carotid artery, internal jugular vein, recurrent laryngeal nerve, and esophagus should be identified and preserved if possible. Owing to the tendency of this tumor to invade vascular structures, it may be necessary to ligate and remove carotid arteries and jugular veins in some cases. Cervical lymph nodes should be examined closely and removed or biopsied, but curative lymph node

excision is unlikely if nodes are enlarged and fixed to surrounding tissues.

If only unilateral thyroid and parathyroid removal is performed, hormone replacement therapy is not required. Since approximately one-third of all carcinomas are bilateral,[7] both lobes of the thyroid gland should be carefully inspected and bilateral thyroidectomy performed if necessary. When bilateral thyroidectomy is performed, it is usually not possible to preserve parathyroid glands and both hypothyroidism and hypoparathyroidism are likely to occur postoperatively. Untreated hypoparathyroidism often results in a life-threatening hypocalcemic crisis.[16] Signs of hypocalcemia in the dog include nervousness, irritability, panting, increased body temperature, muscle tremors, tetany, and convulsions. Emergency treatment of hypocalcemia should be intravenous 10% calcium gluconate 1.0 to 1.5 ml/kg administered over 10 to 20 minutes. Concurrent electrocardiographic monitoring is desirable, and if bradycardia or shortening of the Q–T interval occurs, calcium infusion should be stopped. After emergency treatment has been completed, 2.5 ml/kg of 10% calcium gluconate should be added to the dog's intravenous fluids every 6 to 8 hours. Additionally, oral vitamin D and calcium therapy should be initiated. In the initial management of a hypoparathyroid patient, large loading doses of the vitamin D preparation

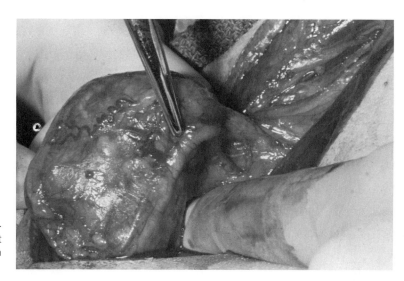

Figure 22-5. Encapsulated non-invasive thyroid carcinoma at surgery. (Same patient as in Fig. 22-3.)

dihydrotachysterol (Hytakerol) shortens the time necessary to achieve normocalcemia. For the first 2 days of therapy, give 0.05 mg/kg/day, followed by 0.02 mg/kg/day for 2 days, and then start maintenance therapy at a dose of 0.01/mg/kg/day. During the initial 4-day loading period, oral calcium gluconate should be given at a dosage of 0.5 to 1.0 g/kg divided into 3 or 4 doses per day. Usually, parenteral calcium can be discontinued after 2 to 3 days of oral vitamin D and calcium loading. For maintenance therapy the dosage of oral vitamin D and calcium should be adjusted according to weekly serum calcium and phosphorus determinations. Hypercalcemia secondary to hypervitaminosis D causes severe nephrotoxicity; therefore, the dosage of vitamin D should be reduced if either hypercalcemia or hyperphosphotemia are detected. Hypothyroidism should be treated with L-thyroxine 20 to 30 μg/kg given once daily. Finally, if bilateral thyroidectomy is performed, the dog should be closely monitored for laryngeal paralysis (secondary to recurrent laryngeal nerve injury) in the postoperative period.

Invasive thyroid carcinomas are virtually impossible to completely excise surgically.[5] It is not recommended that complete excision be attempted in cases of invasive tumors because the surgical procedure carries a high morbidity and may irreparably damage vital structures in the neck. Instead, these tumors should be biopsied and alternative forms of therapy considered. Doxorubicin given at a dosage of 30 mg/m² intravenously over 5 to 15 minutes, every 3 weeks, for a total of five treatments has been reported to result in a partial regression in about one-half of all cases.[5,6] At least two treatments with doxorubicin should be done prior to assessing the efficacy of chemotherapy.[6] Some tumors may be surgically removable after a partial regression is achieved. Doxorubicin therapy has also been recommended as adjuvant therapy for incompletely excised carcinomas, or tumors with a volume greater than 20 cm³, because metastatic disease is likely in these cases. Recently, the efficacy of doxorubicin for the treatment of malignant thyroid tumors has been questioned. In a review of 64 cases, no beneficial effects were seen in affected dogs treated with doxorubicin compared to dogs not receiving it.[17]

Completely excised tumors displaying vascular invasion may also benefit from adjuvant chemotherapy with doxorubicin. However, in one study, survival was not improved when doxorubicin was given following surgery when compared to surgery alone.[17] External beam radiotherapy should be considered for treatment of local disease if chemotherapy is unsuccessful and no metastatic disease is present. Controlled trials of radiation treatment of thyroid carcinomas have not been reported. A flow chart summarizing suggested treatment of thyroid carcinoma is shown in Figure 22-6.

PROGNOSIS

The prognosis for adenomas is excellent with surgical excision. For small, noninvasive, encapsulated carcinomas, the prognosis is also good; survival times of 1 to 4 years are re-

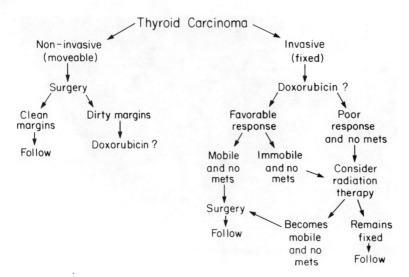

Figure 22-6. Flow diagram outlining treatment for thyroid carcinoma in the dog.

ported.[2,3] Median survival of 21 dogs with non-fixed and surgically excised tumors (regardless of size) was 36 months.[17] In this study mobility and therefore excisability was more important than tumor volume in predicting outcome. Larger invasive tumors have a poor prognosis due to the inability to completely remove the tumor at surgery and the greater likelihood of metastasis. In one study, 80% of all dogs with thyroid carcinomas less than 5 cm in diameter were free of disease 7 months postoperatively, while only 27% of those with tumor diameter greater than 5 cm remained free of disease over the same period of time.[4,5] It should be pointed out that few of the dogs with larger tumors received any treatment other than surgery. More aggressive treatment with chemotherapy and radiation therapy may improve the prognosis.

COMPARATIVE ASPECTS

The incidence, clinical behavior, treatment, and prognosis of thyroid tumors is much different in the dog than in the cat (Table 22-1). Papillary carcinomas are the most common thyroid tumor type in humans but are rare in dogs.[18] In humans, thyroid tumors are more common in women than men. Previous radiation to the cervical area has been associated with the development of tumor. Medullary carcinoma is also more common in humans, and although high concentrations of calcitonin are seen, affected people are not usually hypocalcemia or hypophosphotemic. Medullary carcinoma has only rarely been reported in the dog, and like affected humans, these dogs tend to have normal serum calcium and phosphorus values. Humans

Table 22-1. Comparison of Canine and Feline Thyroid Tumors

	CANINE	FELINE
Incidence rate	Low	Moderate
Geographical incidence	None	Higher on East and West Coasts
Malignancy %	63–87.5%	<1%
Local invasion	Common	Rare
Metastatic behavior	Common with larger tumors	Rare
Association with hyper-thyroidism	<1%*	>99%
Association with cardiac disease	None	10–20%
Appropriate therapeutic modalities	Surgery, doxorubicin? radiation?	Antithyroid drugs, surgery, [131]I

* One report claimed a 20% incidence of hyperthyroidism in dogs with thyroid tumors. In my opinion, this seldom occurs.

with medullary carcinomas may have diarrhea secondary to excess serotonin or prostaglandin production. Diarrhea has been noted in one dog with a medullary carcinoma.[13b]

FELINE HYPERTHYROIDISM

INCIDENCE AND RISK FACTORS

Although feline hyperthyroidism has only been recognized since the late 1970s, it is now diagnosed frequently and is probably the most common endocrinopathy in the cat. It appears that the incidence of the disease is greater on the East and West Coasts then in the central region of the United States, though the reason for this geographical difference is unknown. There appears to be no breed or sex predilection for the disease. There is no known etiology for hyperthyroidism in cats. The average age of cats with hyperthyroidism is 13 years, and a range of 6 to 20 years is reported.[19]

PATHOLOGY AND NATURAL BEHAVIOR

Feline hyperthyroidism usually results from a functional thyroid adenoma (adenomatous hyperplasia) involving one or both lobes of the thyroid. In about 70% of cases both lobes are involved, while in the remaining 30% only one lobe is involved. Thyroid carcinoma has only rarely been reported to be the cause of hyperthyroidism in the cat.[20,20a] Most carcinomas are mixed compact and follicular, with follicular and papillary being less common. Infrequently, adenomas arising from accessory thyroid tissue located in the mediastinum have been reported.[21] Histologically, thyroid adenomas in the cat are characterized by a proliferation of well-differentiated thyroid epithelial cells without evidence of stromal or vascular invasion. These tumors are not metastatic.

HISTORY AND CLINICAL SIGNS

Since thyroid hormones affect many different organ systems, hyperthyroid cats may present with a wide variety of signs. However, signs referable to a single organ system may predominate. The severity of clinical signs can vary from mild to severe, depending on the duration of hyperthyroidism and the presence of concur-

rent organ system disfunction. In a review of 131 cases of hyperthyroidism, the most commonly reported signs were weight loss, polyphagia, increased activity, polydipsia, polyuria, and vomiting.[19] Diarrhea, increased fecal volume, anorexia, panting, heat intolerance, muscle weakness, muscle tremor, increased nail growth, dyspnea, alopecia secondary to excessive grooming, and ventral neck flexion were less frequently seen. While most hyperthyroid cats are hyperexcitable and polyphagic, approximately 10% are depressed and anorexic. These cats are described as having apathetic or masked hyperthyroidism and also usually have concurrent cardiac abnormalities.

On physical examination, unilateral or bilateral thyroid lobe enlargement is detected in about 90% of all affected cats. Enlarged lobes may descend ventrally towards the thoracic inlet. Since these enlarged lobes may range in size from a few millimeters to 3 cm in diameter, careful palpation is required. Shaving and wetting the neck may facilitate palpation and visualization of small tumors. Signs referable to the cardiovascular system, including tachycardia, gallop rhythm, systolic murmur, and bounding rapid pulse are also common. Approximately 10% of the cases present in congestive heart failure. In these cats, muffled heart sounds and dyspnea due to pleural effusion can be seen.

DIAGNOSTIC TECHNIQUES AND WORK-UP

Routine laboratory testing should be performed in cases of suspected feline hyperthyroidism. The most commonly observed hematologic abnormalities are a stress leukogram (leukocytosis, eosinopenia, and lymphopenia), mild to moderate erythrocytosis (increased PCV, RBC, hemoglobin), and macrocytosis.[19,20] It is postulated that the erythroid abnormalities result from a direct stimulatory effect of thyroid hormones on the bone marrow and also from an increased production of erythropoietin. Macrocytosis may occur owing to premature release or erythroid precursors from the bone marrow secondary to thyroid hormone excess. Increases in the liver enzymes, serum alkaline phosphatase (SAP), lactate dehydrogenase (LDH), alanine aminotransferase (ALT or SGPT), and aspartate aminotransferase (AST or SGOT) are commonly seen in cases of hyperthyroidism. Elevated total serum bilirubin may also be seen. Histopathology of the liver usually reveals nonspecific changes such as centrolobular fatty infiltration and mild hepatic necrosis. While the exact cause of the hepatic abnormalities seen in hyperthyroidism remains unknown, it has been demonstrated that these abnormalities are entirely reversible once the cat is converted to a euthyroid state. Increased serum phosphorus is seen in about 20% of all cases. Hyperphosphotemia may be secondary to renal insufficiency or to increased bone resorption mediated by thyroid hormone excess.

Thoracic radiographs commonly show abnormalities in cases of feline hyperthyroidism. Approximately 50% of cases have radiographic evidence of cardiomegaly. Less commonly, extracardiac signs of congestive heart failure such as pulmonary edema and pleural effusion may be seen. Approximately 80% of affected cats have electrocardiographic abnormalities.[22] A reversible form of hypertrophic cardiomyopathy can be induced in normal cats by the chronic administration of excessive thyroid hormones.[23] Sinus tachycardia, increased QRS complex amplitude, and atrial and ventricular arrhythmias are most commonly seen. Since similar clinical, radiographic, and electrocardiographic signs may be seen in cats with primary hypertrophic cardiomyopathy, the possibility of hyperthyroidism should be entertained in all cats presenting for cardiac abnormalities. However, the cats affected with hyperthyroidism and secondary cardiac disease are usually underweight, while those with primary heart disease tend to be overweight. The cardiomyopathy associated with hyperthyroidism in cats is usually reversible once euthyroidism is restored.

Definitive diagnosis requires radioimmunoassay of serum thyroid hormones. Nearly all hyperthyroid cats show elevations in serum T_4 and T_3.[19] TSH testing is not usually required to establish the diagnosis and may be detrimental to the animal in that thyroid storm, resulting in life-threatening cardiac arrhythmias, may occur. Nuclear scans using either ^{123}I or sodium pertechnetate (technetium [99]m) are helpful in establishing whether bilateral (70% of cases) or unilateral (30% of cases) involvement is present.[19,20] Scanning is also very helpful in cases where no cervical enlargement is palpable. Usually the scan will demonstrate the occasional affected lobe that has descended through the thoracic inlet into the mediastinum, but aden-

omas arising from ectopic thyroid tissue inside the chest have also been described. Finally, nuclear scans may also be valuable in identifying metastases in rare cases of functional thyroid carcinomas.[20a]

THERAPY

There are three possible therapies for hyperthyroid cats: chronic antithyroid drug administration, surgical thyroidectomy, and ^{131}I radiotherapy. Two antithyroid drugs, propylthiouracil (PTU) and methimazole, have been used in treatment of hyperthyroid cats. Both drugs inhibit thyroid hormone synthesis, but methimazole is at least 10 times more potent than PTU. Therefore the initial dose of PTU is 50 mg PO TID, while methimazole is given at 5 mg PO TID. More important, PTU is associated with a much higher incidence of mild and serious side-effects than is methimazole. Mild side-effects include anorexia, vomiting, and lethargy. Serious side-effects seen with PTU include life-threatening immune-mediated hemolytic anemia and thrombocytopenia.[24] Since methimazole is better tolerated and safer to use, PTU therapy is not recommended. Side-effects with methimazole are uncommon; they include anorexia, vomiting, and lethargy.[24a] In most cats, these effects resolve despite continued drug administration; however, continued adverse gastrointestinal side-effects may necessitate discontinuation of therapy. Rarely, skin rashes and pruritus have been reported. Finally, although serious hematologic side-effects are uncommon with methimazole, agranulocytosis (severe leukopenia with WBC <250/mm^3 and thrombocytopenia with platelets <75,000/mm^3) have been reported. Agranulocytosis is most likely to occur between the second and twelfth weeks following initiation of therapy. If seen, drug therapy should be discontinued and supportive care administered. Most cases resolve within 5 days. More commonly a transient mild leukopenia with a normal differential, eosinophilia, and lymphocytosis may occur with methimazole therapy. Unlike agranulocytosis, this condition is usually self-limiting and is not an indication to discontinue methimazole therapy. Conversion to a positive antinuclear antibody (ANA) titer is commonly seen in cats on chronic methimazole therapy, but clinical signs of systemic lupus are rare. Initially, methimazole should be given at 5 mg PO TID. Upon initiating treatment, a CBC and platelet count should be performed biweekly to monitor for agranulocytosis. After 2 weeks, serum T_4 should be rechecked. In most cases it will have normalized and methimazole may be reduced to 5 mg BID for maintenance therapy. True resistance to the antithyroid effects of the drug is rare. The owner's noncompliance in giving medication or difficulty in administration is more often the problem. Cats maintained on methimazole chronically should have CBC, ANA titer, T_3, and T_4 rechecked at 3-month intervals. If ANA titer reverts to positive, serum chemistry panel and urinalysis should also be performed every 3 months. If clinical or laboratory signs of systemic lupus develop, methimazole therapy should be stopped.

Surgery is the most common form of therapy. However, in order to avoid anesthetic complications, it is essential that cats be converted to a euthyroid state prior to surgical thyroidectomy. This is most easily accomplished with methimazole, but propranolol with or without concurrent iodine therapy may also be used.[19] Propranolol given at 2.5 to 5.0 mg TID will not decrease serum concentrations of thyroid hormones, but it will help reverse the cardiac and neuromuscular abnormalities seen in hyperthyroidism. Propanolol therapy should be instituted for all cats with hypertrophic cardiomyopathy. Oral potassium iodine given at 50 to 100 mg/day for

7 to 14 days prior to surgery will decrease serum thyroid hormones. Unfortunately the antithyroid effect of iodine is lost within a few weeks. Iodine should never be used alone but only in conjunction with propranolol because thyroid hormones do not usually return to entirely normal levels.

At surgery, both lobes of the thyroid gland should be inspected carefully. As previously stated, in approximately 70% of cases involvement is bilateral. Usually this is easily recognized at surgery as bilateral enlargement, and bilateral thyroidectomy without removal of cranial parathyroid glands may be performed (Fig. 22-7). With unilateral tumors, there should be atrophy of the contralateral lobe. In this case, only the affected lobe should be removed. With unilateral thyroidectomy, it is not necessary to save the cranial parathyroid gland on the affected lobe (Fig. 22-8). However, in some cases one lobe may only be slightly enlarged and may be misjudged as being normal at the time of surgery. Preoperative nuclear scans are helpful in avoiding this dilemma. If preoperative scans are not available it is recommended that the obviously enlarged lobe be removed with every attempt to preserve the cranial parathyroid gland and that thyroid hormones be evaluated every 3 months for possible recurrence (Fig. 22-9).

If hyperthyroidism recurs, it will usually do so within 12 months following surgery. However, recurrence as late as 44 months later has

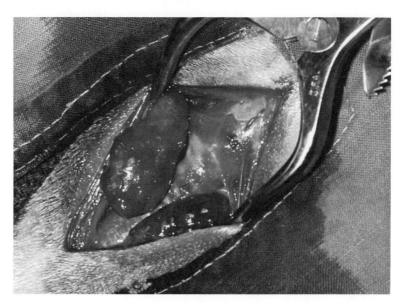

Figure 22-7. Bilaterally enlarged thyroids in a cat at surgery. Bilateral thyroidectomy is indicated in this case.

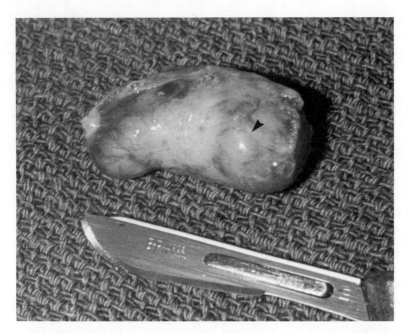

Figure 22-8. Unilateral thyroid tumor following extracapsular surgical removal from a cat. Arrow indicates cranial parathyroid gland. Since the contralateral thyroid lobe and associated parathyroid tissue were not removed, it was not necessary to dissect out the cranial parathyroid gland on the affected lobe.

been reported. Postoperatively, Horner's syndrome and laryngeal paralysis are possible complications. After bilateral thyroidectomy, hypoparathyroidism may occur; in this case, calcium should be monitored daily. The animal should be closely watched for signs of hypocalcemia (restlessness, panting, irritability, elevated body temperature tremor, tetany, and seizures). Hypoparathyroidism is usually seen within 3 days of surgery; treatment of it is discussed earlier

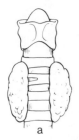 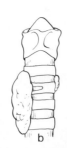 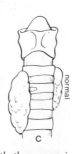

Figure 22-9. The surgeon is faced with three possibilities. *(A)* Obvious bilateral thyroid enlargement. Bilateral thyroidectomy is indicated. *(B)* Unilateral enlargement with atrophy of the contralateral lobe. Unilateral thyroidectomy of the enlarged lobe is indicated. *(C)* Unilateral thyroid enlargement with a normal size contralateral lobe. Unilateral thyroidectomy is indicated, but serum T_4 assay should be performed every 3 months to check for recurrence of hyperthyroidism.

in this chapter. In many cases hypoparathyroidism is transient and therapy can be discontinued in 2 to 3 months.[19] To avoid these complications, the surgeon should always attempt to avoid removal of the cranial parathyroid glands when performing bilateral thyroidectomy. Intracapsular removal makes it easier to leave the parathyroid gland but may carry the risk of incomplete thyroid gland removal. Also, care should be exercised to avoid traumatizing the recurrent laryngeal nerve. Following unilateral thyroidectomy, thyroxine supplementation is not required. Starting at 1 to 2 days following bilateral thyroidectomy, 0.1 mg thyroxine should be given daily to prevent hypothyroidism from occurring. Since remnants of abnormal thyroid tissue may remain following surgery, hyperthyroidism can recur in cats even following bilateral thyroidectomy. Serum thyroid hormones should be checked every 6 months to monitor for recurrence.

Radioiodine therapy involves a single administration of [131]I.[20a,25,26] Because the ^{131}I is rapidly taken up by the hyperfunctioning tissue, normal thyroid tissue is protected. Persistent hyperthyroidism occurs in 10% to 18% of cases, while hypothyroidism occurs in 2% to 18% of cases following treatment with [131]I. Hypoparathyroidism has not been reported following ^{131}I therapy. Once ^{131}I is taken up by adenomatous thyroid tissue, beta particles, which destroy the abnormal tissue, are emitted. With underdosage, radioiodine treatment may need to be repeated for residual hyperthyroidism. Although radioiodine therapy is the safest form of treatment, it has the disadvantage of requiring special handling of cats and their excrement for 2 to 3 weeks following treatment. It also requires special licensing, making it available only at referral centers.

PROGNOSIS

Since hyperthyroidism in most cats is due to adenomatous hyperplasia, the prognosis is good for cure (Fig. 22-10) or at least for control with appropriate therapy. Operative mortality has been reported to be 9%,[27] but in many cases thyroid function was not normalized prior to surgery in cats that died. With appropriate preoperative treatment, mortality should be much lower. Even cats with cardiac abnormalities can usually be stabilized effectively with appropriate cardiac medications before treatment for their underlying hyperthyroid state. In the rare cases of feline hyperthyroidism secondary to thyroid carcinomas, prognosis is guarded owing to the underlying malignant condition. However, in one study of 12 cats treated with ^{131}I, the mean survival times ranged from 450 to 600 days.[20a]

COMPARATIVE ASPECTS

As mentioned previously, there is a marked contrast between canine and feline thyroid tumors (Table 22-1). In humans, the most common cause for hyperthyroidism is Grave's disease, an

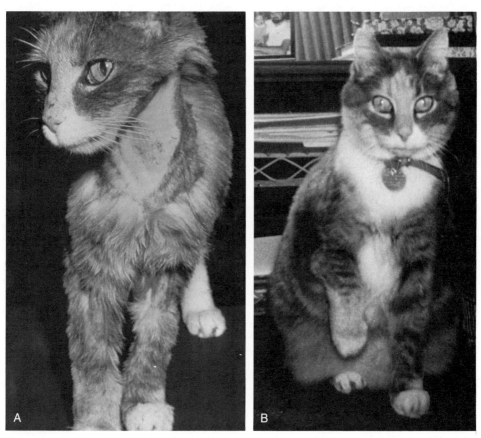

Figure 22-10. Hyperthyroid cat shown *(A)* at presentation and *(B)* 2 years following bilateral thyroidectomy. This 17-year-old cat demonstrates that with appropriate therapy, all clinical signs are reversible and prognosis is good.

autoimmune disorder most commonly seen in young women in which circulating autoantibodies stimulate excessive thyroid hormone secretion. Exophthalmos is also commonly seen in this disorder. Autoantibodies and exophthalmos have not been detected in feline hyperthyroidism. The histologic changes seen in cats most closely resemble toxic nodular goiter in humans, which most commonly occurs in old age and is characterized by one or more hyperfunctioning adenomatous thyroid nodules.

HYPERADRENOCORTICISM

Hyperadrenocorticism is a systemic disease resulting from excessive circulating cortisol. This disorder can occur secondary to pituitary abnormalities (pituitary-dependent hyperadrenocorticism [PDH]) or adrenocortical tumors (AT). Since the resulting disease states are similar, the two etiologies for hyperadrenocorticism will be discussed together.

INCIDENCE AND RISK FACTORS

Hyperadrenocorticism is probably the most common endocrinopathy in the dog, with 85% to 90% of cases occurring secondary to pituitary abnormalities and 10% to 15% secondary to adrenocortical tumors. This disorder is rare in the cat, although both PDH, adrenal adenoma, and bilateral adrenocortical hyperplasia have been described.[28–30,30a,30b] Dogs with PDH are usually middle-aged to older (>6 years), although dogs as young as 1 year may be affected. Poodles, dachshunds, and boxers appear to be at increased risk, but no sex predilection exists.[31] In a recent review of 25 dogs with AT, the mean age was 10.5 years with a range from 5 to 14 years. Larger breeds (body weight >20 kg) are more commonly affected than small breeds.[32] Seventy to 75% of affected dogs are female. No risk factors for either PDH or AT have been identified.

PATHOLOGY AND NATURAL BEHAVIOR

In PDH there is excessive production and secretion of ACTH by the pituitary, which results in bilateral adrenocortical hyperplasia and excessive adrenocortical cortisol production. The reported incidence of pituitary tumors in this disease has ranged from 20% to 100%. Adenomas arising from the pars distalis are most common, but pars intermedia tumors have also been described.[33] Either pituitary hyperplasia or failure of the pituitary corticotrophs to decrease ACTH secretion in response to elevated serum cortisol concentrations has been theorized to occur in cases where pituitary tumors have not been identified.

In AT there is excessive production of cortisol by adrenocortical neoplasms. Since the hypothalamic-pituitary-adrenal axis is normal, elevated cortisol results in decreased pituitary ACTH production and atrophy of the contralateral adrenal cortex. Adenomas and carcinomas occur with equal frequency, and the right and left adrenal glands are affected equally. Bilateral adrenocortical tumors causing hyperadrenocorticism are extremely rare. Concurrent adrenal and pituitary neoplasia is also extremely rare but has been described.[34] While adenomas remain confined to the adrenal gland, carcinomas may show both metastatic and invasive behavior. About 50% of adrenal carcinomas have gross evidence of liver metastasis. Invasion of the caudal vena cava, renal vein, and phrenicoabdominal vein can also occur.

In cats, approximately 50% will have AT and 50% will have pituitary tumors.[30a,30b]

HISTORY AND CLINICAL SIGNS

The signs of hyperadrenocorticism are due to excess circulating glucocorticoids, and similar signs are seen in PDH and AT. The most common clinical sign is polyuria/polydipsia, which occurs in about 85% of cases. Pendulous abdomen (pot-bellied appearance), hepatomegaly, skin atrophy, hair loss, lethargy, polyphagia, muscle weakness, anestrus, and obesity are also commonly seen. Less frequently, muscle atrophy, comedones, increased panting, testicular atrophy, hyperpigmentation, calcinosis cutis, facial dermatosis, and facial nerve palsy may be seen. Central nervous system signs, such as seizures, blindness, and dementia due to the compressive effects of large pituitary neoplasms, may occur but are uncommon. Affected dogs are predisposed to bacterial infections of the skin, lungs, and urinary tract owing to the immunosuppressive effects of cortisol. Acute dyspnea rapidly progressive to death may occur with fulminating pneumonia, but pulmonary thromboembolism resulting in similar clinical signs has also been described.[32,35] Diabetes has been shown to occur in about 20% of affected dogs.[36] It probably results from the antagonistic effects of excessive cortisol on insulin. In most cases there is an insidious onset and slow progression of signs. However, dogs with adrenal carcinomas may display a rapid onset and progression of signs, often without the prominent dermatologic signs usually seen in hyperadrenocorticism. Cats with hyperadrenocorticism appear to be predisposed to hyperglycemia and diabetes mellitus. The most common clinical signs are polyuria, polydipsia, and patchy endocrine alopecia involving the trunk and flanks.[28–30]

DIAGNOSTIC TECHNIQUES AND WORK-UP

Dogs affected with hyperadrenocorticism frequently show abnormalities on routine laboratory testing. An absolute eosinopenia is the most common hematologic abnormality, occurring in about 85% of cases.[31] A mature leukocytosis; eosinopenia and lymphopenia; and increases in hemoglobin, packed cell volume, and red blood cell count can also be seen but are not consistent findings. Increased serum alkaline phosphatase (SAP), due to induction of a specific hepatic isoenzyme, is the most consistent abnormality seen on serum chemistries; it occurs in about 85% of all cases. Increased cholesterol, alanine aminotransferase (ALT or SGPT), glucose, and total CO_2 can also be seen. Urinalysis frequently reveals a specific gravity in the isosthenuric range, but unless there is concurrent renal disease, the animal can concentrate urine if deprived of water. Signs of urinary tract infection such as bacteriuria, hematuria, proteinuria, and increased numbers of white blood cells may also be seen. In some cases, cystitis may be present without evidence of pyuria on the urinalysis. Routine chest and abdominal radiographs may reveal abdominal distention, hepatomegaly, osteopenia of vertebrae, and mineralization of tracheal rings, skin (calcinosis cutis), subcutaneous tissues, and vasculature.[31a,31b] Calcification in the adrenal gland is reported in 25% to 40% of cases of AT.[31,32] Both adenomas and carcinomas may show radiographic evidence of calcification.

Although history, physical exam, and routine laboratory findings may be highly suggestive of hyperadrenocorticism, specific diagnostic tests are required to establish the diagnosis. It is vital that the diagnosis be confirmed because both medical and surgical treatments for hyperadrenocorticism are expensive and not without risk.

Screening tests for hyperadrenocorticism include serum cortisol, ACTH stimulation, low-dosage dexamethasone suppression, glucagon tolerance, and determination of urinary corticoids. Unfortunately, determination of single serum cortisol concentration is not reliable in differentiating normal dogs from those with hyperadrenocorticism and is not recommended as a screening test. Both normal and affected dogs display episodic secretion of cortisol, and about 50% of affected dogs have serum cortisol concentrations within the normal range when a single sample is assayed.[37]

The ACTH stimulation test is a valuable screening test and is performed by either sampling before and 2 hours after giving 2.2 U/kg (up to a maximum dose of 20 U) of ACTH gel IM or sampling before and 1 hour after giving 0.5 U/kg of aqueous ACTH IV. A diagnosis of hyperadrenocorticism is confirmed when there is an excessive increase in serum cortisol concentrations. Absolute ranges for normal dogs must be established by the laboratory performing the cortisol assays in order for the test to be interpretable. About 85% of PDH cases, but only about 50% of AT, show a diagnostic hyperresponse with the ACTH stimulation test.[31,38,39] Low-dosage dexamethasone suppression testing appears to be the most accurate screening test for hyperadrenocorticism in the dog. This test is performed by sampling before and 3 and 8 hours after giving 0.01–0.015 mg/kg dexamethasone IV or IM. Serum cortisol concentrations following dexamethasone are less than 1.0 µg/dl in normal dogs. Dogs with hyperadrenocorticism may show some decrease in serum cortisol concentration following dexamethasone, but should not suppress to less than 1.0 µg/dl. This test is diagnostic for 100% of dogs with AT and for 96% with PDH.[39]

Measurement of urinary corticoids in unextracted urine has been shown to be a valid screening test for hyperadrenocorticism in the dog.[40] This test differentiated normal from affected dogs when urinary corticoids were indexed either to 24-hour urine production or to urine creatinine. Using the urinary corticoids-to-creatinine ratio has the advantage of requiring only a single urine sample rather than all urine produced over 24 hours. Unfortunately, at the present time, this test is not widely available.

The glucagon tolerance test is another new screening test for hyperadrenocorticism.[41] To perform this test, blood samples are collected before and at 15, 30, 45, and 60 minutes following IV administration of 0.03 mg/kg glucagon. Collected samples are then analyzed for glucose. A diagnosis of hyperadrenocorticism is established if peak serum glucose exceeds 300 mg/dl. Normal dogs display peak glucose values of about 200 mg/dl. The advantage of this screening test is that expensive cortisol radioimmunoassay is not required. Its disadvantage is that exogenous steroids lead to a false positive result.[42]

To differentiate PDH from AT the high-dosage dexamethasone suppression test should be performed. Serum samples are obtained before and 3 and 8 hours following IV administration of 1.0 mg/kg dexamethasone. Suppression of serum cortisol concentrations to below 1.5 μg/dl is diagnostic for PDH and rules out AT. Unfortunately, 15% of dogs affected with PDH do not show cortisol suppression with this test[31] and must be further tested. If calcification in the area of the adrenal gland is seen on abdominal radiographs, a diagnosis of AT can be made and no further testing is necessary. If calcification is not seen, determination of plasma ACTH, corticotrophin-releasing hormone (CRH) stimulation testing, exploratory laparotomy, adrenal gland scintigraphy, or computed tomography (CT) should be performed to establish the etiology of the disease.[42a] Plasma ACTH is normal to elevated (>40 pg/ml) in dogs with PDH, and is low to low-normal (<20 pg/ml) in dogs with AT.[43] ACTH is a highly labile peptide, and blood samples must be immediately placed on ice and centrifuged (preferably in a cold centrifuge) and the plasma frozen. Samples should be allowed to contact only plastic because ACTH will bind to glass. Finally, only ACTH assays validated for the dog provide reliable results. A human ACTH assay should not be used.

To perform the CRH stimulation test, samples are collected before and 15 to 30 minutes following IV administration of 1.0 μg/kg of CRH, and plasma samples are assayed for ACTH. Increases are seen in both normal dogs and dogs with PDH, but no increase is seen in dogs with AT.[31] Unfortunately, CRH is not readily available. Because the contralateral adrenal gland is atrophied in AT but bilateral enlargement is seen in PDH, assessing adrenal gland size by exploratory laparotomy, adrenal scintigraphy, or CT scan can be used to differentiate PDH from AT.

THERAPY

The therapy for PDH is quite different from that for AT. For PDH, surgical hypophysectomy and bilateral adrenalectomy have been successful.[44,45] However, excellent surgical skills, close postoperative monitoring, and lifelong hormonal supplementation are required with either of these approaches, and medical therapy is therefore preferred. Cyproheptadine and bromocriptine can be used to reduce pituitary ACTH secretion but have not been demonstrated to be clinically effective and have adverse side-effects in dogs.[31,46]

At present, the medical therapy of choice for PDH is o,p'-DDD (mitotane, Lysodren).[31] This drug causes necrosis and atrophy of the portion of the adrenal cortex that secretes glucocorticoids (zona fasciculata and zona reticularis) while in most cases sparing the portion that secretes mineralocorticoids (zona glomerulosa). During the initial 10-day loading period, the animal should be treated with 50 mg/kg divided BID. Administration of o,p'-DDD usually results in a rapid decline in serum cortisol concentrations. Even if cortisol remains in the normal range, adverse side-effects of anorexia, weakness, vomiting, and diarrhea, which reflect a hypoglucocorticoid state, may be seen. To avoid these effects, maintenance dosages of either oral prednisone or prednisolone (0.2 mg/kg q 24 hr) or cortisone (1.0 mg/kg q 24 hr) may be administered during the loading period.

If the dog displays signs of glucocorticoid deficiency during the loading period, o,p'-DDD therapy should be discontinued and twice the maintenance dosage of prednisone, prednisolone, or cortisone administered. If the patient is not dramatically improved in 3 hours, the animal should be examined immediately and a cause other than glucocorticoid deficiency suspected. Dogs with concurrent diabetes mellitus and hyperadrenocorticism should be treated with a less aggressive protocol during the loading to avoid drastic decreases in insulin requirement, which frequently lead to insulin overdosage and life-threatening hypoglycemia.[36] These dogs should receive 25 mg/kg divided BID and twice the maintenance dosage of glucocorticoids during loading.

Either following the 10-day loading period or if o,p'-DDD loading is discontinued for signs relating to a hypoglucocorticoid state, adrenal function should be reevaluated with an ACTH stimulation test to assess treatment efficacy. Exogenous glucocorticoid therapy should be discontinued for at least 24 and preferably 48 hours prior to repeating the ACTH stimulation test because these substances cross-react with cortisol assays. It has been demonstrated that serum ACTH concentrations increase following o,p'-DDD therapy owing to decreased negative feedback on the pituitary by cortisol. The goal of loading therapy is to suppress adrenocortical function so that both the pre- and post-ACTH serum cortisol concentrations are in the normal resting (i.e., pre-ACTH) range so that supra-physiologic amounts of cortisol are not secreted in response to high serum ACTH concentrations. If the ACTH stimulation test reveals pre- and post-cortisol concentrations in the range seen in normal dogs, the patient requires further o,p'-DDD loading.[31]

About 15% of treated dogs require supplemental loading, which consists of 5 more days of o,p'-DDD and supplemental glucocorticoid therapy given at the same dosages used during initial loading. Following supplemental loading, adrenocortical function should again be reevaluated with an ACTH stimulation test. If adequate suppression is not observed, the dog should undergo another 5-day loading period and then be reevaluated with ACTH stimulation testing. In rare cases, 30 to 60 days of loading are required. About one-third of dogs display oversuppression of adrenocortical function as evidenced by pre- and post-ACTH cortisol concentrations less than low-normal resting values.[31] These animals should be continued on maintenance glucocorticoid therapy and reassessed with ACTH stimulation in 2 to 6 weeks. Most dogs will be adequately suppressed at that time, but some may remain oversuppressed for months.

Once adequate loading had been achieved, maintenance therapy with o,p'-DDD given at a dosage of 50 mg/kg/wk divided into 2 or 3 weekly doses should be initiated. Exogenous glucocorticoids should only be given during periods of stress or illness. If signs of glucocorticoid deficiency are observed, o,p'-DDD should be discontinued and twice the maintenance dosage of glucocorticoids started. Again, if the animal is not dramatically improved in 3 hours, it should be immediately evaluated for another underlying illness. Dogs that respond to exogenous glucocorticoids should be continued on maintenance glucocorticoids for 2 to 6 weeks. After that time maintenance o,p'-DDD can be restarted. Irreversible combined glucocorticoid and mineralocorticoid insufficiency (Addison's disease) requiring lifelong glucocorticoid and mineralocorticoid supplementation has been reported[47] but is an uncommon complication of o,p'-DDD therapy. O,p'-DDD therapy usually results in resolution of clinical signs in 3 to 5 months. Repeat ACTH stimulation testing should be performed at 4, 8, and 12 months and every 6 months thereafter. It is common for dogs with PDH to come out of remission during maintenance therapy. When this occurs, the dog should undergo a standard 5-day loading treatment and the maintenance dosage of o,p'-DDD should be increased by 50%.

Other nonsurgical therapies for PDH include ketaconazole or radiation. Ketoconazole is an antifungal agent that has recently been shown to be effective in the treatment of both PDH and AT. In a preliminary study, ketaconazole given at a dosage of 15 mg/kg BID per os resulted in rapid normalization of serum cortisol and remission of clinical signs in seven of eight dogs with PDH and two of three dogs with AT.[48] The drug should be administered with food to facilitate absorption. Ketaconazole may cause vomiting in some dogs, requiring therapy to be discontinued. Unfortunately, maintenance ketoconazole therapy is approximately 7 times more costly than maintenance therapy with o,p'-DDD.

Therapy with o,p'-DDD can result in accelerated growth of pituitary neoplasms and is therefore not recommended for space-occupying pituitary adenomas. This possibility should be suspected if CNS signs or non-dexamethasone-suppressible PDH is present.

Radiation therapy is the therapy of choice in these cases and results in a rapid decrease in tumor size.[49] However, because ACTH production does not normalize for at least 6 months following radiation, affected dogs should initially receive concurrent o,p'-DDD or ketaconazole.

Surgical removal is the treatment of choice for adrenal tumors. In order to examine both adrenal glands and do a thorough abdominal exploratory to detect metastatic disease, a ventral midline approach is preferred. Atrophy of the contralateral adrenal gland is a consistent finding with AT. Exogenous glucocorticoids are required until the contralateral gland regains function.[31] On the morning prior to surgery, it is recommended that large dosages of IV corticosteroids be given (5 mg/kg soluble hydrocortisone, 2.0 mg/kg prednisolone sodium succinate or 0.1–0.2 mg/kg dexamethasone). Following surgery the preoperative dosage of steroids should be repeated. On the first postoperative day, 0.5 mg/kg prednisolone or prednisone BID, 2.5 mg/kg cortisone BID, or 0.1 mg/kg dexamethasone q 24 should be given. The dosage of steroids can be tapered to maintenance by 7 to 10 days and can usually be discontinued by 2 months. If both adrenal glands are enlarged, non-dexamethasone-suppressible PDH should be suspected, and only a biopsy of an adrenal gland should be performed to confirm the diagnosis. In a recent review of 25 dogs undergoing surgery for AT,[32] 50% of dogs not euthanized at the time of surgery developed serious complications, including cardiac arrest, pneumonia, pulmonary artery thromboembolism, pancreatitis, and acute renal failure. However, in another review of 10 dogs with AT,[45] complications following surgery were minimal. It is recommended that prior to surgery dogs with AT be pretreated with 15 mg/kg ketaconazole BID for 7 to 10 days to normalize adrenocortical function and thereby improve surgical outcome. High dosages of o,p'-DDD (50 to 150 mg/kg/day) may be attempted to treat metastatic or recurrent disease but have generally not been successful. Ketoconazole has not yet been evaluated for the treatment of metastatic or recurrent disease, but it could be considered for these uses. Hypophysectomy is another effective treatment for pituitary dependent hyperadrenocorticism, but it is a technically demanding surgical procedure.[44]

In cats adrenalectomy is reported to be the only successful treatment for hyperadrenocorticism.[30a,30b] The use of o,p'-DDD requires further study in the cat before it can be recommended.

PROGNOSIS

Without treatment dogs with hyperadrenocorticism deteriorate and die. Excess circulating glucocorticoids can lead to hypertension, cardiovascular disease, thromboembolism, diabetes mellitus, or serious bacterial infections that may result in death. Alternatively, death may result from metastasis of adrenal carcinomas or enlargement of pituitary tumors. With surgical removal, the prognosis for adrenal adenomas is excellent. Even with treatment, the prognosis for adrenal carcinoma is poor. Medical treatment of PDH prolongs life and improves its quality, with most dogs dying from disease involving other organ systems. About 10% of dogs with PDH can be successfully managed for periods greater than 4 years.[31]

COMPARATIVE ASPECTS

Hyperadrenocorticism is much less common in humans than in dogs.[18] However, as in dogs, PDH is much more common than AT. Adrenal adenomas and carcinomas occur with approximately equal incidence in humans, as in the case with dogs.

PANCREATIC INSULIN-SECRETING NEOPLASMS

Pancreatic insulin-secreting neoplasms are also termed insulinomas, insulin-producing islet cell neoplasms, beta cell tumors, islet cell tumors, and insulin-producing pancreatic tumors. Beta cells belong to a larger family of tissues that originate from the embryonic neural crest and function to secrete a variety of polypeptide hormones. APUD is an acronym for amine, precursor, uptake, and decarboxylation which describes certain characteristics of these cells. Tumors derived from beta cells are termed APUDomas. Pancreatic insulin-secreting tumor is one type of APUDoma.

INCIDENCE AND RISK FACTORS

Pancreatic insulin-secreting neoplasms are uncommon in the dog and are extremely rare in the cat.[50,51] This tumor has also been reported to occur in the ferret.[52] The average age of affected dogs is about 9 years with a range of 3.5 to 15 years reported.[53–56] The tumor does not appear to have a sex predilection. Canine breeds in which this tumor is more prevalent include the boxer, German shepherd, Irish setter, standard poodle, collie, Labrador retriever, and fox terrier. Functional pancreatic tumors are more commonly seen in medium to larger breeds but can also be seen in smaller breeds. The etiology of these tumors in the dog and cat is unknown.

PATHOLOGY AND NATURAL BEHAVIOR

Insulin-secreting neoplasms are usually single nodular masses (Fig. 22-11), but multiple pancreatic masses and diffuse microscopic infiltration of neoplastic beta cells have been described. The lobes of the pancreas are affected with about equal frequency. Almost all insulinomas are malignant and metastasize by way of lymphatics to local lymph nodes and liver, as evidenced at abdominal exploratory in about 50% of cases. Metastatic spread to mesentery, omentum, portal vessels, lung, spleen, myocardium, or spinal meninges has been described but is uncommon. It is very difficult to predict the biologic behavior of these tumors on the basis of their histologic appearance. Even tumors diagnosed as "benign" adenomas have shown metastatic behavior following surgical removal. For this reason, many pathologists classify these tumors as islet cell tumors but do not identify them as malignant or benign. Canine pancreatic islet cell tumors are usually of B-cell origin but gastrin secreting islet cell tumors producing the Zollinger-Ellison syndrome have been rarely reported.[56a]

HISTORY AND CLINICAL SIGNS

Dogs with insulinomas have the clinical signs of hypoglycemia rather than physical evidence of the tumor or metastases. Frequently reported clinical signs include seizures, hindlimb weakness, collapse, generalized weakness or ataxia, and muscle tremors.[53-56] Evidence of peripheral nervous system involvement is less likely because the peripheral nervous system is not dependent on glucose and has the ability to use amino acids or fatty acids to supplement its energy needs.[61a] Less frequently reported signs include exercise intolerance, depression, bizarre behavior or hysteria, irritability, polyphagia, and polydipsia/polyuria. The clinical course is progressive, with signs becoming more severe and frequent with time. Signs are episodic and last for only seconds to minutes, but intraictal CNS signs, especially focal facial twitching, have been reported. Most dogs display multiple clinical signs. The signs are the result of increased sympathetic discharge (*e.g.*, muscle tremors and irritability) or of neuroglucopenia (*e.g.*, seizures, collapse, and generalized muscle weakness). The rate of decline of serum glucose probably affects the type of clinical signs seen. With a rapid fall in glucose there is activation of hypothalamic glucoreceptors resulting in increased sympathetic discharge and associated clinical signs, but with a slow decline only signs of neuroglucopenia appear. With chronicity, adaptation may take place and the dog may be asymptomatic despite a profoundly subnormal blood glucose. Stimuli reported to induce hypoglycemia are fasting (decreased nutrient intake without a decrease in insulin); exercise, excitement, or

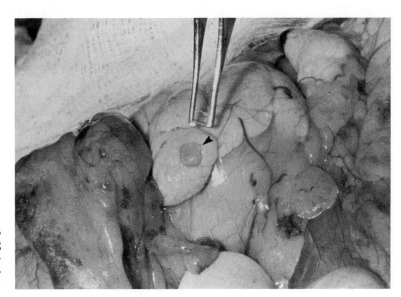

Figure 22-11. Arrow indicates a nodular insulin-secreting pancreatic mass in a dog. Surgical removal resulted in remission of signs for 32 months.

stress (increased glucose utilization by tissues without a decrease in insulin); and feeding (exaggerated insulin secretion in response to postprandial increases in blood glucose). Some reports have not associated clinical signs with feeding. Also, glucose tolerance testing in histologically confirmed cases has shown these tumors to be poorly responsive to exogenous glucose, supporting the claim that feeding is not a stimulus to hypoglycemia. The duration of clinical signs prior to diagnosis varies between 1 day and 3 years, but averages 3 months in most studies.[53-56] In one study, 29% of dogs were misdiagnosed initially and placed on anticonvulsant therapy.[56] Physical examination is usually unremarkable unless the clinician is able to observe the animal during a hypoglycemic episode. It is uncommon for dogs with insulinomas to be thin, and insulin-induced lipogenesis may predispose them to obesity.

DIAGNOSTIC TECHNIQUES AND WORK-UP

Glucose test strips* are valuable for screening patients for hypoglycemia. However, since these methods produce results 15% lower than standard laboratory methods, suspicious values should always be verified with standard methods. In retrospective studies, about 95% of dogs with insulinomas were hypoglycemic upon presentation.[53-57] The remaining animals demonstrated hypoglycemia following short periods of fasting (8–12 hours). Dogs with insulinomas usually display Whipple's triad: clinical signs (i.e., neurologic signs) associated with hypoglycemia; fasting blood glucose ≤40 mg/dl; and disappearance of clinical signs with dextrose administration. However, since Whipple's triad is consistent with any cause of hypoglycemia, other differentials must be considered. Differential diagnoses for hypoglycemia in mature dogs includes improper sample handling (i.e., failure to separate serum from clotted blood), hypoadrenocorticism, sepsis, end-stage liver disease, "hunting dog" hypoglycemia, starvation, extrapancreatic tumors (especially hepatocellular carcinomas), renal failure, heart failure, congenital hepatic enzyme deficiencies resulting in glycogen storage diseases (rare), exogenous insulin, oral hypoglycemic agents (e.g., sulfonylurea com-

* Dextrostix (Ames, Elkhardt, IN) or Chemstrip BG (Boehninger Mannheim, Indianapolis, IN)

pounds), toxicities (e.g., ethanol, salicylate, and propranolol), and laboratory error.[57,58]

CBC, serum chemistries, and urinalysis are usually normal in affected dogs. Elevations in alanine amino transferase (ALT or SGPT) and serum alkaline phosphatase (SAP) have been reported in affected dogs, but do not appear to be predictive for liver metastases. About 20% of the dogs in one study[55] displayed mild hypokalemia, which did not require treatment. Routine thoracic and abdominal radiographs are normal unless other concurrent diseases are present. In two studies serum insulin concentration was elevated in 76.1% and 66.9% of affected dogs.[55,56] Increased serum insulin with concurrent hypoglycemia is very reliable for diagnosing insulinomas.

An insulin-glucose ratio greater than 0.3 μU/mg and- glucose-insulin ratio of less than 2.5 are also very suggestive of insulinoma. The ratios appear to be of equal diagnostic value, but false negatives have been reported with both tests. The amended glucose-insulin ratio (AGIR) is defined by the following formula:

$$AGIR = \frac{\text{serum insulin } (\mu U/ml) \times 100}{\text{plasma glucose } (mg/dl) - 30}$$

When plasma glucose is ≤30, a value of 1 should be used for the denominator. Ratios above 30 are indicative of insulin-secreting tumors.[53] Although nearly all dogs with insulinoma have an elevated AGIR, an elevation has also been documented in dogs with hypoglycemia from sepsis or nonpancreatic tumors.[58,59] In most cases a high degree of suspicion of an insulin-secreting tumor can be made on the basis of the signalment, history, physical exam, and demonstration of Whipple's triad, along with ruling out other differential diagnosis for hypoglycemia by laboratory testing and radiographic studies. Serum insulin determination can be helpful, but is not always required to establish the diagnosis. Provocative testing including high-dosage IV glucose, glucagon, L-leucine, and tolbutamide tolerance testing has been described, but the diagnostic value of provocative testing is limited and the risk of inducing symptomatic hypoglycemia is significant. For these reasons, provocative testing is not recommended.

Insulinoma has been associated with polyneuropathy in the dog.[60,61,61a] Undoubtedly, if this possibility were investigated in all cases, the incidence of polyneuropathy would be higher.

A complete neurologic exam should be performed in all dogs suspected of having insulinoma. If hyporeflexia or decreased conscious proprioception is seen, electromyography, nerve conduction velocity testing, and nerve and muscle biopsies should be considered in order to establish a diagnosis of polyneuropathy.

THERAPY

Surgery is indicated in order to obtain a biopsy (excisional) to histologically confirm the diagnosis, reduce the tumor burden, and clinically stage the extent of disease for prognostic purposes. Although surgery is rarely curative, it prolongs survival and improves the quality of life. Surgery has been shown to result in longer survival than either medical management or chemotherapy for insulin-secreting pancreatic tumors.[55,56]

Rather than fasting the animal overnight, it is recommended that small feedings be administered every 4 hours through the night and up until 4 hours prior to surgery in order to avoid hypoglycemic seizures. Alternatively, the animal may be fasted overnight while maintained on dextrose-containing intravenous fluids. Although blood glucose should be monitored frequently with glucose test strips while the patient is under general anesthesia to detect intraoperative hypoglycemia, in most cases glucose increases intraoperatively owing to stress-induced glycogenolysis and gluconeogenesis, making the addition of dextrose to intravenous fluids unnecessary.

A ventral midline incision should be made from the xiphoid to the pubis so that a thorough abdominal exploratory may be performed. The entire pancreas should be visually inspected and palpated. Intrapancreatic tumor masses palpate firmer than normal pancreatic tissue. Most tumors appear as single discrete nodular masses 0.5 to 2 cm in diameter (Fig. 22-11), but multiple nodular masses and diffuse infiltration of the pancreas have been reported. Tumors occur with equal incidence in the right and left lobes of the pancreas. Even if no discrete tumor is detected, a pancreatic biopsy should be taken to rule out diffuse infiltrative disease. A partial pancreatectomy should be performed if possible. If it is not possible to save at least one pancreatic duct, a total pancreatectomy should be performed. The liver should be closely inspected for metastatic disease. Since the duodenal, splenic,

hepatic, and greater mesenteric lymph nodes all receive drainage from the pancreas, they should also be visually inspected and palpated. Suspicious nodes should be excised and examined histologically. Even if all nodes appear normal, a lymph node and the liver should be biopsied for staging purposes. Since dogs with diffuse metastatic disease have been managed for over 1 year medically, euthanasia is not mandatory if the tumor cannot be totally resected. Because pancreatitis can occur postoperatively, dogs displaying vomiting should be given nothing by mouth and maintained on intravenous fluids until the problem resolves. Following surgery dogs may have normal, low, or elevated blood glucose concentrations. If hypoglycemia persists past 2 days following surgery, residual tumor should be suspected. Persistent hyperglycemia can occur owing to atrophy of the normal islet tissue from chronic hypoglycemia and may require insulin therapy.

Medical management is indicated for insulinomas that are incompletely resected or that recur following surgery. Acute episodes of hypoglycemia can be treated by owners by applying corn syrup to the dog's gums. If the owner is unable to control clinical signs, the animal should be seen by a veterinarian as soon as possible. Neurologic signs should be treated immediately with 0.1 to 0.5 g/kg dextrose given intravenously as a 25% dextrose solution. If the animal is not responsive to dextrose, cerebral laminar necrosis secondary to profound hypoglycemia should be suspected. These cases may require anticonvulsant therapy. Once the dog is recovered and able to swallow, a small meal should be fed. Then small feedings of a diet high in protein and fat should be given frequently. Carbohydrates should be in the form of complex carbohydrates rather than simple sugars. Semimoist diets are high in simple sugars and therefore should be avoided. Since exercise and stress can initiate hypoglycemic episodes, they should be minimized.

Once dietary management practices no longer control clinical signs, drug therapy should be initiated. Prednisone is useful in preventing hypoglycemia and acts by increasing hepatic gluconeogenesis and inhibiting and action of insulin on peripheral tissues. Initially, prednisone should be given as a dosage of 0.25 mg/kg BID but can be increased up to 2 mg/kg BID if needed. Side-effects of prednisone include polydipsia/polyuria, polyphagia, muscle weakness, alopecia, episodic panting (especially at high dosages), and mild to moderate immunosuppression. Diazoxide may also be used to manage hypoglycemia, either alone, or in combination with prednisone. Diazoxide is a nondiuretic benzothiadiazide that increases serum glucose by inhibiting insulin secretion, decreasing peripheral uptake of glucose by a direct action and through increased adrenergic stimulation and increasing hepatic glycogenolysis and gluconeogenesis by means of adrenergic stimulation. Initially, diazoxide should be given at a dosage of 5 mg/kg BID, but this may be increased up to 40 mg/kg BID if necessary. Anorexia, vomiting, and diarrhea are commonly seen adverse side-effects. Giving diazoxide with food will decrease gastrointestinal side-effects. Other less commonly reported adverse effects include diabetes mellitus, cataracts, sodium and fluid retention, bone marrow suppression, and tachycardia. Since the drug is metabolized by the liver, increased toxicity is seen with hepatic dysfunction. Phenytoin, propranolol, and L-asparaginase have been recommended for the medical treatment of insulinomas, but they do not appear to be effective.

Streptozotocin and alloxan have been used to create insulinopenic dogs for research purposes. Unfortunately, both agents are nephrotoxic. Acute renal failure resulting in death occurred in the two reported cases of insulinomas in dogs treated with streptozotocin.[62,63] Feldman reported some success in treating 50 dogs with metastatic insulinoma with 65 mg/kg alloxan given once intravenously.[64] Until further experimental work has been performed, treatment with either streptozotocin or alloxan is not recommended.

PROGNOSIS

The long-term prognosis for affected dogs is poor. However, the average survival time in dogs following surgery is approximately 10 to 14 months.[53-56] Survival does not correlate with breed; body weight, type, severity, frequency, or duration of clinical signs; preoperative serum glucose concentrations; or tumor location within the pancreas.[56] However, higher serum insulin concentrations were associated with a shorter survival, and younger dogs have been shown to have significantly shorter survival times than older dogs.[56] Dogs with metastasis to organs beyond the regional lymph nodes (clinical stage 3; T_1, N_0, M_1 or N_1, N_0) have been shown to have significantly shorter survival times (Fig. 22-12).[56] Interestingly, dogs with metastasis to regional lymph nodes only (clinical stage 2; T_1, N_1, M_0) appear to have similar survival times when compared to dogs with tumor that appears to be confined to the pancreas (clinical stage 1; T_1, N_0, M_0) at the time of surgery.[56] However, dogs presenting in clinical stage 1 have a significantly longer disease-free interval (i.e., period of normoglycemia) following surgery than dogs presenting in clinical stage 2 or 3 (Fig. 22-13).[56] There is approximately a 50% chance that a dog with clinical stage 1 will be normoglycemic

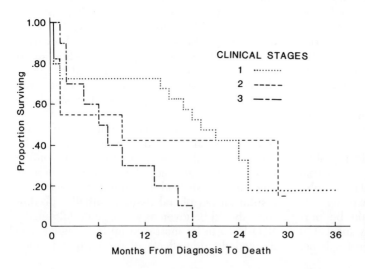

CLINICAL STAGES

1 ··········
2 - - - - -
3 — · — ·

Figure 22-12. Survival curve following surgery in 52 dogs with insulin-secreting islet cell tumors based on clinical stage. Dogs with metastasis of the tumor beyond regional lymph nodes (clinical stage 3; T_1, N_0, M_1, or N_1, M_1) have significantly ($p < 0.0052$) shorter survival times when compared to dogs with metastasis to regional lymph nodes only (clinical stage 2; T_1, N_1, M_0) or dogs with tumor confined to the pancreas (clinical stage 1; T_1, N_0, M_0) at the time of surgery.[56]

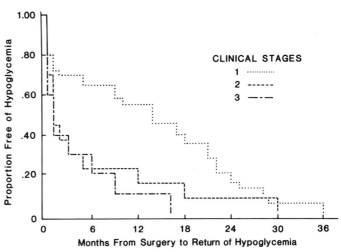

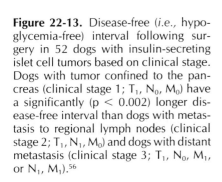

Figure 22-13. Disease-free (*i.e.*, hypoglycemia-free) interval following surgery in 52 dogs with insulin-secreting islet cell tumors based on clinical stage. Dogs with tumor confined to the pancreas (clinical stage 1; T_1, N_0, M_0) have a significantly ($p < 0.002$) longer disease-free interval than dogs with metastasis to regional lymph nodes (clinical stage 2; T_1, N_1, M_0) and dogs with distant metastasis (clinical stage 3; T_1, N_0, M_1, or N_1, M_1).[56]

for 14 months following surgery, but only a 20% chance that a dog in clinical stage 2 or 3 will be normoglycemic for the same period of time.

COMPARATIVE ASPECTS

In contrast to the statistics for dogs, benign tumors account for about 90% of all insulin-secreting tumors in humans.[18] As in the dog, the anatomic distribution of these tumors in humans is equal throughout the pancreas.

OTHER TUMORS OF THE ENDOCRINE SYSTEM

Other tumors of the endocrine system that occur less frequently include non-ACTH-secreting pituitary tumors, parathyroid tumors, Zollinger-Ellison syndrome, pheochromocytoma, and multiple endocrine neoplasia. These tumors along with chemodectoma will be reviewed in this section.

PITUITARY TUMORS

Non-ACTH-producing pituitary tumors have been described in the dog and the cat. Craniopharyngioma occurs in younger dogs and results in hypopituitarism.[65] Since the diaphragma sellae is incomplete in dogs, these tumors can invade dorsally to involve cranial nerves, hypothalamus, and thalamus. Resulting clinical signs reflect abnormalities in pituitary/hypothalamic and central nervous system function. Decreased long bone growth resulting in dwarfism can occur secondary to decreased growth hormone secretion prior to closure of physeal plates. Diabetes insipidus can occur owing to interference with antidiuretic hormone release; it results in polyuria and compensatory polydipsia. Due to decreased secretion of ACTH and TSH, hypo-adrenocorticism and hypothyroidism can also occur. Because hypo-adrenocorticism does not disrupt mineralocorticoid production, serum electrolytes are normal. Blindness, behavior change, depression, and seizures can occur with involvement of the central nervous system.

Other nonfunctional tumors in the dog include adenoma, acidophil adenoma, and basophil adenoma of the pars distalis and pituitary chromophobe carcinoma. These tumors occur in older animals and give rise to the clinical signs described for craniopharyngioma except that dwarfism is not seen. Metastatic pituitary tumors include lymphoma, mammary gland adenocarcinoma, and malignant melanoma. Additionally, local invasion of the pituitary from meningioma, osteosarcoma, neurofibroma, and ependymoma arising from adjacent structures has also been described.

In the cat, a pituitary tumor associated with elevated serum concentrations of growth hormone and acromegaly has been described.[66] It was accompanied by diabetes mellitus and features consistent with acromegaly, including a large head, paws, and prognathia inferior and an enlarged abdomen. Nonfunctional pituitary tumors are uncommon in the cat, but chromophobe adenoma and pituicytoma of the neurohypophysis have been described.[67,68] See Chapter 27 for further information on diagnosis and treatment of pituitary tumors.

PARATHYROID TUMORS

Parathyroid tumors are rare in the dog and have not yet been reported in the cat. In one series, affected dogs were middle-aged to older (7 to 13 years).[69] Keeshounds appeared to be overly represented, but no sex predilection was evident. Primary hyperparathyroidism has been described in two German shepherd pups from a litter of four females and was postulated to be inherited in an autosomal recessive manner.[70] Parathyroid adenomas are more common, and carcinomas are infrequently described. Parathyroid tumors are usually cervical in location, but a tumor arising from mediastinal accessory parathyroid tissue has been described.[71]

Hypercalcemia is consistently reported with hyperparathyroidism. Other differentials for hypercalcemia include hyperproteinemia, cancer-associated hypercalcemia (especially lymphoma, adenocarcinoma of the apocrine gland of the anal sac, and multiple myeloma), hypoadrenocorticism, renal failure, hypervitaminosis D, and skeletal disorders (primary and metastatic bone tumors, septic osteomyelitis, and disuse osteoporosis).[72] To correct for the effect of albumin and total serum protein concentrations on serum calcium measurement, the following formulas should be used:[73]

$$\text{corrected Ca} = \text{measured Ca (mg/dl)} - \text{albumin (gm/dl)} + 3.5$$
or
$$\text{corrected Ca} = \text{measured Ca (mg/dl)} - 0.4\ [\text{total protein (gm/dl)}] + 3.3$$

If the corrected calcium is elevated, a second serum sample should be submitted for calcium determination to document hypercalcemia. Serum lipemia will falsely elevate the measured calcium value. Because primary hyperparathyroidism is rare, once hypercalcemia is documented, other etiologies should be ruled out.

A medical work-up consisting of a good history, careful physical exam, serum chemistry panel, chest and abdominal radiographs, and lymph node aspirate or biopsy rules out most of the other differentials. The owners should be questioned concerning exogenous vitamin D supplementation. Since lymphoma is the most common etiology for hypercalcemia in the dog, physical examination should include palpation of lymph nodes and the abdomen for liver or splenic enlargement and abdominal masses. Enlarged peripheral nodes should be aspirated or biopsied to rule out underlying lymphoma. Unfortunately, cervical palpation does not detect most parathyroid tumors. A careful rectal exam should be done to detect possible adenocarcinoma of the apocrine gland of the anal sac. This tumor is most commonly seen in older female dogs (see Chapter 19). If serum chemistries reveal normal values for sodium and potassium and no azotemia, underlying hypoadrenocorticism can be ruled out. Similarly, a normal BUN and creatinine will rule out renal failure as an underlying cause for hypercalcemia. Chest and abdominal radiographs should be carefully examined for hepatomegaly, splenomegaly, internal lymph node and thymic enlargement, and possible tumor masses. Lytic bone lesions on radiographs may indicate underlying multiple myeloma, and soft tissue mineralization may indicate hypervitaminosis D. Since skeletal lesions are an uncommon cause for hypercalcemia, in the absence of clinical signs referable to the skeletal system, routine radiographs of the skeleton are not indicated. Once other causes for hypercalcemia can be ruled out, hyperparathyroidism should then be considered.

Most dogs with parathyroid tumors are presented for polyuria/polydipsia, listlessness, and muscle weakness. Less commonly, inappetence or anorexia and episodic shivering have been described. Affected dogs have a normal CBC, while urinalysis may reveal an inflammatory sediment because these dogs may be predisposed to lower urinary tract infection and urolithiasis. Serum phosphorus is usually decreased or normal but can be elevated if concurrent renal insufficiency is present. Serum alkaline phosphatase may be elevated.

Once other etiologies have been ruled out, cervical exploratory surgery should be performed to remove possible neoplastic parathyroid glands. If cervical exploration is negative, serum should be submitted for assay to a laboratory with a validated canine parathormone radioimmunoassay. If the serum parathormone concentration is elevated, a diagnosis of hypercalcemia secondary to hyperparathyroidism is confirmed. A second surgery should then be performed to re-explore the cervical region. If the second cervical exploration is negative, while the animal is under the same anesthesia a sternal split should be performed and the anterior mediastinum carefully examined for ectopic parathyroid tumors. Following removal of parathyroid tumor, the remaining parathyroid tissue will be atrophied secondary to chronic hypercalcemia. The dog should be treated for hypoparathyroidism as outlined previously in this chapter (see "Canine Thyroid Tumors"). Because the remaining parathyroid tissue will regain function, treatment is usually required for only 2 to 3 months. The prognosis following surgical removal is good.

ZOLLINGER–ELLISON SYNDROME

Zollinger–Ellison syndrome is characterized by gastrin-secreting tumor of the delta (D) cells of the pancreatic islets. This tumor, also termed gastrinoma, is another example of an APUDoma. The syndrome is well described in humans but is rare in small animals, having been documented in only a few dogs and one cat.[74–77,77a,77b] The etiology in dogs and cats is unknown. Like insulinomas, these tumors tend to be discrete and only 1 to a few centimeters in diameter. In the few documented cases, tumors were malignant, and metastasis to regional lymph nodes and liver was described. In one case myelofibrosis was associated with this syndrome.[77b]

As with insulin-secreting islet cell tumors, clinical signs result from the secretory product of the tumor rather than from its physical presence. Hypergastrinemia stimulates increased hydrochloric acid secretion by the parietal cells of the stomach. This increased gastric acid secretion causes ulceration in the stomach or proximal intestine. Esophagitis secondary to reflux of gastric acid has also been described. Because gastrin has a trophic effect on the gastric mucosa, mucosal hypertrophy also occurs. Most affected animals are middle-aged to older and present for chronic vomiting and weight loss. The vomitus may contain fresh or digested blood, and melena can occur. Diarrhea, polydipsia, and depression also occur. Diarrhea is usually characterized by steatorrhea due to inactivation of pancreatic lipase and bile salts and irritation of the intestinal mucosa by gastric acid. If an ulcer perforates, acute peritonitis can occur.

Routine laboratory testing can reveal evidence of iron deficiency anemia secondary to gastrointestinal bleeding. Serum chemistries may show hypochloremia, hypokalemia, and metabolic alkalosis due to excessive gastric acid secretion. Liver enzymes may be increased if metastasis to the liver occurs. Hypocalcemia can occur secondary to gastrin-induced hyperplasia of thyroid C cells and elevated calcitonin levels. Prominent gastric rugal folds and ulcers can be seen with contrast radiography. Endoscopy may reveal esophagitis, gastritis, and ulcerative lesions in the pyloric antral region or proximal duodenum. Gastric mucosal biopsy reveals gastric mucosal hypertrophy and chronic gastritis. Fasting concentrations of gastrin in serum are usually very elevated in affected dogs. However, since other disease conditions can also show pronounced elevations, provocative testing is indicated. Since gastric acid secretion is already maximally stimulated, stimulation with pentagastrin, results in little change. In the normal dog, pentagastrin causes marked increase in gastric acid secretion. A more detailed discussion of this testing procedure is available elsewhere.[77]

There are only limited reports regarding therapy of Zollinger-Ellison syndrome in small animals. Surgery is indicated to establish the diagnosis and to remove large ulcers. Regional lymph nodes and the liver should be biopsied for staging purposes. In humans, total gastrectomy is performed to remove the target organ for gastrin. Cimetidine or ranitidine, H_2 blockers, should be used preoperatively to decrease gastric acid secretion; they are also indicated postoperatively if residual tumor remains. Additionally, anticholinergic agents may also help decrease gastric acid secretion. The prognosis for cases previously described in the literature has been poor, because most have metastasized by the time of diagnosis.

PHEOCHROMOCYTOMA

Pheochromocytomas, or chromaffin cell tumors, are functional tumors arising from the adrenal medulla; they secrete catecholamines. Pheochromocytoma is another example of an APUDoma. This tumor is rare and has only been described in a few dogs.[78,79,81a] It has not been described in the cat. Affected dogs tend to be older, but no breed or sex predilection exists. Pheochromocytomas are generally large and are locally invasive into the vena cava, liver, and kidney. Increased circulating catecholamines result in hypertension, which may be paroxysmal or sustained, depending on the secretory characteristics of the tumor. In dogs, as with affected humans, episodic hypertension resulting from paroxysmal secretion appears to be more common.[80] The length of the episodes is quite variable and the duration of signs prior to diagnosis ranges from days to years. The clinical signs in affected dogs are vague and result from both the physical presence of the tumor and also its production of increased amounts of catecholamines. Respiratory signs characterized by episodic panting or dyspnea are commonly seen. Tachycardia and cardiac arrythmias are common.[81a] Episodic weakness, muscle tremors, polydipsia, polyuria, anorexia, restlessness, and reluctance to sleep may also be reported. Severe hypertension can also cause epistaxis, seizures, and cerebrovascular accidents. Dogs may also be presented for acute collapse and hypovolemic shock secondary to intra-abdominal hemorrhage from a ruptured tumor. Findings on physical examination are relatively nonspecific and frequently unrewarding in the diagnosis. Because of the episodic pattern of catecholamine secretion, neither hypertension nor the resulting clinical signs may be present during the physical examination. Complete or partial obstruction of the vena cava by the tumor thrombus (Fig. 22-14) may produce ascites, edema of the rear legs, or distention of the caudal superficial epigastric veins. The tumor may be large enough to be palpated. Cardiac auscultation may reveal tachy-cardia, arrhythmias, or cardiac murmurs. Pupils may be dilated secondary to excess sympathetic input.

Routine laboratory tests reveal no consistent abnormalities, although hemoconcentration, anemia, neutrophilia, and proteinuria may be found. Plain abdominal radiographs may reveal an adrenal mass, but the most diagnostic radiographic procedure in this disease is caudal vena caval venography. This study is performed by a rapid hand injection of contrast media into the lateral saphenous vein, followed by a series of abdominal films. Since tumor thrombus invading the posterior vena cava is common in pheochromocytomas, demonstrating such a thrombus supports a presumptive diagnosis. Abdominal ultrasonography has been very helpful in the diagnosis and extent of disease.[81a] Blood pressure measurement can be normal owing to the episodic secretory pattern of pheochromocytomas. Provocative testing with phentolamine, an alpha-adrenergic blocking agent, results in a significant and sustained fall in blood pressure in hypertensive dogs with pheochromocytoma but has little effect in normal dogs. Details concerning this and other provocative tests are covered elsewhere.[80] Demonstration of high circulating concentrations of catecholamines or increased urinary excretion of catecholamines and their breakdown products can also be helpful in establishing the diagnosis. Again, detailed discussions of these tests are available elsewhere.[80]

The therapy of choice for pheochromocytoma is surgery. The major role of medical therapy in this disease is to normalize the cardiovascular

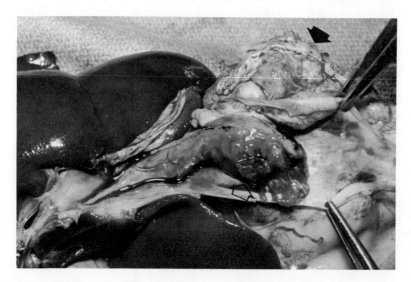

Figure 22-14. Pheochromocytoma (indicated by closed arrow) with local invasion into the caudal vena cava by tumor thrombus (indicated by open arrow).

and metabolic status of the patient prior to surgery in order to reduce the risk involved with anesthesia and surgery. Phenoxybenzamine hydrochloride, an alpha-adrenergic blocking agent, should be administered at a dosage of 0.2 to 1.5 mg/kg orally twice daily for 10 to 14 consecutive days prior to surgery. It is suggested that phenoxybenzamine be initiated at the low end of the dosage range and gradually increased until the desired reduction in blood pressure is obtained. Beta-adrenergic blocking agents, such as propranolol given at a dosage of 0.15 to 0.5 mg/kg orally three times a day, are indicated to control cardiac arrhythmias and hypertension that persist despite phenoxybenzamine therapy. Propranolol should not be initiated without concurrent phenoxybenzamine therapy; propranolol alone could precipitate severe hypertension.

Care must be taken when planning the anesthetic regimen for these patients. Phenothiazines, such as acepromazine, should be avoided because they possess alpha-blocking affects and could result in hypotensive crisis. Narcotic agents may be used as preanesthetics. Because dogs with pheochromocytomas may show a pronounced tachycardia after treatment with atropine, this agent should be avoided as a preanesthetic. If an anticholinergic must be used, glycopyrrolate is preferred because it is less likely to cause severe tachyarrythmias. Narcotic agents or mask inductions are preferred over ultra-short-acting barbiturates for induction because they are less arrythmogenic. Isoflurane is the maintenance agent of choice. It is recommended that a direct arterial line and central venous catheter be placed so that arterial blood pressure and central venous pressure (CVP) can be monitored during surgery. Intraoperative hypertensive episodes should be treated with repeated intravenous boluses of phentolamine (0.02 to 0.1 mg/kg). Intraoperative hypotension should be treated with vigorous fluid administration rather than the pressor administration. Intraoperative arrhythmias should be treated with intravenous propranolol (0.03 to 0.1 mg/kg).

The potential for surgical success is dependent on the invasive nature of the tumor. Tumors without local invasive spread can often be completely resected. However, recurrences are common due to the rich venous network associated with these tumors. Approximately half the dogs will have distant metastases to the liver, lung, spleen, and regional lymph nodes.[81b,81c] Great care must be taken in the dissection of the tumor mass, since it is quite vascular and can bleed profusely when incised. Invasive tumors, especially those involving thrombus growth into the vena cava, require sophisticated surgical techniques. For optimal histologic characterization of the tumor, biopsy specimens should be placed in Zenker's fixative without acetic acid rather than in formalin. Following surgery, if the patient remains hypertensive, residual tumor is likely present. With complete resection of the tumor, prognosis is fair, but if complete resection is not possible, prognosis is poor.

MULTIPLE ENDOCRINE NEOPLASIA

In humans, multiple endocrine neoplasia (MEN) syndromes occur in which there is neoplasia or hyperplasia of two or more endocrine glands.[18] In humans, three distinct types of MEN have been recognized. In MEN I there is parathyroid hyperplasia associated with pancreatic islet cell adenoma or carcinoma or hyperplasia of the anterior pituitary. In MEN II or IIa, there is medullary carcinoma of the thyroid associated with pheochromocytoma or parathyroid hyperplasia. In MEN III or IIb, there is medullary carcinoma of the thyroid associated with pheochromocytoma or multiple mucosal neuromas. A dog with medullary carcinoma of the thyroid gland, pheochromocytoma, and parathyroid hyperplasia consistent with MEN IIa in humans has been described.[81]

CHEMODECTOMA

The term chemodectoma is synonymous with nonchromaffin paraganglioma. The two most common types of chemodectomas are aortic body tumors (Fig. 22-15) and carotid body tumors. Although both tumors have been described in the cat they are very uncommon.[82,83] They are also uncommon in the dog. In two reviews of chemodectoma in the dog, aortic body tumors accounted for 80% to 90%, and carotid body tumors for the remainder.[84,85] Affected dogs were usually between 10 and 15 years of age, and boxers and Boston terriers were most commonly affected. Dogs appear to have no sex predisposition for carotid body tumors, but male dogs appear to be predisposed to aortic body tumors. Tumors can range in size from 1 to 13

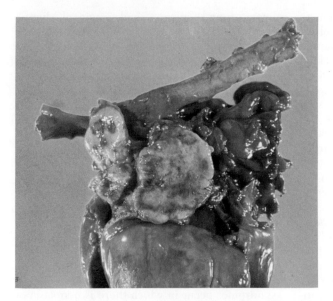

Figure 22-15. Invasive aortic body tumor at the heart base of a dog.

cm. Larger aortic body tumors may result in congestive heart failure. Dogs with carotid body tumors usually present for neck masses, dysphagia, or dyspnea. In about one-fifth of cases metastasis to the lungs, liver, myocardium, kidney, lymph node, adrenal gland, brain, and bone may occur. Local invasion, especially into blood vessels, occurs in about one-half of all cases. Local invasion into the first thoracic vertebra has been described in a dog with an aortic body tumor.[86] Arteriovenous fistula has also been associated with carotid body tumor in a dog.[87] It is suspected that chronic hypoxemia may be important in the etiology of chemodectomas in humans.[88] This would explain the brachycephalic breed predisposition for these tumors. Treatment of these tumors is not well described in the literature, but owing to their invasive nature, they are difficult to remove surgically. Mobile masses in the neck, or rarely on the heart, can be surgically excised with good outcomes. One paper described 11 cases of carotid body tumors in dogs. Ten were treated surgically, with 4 dying perioperatively. The median survival of the other 6 dogs was 22 months. Two dogs suffered a local recurrence and 4 dogs developed metastatic disease.[89] On the basis of a limited number of cases, radiation therapy may be effective in the treatment of these tumors.*

* Gillette EL: Colorado State University, personal communication, 1986

REFERENCES

1. Birchard SJ, Roesel OF: Neoplasia of the thyroid gland in the dog: A retrospective study of 16 cases. J Am Anim Hosp Assoc 17:369–372, 1981

2. Brodey RS, Kelly DF: Thyroid neoplasms in the dog. Cancer 22:406–416, 1968

3. Harari JR, Patterson JS, Rosenthal RC: Clinical and pathologic features of thyroid tumors in 26 dogs. J Am Vet Med Assoc 188:1160–1164, 1986

4. Mitchell M, Hurov LI, Troy GC: Canine thyroid carcinomas: Clinical occurrence, staging by means of scintiscans, and therapy of 15 cases. Vet Surg 8:112–118, 1979

5. Loar AS: Canine thyroid tumors. In Kirk RW (ed): Current Veterinary Therapy IX, pp. 1033–1039. Philadelphia, W.B. Saunders, 1986

6. Jeglum KA, Whereat A: Chemotherapy of canine thyroid carcinoma. Comp Cont Educ 5:96–98, 1983

7. Leav I, Schiller AL, Rijnberk A, et al: Adenomas and carcinomas of the canine and feline thyroid. Am J Pathol 83:61–93, 1976

8. Zarrin KH, Hanichen T: Comparative histopathological study of the canine thyroid gland in London and Munich. J Small Anima Pract 15:329–342, 1974

9. Axelrad AA, Leblond CP: Induction of thyroid tumors in rats by a low iodine diet. Cancer 8:339–367, 1955

10. Pendergast WJ, Milmore BK, Marcus SC: Thyroid cancer and thyrotoxicosis in the United

States: Their relation to endemic goiter. J Chronic Dis 13:22–38, 1961

11. Belshaw BE, Becker DV: Necrosis of follicular cells and discharge of thyroidal iodine induced by administering iodide to iodine-deficient dogs. J Clin Endocrinol Metab 36:466–474, 1973

12. Belshaw BE, Cooper TB, Becker DV: The iodine requirement and influence of iodine intake on iodine metabolism and thyroid function in the adult beagle. Endocrinol 96:1280–1291, 1975

13. Walsh KM, Diters RW: Carcinoma of ectopic thyroid in a dog. J Am Anim Hosp Assoc 20:665–668, 1982

13a. Holscher MA, Davis BW, Wilson, RR: Ectopic thyroid tumor in a dog: Thyroglobulin, calcitonin, and neuron-specific enolase immunochemical studies. Vet Pathol 23:778–779, 1986

13b. Patnaik AK, Lieberman PH, Erlandson RA: Canine medullary carcinoma of the thyroid. Vet Pathol 15:590–599, 1978

14. Rijnberk A: Iodine Metabolism and Thyroid Diseases in the Dog, PhD thesis, Utrecht, Drukkerj Elinkwijk, 1971

15. Branum JE, Leighton RL, Hornoff WJ: Radioisotope imaging for the evaulation of thyroid neoplasia and hypothyroidism in the dog. J Am Vet Med Assoc 180:1077–1079, 1982

16. Peterson ME: Hypoparathyroidism. In Kirk RW (ed): Current Veterinary Therapy IX, pp. 1039–1045. Philadelphia, W.B. Saunders, 1986

17. Klein MK, Powers BE, Withrow SJ: Canine thyroid carcinoma: A retrospective review of 64 cases. Submitted for publication, 1988

18. Brennan MF, Macdonals JS: Cancer of the endocrine system. In DeVita VT Jr et al (eds): Cancer: Principles and Practice of Oncology, 2nd ed, pp. 1179–1241. Philadelphia, J.B. Lippincott, 1985

19. Peterson ME, Kintzer PP, Cavanagh PG, et al: Feline hyperthyroidism: Pretreatment clinical and laboratory evaluations of 131 cases. J Am Vet Med Assoc 183:103–110, 1983

20. Peterson ME, Turrel JM: Feline hyperthyroidism. In Kirk RW (ed): Current Veterinary Therapy IX, pp. 1026–1033. Philadelphia, W.B. Saunders, 1986

20a. Turrel JM, Feldman EG, Nelson RW et al: Thyroid carcinoma causing hyperthyroidism in cats: 14 cases (1981–1986). J Am Vet Med Assoc 193:359–364, 1988

21. Noxon JO, Thornburg LP, Dillender MJ, et al: An adenoma in ectopic thyroid tissue causing hyperthyroidism in a cat. J Am Anim Hosp Assoc 19:369–372, 1983

22. Peterson ME, Keene B, Ferguson DC, et al: Electrocardiographic findings in 45 cats with hyperthyroidism. J Am Vet Med Assoc 180:934–938, 1982

23. Lui SK, Peterson ME, Fox PR: Hypertrophic cardiomyopathy and hyperthyroidism in the cat. J Am Vet Med Assoc 185:52–57, 1984

24. Peterson ME, Hurvitz AI, Leib MS, et al: Propylthiouricil-associated hemolytic anemia, thrombocytopenia, and antinuclear antibodies in cats with hyperthyroidism. J Am Vet Med Assoc 184:806–808, 1984

24a. Peterson ME, Kintzer PP, Hurvitz AI: Methimazole treatment of 262 cats with hyperthyroidism. J Vet Int Med 2:150–157, 1988

25. Meric SM, Hawkins EC, Washabau RJ, et al: Serum thyroxine concentrations after radioactive iodine therapy in cats with hyperthyroidism. J Am Vet Med Assoc 188:1038–1040, 1986

26. Turrel JM, Feldman ED, Hays M, et al: Radioactive iodine therapy in cats with hyperthyroidism. J Am Vet Med Assoc 184:554–559, 1984

27. Birchard SJ, Peterson ME, and Jacobson A: Surgical treatment of feline hyperthyroidism: Results of 85 cases. J Am Anim Hosp Assoc 20:705–709, 1984

28. Meijer JC, Lubberick AAME, Gruys E: Cushing's syndrome due to adrenocortical adenoma in a cat. Tijdschr Diergeneeskd 103:1048–1051, 1978

29. Peterson ME, Steele P: Pituitary-dependent hyperadrenocorticism in a cat. J Am Vet Med Assoc 189:680–683, 1986

30. Fox FG, Beaty DO: A case of complicated diabetes mellitus in a cat. J Am Anim Hosp Assoc 11:129–134, 1975

30a. Nelson RW, Feldman EG, Smith MC: Hyperadrenocorticism in cats: Seven cases (1978–1987). J Am Vet Med Assoc 193:245–250, 1988

30b. Zerbe CA, Nachreiner RF, Dunstan RW et al: Hyperadrenocorticism in a cat. J Am Vet Med Assoc 190:559–563, 1987

31. Peterson ME: Canine hyperadrenocorticism. In Kirk RW (ed): Current Veterinary Therapy IX, pp. 963–972. Philadelphia, W.B. Saunders, 1986

31a. Penninck DG, Feldman EG, Nyland TG: Radiographic features of canine hyperadrenocorticism caused by autonomously functioning adrenocortical tumors: 23 cases (1978–1986). J Am Vet Med Assoc 192:1604–1608, 1988

31b. Huntley K, Frazer J, Gibbs C et al: The radiographical features of canine Cushings' syndrome: A review of 48 cases. J Small An Pract 23:369–380, 1982

32. Scavelli TD, Peterson ME, Mattheisen DT: Results of surgical treatment for hyperadrenocorticism caused by adrenocortical neoplasia in the dog: 25 cases (1980–1984). J Am Vet Med Assoc 189:1360–1364, 1986

33. Peterson ME, Drieger DT, Drucker WD, et al: Immunocytochemical study of the hypophysis in 25 dogs with pituitary-dependent hyperadrenocorticism. Acta Endocrinol 101:15–24, 1982

34. Cohen SJ, Knieser M: Hyperadrenocorticism in a dog with adrenal and pituitary neoplasia. J Am Anim Hosp Assoc 16:259–262, 1980

35. Burns MG, Kelly AB, Hornoff WJ, et al: Pulmonary artery throbosis in 3 dogs with hyperadrenocorticism. J Am Vet Med Assoc 178:388–393, 1981

36. Peterson ME, Nesbitt GH, Schaer M: Diagnosis and management of concurrent diabetes mellitus and hyperadrenocorticism in thirty dogs. J Am Vet Med Assoc 179:66–69, 1981

37. Peterson ME, Drucker WD: Advances in the diagnosis and treatment of canine Cushing's syndrome. In Proceedings of the 37th Gaines Veterinary Symposium, Louisiana State University, 1981, pp. 17–24

38. Peterson ME, Gilbertson DR, Drucker WD: Plasma cortisol response to exogenous ACTH in 22 dogs with hyperadrenocorticism caused by adrenocortical neoplasia. J Am Vet Med Assoc 180:542–544, 1982

39. Feldman EC: Comparison of ACTH response and dexamethasone suppression as screening tests in canine hyperadrenocorticism. J Am Vet Med Assoc 182:506–510, 1983

40. Stolp R, Rijnberk A, Meijer JC, et al: Urinary corticoids in the diagnosis of canine hyperadrenocorticism: Res Vet Sci 34:141–144, 1983

41. Kaufman J, Macy DW: The glucagon tolerance test as a screening method for canine hyperadrenocorticism. In Proceedings of the Second Annual Veterinary Medical Forum, American College of Veterinary Internal Medicine, Washington, D.C., p. 30. 1984

42. Roberts SM, Lavach JD, Macy DW, et al: Effect of ophthalmic prednisolone acetate on the canine adrenal gland and hepatic function. Am J Vet Res 45:1711–1714, 1984

42a. Voohout G, Stolp R, Lubberink AAME: Computed tomography in the diagnosis of canine hyperadrenocorticism not suppressible with dexamethasone. J Am Vet Med Assoc 192:641–646, 1988

43. Feldman EC: Effect of functional adrenocortical tumors on plasma cortisol and corticotropin concentrations in dogs. J Am Vet Med Assoc 178:823–826, 1981

44. Lubberink AAME: Therapy for spontaneous hyperadrenocorticism. In Kirk RW (ed): Current Veterinary Therapy VIII, pp. 979–983. Philadelphia, W.B. Saunders, 1980

45. Enns SG, Johnston DE, Eigenmann JE, et al: Adrenalectomy in the management of canine hyperadrenocorticism. J Am Anim Hosp Assoc 23:557–564, 1987

46. Stolp R, Croughs RJM, Rijnberk A: Results of cyproheptadine treatment in dogs with pituitary-dependent hyperadrenocorticism in a dog. J Am Vet Med Assoc 187:276–278, 1985

47. Willard MD, Schall WD, Nachreiner RF, et al: Hypoadrenocorticism following therapy with o,p'-DDD for hyperadrenocorticism in four dogs. J Am Vet Med Assoc 180:638–641, 1982

48. Bruyette DS, Feldman EC: Efficacy of ketoconazole in the management of spontaneous canine hyperadrenocorticism. In Proceedings of the Fifth Annual Veterinary Medical Forum, American College of Veterinary Internal Medicine, San Diego, California, p. 885, 1987

49. Dow SW, LeCouteur RA, Rosychuck RAW, et al: Treatment of functional pituitary neoplasms of dogs by means of irradiation. Submitted, J Small An Prac

50. McMillan FD, Barr B, Feldman EC: Functional pancreatic islet cell tumor in a cat. J Am Anim Hosp Assoc 21:741–746, 1985

51. Priester WA: Pancreatic islet cell tumors in domestic animals. Data from 11 colleges of veterinary medicine in the United States and Canada. J Natl Cancer Inst 53:227–229, 1974

52. Kaufman J, Schwarz P, Mero K: Pancreatic beta cell tumor in a ferret. J Am Vet Med Assoc 185:998–1000, 1984

53. Kruth SA, Feldman EC, Kennedy PC: Insulin-secreting islet cell tumors: Establishing a diagnosis and the clinical course for 25 dogs. J Am Vet Med Assoc 181:54–58, 1982

54. Mehlhaff CJ, Peterson ME, Patnaik AK, et al: Insulin-producing islet cell neoplasms: Surgical considerations and general management in 35 dogs. J Am Anim Hosp Assoc 21:607–612, 1985

55. Leifer CE, Peterson ME, Matus RE: Insulin-secreting tumor: Diagnosis and medical and surgical management in 55 dogs. J Am Vet Med Assoc 188:60–64, 1986

56. Caywood DD, Klausner JK, O'Leary TP, et al: Pancreatic insulin-secreting neoplasms: Clinical, diagnostic, and prognostic features in

73 dogs. J Am Anim Hosp Assoc 24:577–584, 1983

56a. Hawkins KL, Summers BA, Kuhajda FP et al: Immunocytochemistry of normal pancreatic islet and spontaneous islet cell tumors in dogs. Vet Path 24:170–179, 1987

57. Leifer CE: Hypoglycemia. In Kirk RW (ed): Current Veterinary Therapy IX, pp. 982–987. Philadelphia, W.B. Saunders, 1986

58. Leifer CE, Peterson ME, Matus RE, et al: Hypoglycemia associated with nonislet cell tumor in 13 dogs. J Am Vet Med Assoc 186:53–55, 1985

59. Breitschwerdt EB, Loar AS, Hribernik TN, et al: Hypoglycemia in four dogs with sepsis. J Am Vet Med Assoc 178:1072–1076, 1981

60. Chrisman CL: Postoperative results and complication of insulinomas in dogs. J Am Anim Hosp Assoc 16:677–684, 1980

61. Shahar R, Rousseaux C, Steiss J: Peripheral polyneuropathy in a dog with functional islet B-cell tumor and widespread metastasis. J Am Vet Med Assoc 187:175–176, 1985

61a. Braund KG, Sterss JE, Amling KA et al: Insulinoma and sublicinical peripheral neuropathy in two dogs. J Vet Intern Med 1:86–90, 1987

62. Meyer DJ: Pancreatic islet cell tumor in a dog treated with streptozotocin. Am J Vet Res 37:1221–1223, 1976

63. Huxtable CR, Farrow BRH: Functional neoplasms of the canine pancreatic-islet beta-cells: A clinico-pathological study of three cases. J Small Anim Pract 20:7373–748, 1979

64. Feldman EC, Nelson RW: Canine and Feline Endocrinology and Reproduction, p. 325. Philadelphia, W.B. Saunders, 1987

65. Capen CC, Martin SC, Koestner A: Neoplasms in the adenohypophysis of dogs. Vet Pathol 4:301–325, 1967

66. Eigenmann JE, Wortman JA, Haskins ME: Elevated growth hormone levels and diabetes mellitus in a cat with acromegalic features. J Am Anim Hosp Assoc 20:747–752, 1984

67. Zaki FA, Harris JM, Budzilovich G: Cystic pituicytoma of the neurohypophysis in a siamese cat. J Comp Pathol 85:467–471, 1975

68. Zaki FA, Lui SK: Pituitary chromophobe adenoma in a cat. Vet Pathol 11:232–237, 1973

69. Berger B, Feldman EC: Primary hyperparathyroidism in dogs: 21 cases (1976–1986). J Am Vet Med Assoc 191:350–356, 1987

70. Thompson KG, Jones LP, Smylie WA, et al: Primary hyperparathyroidism in German shepherd dogs: A disorder of probable genetic origin. Vet Pathol 21:370–376, 1984

71. Patnaik AK, MacEwen EG, Erlandson RA, et al: Mediastinal parathyroid adenocarcinoma in a dog. Vet Pathol 15:55–63, 1978

72. Meuten DJ: Hypercalcemia. Vet Clin North Am 14:891–910, 1984

73. Meuten DJ, Cew DJ, Kociba GJ, et al: Relationship of calcium to albumin and total proteins in dogs. J Am Vet Med Assoc 180:63–67, 1982

74. Happe HP, Van Der Gaag I, Lamers CRHW, et al: Zollinger-Ellison syndrome in three dogs. Vet Pathol 17:117–186, 1980

75. Jones BR, Nicholls MR, Badman R: Peptic ulceration in a dog associated with an islet cell carcinoma of the pancreas and an elevated plasma gastrin level. J Small Anim Pract 17:593–598, 1976

76. Middleton DJ, Watson ADJ: Duodenal ulceration associated with gastrin-secreting pancreatic tumor in a cat. J Am Vet Med Assoc 183:461–462, 1983

77. Straus E, Johnson GF, Yalow RS: Canine Zollinger-Ellison syndrome. Gastroenterology 72:380–381, 1977

77a. Breitschwerdt EB, Turk JR, Turnwald GH et al: Hypergastrinemia in canine gastrointestinal disease. J Am An Hosp Assoc 22:585–592, 1986

77b. English RV, Breitschwerdt EB, Grindem CB et al: Zollinger-Ellison syndrome and myelofibrosis in a dog. J Am Vet Med Assoc 192:1430–1434, 1988

78. Twedt DC, Tilley LP, Ryan WW, et al: Grand rounds conference: Pheochromocytoma in a canine. J Am Anim Hosp Assoc 11:491–496, 1975

79. Schaer M: Pheochomocytoma in a dog: A case report. J Am Anim Hosp Assoc 16:583–587, 1980

80. Wheeler SL: Canine pheochromocytoma. In Kirk RW (ed): Current Veterinary Therapy IX, p. 977–981. Philadelphia, W.B. Saunders, 1986

81. Peterson ME, Randolph JF, Zaki FA, et al: Multiple endocrine neoplasia in a dog. J Am Vet Med Assoc 180:1476, 1982

81a. Bouayad H, Feeney DA, Caywood DD et al: Pheochromocytoma in dogs: 13 cases (1980–1985). J Am Vet Med Assoc 191:1610–1614, 1987

81b. Capen CC. Adrenal medulla. In Jabb KUF, Kennedy CP, Palmer N, eds: Pathology of Domestic Animals, 3rd ed, vol. 3, pp. 392–394. Orlando, Academic Press Inc, 1985

81c. Capen CC. Tumors of the adrenal medulla. In Moulton J, ed: Tumors of Domestic Animals, 2nd ed, pp. 393–404. Berkeley, University of California Press, 1978

82. Buergelt CD, Das KM: Aortic body tumor in a cat, a case report. Vet Pathol 5:84–90, 1968

83. Collins DR: Thoracic tumor in a cat. Vet Med/ Small Anim Clin 59:459, 1964

84. Hayes HM: An hypothesis for the etiology of canine chemoreceptor system neoplasms, based upon an epidemiological study of 73 cases among hospital patients. J Small Anim Pract 16:337–343, 1975

85. Patnaik AK, Liu SK, Hurvitz AI, et al: Canine chemodectoma (extra-adrenal paragangliomas)—A comparative study. J Small Anim Pract 16:785–801, 1975

86. Blackmore J, Gorman NT, Kagan K, et al: Neurologic complications of a chemodectoma in a dog. J Am Vet Med Assoc 184:475–478, 1984

87. Hopper PE, Jongeward SJ, Lammerding JJ, et al: Carotid body tumor associated with an arteriovenous fistula in a dog. Comp Cont Educ 5:68–72, 1983

88. Arias–Stella J: Human carotid body at high altitudes. Am J Pathol 55:82a, 1969

89. Obradovich JE, Withrow SJ, Ogilvie GK et al: Carotid body tumors in the canine: 11 cases. The 8th Annual Conference of the Veterinary Cancer Society, Estes Park, Colorado, 8:25, 1988

23

TUMORS OF THE FEMALE REPRODUCTIVE SYSTEM

Mary Kay Klein

OVARIAN TUMORS

INCIDENCE

Ovarian tumors are uncommon in dogs and cats. The reported incidence in the intact female dog is 6.25%,[1] comprising 0.5% to 1.2% of all canine tumors.[2,3] Incidence rates in the cat range from 0.7% to 3.6%.[4] The low incidence rate in both species is undoubtedly biased by the large segment of the population that is surgically neutered at an early age. With the exception of teratomas,[5,6,7] the tumors occur most commonly in middle aged to older animals and without an identified breed predilection.

PATHOLOGY AND NATURAL BEHAVIOR

Canine Ovarian Tumors

Three general categories of canine ovarian tumors are described according to cell of origin: epithelial cell, germ cell, and sex-cord stromal cell (Table 23-1). Epithelial and sex-cord stromal tumors account for the majority of recorded cases (80–90%).[3,8–10]

Epithelial Cell Tumors. Epithelial tumors include the papillary adenoma, papillary adenocarcinoma, cystadenoma, and undifferentiated carcinoma; they account for 40% to 50% of reported canine ovarian neoplasms.[3,8–10] On the basis of size, location, mitotic index, and morphology, epithelial tumors are divided into malignant and benign classifications.

Papillary adenomas and adenocarcinomas can be bilateral.[8,10,11] Differentiation between the two forms can be difficult and is usually based on the following considerations:

1. The malignant tumor is generally large.
2. A higher mitotic index is noted in the adenocarcinoma.
3. Invasion of the ovarian stroma indicates malignant potential.
4. Extension into the ovarian bursa and adjacent peritoneum also indicates malignant potential.[9,11]

283

Table 23-1.   Classification of Canine Ovarian Tumors

	EPITHELIAL CELL TUMORS	GERM CELL TUMORS	SEX-CORD STROMAL TUMORS
Histologic classifications	Papillary adenoma Papillary adenocarcinoma Cystadenoma Undifferentiated carcinoma	Dysgerminoma Teratocarcinoma Teratoma	Thecoma Luteoma Granulosa cell tumor
% of cases	40–50	6–20	35–50
Bilateral incidence	frequent	rare	rare
Functional incidence	rare	rare	<50%
Metastatic rate	~10%	10–20%	<20%

Classically the papillary adenocarcinoma is associated with widespread peritoneal implantation and formation of malignant effusion. Malignant effusions may develop by means of several mechanisms:

1. Edema within the ovarian tumor may cause leakage of fluid through the tumor capsule.
2. If the tumor exfoliates cells resulting in transcoelomic metastasis, these tumor implants can exert pressure and obstruct peritoneal and diaphragmatic lymphatics.
3. Secretions from metastatic peritoneal implants can also occur.[2,12]

Papillary adenocarcinomas have been noted to metastasize to the renal and para-aortic lymph nodes, omentum, liver, and lungs.[3]

The cystadenoma appears to originate from the rete ovarii, is generally unilateral, and consists of multiple thin-walled cysts containing clear, watery fluid.[8,11]

Undifferentiated carcinoma is the term used to denote tumors whose embryonic morphology and absence of hormonal secretion does not allow identification of a specific epithelial cell of origin.

Germ Cell Tumors. The primordial germ cells of the ovary are thought to be the origin of dysgerminomas, teratomas, and teratocarcinomas. Germ cell tumors comprise 6% to 12% of canine ovarian tumors.[3,10] Dysgerminomas arise from undifferentiated germ cells and so closely resemble their testicular counterparts that they have been referred to as "ovarian seminomas."[3,8,11–13] Dysgerminomas are generally unilateral, grow by expansion,[11,12] and have a reported metastatic rate of 10% to 20%.[3,6,8–11] The most common metastatic site is the abdominal lymph nodes; however, involvement of the liver, kidney, omentum, and adrenal glands has been reported.[3,6,11]

By definition, teratomas are composed of cells arising from more than one germ cell layer. Any combination of ectodermal, mesodermal, and endodermal tissues can be seen. In the teratoma, these tissues are noted to be well-differentiated. Teratocarcinomas have both mature elements and undifferentiated elements resembling those of the embryo.

A cumulative review[6] of the literature revealed a 32% metastatic rate in canine teratomas/teratocarcinomas. Metastases were noted in multiple abdominal sites as well as lungs, anterior mediastinum, and bone. The metastatic lesions were noted to be composed predominantly of undifferentiated elements.

Sex-cord Stromal Tumors. The most common sex-cord stromal tumor is the granulosa cell tumor, which accounts for approximately 50% of ovarian tumors in several reviews.[3,8,10,11] Because the sex-cord stromal tumor arises from the specialized gonadal stroma of the ovary, which is responsible for estrogen and progesterone production, all of these tumors have the potential to elaborate hormones that may manifest clinical signs.

Granulosa cell tumors are usually unilateral and tend to be firm and lobulated, although cysts are commonly apparent on cross-section. These tumors can be quite large.[3,10] Tumors of the Sertoli-Leydig classification have been included collectively with granulosa cell tumors in the past. Sertoli-Leydig cell tumors can occur bilaterally.[10] Up to 20% of granulosa cell tumors demonstrate malignant behavior in the dog,[3,8–11,13,14] with metastasis to sublumbar lymph nodes, liver, pancreas, and lung[3] as well as peritoneal carcinomatosis.[14]

Thecomas are generally benign in their behavior, growing by expansion without metastasis.[8,9] Luteomas are rarely seen but have been reported in the dog[8,9] and are considered benign.

Thecomas and luteomas arise from ovarian stromal cells.[9]

Tumorlike Conditions and Metastatic Involvement. Numerous tumorlike conditions can exist and often must be differentiated histologically. Ovarian cysts are common in the dog and can be very large and easily confused with a neoplastic process.[1] Paraovarian cysts, arising from mesonephric tubules, can be single or multiple. Less common conditions include cystic rete tubules, vascular hematomas, and adenomatous hyperplasia of the rete ovarii.[8,9]

The ovary is rarely a site for metastatic disease; however, ovarian metastasis has been recorded in cases of mammary, intestinal, and pancreatic carcinomas and lymphomas.[1,8]

Feline Ovarian Tumors

Feline ovarian tumors are also defined as epithelial, germ cell, or sex-cord stromal tumors. The latter category is by far the most common. Epithelial tumors are extremely rare in the cat,[15,16,17] although bilateral cystadenomas and ovarian adenocarcinomas have been reported.[16,17] Metastasis to lungs, liver, pelvic, and abdominal peritoneum was seen in one case of ovarian adenocarcinoma.[17]

Approximately 15% of feline ovarian neoplasms are dysgerminomas.[13,15] In one study, two of six occurrences were noted to be bilateral.[16] Dysgerminomas are generally considered to be hormonally inactive and slow to metastasize; yet metastasis has been reported in 20%[13] to 33%[16] of cases. These tumors tend to be encapsulated, smooth, dense tissue masses that not uncommonly attain a large size within the ovary.[13,17] Teratomas are reported only rarely[15-17] and in at least one case demonstrated malignant behavior.[17]

Over half of granulosa cell tumors in cats are malignant.[11,13,15-18] As is true in the dog, they often show evidence of hormonally induced changes and are most commonly unilateral.[15-17] Reported metastatic sites include the peritoneum, lumbar lymph nodes, omentum, diaphragm, kidney, spleen, liver, and lungs.[15-18]

In one series of 14 sex-cord stromal tumors, the author classified 5 as interstitial gland tumors (luteomas). All were benign in behavior.[16] A similarly described tumor appeared to have virilizing effects in a 9-year-old cat.[17]

Lymphomas and endometrial carcinomas have been noted to secondarily involve the ovaries in the cat.[15]

HISTORY AND CLINICAL SIGNS

Canine Ovarian Tumors

The history and clinical signs of canine ovarian tumors can be quite variable depending on their tissue of origin. Granulosa cell tumors are most commonly unilateral and have been reported in dogs ranging in age from 14 months to 16 years.[3,10,11,14] No breed predilection or consistently abnormal laboratory findings are noted.

Sex-cord stromal tumors are well documented to have the ability to produce steroid hormones (estrogen and progesterone).[3,8,10,11,13,14] Animals may present with clinical signs of anestrus or persistent to prolonged heat periods. At least half the recorded cases have had concurrent pyometra, cystic ovarian disease or cystic endometrial hyperplasia,[3,8,10,11,13,14] presumably secondary to elevated estrogen and/or progesterone activity. Occasionally gynecomastia and a bilaterally symmetrical alopecia are noted.[11] Rarely, thecomas may produce estrogens, and luteomas can have secondary masculinizing effects. Regardless of whether or not they are functional, most sex-cord stromal tumors are large enough to be palpable by the time of presentation.[10,11,14]

Most epithelial cell tumors are asymptomatic until signs referable to a space-occupying mass occur.[11-13] Epithelial tumors may present with malignant ascites.[11,12] Pleural effusions have also been noted secondary to thoracic metastasis.[12] Cytologic analysis of fluid may reveal signet ring and rosette cellular patterns suggestive of adenocarcinoma.[11,12]

Germ cell tumors have been associated with evidence of hormonal dysfunction, but more commonly are associated with clinical signs of a space-occupying mass. Teratomas in particular can attain large proportions,[5,11] and areas of calcification are often seen on routine abdominal radiographs.[5,6,11] Teratomas have been reported in animals ranging in age from 20 months to 9 years, with the majority of animals 6 years old or younger.[5,6,10]

Feline Ovarian Tumors

Ovarian tumors have been reported in cats ranging from 2 months to 20 years of age with a mean of 6.7 years.[16] The granulosa cell tumor is most commonly recognized.[9,15-17] Clinical signs of hyperestrogenism are commonly reported, including persistent estrus, alopecia, and cystic or adenomatous hyperplasia of the endometrium.[5-18] Granulosa cell tumors are generally unilateral and large enough to be detected on palpation at presentation.[9,15,17,18] In at least one case, a functional androgenic interstitial gland tumor resulted in virilizing clinical signs.[17]

Dysgerminomas can be found bilaterally and may attain great size.[15-17] Signs of depression, vomiting, abdominal distention, and ascites are usually referable to the mass lesion.[15] The reported mean age of occurrence is 7 years.[17]

Teratomas have also been reported on rare occasions, and the clinical signs noted were referable to their large size.[16,17] Epithelial tumors are reported only rarely and can be found bilaterally.[16,17]

DIAGNOSTIC TECHNIQUES AND WORK-UP

There are no consistently abnormal laboratory findings with ovarian tumors. The presence of an abdominal mass in an intact female animal with or without signs referable to the reproductive tract should place an ovarian tumor on the list of differentials. Small tumors are in proximity to the caudal pole of the kidney, while larger tumors are pendulous and mimic any midabdominal mass in location. Intravenous pyelography can be of benefit in differentiating ovarian from renal masses. Ultrasonography may aid in defining the size and location of the tumor. Cytologic evaluation of abdominal or pleural fluid may be suggestive of malignant effusions. Radiographic evidence of calcification within the mass is suggestive of teratomas; however, definitive diagnosis rests with histopathologic sampling at the time of exploratory laparotomy. Thoracic radiographs should be evaluated for any evidence of metastatic disease, but they only rarely are positive at the time of diagnosis.

THERAPY

Surgery remains the mainstay of treatment for ovarian tumors. A complete ovariohysterectomy is recommended, although oophorectomy alone is possible. Gentle handling of tissues to minimize transcoelomic spread is warranted. Careful examination of all surfaces and removal or biopsy of any lesions suspected of metastatic disease is recommended for staging purposes. One case of metastatic granulosa cell tumor was successfully treated with immunotherapy,[2] and one case of ovarian cystadenocarcinoma was successfully treated with serial and combination use of cyclophosphamide, chlorambucil, CCNU, and bleomycin.[12] Intracavity instillation of thiotepa may be of benefit in controlling malignant effusions. Radiation therapy is rarely indicated or used because animals with disease confined to the ovary (amenable to radiation) are usually successfully treated with surgery.

PROGNOSIS

The prognosis for all ovarian tumors is virtually the same, regardless of histology. The prognosis is good when single tumors are completely excised at surgery. If there is any evidence of metastatic disease, the prognosis must be considered poor. In a very limited number of cases, chemotherapy or possibly immunotherapy would appear to have the potential to lengthen survival times in patients with evidence of metastatic disease.

COMPARATIVE ASPECTS

Ovarian cancer is the eighth most common cancer in women.[20] Most human patients also present with advanced, disseminated disease. Ovarian tumors are localized to the reproductive system in only 25% of women at the time of diagnosis.[20,21] Human and canine tumors share many characteristics:

1. a similar incidence rate: 4% of human female tumors),[20] 6.25% of intact female canine tumors[1]
2. an increasing incidence with age[20]
3. a tendency for transcoelomic metastasis and bilateral frequency of epithelial tumors[8,20]
4. epithelial and stromal tumors accounting for approximately 90% of cases seen[8,20]

Several prognostic factors have been elucidated in human clinical studies, including histologic grade, the extent of residual disease postoperatively, the stage of the disease at presentation, and the age of the patient.[21-23] Prognostic indices have not been determined for animal tumors. In the human literature, epithelial tumors are well documented to be chemoresponsive; however, long-term patient survival is still infrequent.[20–22]

Single chemotherapeutic agents that have demonstrated efficacy against human ovarian tumors include doxorubicin, *cis*-platinum, and melphalan. Combination regimens have demonstrated significantly improved response rates over melphalan and cyclophosphamide singly[22,23] and would appear to be feasible in veterinary medicine. "Cure" rates are still less than 10%, and such measures must be considered palliative. *Cis*-platinum combinations are generally best at salvage in cases failing initial therapy, but the vast majority of responses are partial and of short duration.[22] Radiation therapy is also of benefit in some cases.[23]

In human granulosa cell tumors, the granulosa cells are thought to be nonfunctional and the thecal cells capable of steroidogenic activity.[17] In the cat and dog, granulosa cells themselves appear to be steroidogenic. The granulosa cell tumor in cats appears to be much more aggressive than its human counterpart.[17]

Teratomas and dysgerminomas are most commonly reported in women less than 35 years of age.[20] Teratomas are most commonly reported in young dogs, and show evidence of being more malignant than their human counterparts.[6,10,24]

UTERINE TUMORS

INCIDENCE

Uterine tumors are rare in both the dog and the cat; reported incidence rates are 0.3% to 0.4% of all canine tumors.[11,13,19,25] Incidence rates are not reported in the cat. Middle-age to older animals are most commonly affected, and no breed predilections have been reported in either species.[13,15,25]

PATHOLOGY AND NATURAL BEHAVIOR

Leiomyomas account for 85% to 90% and leiomyosarcomas for 10%, of canine uterine tumors.[13,19] On rare occasions adenomas, adenocarcinomas, fibromas, fibrosarcomas, and lipomas have been reported.[11,19,27]

Leiomyomas are generally noninvasive, nonmetastatic and slow growing.[11] Grossly, it is difficult to distinguish them from their malignant counterparts, leiomyosarcomas.[19] A syndrome characterized by multiple uterine leiomyomas, bilateral renal cystadenocarcinomas and nodular dermatofibrosis has been characterized in German shepherd dogs and noted to have a hereditary component.[26]

In the cat, uterine adenocarcinomas account for the majority of cases and arise from the endometrium.[15,28] The uterus appears thickened and nodular. Metastases to the cerebrum, eyes, ovaries, adrenal glands, lungs, liver, kidneys, bladder, colon, diaphragm, and regional lymph nodes have been reported. Other uterine neoplasms reported less commonly in the cat include leiomyoma, leiomyosarcoma, fibrosarcoma, lymphosarcoma, fibroma, and lipoma.[15]

HISTORY AND CLINICAL SIGNS

Leiomyomas and leiomyosarcomas are rarely associated with clinical signs, and in fact, many are incidental findings at the time of necropsy or ovariohysterectomy.[11,19,25,26] They can on occasion gain sufficient size to compress adjacent viscera.[11,19] Vaginal discharge and pyometra may accompany malignant or benign uterine tumors.[11,19,25]

Uterine adenocarcinomas are generally seen in cats more than 8 years of age. Clinical signs may not be seen until the tumor gains large proportions. A vaginal discharge is common and can vary from purulent to mucoid to darkly hemorrhagic. Other reported clinical signs include abnormal estrous cycles, polydipsia, polyuria, vomiting, and abdominal distention.[15,28]

DIAGNOSTIC TECHNIQUES AND WORK-UP

No consistent laboratory abnormalities are noted, and abdominal radiographs only confirm the presence of an abdominal or uterine mass. A definitive diagnosis is usually attained upon histologic examination of surgically excised specimens.

THERAPY

A complete ovariohysterectomy is recommended, and attempts should be made to remove all tumors and metastatic foci. Chemotherapy and radiation therapy have been largely unreported in veterinary cases.

PROGNOSIS

The prognosis associated with leiomyomas and other benign tumors is excellent as surgery is nearly always curative. In the case of leiomyosarcomas and other malignant tumors, the prognosis remains good if there is no evidence of metastatic disease at the time of surgery and complete excision is possible. Nonresectable or metastatic disease warrants a grave prognosis.

As feline uterine adenocarcinomas have well-documented metastatic potential, the prognosis must be considered guarded.[15,28] Again, the presence of metastatic disease indicates a grave prognosis.

COMPARATIVE ASPECTS

In women, carcinoma of the endometrium is the most common malignant tumor in the genital tract, comprising approximately 13% of all malignant tumors. Most cases are diagnosed in the 60- to 70-year-old age group. The pathology and natural behavior of the disease in humans most closely resembles the disease in the cat. Radiotherapy is used extensively in human cases. Chemotherapy has not been studied in any detail. Doxorubicin has been well evaluated in adequate numbers of patients, and results in one study indicate a 37% response rate.[29]

VAGINAL AND VULVAR TUMORS

CANINE OCCURRENCES

Incidence and Risk Factors

Vulvar and vaginal tumors account for 2.4% to 3% of canine neoplasms.[25,30] The vast majority are benign, are found in intact female dogs, and affect dogs from 2 to 18 years of age, with an average of 10.8 years.[13,25,30,31] One study found the boxer to be at an increased risk over other breeds.[30]

Pathology and Natural Behavior

Tumors of smooth muscle origin predominate. In endemic areas, transmissible venereal tumors are common (see Chapter 30). Smooth muscle tumors called leiomyoma, fibroleiomyoma, fibroma, and polyp vary only in the amount of connective tissue present. Because the clinical course of the tumor does not appear to be affected by histologic variations,[25,30] it is justified to consider these tumors collectively. As many as 86% of vulvar and vaginal tumors are reported to be benign smooth muscle tumors.[30,31]

Most leiomyomas arise from the vestibule of the vulva rather than from the vagina.[25,30] Extra- and intraluminal forms are described. Extraluminal forms present as a slow-growing perineal mass. On cut section these tumors are gray to white to tan in color, well encapsulated, and poorly vascularized.[11,19,25]

Intraluminal tumors are attached to the vestibular or vaginal wall by a thin pedicle. They are often firm and ovoid, and although their mucosa is generally intact, ulceration may occur with exposure or irritation.[19,30] Intraluminal tumors can be multiple.[30,31] All pedunculated or polypoid tumors were found to be benign in one study.[30]

Subjective data indicate that leiomyomas are hormonally controlled. In two studies, none of the dogs diagnosed with leiomyoma, fibroma, or polypoid tumors had prior ovariohysterectomies.[30,31] There was a 15% recurrence rate in dogs left intact after treatment and no recurrences in dogs ovariohysterectomized at that time.[30] In another study, leiomyomas were not seen in bitches ovariectomized prior to 2 years of age.[25] Concurrent uterine, ovarian, and mammary gland changes, including cystic glandular hyperplasia, ovarian cysts, hemorrhage, and mammary gland tumors, were present in approximately one-third of the cases.[25,31] At the present time it is impossible to state whether hormonal influences are a definitive control, but evidence such as the above makes it highly likely that they are.

Other benign vaginal and vulvar tumors that have been reported include lipomas, sebaceous adenomas, fibrous histiocytomas, benign melanomas, myxomas, and myxofibromas.[11,13,25,30]

The most common malignant tumor seen is the leiomyosarcoma.[11,19,25,30] Distant metastases have been reported.[25]

Other tumors with malignant potential that have been reported include transmissible venereal tumor, adenocarcinoma, squamous cell carcinoma, hemangiosarcoma, osteosarcoma, mast cell tumor, and epidermoid carcinoma.[11,13,19,25,30] The labia of the vulva may be the site for any tumor associated with cutaneous tissues. Carcinomas arising from the bladder or urethra may also present with palpable vaginal masses near the urethral papilla[31,32] (see Chapter 26).

History and Clinical Signs

Leiomyomas can be characterized as a disease of older, sexually intact dogs. The incidence rate of these tumors is significantly higher in nulliparous bitches.[25] There is no difference between malignant and benign cases as to age or breed; however a greater proportion of malignancy is noted in intact females as are frequent recurrence and a lack of pedunculation.[25]

The duration of clinical signs tends to be longer in cases of extraluminal tumors.[25] The presenting clinical sign is generally a slow-growing perineal mass (Fig. 23-1). Intraluminal tumors, by virtue of their tendency toward pedunculation, often appear externally when straining causes the mass to extrude through the vulvar lips, especially at the time of estrus

(Fig. 23-2). The most common owner complaint recorded is that of a mass "popping out" of the vulva. Clinical signs seen less frequently include vulvar bleeding or discharge, an enlarging vulvar mass, dysuria, hematuria, tenesmus, excessive vulvar licking, and dystocia.[25,30,31]

Lipomas tend to occur in younger dogs with an age range of 1 to 8 years and a mean of 6.3 years.[25] The only clinical sign reported is that of a slow-growing mass and subsequent impingement on adjacent structures. The tumors can arise from the perivascular and perivaginal fat and lie within the pelvic canal. They may attach to the tuber ischium. All are reported to be well circumscribed and relatively avascular.[19,25]

Diagnostic Techniques and Work-Up

Although the older, intact female signalment of the animal combined with the location and gross appearance are suggestive, a definitive diagnosis

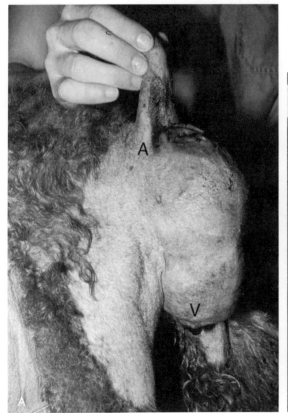
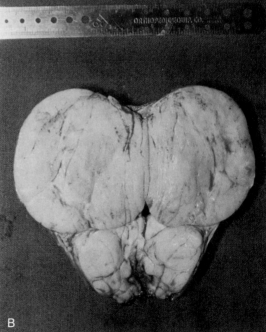

Figure 23-1. *(A)* Slow-growing perineal mass typical of an extraluminal leiomyoma (anus A, vulva V). *(B)* A midline perineal incision allowed the removal of this well-encapsulated mass. Histology confirmed a benign leiomyoma.

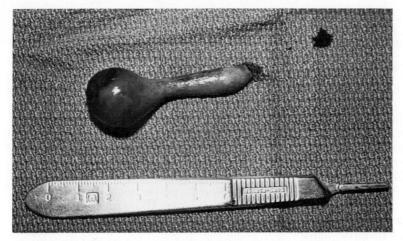

Figure 23-2. Pedunculated intraluminal vaginal leiomyoma. This tumor often prolapses during estrus, and exposed surface may ulcerate when traumatized. Treatment included removal by simple ligation of the pedicle and concomitant ovariohysterectomy.

rests upon histopathologic examination of excised tissue. Caudal abdominal radiographs may be indicated for an extraluminal mass with extension cranially.

Therapy

In light of the evidence of hormonal dependence and high incidence of disease associated with an intact reproductive system in an aging bitch, it would appear prudent to perform an ovariohysterectomy at the time of treatment. This also permits examination of abdominal organs for evidence of metastatic disease. Conservative surgical excision combined with ovariohysterectomy is usually curative for benign tumors. Intraluminal tumors can be easily removed by placing one or more sutures in the pedicle. Wide removal is not necessary if ovariohysterectomy is performed, even though these tumors probably arise in the smooth muscle of the vaginal wall. If the pedicle or urethral papilla cannot be adequately visualized, a dorsal episiotomy ensures complete resection and avoids any damage to the urethra.

Surgical removal of extraluminal tumors can also be readily accomplished through a dorsal episiotomy. Because they tend to be well encapsulated and poorly vascularized, blunt dissection generally removes them entirely. On rare occasions, a perineal approach or pelvic split may be required. Catheterization of the urethra aids in preventing accidental damage to that tissue. If complete excision of the primary tumor and metastatic foci cannot be accomplished, local radiation therapy may be of benefit.[19]

Prognosis

Surgery for benign lesions is nearly always curative, and vulvo-vaginal tumors are rarely identified as a cause of death. Many are incidental findings at necropsy. The prognosis associated with adenocarcinomas and squamous cell carcinomas is generally poor due to high local recurrence and metastatic rates.[19,30]

Comparative Aspects

Uterine fibroids affect 20% of all women over 30 years of age but are very uncommon in the canine uterus.[24] Conversely, vaginal fibroids are rare in women but common in the dog. Why such differences exist is not known. Human genital leiomyomas typically cease growth after menopause and resume growth if estrogens are administered. However, the majority of women with these tumors have normal ovarian function, and there is no objective data to indicate that an endocrine imbalance precedes their formation.[29]

FELINE OCCURRENCES

The only reported vulvar and vaginal tumors in the cat are benign and include leiomyomas and a pedunculated fibroma.[15,33] The tumor masses are generally quite firm and the clinical signs are secondary to the presence of a space-occupying mass. Constipation due to dorsal compression of the rectum and dilation of the colon anterior to the tumor was noted in two older intact queens with vaginal leiomyomas.[33] One cat also had cystic ovaries and a mammary adenocarcinoma. Again, surgery along with ovariohysterectomy was curative, and no recurrence was noted.

REFERENCES

1. Dow C: Ovarian abnormalities in the bitch. J Comp Pathol 70:59–69, 1960

2. Hayes A, Harvey HJ: Treatment of metastatic granulosa cell tumor in a dog. J Am Vet Med Assoc 174:1304–1306, 1979

3. Cotchin E: Canine ovarian neoplasms. Res Vet Sci 2:133–142, 1961

4. Cotchin E: Some tumours of dogs and cats of comparative veterinary and human interest. Vet Rec 71:1041, 1959

5. Wilson RB, Cave JS, Copeland JS, Onks J: Ovarian teratoma in 2 dogs. J Am Anim Hosp Assoc 21:249–253, 1985

6. Greenlee PG, Patnaik AK: Canine ovarian tumors of germ cell origin. Vet Pathol 22:117–122, 1985

7. Jergens AE, Knapp DW: Ovarian teratoma in a bitch. J Am Vet Med Assoc 191:81–83, 1987

8. Nielsen SW, Misdorp W, McEntee K: Tumours of the ovary. Bull WHO 53:203–215, 1976

9. Nielsen SW: Classification of tumors in dogs and cats. J Am Anim Hosp Assoc 19:13–52, 1983

10. Patnaik AK, Greenlee PG: Canine ovarian neoplasms: A clinicopathologic study of 71 cases, including histology of 12 granulosa cell tumors. Vet Path 24:509–514, 1987

11. Herron MA: Tumors of the canine genital system. J Am Anim Hosp Assoc 19:981–994, 1983

12. Greene JA, Richardson RC, Thornhill JA, Boon GD: Ovarian papillary cystadenocarcinoma in a bitch. Case report: literature review. J Am Anim Hosp Assoc 15:351–356, 1979

13. Theilen GH, Madewell BR: Tumors of the urogenital tract. In Veterinary Cancer Medicine, pp. 367–373. Philadelphia, Lea & Febiger, 1979

14. Anderson GL: Granulosa cell tumor in a dog. Comp Cont Educ 8:158–168, 1986

15. Stein BS: Tumors of the feline genital tract. J Am Anim Hosp Assoc 17:1022–1025, 1981

16. Gelberg HB, McEntee K: Feline ovarian neoplasms. Vet Pathol 22:572–576, 1985

17. Norris HJ, Garner FM, Taylor HB: Pathology of feline ovarian neoplasms. J Pathol 97:138–143, 1969

18. Arnberg J: Extra-ovarian granulosa cell tumor in a cat. Fel Pract 10:26–32, 1980

19. Withrow SJ, Susaneck SJ: Tumors of canine female reproductive tract. In Morrow DA (ed): Current Therapy in Theriogenology 2. Philadelphia, W.B. Saunders, 1986

20. Barber HRK: Ovarian cancer.CA–A Cancer Journal for Clinicians 36:149–184, 1986

21. Kerstin S, Silfversward C, Einhorn M: Ovarian cancer: The challenge of local tumor control: Its impact on survival. Int J Radiat Oncol Phys 12:567–571, 1986

22. Ozols RF, Young RC: Chemotherapy of ovarian cancer. Semin Oncol 11:251–263, 1984

23. Dembo AJ: Radiotherapeutic management of ovarian cancer. Semin Oncol 11:238–250, 1984

24. Patnaik AK, Schaer M, Parks J, Liu SK: Metastasizing ovarian teratocarcinoma in dogs. J Small Anim Pract 17:235–246, 1976

25. Brodey RS, Roszel JF: Neoplasms of the canine uterus, vagina, vulva: A clinicopathologic survey of 90 cases. J Am Vet Med Assoc 151:1294–1307, 1967

26. Lium B, Moe L: Hereditary multifocal renal cystadenocarcinomas and nodular dermatofibrosis in the German shepherd: Macroscopic and histopathologic changes. Vet Pathol 22:447–455, 1985

27. Wardrip SJ, Esplin DG: Uterine carcinoma with metastasis to the myocardium. J Am Anim Hosp Assoc 20:261–264, 1984

28. O'Rourke MD, Geib L: Endometrial adenocarcinoma in a cat. Cornell Vet 60:598, 1970

29. Perez CA, Knapp RC, Young RC: Gynecologic tumors. In DeVita VT Jr, Hillman S, Rosenberg SA (eds): Cancer: Principles and Practic of Oncology, pp. 849–860. Philadelphia, J.B. Lippincott, 1982

30. Thacher C, Bradley RL: Vulvar and vaginal tumors in the dog: A retrospective study. J Am Vet Med Assoc 183:690–692, 1983

31. Kydd DM, Burnie AG: Vaginal neoplasia in the bitch: A review of 40 clinical cases. J Sm Anim Pract 27:255–263, 1986

32. Magne ML, Hoopes PJ, Kainer RA, Olson PN, Husted PW, Allen TA, Wykes PM, Withrow SJ: Urinary tract carcinomas involving the canine vagina and vestibule. J Am Anim Hosp Assoc 21:767–772, 1985

33. Wolke RE: Vaginal leiomyoma as a cause of chronic constipation in the cat. J Am Vet Med Assoc 143:1103, 1963

24

TUMORS OF THE MAMMARY GLAND

E. Gregory MacEwen
Stephen J. Withrow

INCIDENCE AND RISK FACTORS

Mammary neoplasms are the most common tumors of the female dog and are estimated to occur in 198.8 per 100,000 animals at risk.[1] Mammary gland tumors have been historically reported to comprise 52% of all neoplasms in the bitch, but the incidence is declining owing to the increased frequency of ovariohysterectomy in young dogs. The median age is between 10 and 11 years. The breeds with the highest incidence are the poodle, English spaniel, Brittany spaniel, English setter, pointer, fox terrier, Boston terrier, and cocker spaniel.[2] Boxers and Chihuahuas are considered to have a decreased risk.[2,3]

Canine mammary tumors are clearly hormone-dependent tumors. The risk for dogs spayed prior to the first estrus is 0.05%; for those spayed after the second estrus the risk increases to 26%.[4] Additional evidence for a hormonal component with this disease is based on the fact that both estrogen and progesterone receptors have been identified in mammary gland tumors. Most studies indicate that between 50% and 60% of all malignant mammary tumors contain either estrogen or progesterone receptors, and these receptors are present in about 70% of benign mammary tumors.[5,6]

The prevalence of feline mammary tumors is reported to be 25 per 100,000 female cats at risk.[1] Skin tumors and lymphomas are the only tumors more commonly observed. Siamese cats have an increased risk of developing mammary tumors. Mammary gland tumors have been reported in cats between the ages of 9 months and 19 years of age. The average age of development of mammary tumors is between 10 and 14 years.

The etiology of feline mammary tumors is unknown. C-type viral particles have been identified in neoplastic tissue, but the significance of these is unknown. Early ovariohysterectomy may have some protective effect on the development of feline mammary tumors, although the effect is not as great as that seen in the dog.[1] The annual incidence of mammary tumors in intact female cats has been reported to be

31.8 per 100,000 cats, and 20.4 per 100,000 ovariohysterectomized female cats.

Progestins such as megestrol acetate have been associated with mammary tumor development. Progesterone receptors have been identified on feline mammary tissue, although the levels have been very low.[7,8] Estrogen receptors are rarely detected.

PATHOLOGY AND NATURAL BEHAVIOR

CANINE MAMMARY TUMORS

Between 41% and 53% of the mammary tumors that occur in the bitch are considered malignant (Table 24-1).[9] Histologic evidence of malignancy does not invariably imply a malignant clinical course. In some studies, histologic malignancy may be under-reported, and in other studies it may be over-reported. A major problem with canine mammary tumors lies in the fact that a number of histologic criteria are used to define malignancy, and the criteria differ from one institution to another and often among individual pathologists in the same institution. Additionally, histologic appearance may vary markedly within the same mass. Most malignant mammary tumors are classified as epithelial tumors or carcinomas. Depending upon the classification system used, the carcinomas may be further subdivided into simple carcinoma, complex carcinoma, adenocarcinoma, and solid carcinoma (Table 24-1). A tumor composed of malignant cells morphologically resembling the epithelial and connective tissue components is termed a malignant mixed tumor or carcinosarcoma. Most histologic classification systems are based on recognition of histologic tissue patterns with little, if any, reference to disease behavior. A new classification system has recently been published;[10] it is based on the biologic behavior of mammary gland tumors in 232 dogs. In this study tumors were assigned to one of four histologic stages:

Histologic Stage 0—malignant proliferation limited to the anatomic borders of the mammary duct system, *i.e.*, *in situ* carcinoma
Histologic Stage 1—malignant proliferations extending beyond the anatomic borders of the mammary duct system into the surrounding stroma, *i.e.*, invasive carcinoma without identifiable vascular or lymphatic invasion
Histologic Stage 2—invasive carcinoma with vascular or lymphatic invasion or metastasis to regional lymph nodes
Histologic Stage 3—evidence of distant metastasis

Mammary tumors can also be evaluated on the basis of their degree of nuclear differentiation: poorly differentiated, moderately differ-

Table 24-1. Distribution of Canine Mammary Neoplasms Based on Histologic Examination

TUMOR TYPE	RELATIVE FREQUENCY	%
BENIGN		
Fibroadenomas (benign mixed tumor)	45.5	47–59%
Simple adenomas	5.0	
Benign mesenchymal tumors	0.5	
MALIGNANT		
Solid carcinomas	16.9	41–53%
Tubular adenocarcinomas	15.4	
Papillary adenocarcinomas	8.6	
Anaplastic carcinomas	4.0	
Sarcomas	3.1	
Carcinosarcoma (malignant mixed tumors)	0.6	

Figures were obtained from an unselected series of 1625 canine mammary tumors sent by general practitioners to the Department of Clinical Veterinary Medicine, Cambridge, England, for diagnosis.
(Reproduced with permission of WB Saunders, Philadelphia, from Bostock R: Neoplasia of the skin and mammary glands in dogs and cats. In Kirk (ed): Current Veterinary Therapy, VI, Small Animal Practice, pp 493–496, 1977)

entiated, and well differentiated. The degree of differentiation is usually inversely related to the tumor's aggressiveness.

Sarcomas comprise less than 5% of all mammary tumors and are much less common than carcinomas. It is uncertain whether they arise from myoepithelial cells that have undergone neoplastic change or from the intralobular connective tissue. There is no evidence that sarcomas arise from pre-existing mixed cell tumors. They can be subdivided into various groups, including osteosarcoma, fibrosarcoma, and chondrosarcoma. The sarcomas tend to have a much higher incidence of metastasis than carcinomas have, and the overall prognosis is quite poor.

Another histologic form of malignant mammary tumors is termed the inflammatory carcinoma.[11] This neoplasm grows with extreme rapidity and invades lymphatics in the skin resulting in marked edema and inflammation (Fig. 24-1). Histologically there is evidence of a poorly differentiated carcinoma with extensive evidence of both mononuclear and polymorphonuclear cellular infiltrate. These tumors have an extremely poor prognosis.

FELINE MAMMARY TUMORS

Among feline mammary tumors, 80% to 90% are considered malignant.[12] Adenocarcinoma predominates among malignant tumors; carcinoma and sarcoma are second and third in prevalence. Feline mammary tumors tend to grow rapidly and to metastasize to local lymph nodes and lungs.

There are two basic types of noninflammatory hyperplasia of the feline mammary gland—lobular hyperplasia and fibroepithelial hyperplasia.

Lobular Hyperplasia[12]

Lobular hyperplasia takes the form of palpable masses in one or more glands. It has been reported in cats from 1 to 14 years of age; most were about 8 years old. Most cats were intact females. The most common lobular hyperplasia involves one or more enlarged lobules with a cystic or dilated ductal component.

Fibroepithelial Hyperplasia[12]

Fibroepithelial hyperplasia usually occurs in young, cycling or pregnant female cats and has even been seen in litters prior to their first estrus. Old unspayed females and males given megestrol acetate have developed the condition. Most cats affected exhibit hyperplasia one or two weeks after their first estrus. The tremendously enlarged glands may appear erythematous and some of the skin may be necrotic. Edema of skin, subcutis, and both rear legs is common. This condition can be easily confused with an acute mastitis.

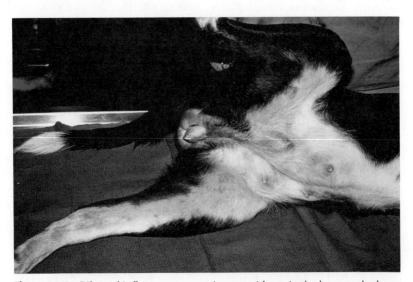

Figure 24-1. Bilateral inflammatory carcinoma with vaginal edema and edema of the leg in a dog. Vaginal cytology and fine needle cytology of the popliteal lymph node were positive for cancer.

These conditions are thought to be associated with hormonal stimulation of the glandular tissue. In acute cases, ovariohysterectomy should be avoided until some of the swelling, edema, and inflammation subside. Combinations of diuretics, corticosteroids, and testosterone have been advocated, but the results are variable. Necrosis and ulceration may be associated with bleeding and localized infection. Systemic infection and pulmonary embolism are not uncommon.

If an ovariohysterectomy is to be performed while the glands are still greatly enlarged, a flank incision should be used. In time, the glands regress, and the ovariohysterectomy should prevent recurrence.

HISTORY AND SIGNS

Mammary tumors are characterized clinically as single (~75%) or multiple (~25%) nodules located within the mammary gland. They may be associated with the nipple or with the glandular tissue itself. In many animals with benign mammary tumors, such as an adenoma, the tumor is small, well circumscribed, and firm on palpation. The dog has five pairs of glands, all of which can develop one or more benign or malignant tumors. Roughly 66% of canine tumors occur in glands 4 and 5, probably owing to greater volume of breast tissue in these glands. Cats have a more or less equal distribution of tumors in all glands. In some animals the tumor may have undergone ulceration and may present with inflammation (Fig. 24-2).

As previously mentioned, the inflammatory carcinomas tend to be diffusely swollen, and there is poor demarcation between normal and abnormal tissue. All or part of one mammary chain may be involved, or bilateral involvement may be observed. Extensive lymph edema of a limb or limbs adjacent to this type of mammary cancer may also occur. Such edema is due to occlusion of affected lymphatics with accompanying retrograde growth down the limb. Inflammatory carcinomas many times are initially misdiagnosed as acute mastitis and are treated as such with antibiotics and corticosteroids. It is important to differentiate this type of malignancy from inflammatory mastitis. The inflammatory carcinomas tend to be quite firm and to have a diffuse type of swelling, whereas mastitis tends to be more localized and is usually seen after estrus or false pregnancy.

Feline mammary tumors tend to present as either single solitary lesions in one breast or multiple lesions in more than one breast. They tend not to be as well circumscribed as in the dog, and their consistency is slightly firm. Ulceration is common, particularly for tumors that are greater than 3 cm in diameter.

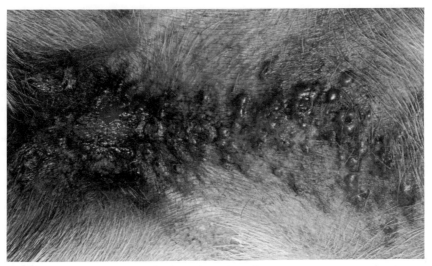

Figure 24-2. Cutaneous involvement in a dog of a recurrent mammary carcinoma with ulceration and nodular plaque formation. This is a poor prognostic sign.

DIAGNOSTIC TECHNIQUES AND WORK-UP

For both the dog and the cat, clinical evaluation should include a thorough physical examination, and a routine hematologic and chemistry profile prior to anesthesia. A coagulogram may be necessary in dogs with inflammatory carcinoma because of the concurrent association with disseminated intravascular coagulation. Thoracic radiographs should be taken prior to surgery to evaluate the lungs for possible metastasis. In some cases if the mammary tumors involve the two caudal glands, it is desirable to evaluate with abdominal radiographs the sublumbar region for metastatic lymphadenopathy. A rectal exam may also reveal palpable evidence of sublumbar lymphadenopathy. Fine-needle aspiration and cytology to differentiate benign from malignant tumors has been reported to be an insensitive method.[13]

The most definitive way to obtain a diagnosis is to take a biopsy of one of the lesions or to excise the tumor and submit it for histopathologic analysis. Because treatment is not altered by knowledge of tumor type, excisional biopsy is preferred for both diagnosis and treatment.

If lymph node metastasis is suspected, cytology can be used to assess the nodes. A fine-needle aspiration for cytologic evaluation has also been proven to be very beneficial in the diagnosis of inflammatory carcinomas.[11]

TREATMENT OF CANINE MAMMARY TUMORS

Surgery remains the treatment of choice for all dogs with mammary gland tumors with the exception of those with inflammatory carcinomas or distant metastasis. The type of surgery depends on the extent of disease.

SURGICAL TECHNIQUE

No prospective clinical trial has shown an improved survival for canine patients undergoing "radical" mastectomy versus local mass removal. The theoretical and practical pros and cons of radical versus local excision have been extensively debated.[14] In a recently published prospective clinical trial to compare simple with radical mastectomy, there was no difference in recurrence rate and survival time between the two procedures.[15] Proponents of radical removal argue that it is the procedure most likely to remove all tumor (unknown or occult) and that it reduces future risk by reducing the volume of breast tissue at risk. Those opposed to routine radical resection argue that it is too much surgery when over 50% of canine breast masses are benign and no published data exists to prove that benign lesions transform to malignancies; a radical procedure can always be performed later on the 40% to 50% of patients with a malignant histology; radical surgery increases the morbidity, time, and expense of the treatment; and most compelling, radical mastectomy does *not* improve survival over lesser procedures.[15]

The goal of surgery in canine breast cancer is to remove all tumor by the simplest procedure. More surgery is not better surgery for the dog.

A variety of procedures exist for removing canine breast tumors, and the choice of procedure is determined by size, fixation, and number of lesions rather than by an anticipated effect on survival. Definitions of the various procedures and their indications are described below.

Lumpectomy or Nodulectomy

A lumpectomy or nodulectomy is indicated for small (<5mm), firm, nonfixed nodules that are generally benign. The skin is incised and the nodule bluntly dissected from the breast tissue with a small rim of normal tissue surrounding the tumor nodule.

Mammectomy

Removal of one gland is indicated for lesions centrally located within the gland, larger than 1 cm, and exhibiting any degree of fixation to skin or fascia. Skin or abdominal wall fascia, if involved, should be removed with the mass. Glands 4 and 5 are often so confluent that removal of the combined glands is easier than removal of either one alone. Occasionally glands 1, 2, and 3 are also confluent, requiring *en bloc* removal.

Regional Mastectomy

Regional mastectomy was originally proposed on the basis of the known venous and lymphatic drainage of the breast tissue. Simply stated, this drainage is gland 3 to gland 2 to gland 1 to lymph node and beyond, or gland 4 to gland 5 to lymph node and beyond. In patients with several masses, the theory is predicated on the presumption that the tumor spreads from one gland to another The opposing theory is that the tumor starts at synchronous primary sites. Although both theories are hard to prove, the latter is more likely, and regional mastectomy is therefore more a theoretical consideration than a necessity.

Unilateral or Bilateral Mastectomy

Gland 1 through 5 can be removed as a unit if multiple tumors or several large tumors preclude rapid and wide removal by lesser procedures. Simultaneous bilateral mastectomy has also been proposed and can be accomplished in dogs and cats with pendulous mammae.[14] These procedures are done because they may be faster than multiple lumpectomies or mammectomies, not because they improve survival in the dog.

For feline mammary tumors, a radical mastectomy is the preferred procedure because local recurrence is common with lesser procedures.

Lymph Node Removal

The axillary lymph nodes are rarely involved with cancer in the dog and should not be removed prophylactically. Axillary node involvement is more common in the cat, and these nodes should be removed if they are mobile. Fixed, adherent, and large axillary nodes can only rarely be removed completely. The inguinal lymph node should be removed when it is enlarged and cytologically positive for cancer, or whenever gland 5 is removed because it is intimately associated with this gland.

In conclusion, mammary cancer in the dog should be removed by the simplest procedure that removes known cancer in the breast. This does not mean that sloppy or debulking surgery is acceptable. With this philosophy it is unusual for any recurrent disease to be inoperable or for dogs to be euthanatized for regionally inoperable disease. The situation in the cat is very different.

CHEMOTHERAPY

No therapeutic or adjuvant chemotherapy protocol has been reported to be effective in the dog. We have evaluated two chemotherapeutic combinations and have found minimal antitumor activity with both. One approach was a combination of cyclophosphamide, vincristine, and methotrexate, and the other a combination of doxorubicin and cyclophosphamide. We found some antitumor activity in dogs with mammary adenocarcinoma when doxorubicin and cyclophosphamide were administered at high doses; however, toxicity was severe. The cyclophosphamide was given orally on days 3, 4, 5, and 6 after the doxorubicin. This combination chemotherapy protocol was quite suppressive of bone marrow, and there was significant toxicity. At this time we do not recommend primary or adjuvant chemotherapy in treating dogs with malignant mammary tumors. Cisplatin chemotherapy, at 60 mg/m^2 I.V. has not been reported to be effective in dogs with mammary adenocarcinoma.[14a]

RADIATION THERAPY

As with chemotherapy, no reliable information on the value of radiation is yet available. Radiation therapy, like surgery, is mainly limited by the extent of the tumor and may only be considered useful in dogs that have tumors too extensive for surgery. Radiation therapy has been tried in a few inoperable patients and in inflammatory carcinoma, but the short-term morbidity is high, and accentuation of already present inflammatory disease is a complication. More carefully designed studies are needed before any efficacy can be attributed to radiation for canine mammary tumors.

BIOLOGIC RESPONSE MODIFIERS

Studies with nonspecific immunomodulation using levamisole[15] and C. parvum with BCG have little effectiveness over surgery;[16,16a] however, one study reported that intratumoral injection of BCG cell walls when combined with surgery increased survival time over surgery alone.[17] Another study reported that mammary tumor cells treated with neuraminidase and used as a vaccine had antitumor activity in the dog.[18,18a] These approaches, though, are still considered experimental and have questionable therapeutic effectiveness.

HORMONAL THERAPY

No published reports are available regarding the effectiveness of the anti-estrogen tamoxifen therapy in canine mammary tumors. The issue of ovariohysterectomy as a treatment for mammary tumors remains unsolved. In one study of 154 dogs treated with mastectomy and ovario-hysterectomy, the mean survival time was reported to be 8.4 months;[19] this compares to mean survival times of 10 and 8 months in other studies treated by mastectomy alone.[9] There have been no well-designed prospective studies to clearly address the issue of ovariohysterectomy as an adjunctive treatment for dogs with malignant mammary tumors.

TREATMENT OF FELINE MAMMARY TUMORS

For feline mammary tumors, surgery remains the treatment of choice.[20] Studies have shown that radical mastectomy—that is, removal of all glands on the involved side—significantly reduces local recurrence.[21] Because tumor size appears to be the most significant prognostic factor,[21,22] early detection and diagnosis are vitally important to the successful therapeutic management of feline mammary tumors.

CHEMOTHERAPY

Combination chemotherapy using doxorubicin (25-30 mg/m² IV slowly) and cyclophosphamide (50–100 mg/m²/os days 3, 4, 5, and 6 after doxorubicin) has been shown to induce short-term partial and complete response in 50% of cats with metastatic or nonresectable local disease.[23,23a] The chemotherapy protocol can be repeated every 3–5 weeks. We have found that the major side-effect with this protocol has been profound anorexia and mild myelosuppression. Five-week intervals between treatments seem to be better tolerated than shorter ones. In addition, it has been reported that doxorubicin can be nephrotoxic to the cat.[24] Prospective studies using combined chemotherapy and mastectomy in the cat have yet to be performed, and at this writing, we are not recommending cyclophosphamide and doxorubicin as an adjunct to surgery.

BIOLOGIC RESPONSE MODIFIERS

Studies using nonspecific biologic response therapy such as levamisole[25] and bacterial vaccines[20] combined with surgery have shown minimal effects on reducing recurrence or prolonging

survival time in cats. In a very recent study of an autogenous tumor cell vaccine combined with BCG there was no effect on recurrence and survival times in cats.[26] To date, no effective biologic response modifier is available that has been shown to be efficacious in the cat with mammary cancer.

PROGNOSIS

In canine mammary tumors the significant prognostic factors have been histologic type, degree of invasion, degree of nuclear differentiation, evidence of lymphoid cellular reactivity in the tumor vicinity, tumor size, lymph node involvement, hormone receptor activity, ulceration, and fixation.[6,9,10,27] Factors that do not seem to be associated with prognosis are tumor location, type of surgery, ovariohysterectomy at surgery, age of patient, and number of tumors present.[15,27–31]

In the study published by Gilbertson et al.,[10] histologic stage was correlated with disease-free interval after mastectomy in 232 dogs with mammary cancer (Table 24-2). In their study only 19% of the dogs with Stage 0—that is, malignant proliferation limited to the anatomic borders of the mammary duct system—had 20% recurrence within 2 years after initial mastectomy, compared to 60% recurrence in dogs with Stage 1 disease—that is, malignant proliferations extending beyond the anatomic borders of the mammary duct system into the surrounding stroma—and 95% recurrence in dogs with Stage 2 disease—that is, invasion into vascular or lymphatic vessels. Thus, prognosis is very good for dogs with preinvasive carcinoma (Table 24-2). Another factor evaluated that has been shown to be important for prognosis is degree of nuclear differentiation, which can be categorized as poorly differentiated, moderately differentiated, or well differentiated. The degree of differentiation is usually inversely related to tumor aggressiveness. Dogs with poorly differentiated tumors have a greater than 4-fold increased risk of developing recurrent carcinoma in less than 2 years after mastectomy, with an overall 90% rate compared to 68% for those with moderately differentiated tumors. Dogs with well-differentiated tumors have only a 24% recurrence rate within 2 years of their mastectomy. Another factor that has been shown to correlate

Table 24-2. Prognosis Related to Clinical and Histologic Features[10]

	% RECURRENCE AT	
	12 mos	24 mos
TUMOR SIZE		
< 3 cm	30	40
≥ 3–5 cm	70	80
> 5 cm	70	80
HISTIOLOGICAL GRADE		
Stage 0	10	20
Stage 1	40	60
Well-differentiated		40
Moderately differentiated		63
Poorly differentiated		77
Stage II	85	95
LYMPH NODE STATUS		
Negative	20	30
Positive	90	100
LYMPHOID CELLULAR REACTIVITY (STAGE I)		
Positive		45
Negative		83

The sarcomas are considered to have a very poor prognosis.[29] Most dogs with sarcomas die of their disease within 9–12 months. The inflammatory carcinomas also have a very poor prognosis.[11] Most of them cannot be resected surgically, and if they are resected, they tend to recur within weeks to a month after surgery. In addition, dogs with inflammatory carcinomas also can have a low-grade disseminated intravascular coagulation (DIC), and we have observed DIC that manifested itself by excessive bleeding at the time of surgery.

Tumor size is also a very important prognostic factor (Figs. 24-3 and 24-4). The most recent World Health Organization (WHO) clinical staging system categorizes canine mammary cancer according to the diameter of the largest tumor. T_1 is a tumor less than 3 cm in diameter; T_2 is a tumor 3–5 cm in diameter; and T_3 is a tumor greater than 5 cm in diameter. In dogs with locally invasive disease, significant differences have been found between T_1 and T_2, and between T_1 and T_3, tumors. Thus, dogs with invasive cancer having malignant tumors of a diameter less than 3 cm have a significantly better prognosis than dogs with malignant tumors of 3 cm or greater in diameter[28] (Fig. 24-4). In a recent study of dogs with invasion of lymphatic vessels or lymph node metastasis, no significant differences were found between T_1, T_2, and T_3 tumors.[28]

There has been some controversy in the literature regarding the influence of lymph node metastases on survival. In one study, lymph node involvement was not associated with sig-

with prognosis is lymphoid cell reactions observed in the tumor vicinity. Dogs with mammary cancer that did not have evidence of lymphoid cell activity at the time of initial mastectomy have a 3-fold increased risk of developing recurrence within 2 years compared to those that showed lymphoid reactivity. Dogs with lymphoid reactivity had a 45% recurrence within 2 years, and dogs without lymphoid reactivity had an 83% recurrence within 2 years. In another study of beagle dogs alone, dogs treated by mastectomy had a median survival time of 10 months. Metastasis was found in 77% of the dogs with carcinomas.[31a]

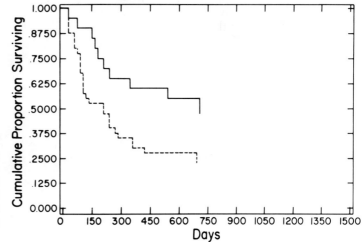

Figure 24-3. A comparison of the cancer-free interval in dogs with malignant WHO Stage II tumors (3–5 cm) as opposed to those with WHO Stage III tumors (>5 cm). All dogs were treated with mastectomy alone (p <0.05).

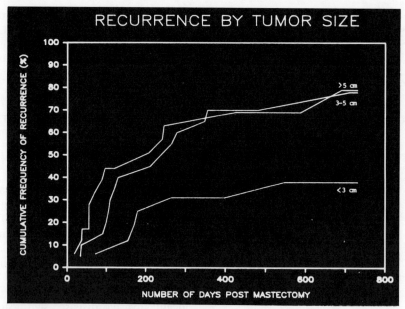

Figure 24-4. A comparison of the cancer-free interval (time from mastectomy to recurrence) based on tumor size. Forty-one dogs with a tumor diameter of 1–3 cm (n = 41) versus 64 dogs with a tumor diameter of >3 cm (n = 64) (p <0.05).[28]

nificant differences in survival.[27] A more recent study found a significant difference in disease-free interval between dogs with and those without lymph node involvement.[28] In this study,

80% of the dogs with lymph node involvement had recurrence within 6 months. Dogs with negative lymph nodes usually have 30% recurrence within 2 years of surgery (Fig. 24-5).

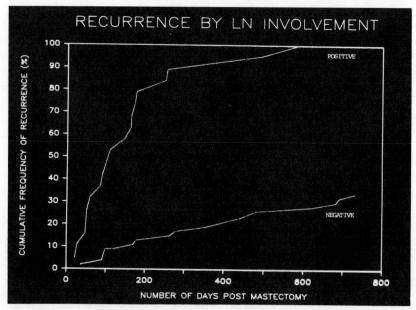

Figure 24-5. A comparison of lymph node metastasis (positive or negative) to recurrence in dogs treated by mastectomy alone.[28]

A recent study shows that dogs with either estrogen or progesterone receptors have a better prognosis following surgery.[6] The presence of these receptors has been correlated with well-differentiated tumors. Unfortunately the availability of receptor analysis for canine tumors is limited.

The most significant prognostic factors affecting recurrence and survival for feline malignant mammary tumors are tumor size[21,22] (Fig. 24-6), extent of surgery[21] (Fig. 24-7), and histologic grading.[22] Tumor size is the single most important prognostic factor. Cats with tumors greater than 3 cm in diameter have a median survival of 6 months after surgery. Cats with tumors 2–3 cm in diameter have a significantly better survival; the median is about 2 years. Cats with tumors less than 2 cm in diameter have a median survival of about 3 years. Thus,

early diagnosis and treatment is a very important prognostic factor for malignant feline mammary tumors.

Very few studies have been performed to evaluate the effectiveness of the extent of local therapy in malignant feline mammary tumors. One study showed that radical mastectomy reduces local recurrence but does not increase overall survival time.[21] The final prognostic factor is the degree of nuclear differentiation. Cats with well-differentiated tumors with few mitotic figures have been shown to have increased survival times.[22]

COMPARATIVE FACTORS

Breast cancer is the most common malignant neoplasm in women. In the United States 1 out

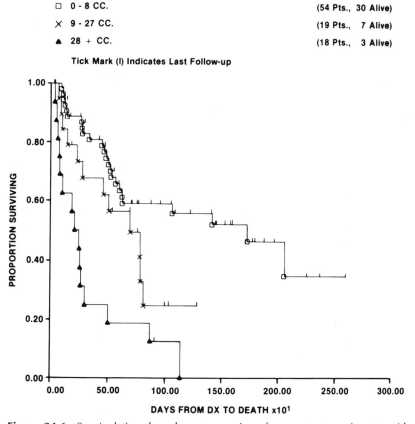

□ 0 - 8 CC.   (54 Pts., 30 Alive)

× 9 - 27 CC.   (19 Pts.,   7 Alive)

▲ 28 + CC.   (18 Pts.,   3 Alive)

Tick Mark (I) Indicates Last Follow-up

Figure 24-6. Survival time based on tumor size after mastectomy in cats with malignant mammary adenocarcinoma. Tumor volume is statistically highly significant as a prognostic factor.[21]

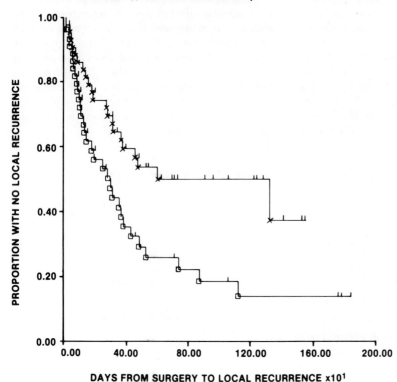

□ 1972 - 1975 Series (Conservative Surgery)   (46 Pts., 15 N.E.D.)

X 1976 - 1980 Series (Radical Surgery)   (44 Pts., 23 N.E.D.)

Tick Mark (I) Indicates Last Follow-up

Figure 24-7. Time to recurrence (remission duration) based on extent of surgery in cats with malignant mammary adeno-carcinoma. Cats undergoing radical mastectomy have a statistically significant remission duration when compared to nonradical mastectomy (conservative surgery).[21]

of every 14 women is likely to develop breast cancer, and 1 out of every 4 women with cancer has breast cancer.[32]

The etiology of breast cancer is unknown. Although there is a familial tendency, the most important factor is hormone status. Early pregnancy and early oophorectomy lower the incidence, whereas late menopause and early menarche are associated with an increased incidence. Other factors that may play a role are fat intake, obesity, body size, and socioeconomic influences.[33]

Pathologically, most breast cancers are infiltrating ductular adenocarcinomas with varying degrees of fibrous tissue reaction. In the majority of women, breast cancer appears to be a systemic disease at the time of diagnosis. Overt metastasis occurs by local infiltration to skin and the opposite breast and lymph nodes and by blood to bone, lungs, liver, and brain. Bone metastases are present in more than 50% of patients with disseminated disease.[34]

Hormonal status plays an important role in the biologic behavior and treatment of breast cancer. Estrogen receptors are present in over 60% of the tumors, progesterone receptors in over 30%, and androgen receptors in over 20%. Receptor-positive tumors have a better prognosis and respond to hormonal therapies, such as oophorectomy and anti-estrogens (tomoxifen).[34]

The management of breast cancer provides a major challenge. Treatment usually involves a combination of mastectomy and radiation therapy. Hormonal therapy (tomoxifen) usually follows surgery in estrogen receptor-positive tumors. Chemotherapy is usually used in patients with more advanced disease (positive lymph nodes, invasive carcinomas) and the useful agents include doxorubicin, alkylating agents, 5-fluorouracil, and methotrexate.

Prognosis for breast cancer patients depends on the histologic tumor type, tumor size, invasiveness, lymph node status, and receptor status.

With surgery alone the 10-year survival rate is around 50%.[35]

REFERENCES

1. Dorn CR, Taylor DON, Schneider R, et al: Survey of animal neoplasms in Alameda and Contra Costa Countries, Calif. II. Cancer morbidity in dogs and cats from Alameda County. J Natl Cancer Inst 40:307–318, 1968
2. Cohen D, Reif JS, Brodey et al: Epidemiological analysis of the most prevalent sites and types of canine neoplasia observed in a veterinary hospital. Cancer Res 34:2859–2868, 1974
3. Priester WA, McKay FW: The occurrence of tumors in domestic animals. NCI Monogr 54:155, 1980
4. Schneider R, Dorn CR, Taylor DON: Factors influencing canine mammary cancer development and postsurgical survival. J Natl Cancer Inst 43:1249–1261, 1969
5. MacEwen EG, Patnaik AK, Harvey HJ, et al: Estrogen receptors in canine mammary tumors. Cancer Res 42:2255–2259, 1982
6. Martin PM, Cotard M, Mialot JP, et al: Animal models for hormone-dependent human breast cancer. Cancer Chemother Pharmacol 2:13–17, 1984
7. Johnston SD, Hayden DW, Kiang DT, et al: Progesterone receptors in feline mammary adenocarcinomas. Am J Vet Res 45:379–382, 1984
8. Elling H, Ungemach FR: Progesterone receptors in feline mammary cancer cytosol. J Cancer Res Clin Oncol 100:325–327, 1981
9. Brodey RS, Goldschmidt MA, Roszel JR: Canine mammary gland neoplasms. J Am Anim Hosp Assoc 19:61–90, 1983
10. Gilbertson SR, Kurzman JD, Zachrau RE, et al: Canine mammary epithelial neoplasms: Biological implications of morphologic characteristics assessed in 232 dogs. Vet Pathol 20:127–142, 1983
11. Susaneck SJ, Allen TA, Hoopes J, et al: Inflammatory mammary carcinoma in the dog. J Am Anim Hosp Assoc 19:971–976, 1983
12. Carpenter JL, Andrews LK, Holzworth J, et al: Tumors and tumor-like lesions. In Holzworth J (ed): Diseases of the Cat. Medicine and Surgery, Vol. 1, pp. 527–538. Philadelphia, W.B. Saunders, 1987
13. Allen SW, Prasse KW, Mahaffey EA: Cytology differentiation of benign from malignant mammary tumors. Vet Pathol 23:649, 1986
14. Ferguson RH: Canine mammary gland tumors. Vet Clin North Am Small Anim Pract 15:501–511, 1985
14a. Knapp DW, Richardson RC, Bonney PL, et al: Cisplatin therapy in 41 dogs with malignant tumors. J Vet Intern Med 2:41–46, 1988
15. MacEwen EG, Harvey HJ, Patnaik AK, et al: Evaluation of effects of levamisole and surgery on canine mammary cancer. J Biol Resp Mod 4:418–426, 1985
16. Parodi AL, Misdorp W, Mialot JP, et al: Intratumoral BCG and Corynebacterium parvum therapy of canine mammary tumors before radical mastectomy. Cancer Immunol Immunother 15:172–177, 1983
16a. Bostock DE, Gorman NT: Intravenous BCG therapy of mammary carcinoma in bitches after surgical excision of the primary tumor. Eur J Cancer 14:879–886, 1978
17. Winters WP, Harris SC: Increased survival and interferon induction by BCG-CW immunotherapy in pet dogs with malignant mammary tumors. Abstract 964, p. 244. Am Assoc Cancer Res, 1982
18. Sedlacek HH, Weise M, Lemmer A, et al: Immunotherapy of spontaneous mammary tumors in mongrel dogs with autologus tumor cells and neuraminidase. Cancer Immunol Immunother 6:47–58, 1979
18a. Sedlacek HH, Hagmayer G, Seiler FR: Tumor therapy of neoplastic diseases with tumor cells and neuraminidases. Cancer Immunol Immunother 23:192–199, 1986
19. Fowler EH, Wilson GP, Koestner AA: Biologic behavior of canine mammary neoplasms based on a histogenetic classification. Vet Pathol 11:212–229, 1974
20. Hayes AA, Mooney S: Feline mammary tumors. Vet Clin North Am Small Anim Pract 15:513–520, 1985
21. MacEwen EG, Hayes AA, Harvey HJ, et al: Prognostic factors for feline mammary tumors. J Am Vet Med Assoc 185:201–204, 1984
22. Weijer K, Hart AAM: Prognostic factors in feline mammary carcinoma. J Natl Cancer Inst 70:709–710, 1983
23. Jeglum KA, DeGuzman E, Young K: Chemotherapy of advanced mammary adenocarcinoma in 14 cats. J Am Vet Med Assoc 187:157–160, 1985
23a. Mauldin GN, Matus RE, Patnaik AK: Efficacy and toxicity of doxorubicin and cyclophosphamide used in the treatment of selected malignant tumors in 23 cats. J Vet Intern Med 2:60–65, 1988
24. Cotter SM, Kanki PJ, Simon M: Renal disease in five tumor-bearing cats treated with Adriamycin. J Am Anim Hosp Assoc 21:405, 1985

25. MacEwen EG, Hayes AA, Mooney S, et al: Evaluation of effect of levamisole on feline mammary cancer. J Biol Resp Med 5:541–546, 1984

26. Jeglum KA, Hanna MG, Hoover HC, et al: A prospectively randomized trial of adjuvant active specific immunotherapy in feline breast cancer. Am J Vet Res (in press) 1989

27. Misdorp W, Hart AMM: Canine mammary cancer. I. Prognosis. J Small Anim Pract 20:285–294, 1979

28. Kurzman ID, Gilbertson SR: Prognostic factors in canine mammary tumors. Semin Vet Med Surg 1:25–32, 1986

29. Misdorp W, Cotchin E, Hampe JF, et al: Canine malignant mammary tumors. I. Sarcomas. Vet Pathol 8:99–177, 1971

30. Misdorp W, Cotchin E, Hampe JF, et al: Canine malignant mammary tumors. II. Adenocarcinomas, solid carcinomas, and spindle cell carcinomas. Vet Pathol 9:447–470, 1972

31. Misdorp W, Cotchin EE, Hampe JF, et al: Canine malignant mammary tumors. III. Special types of carcinomas, malignant mixed tumors. Vet Pathol 10:241–256, 1973

31a. Moulton JE, Rosenblatt LS, Goldman M: Mammary tumors in a colony of beagle dogs. Vet Pathol 23:741–749, 1986

32. Kelsey JL: A review of the epidemiology of human breast cancer. Epidmiol Rev 1:74–109, 1979

33. MacMahon B, Cole P, Brown J. Etiology of human breast cancer: A review. J Natl Cancer Inst 50:21–42, 1973

34. Harris JR, Hellman S, Canellos GP, et al: Cancer of the breast. In DeVita VT, Hellman S, Rosenberg SA (eds): Cancer: Principles and Practice of Oncology, 2nd ed, pp. 1119–1177. Philadelphia, J.B. Lippincott, 1985

35. Haskell CM, Giuliano AE, Thompson RW: Breast cancer. In Haskell CM (ed): Cancer Treatment, 2nd ed, pp. 137–180. Philadelphia, W.B. Saunders, 1985

25

TUMORS OF THE MALE REPRODUCTIVE TRACT

Nancy C. Postorino

CANINE TESTICULAR TUMORS

Testicular tumors are the second most common tumor of the male dog.[1] They are more common in the dog than in any other species, including humans.[2,3] Sertoli cell tumors (SCT), seminomas (SEM), and interstitial cell tumors (ICT), the most common histologic types of testicular tumor, occur with approximately equal frequency in the dog (Table 25-1).[4] Combinations of several tumor types may be found in the same dog. Cryptorchid males have a risk 13.6 times greater of developing SCT or SEM than normal males,[1] and the average age of occurrence in cryptorchid animals is younger.[5] The right testicle is more often affected with tumor than the left.[3,6,7]

INCIDENCE AND RISK

Sertoli Cell Tumors. Approximately 50% of all SCT occur in abdominal or inguinal testicles.[5,7] The average age of occurrence is 9 years,[7] and no breed predilection has been reported.[1]

Seminomas. Two-thirds of SEM occur in descended testicles.[5] The average age of occurrence is 10 years,[4] and there is no reported breed predilection.[1]

Interstitial Cell Tumors. Virtually all ICT occur in descended testicles.[8] ICT are often incidental findings in older, intact male dogs, and they occur more often than they are·clinically detected. The average age of occurrence is 11.5 years.[4] There is no apparent breed predilection for ICT.[1]

PATHOLOGY AND NATURAL BEHAVIOR

Sertoli Cell Tumors. SCT arise from Sertoli cells and are slow growing. Grossly, they are smooth, lobulated, and contained within a well-vascularized intact tunica. Cystic areas filled with a clear brown fluid are often found within the tumor.[4,7–9] SCT are clinically important because of their potential for metastasis and their ability to produce excessive amounts of estrogen. SCT

Table 25-1.   Canine Testicular Tumors

	SCT	SEM	ICT
% of testicular tumors	33	33	33
% retained*	50	33	0
Average age (yrs)	9	10	11.5
% functional (*i.e.*, signs of increased hormone production)	25–50	<5	0
% metastasis	2–14	<5	0

* % occurring in retained testicles

have the highest rate of metastasis of all canine testicular tumors (2% to 15%).[7] Lymphatic spread to the regional lymph nodes is the usual route of dissemination. Metastases to the liver, kidney, spleen, pancreas, and lung have been reported but are quite rare.[7]

Seminomas. SEM arise from the primitive gonadal cells of the testes. They are usually homogenous, white to pinkish gray, and unencapsulated.[4,7–9] The metastatic rate is low.[8]

Interstitial Cell Tumors. ICT arise from the Leydig cells of the testicle. These tumors remain within the testicle and are usually surrounded by a dense, fibrous capsule. ICT are pink or tan

in color and tend to bulge out from the cut surface.[4,7–9] Metastasis does not occur.[6]

HISTORY AND CLINICAL SIGNS

Sertoli Cell Tumors. Scrotal or inguinal enlargement is the most common presenting sign of dogs with SCT, although some affected dogs may present with abdominal distention, feminization, or hematologic abnormalities.[6] Feminization is a direct consequence of increased production of estrogens by the tumor. The magnitude of hormone production is generally proportional to tumor size and is more often increased with a larger abdominal SCT.[7] Of dogs with SCT, 25% to 50% show some sign of hyperestrogenism such as anemia; bilaterally symmetrical alopecia of the ventral abdomen, thorax, caudal and lateral thigh; gynecomastia; and pendulous prepuce (Fig. 25-1).[4,6,7] These dogs may be lethargic and often exhibit a decreased libido. The prostate gland may enlarge owing to squamous metaplasia secondary to increased serum estrogen concentrations.[4,6] Estrogen myelotoxicity is occasionally observed in association with SCT.[10,11] Nonregenerative anemia, granulocytopenia, and thrombocytopenia are the hematologic signs of myelotoxicity.[10,11]

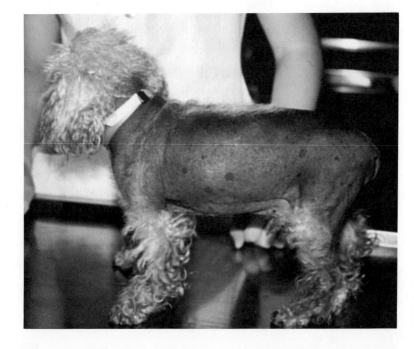

Figure 25-1. Dog with characteristic chronic dermatologic manifestations of Sertoli cell tumor.

Seminomas. Scrotal or inguinal swelling is a sign of SEM. These tumors have occasionally been associated with increased estrogen production,[2] but clinical signs of excessive hormone production are rare.[6]

Interstitial Cell Tumors. ICT are usually incidental clinical or necropsy findings. They have been associated with increased testosterone levels, which have been thought to lead to an increased incidence of perineal hernias and perineal adenomas.[6]

DIAGNOSIS AND WORK-UP

Part of the preoperative workup for SCT and SEM should include a complete blood count (CBC) and platelet count to determine if estrogen myelotoxicity is present. Dogs with large tumors, retained testicles. or clinical evidence of feminization especially need these measures. Lymph nodes should be evaluated for tumor spread (SCT or SEM) either radiographically or at the time of surgery for retained testicles. Thoracic radiographs to assess pulmonary metastases may not be cost effective owing to the low metastatic rate of the tumors. Preoperative tissue biopsy or fine-needle aspiration cytology is rarely performed since the results of these tests will not alter the treatment, which is castration. Thrombocytopenic patients should receive a fresh whole blood transfusion prior to surgery, and extreme care should be taken to attain adequate hemostasis during surgery.

THERAPY

Castration is generally the treatment of choice for all testicular tumors. Large descended testes with fixation to the scrotal skin are best managed with castration and scrotal ablation. Abdominal testicles can become very large and are frequently quite vascular (Fig. 25-2). They may be very friable, requiring care at surgery to avoid exfoliation of viable tumor cells into the abdomen. Regional lymph nodes that are enlarged owing to tumor involvement can occasionally be excised. Radiation therapy has shown promise in control of lymph node metastasis in 4 dogs with seminoma.[11a] Chemotherapy for testicular tumors is rarely attempted because surgery is curative in most cases. Metastatic SCT has been

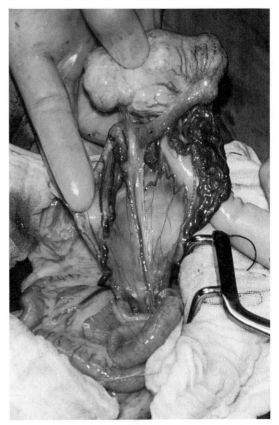

Figure 25-2. Intraoperative view of Sertoli cell tumor in a retained testicle. Note typical engorged vessels.

reported to respond to drugs such as methotrexate, vinblastine, and cyclophosphamide.[8] These drugs should be considered in cases with widespread metastases.

PROGNOSIS

Sertoli Cell Tumors. The prognosis for SCT without metastasis or myelotoxicity is excellent. Improvement of hematologic parameters occurs in most cases within 2 to 3 weeks of surgery; however, full recovery may take up to 5 months. Myelotoxicity can prove fatal in spite of aggressive supportive care. In one study, 8 of 10 dogs died or were euthanatized owing to the myelotoxic effects of estrogen secreted by their tumors.[10] Dogs presented with these complications should be given a very guarded prognosis.

Seminoma and Interstitial Cell Tumors

The prognosis for ICT is uniformly excellent. SEM will occasionally produce estrogen or metastize but the prognosis is still good overall.

FELINE TESTICULAR TUMORS

Testicular tumors are rare in the cat owing in part to the fact that most older male cats are castrated. Several carcinomas,[12] an ICT,[13] a malignant SEM and SCT have been reported.[12] Testicular tumors are so rare in the cat that virtually nothing can be said about their behavior. Castration is the treatment of choice for these tumors.

COMPARATIVE ASPECTS

Testicular tumors account for 1% of all malignant tumors in men. They generally occur in young men and are the leading cause of cancer death in the 20- to 30-year-old age group. SEM constitute 90% of all testicular tumors and are more frequent in the right testicle. Three other histologic types are common: embryonal carcinoma, teratoma, and choriocarcinoma. SEM are very radiosensitive, and because they usually present at a very early stage, the prognosis is good following therapy with surgery, radiation therapy, or combination chemotherapy.[14]

CANINE PROSTATIC TUMORS

INCIDENCE AND RISK

Prostatic tumors are rare in the dog and most often affect older, intact male dogs; the average age of occurrence is 10 years.[15] No particular breed is at increased risk; however middle- to large-breed dogs seem to be over-represented.[16,17] Androgens are known to increase the size and weight of the normal prostate gland[18] and may play a role in the development of prostatic adenocarcinomas. However, a recent publication suggests that prostatic carcinoma in the dog develops independently of hormone status (castrated versus noncastrated).[18a]

PATHOLOGY AND NATURAL BEHAVIOR

Adenocarcinomas (ADC) account for the majority of canine prostatic tumors.[15] Undifferentiated carcinomas, transitional cell carcinomas, squamous cell carcinomas, and leiomyosarcomas have also been reported[8] but are rare. In addition, transitional cell carcinomas of the prostatic urethra can extend into the prostate gland. There are several histologic classifications of prostatic ADC, and complete descriptions of these categories are given elsewhere.[15] Prostatic ADC are highly malignant tumors; 70% to 80% of affected animals have tumor spread at the time of diagnosis.[16] The tumors usually spread by means of the lymphatic system to the external and internal iliac, pelvic and sublumbar lymph nodes, lungs, and skeletal system, especially the lumbar vertebrae. Direct extension of the tumor to the bladder, colon, and surrounding tissues often occurs as well.[15] Owing to the insidious onset of the disease, most tumors are quite advanced at the time of diagnosis. Benign prostatic tumors are very rare in the dog.

HISTORY AND CLINICAL SIGNS

The most common clinical signs associated with prostatic ADC are (in order of decreasing frequency): weight loss (70%), rear limb lameness or weakness (50%), tenesmus (45%), lumbar pain (30%), stranguria (30%), polyuria/polydipsia (30%) and hematuria (25%).[15] The differential diagnosis includes benign prostatic hypertrophy, prostatic cysts, or abscess and prostatitis.

DIAGNOSIS AND WORK-UP

A complete physical examination, including a digital rectal examination of the prostate gland is essential. The malignant gland may feel normal but is usually increased in size and irregular with firm nodular areas. The gland may also extend into surrounding tissues such as the colon, bladder, and pelvic structures. Sublumbar lymph nodes should be evaluated radiographically and by digital examination for tumor spread. Laboratory evaluation should include CBC, serum chemistry panel, and urinalysis. However, the urinalysis is rarely helpful in differentiating neoplasia from other types of prostatic disease. Thoracic and abdominal radiographs should be performed to identify metastasis to lymph nodes or lung. Retrograde urethrocystography is also helpful to diagnose prostatic neoplasia.[18b] Ultrasound examination of the enlarged prostate has been reported to be helpful in differentiating cysts from neoplasia.[17] Although a diagnosis of prostatic ADC can sometimes be made from the prostatic fraction of an ejaculate or a prostatic wash, false negative results are common.[17–19] Diagnosis of prostatic ADC can only be made from tissue biopsy. Prostatic needle biopsy can be performed transabdominally, through the perineum or transrectally (Fig. 25-3).[20] Open biopsy of the prostate and regional lymph nodes (for staging purposes) is the most reliable technique, however.

THERAPY

Most canine patients with prostatic ADC are not diagnosed until late in the course of the disease. Because of this, virtually all attempts at treatment have yielded poor results. Prostatectomy may theoretically be curative; however the high morbidity associated with the procedure as well as the high metastatic rate of these tumors often preclude this form of therapy.[21] Most prostatic cancer has spread into the trigone of the bladder or urethra by the time of diagnosis, making complete resection with preservation of

vascular and nerve supply to the bladder difficult, if not impossible. Castration may theoretically slow the growth of the tumor, but this is temporary and palliative at best. Unfortunately, most animals are euthanatized soon after the diagnosis of prostatic ADC. Chemotherapy with drugs such as estramustine, a combination of estrogen and nitrogen mustard, have had limited success.[22] Radiation therapy is used in humans with localized disease[23] and could be considered in canine patients with comparable disease. The use of intra-operative radiation therapy for localized prostatic neoplasia has had positive and negative results but may be considered in dogs with disease localized to the prostate gland.[24,25]

PROGNOSIS

The prognosis is grave owing to the high metastatic rate and aggressive nature of the local disease in dogs. Most untreated dogs are euthanatized within 1 to 3 months of diagnosis because of local disease extension.

FELINE PROSTATIC TUMORS

Prostatic tumors are very rare in the cat. One fibroadenoma[13] and three carcinomas[12] have been reported. The behavior of these tumors as well as the prognosis for these cats is unknown.

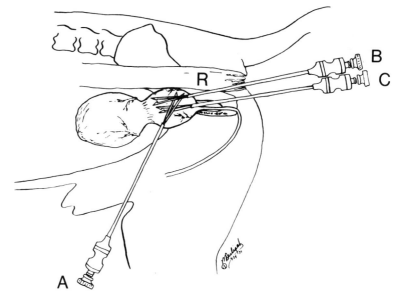

Figure 25-3. Various means of closed prostatic biopsy with needle punch. All penetrations of the prostate should be lateralized to avoid the urethra. Rectum is labeled R. A, Percutaneous punch lateral to prepuce. B, Transrectal route uses punch enclosed in glove on index finger while the prostate is palpated rectally. C, Perineal approach enters skin lateral to rectum and travels in pelvic canal up to prostate.[20]

Aggressive surgical excision of the primary tumor and regional lymph nodes is the recommended treatment.[12]

COMPARATIVE ASPECTS

Prostatic tumors are quite common in men over 50 years of age. ADC is the most common histologic type. Most tumors are diagnosed much earlier than in the dog and, therefore, more treatment options are available. Acid phosphatase is often elevated and serves as a marker for diagnosis and response to therapy. Diagnosis and treatment are often possible by means of transurethral resection. The treatment may also include combinations of surgery, radiation, chemotherapy, and hormonal therapy, depending on the clinical stage of the disease. Prognosis is guarded, although much better results are obtained in men than in dogs owing to earlier detection and the more localized extent of the disease.[23]

CANINE TUMORS OF THE PENIS AND EXTERNAL GENITALIA

Tumors that occur on the prepuce are similar to those affecting other haired regions of the body. Mast cell tumors and squamous cell carcinomas are common. Transmissible venereal tumors are the most frequently encountered type of canine penile tumor (see Chapter 30). Penile squamous cell carcinomas and adenocarcinomas have been reported[8,15] but are rare.

HISTORY AND CLINICAL SIGNS

The appearance of a rapidly growing mass on the penis or prepuce is the usual presenting complaint. Drainage from the prepuce (often bloody) is also common.

DIAGNOSIS AND WORK-UP

Biopsy of the lesion is necessary to arrive at a diagnosis. Radiographs of the caudal abdomen should be taken to evaluate regional lymph nodes.

TREATMENT

Surgical excision of the lesion is the usual treatment for penile tumors. Extirpation of the external genitalia (prepuce and penis) with perineal urethrostomy may be required, depending on the location of the lesion. Radiation therapy may be effective for sensitive tumors types, especially squamous cell carcinoma.

PROGNOSIS

The prognosis for preputial tumors is similar to those of similar histology found elsewhere on the body. Transmissible venereal tumors of the penis have a good prognosis with treatment. The prognosis for squamous cell carcinoma of the penis depends on the tumor's size and location and the ability to completely excise the tumor.

FELINE TUMORS OF THE PENIS AND EXTERNAL GENITALIA

A carcinoma and a sarcoma have been reported.[12]

COMPARATIVE ASPECTS

Squamous cell carcinoma is the most common type of penile tumor in man but is rare, accounting for considerably less than 1% of the malignancies in men of the United States.[23]

REFERENCES

1. Hayes HM, Pendergrass TW: Canine testicular tumors: Epidemiologic features of 410 dogs. Int J Cancer 18:482–487, 1976
2. Comhaire F, Mattheeuws D, et al: Testosterone and oestradiol in dogs with testicular tumours. Acta Endocrinol 77:408–416, 1974
3. Moulton JE: Tumors of the genital system. In Moulton JE (ed): Tumors in Domestic Animals, pp. 309–329. Berkeley, University of California Press, 1978
4. Cotchin E: Testicular neoplasms in dogs. J Comp Pathol 70:232–247, 1960
5. Reif JS, Maguire TG, et al: A cohort study of

canine testicular neoplasia. J Am Vet Med Assoc 175:719–723, 1979

6. Lipowitz AJ, Schwartz A, et al: Testicular neoplasms and concomitant clinical changes in the dog. J Am Vet Med Assoc 163:1364–1368, 1973

7. Pulley LT: Sertoli cell tumor. Vet Clin North Am 9:145–150, 1979

8. Theilen GH, Madewell BR: Tumors of the urogenital tract. In Theilen GH, Madewell BR (eds): Veterinary Cancer Medicine, pp. 357–381. Philadelphia, Lea & Febiger, 1979

9. Dow C: Testicular tumours in the dog. J Comp Pathol 72:247–265, 1962

10. Morgan RV: Blood dyscrasias associated with testicular tumors in the dog. J Am Anim Hosp Assoc 18:971–975, 1982

11. Sherding RG, Wilson GP, et al: Bone marrow hypoplasia in eight dogs with Sertoli cell tumor. J Am Vet Med Assoc 178:497–501, 1982

11a. McDonald RK, Walker M, Legendre AM, et al: Radiotherapy of metastatic seminoma in the dog. J Vet Int Med 2:103–107, 1988

12. Carpenter JL, Andrews LK, Holzworth J: Tumors and tumor-like lesions. In Holzworth J (ed): Disease of the Cat, pp. 517–519. Philadelphia, W.B. Saunders, 1987

13. Cotchen E: Neoplasia. In Wilkinson GT (ed): Diseases of the Cat and Their Management, pp. 366–387. Melbourne, Blackwell Scientific Publications, 1983

14. Paulson DF, Elkhorn LH, et al: Cancer of the testis. In DeVita VT (ed): Cancer: Principles and Practice of Oncology, pp. 786–822. Philadelphia, J.B. Lippincott, 1982

15. Leav I, Ling GV: Adenocarcinoma of the canine prostate. Cancer 22:1329–1345, 1968

16. Hargis AM, Miller LM: Prostatic carcinoma in dogs. Comp Cont Educ Pract Vet 5:647–653, 1983

17. Rogers KS, Wantschek L, Lees GE: Diagnostic evaluation of the canine prostate. Comp Cont Educ Pract Vet 8:11, 799–814, 1986

18. Thrall MA, Olson PN: Cytologic diagnosis of canine prostatic disease. J Am Anim Hosp Assoc 21:95–102, 1985

18a. Obradovich JE, Walshaw R, Goullaud E: The influence of castration on the development of prostatic carcinoma in the dog. J Vet Int Med 1:183–187, 1987

18b. Feeney DA, Johnston GR, Klausner JS, et al: Canine prostatic disease—comparison of radiographic appearance with morphologic and microbiologic findings: 30 cases (1981–1985). J Am Vet Med Assoc 190:1018–1034, 1987

19. Barsanti JA, Finco DR: Evaluation of techniques for diagnosis of canine prostatic diseases. J Am Vet Med Assoc 185:2, 198–200, 1984

20. Withrow SJ, Lowes N: Biopsy techniques for use in small animal oncology. J Am Anim Hosp Assoc 17:889–902, 1981

21. Hardie EM, Barsanti JA, Rawlings CA: Complications of prostatic surgery. J Am Anim Hosp Assoc 20:50–56, 1984

22. Stearns ME, Tew KD: Antimicrotubule effects of estramustine, an antiprostatic tumor drug. Cancer Res 45:3891–3897, 1985

23. Paulson DF, Perez CA, Anderson T: Genitourinary malignancies. In DeVita VT (ed): Cancer: Principles and Practice of Oncology, pp. 732–785. Philadelphia, J.B. Lippincott Co, 1982

24. Turrel JM: Intraoperative radiotherapy of carcinoma of the prostate gland in ten dogs. J Am Vet Med Assoc 190:1,48–52, 1987

25. Withrow SJ, Gillette EL, Hoopes PJ, et al: Intraoperative irradiation of 16 spontaneously occurring canine neoplasms. Vet Surg 18:7–11, 1989

26

TUMORS OF THE URINARY SYSTEM

Stephen J. Withrow

RENAL CANCER

INCIDENCE AND RISK FACTORS

Primary renal cancer accounts for approximately 1% of all cancers; metastatic cancer to the kidney, on the other hand, is common, presumably owing to its high blood flow and rich capillary network. Epithelial malignancies are most common and are seen in older patients with a mean age of 9 years.[1] Male dogs are more commonly affected with epithelial tumors than females; the ratio is 1.5 males to 1 female. Embryonal neoplasms may be seen in younger patients with a mean age of 4 years.[2]

A syndrome of dermal fibrosis, uterine polyps, and concomitant renal cystadenocarcinoma is seen almost exclusively in the German shepherd bitch and may be heritable.[3,4]

PATHOLOGY AND NATURAL BEHAVIOR

Ninety percent of primary renal tumors in the dog and cat are malignant. Over half are epithelial (tubular adenocarcinoma and transitional cell carcinoma), 20% are mesenchymal (fibrosarcoma, chondrosarcoma, and so on) and 10% are derived from embryonal pluripotential blastema (Wilm's tumor, nephroblastoma, embryonal nephroma).[5] Some tumors, especially adenocarcinoma and lymphoma, are often bilateral. Lymphoma is the most common tumor affecting the feline kidney, but it is only occasionally localized to the kidney. The mean age of affected cats is 6 years.[6]

Renal adenocarcinomas usually arise in the cortex or one pole of the kidney. They can be highly invasive to regional structures and may invade the vena cava. Metastasis to regional lymph nodes, lung, liver, and bone occurs in over half the cases.[1] Benign tumors are rare and account for less than 10% of renal tumors.

Transitional cell carcinoma of the kidney usually arises in the renal pelvis; it may be very invasive locally. The metastatic rate appears to be less than that of renal tubular adenocarcinoma.[1]

312

Nephroblastoma is usually not metastatic, but it often attains a large size and may implant the peritoneal cavity if it ruptures.

HISTORY AND CLINICAL SIGNS

The onset of symptoms is generally slow and nonspecific over weeks to months. Signs may include weight loss, depression, fever, abdominal distention, and pain. Gross hematuria is an uncommon finding except with hemangioma[7] and renal pelvic locations (transitional cell car-

cinoma). Hypertrophic osteopathy has been described in association with renal tumors.[8,9]

Slow-growing, firm skin and subcutaneous fibrous nodules in German shepherds should alert the clinician to the possibility of concomitant renal cystadenocarcinoma (Fig. 26-1).[3,4]

DIAGNOSTIC TECHNIQUES AND WORK-UP

Careful abdominal palpation may reveal a mass or pain in the region of the kidneys, presumably from tension on the capsule or ureteral obstruction and secondary hydronephrosis.

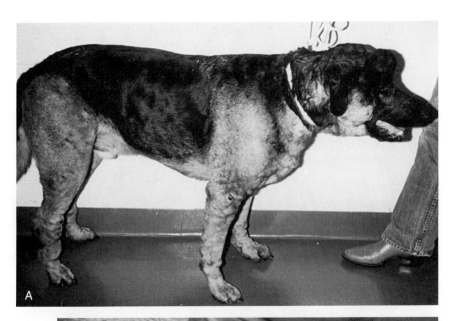

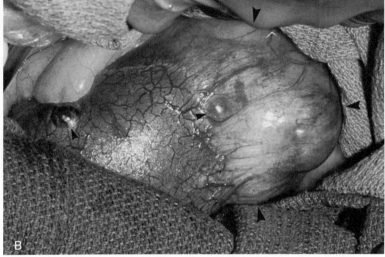

Figure 26-1. (A) Middle-aged German shepherd dog exhibiting numerous firm, fibrous, and painless nodules in the skin and subcutaneous tissues. Note large lesion over frontal sinus area. (B) Operative view of kidney from patient in A. Note several small cystic masses (small arrows) and larger mass (large arrow) on right pole. Diagnosis was confirmed as bilateral renal cystadenocarcinoma. No treatment was performed. This patient survived 18 months after first detection of skin and subcutaneous fibrosis.

Abdominal radiographs may demonstrate renal enlargement and irregularity and, if they are suspicious, should be followed by an intravenous urogram (Fig. 26-2).[1] Further tests such as arteriography and ultrasound may be needed to demonstrate subtle lesions.[5,10] Thoracic radiographs demonstrate metastasis in up to a third of the cases, especially with adenocarcinoma.

Hematologic changes may include a mild to moderate anemia secondary to hematuria. Polycythemia, presumably due to increased erythropoietin production, has been documented on rare occasions in several dogs and at least one cat.[11,12,12a] Extreme neutrophilic leukocytosis (200,0000 to 250,000 WBC/μL) has also been reported.[12b]

Blood chemistries are usually normal but may reveal signs of renal failure (primary or obstructive) if both kidneys or ureters are involved.

Urinalysis will frequently reveal red blood cells, but definite identification of exfoliated tumor cells is rare. Proteinuria is a common but nonspecific finding.[1]

Transabdominal or "closed" renal biopsy has been described[13] but is usually reserved for patients with bilateral involvement (precluding

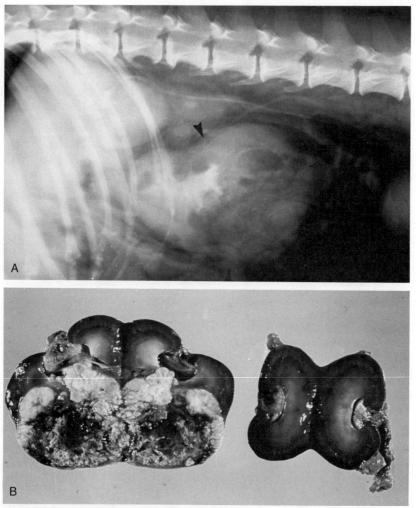

Figure 26-2. *(A)* Lateral abdominal radiograph of a dog during intravenous pyelography. Note irregular filling of caudal pole of left kidney (arrow). Diagnosis was renal adenocarcinoma. *(B)* Gross photo of kidneys from dog in *A*. No treatment was offered owing to metastasis to several bones and lung.

surgical treatment) or suspect lymphoma, when medical treatment would be employed.

Surgical exploration for biopsy, staging, or treatment is preferred for patients with only one kidney involved.

TREATMENT

Unilateral renal cancer is best treated by complete nephrectomy. This includes removal of the ureter and possibly retroperitoneal muscle and tissue if capsular extension has occurred. Early ligation of the renal vein is advisable. Partial nephrectomy is rarely possible or desired, except in cases of bilateral involvement. Regional lymph nodes (para-aortic) should be biopsied if they are visible or enlarged. Some tumors (especially nephroblastomas) can attain very large size (Fig. 26-3) and still be easily operable.

Actinomycin D has been advocated as therapeutic or adjuvant treatment for nephroblastomas in dogs, but unequivocal proof of its efficacy is lacking.[9]

Lymphoma can be effectively treated with chemotherapy, but the prognosis is poor if renal failure is present.[6,14]

Radiation therapy has rarely been attempted for renal cancer.

PROGNOSIS

The literature has few treated cases with long-term follow-up.[1,5,15] Carcinomas are metastatic, bilateral, or locally invasive in over half the cases.[16] Mean survival is 6 to 10 months for canine patients who are deemed operable and who live at least 21 days postoperatively. However, survivals of up to 4 years have been reported.[15,17] Nephroblastoma is less metastatic and complete nephrectomy has the potential to be curative.

Renal lymphoma will respond to chemotherapy but is usually not curable and will usually progress to the generalized form. Central nervous system metastasis is a common sequela in cats with renal lymphoma.[14] Signs of renal failure denote a poor prognosis even with the use of chemotherapy.[6,14]

The German shepherd syndrome of bilateral cystadenocarcinomas is rarely amenable to surgery, but survival may be many months or more without treatment.

COMPARATIVE ASPECTS[18]

Benign and cystic lesions comprise over 85% of space-occupying lesions of the human kidney. Malignant primary cancer is generally adenocarcinoma (hypernephroma), renal pelvic transitional cell carcinoma, or Wilms' tumor (nephroblastoma).

Experimental and clinical carcinogens for hypernephroma include radiation, hormones (especially estrogen), and tobacco products. Transitional cell carcinoma of the renal pelvis is associated with an almost 50% incidence of other urinary cancer that is thought to be due to a common exposure to carcinogens (field defect) rather than to tumor cell reimplantation. Treatment for the above two tumors is generally complete nephroureterectomy. Radiation, chemotherapy, and hormonal treatment play lesser roles. Five-year survivals are 30% to 40%.

Wilm's tumor generally affects children under 7 years of age (30% <1 yr). A dramatic improvement in prognosis with combinations of surgery, radiation, and chemotherapy (vincristine and actinomycin-D) has resulted in 5-year survival rates of 80% or better.

CANCER OF THE URETER

Primary cancer of the ureter is extremely rare. Reported cases have included leiomyoma, leiomyosarcoma, fibropapilloma, and transitional cell carcinoma.[19-22] More commonly, involvement of the ureter is secondary to cancer of the kidney, bladder, or retroperitoneal space. Treatment is generally with nephro-ureterectomy, although for very distal lesions, the proximal ureter could be reimplanted in the bladder or anastomosed to the contralateral ureter. Tension-free end-to-end anastomosis after resection of a segment is difficult. Benign lesions carry an excellent prognosis with resection.[19,21]

URINARY BLADDER CANCER

INCIDENCE AND RISK FACTORS

Bladder cancer is the most common urinary tract cancer, but it accounts for less than 1% of all cancer. It is more common in the dog than the cat. Experimentally, many chemicals are carci-

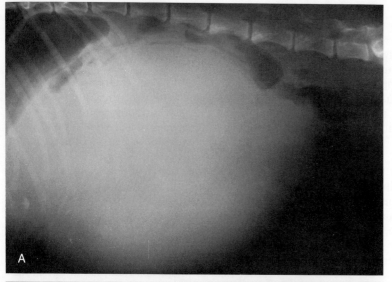

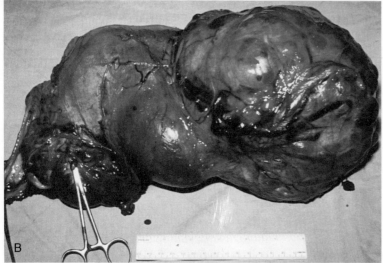

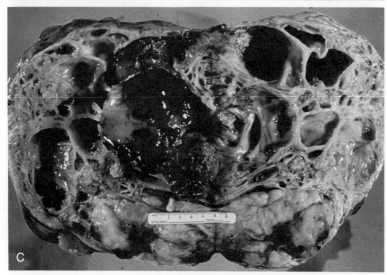

Figure 26-3. *(A)* Lateral radiograph of dog with large mid-abdominal mass. Mass could have arisen from several intra-abdominal structures but was confirmed as nephroblastoma. *(B)* 8-kg renal tumor removed from patient in *A*. *(C)* Cross-section of tumor in *B*. Note multiple cystic areas making accuracy of closed biopsy difficult. Surgical removal resulted in 16-month survival; then patient was lost to further follow-up.

nogenic,[23] and clinically, cyclophosphamide has caused transitional cell carcinoma in the dog.[24,25] That metabolites of tryptophan (a proposed carcinogen) are excreted in higher concentrations in the urine of the dog than that of the cat may account for the higher incidence of the canine.[26] The average age of affected dogs is 10 years and of affected cats, 9.7 years.[27] Female dogs and male cats are at higher risk for development of bladder cancer.[27,28]

PATHOLOGY AND NATURAL BEHAVIOR

Malignant cancers are much more common than are benign lesions. Transitional cell carcinoma is the most common histologic type followed by squamous cell carcinoma and adenocarcinoma.[29] Primary sarcomas (fibrosarcoma, leiomyosarcoma, and hemangiosarcoma) of the bladder are uncommon. A rare cancer of the younger dog is botryoid or embryonal rhabdomyosarcoma.[30] Fibromas, leiomyomas, and papillomas are the most common benign lesions.[30a] Pyogranulomatous or diffuse polypoid cystitis may mimic diffuse uroepithelial cancer.[31]

Malignant carcinomas, especially transitional cell carcinoma, are very locally invasive. They metastasize to regional lymph nodes and lung in more than half the cases.[32]

HISTORY AND CLINICAL SIGNS

Most animals present with signs similar to cystitis (hematuria, dysuria, and increased frequency of urination). Signs may be present for weeks to several months, and apparent short-term response to antibiotics may be observed. Hematuria may be more pronounced than with other bladder disorders. Occasionally hypertrophic osteopathy may be observed secondary to bladder cancer, especially in association with botryoid rhabdomyosarcoma.[30,33] Cystitis or hematuria that is unresponsive to conservative medical treatment warrants further diagnostic evaluation.

DIAGNOSTIC TECHNIQUES AND WORK-UP

Routine blood tests and physical examination rarely help diagnose these tumors. Occasional patients have renal failure secondary to obstruction. Most bladder cancer is not detectable by abdominal palpation.

A urinalysis often reveals white blood cells, red blood cells, and protein compatible with routine cystitis. Secondary bacteriuria may also be noted. Neoplastic cells may be exfoliated into the urine[29] but are often difficult to distinguish from reactive transitional cells.

Radiography is a valuable tool in the diagnosis and localization of bladder lesions. Positive or negative contrast cystograms usually reveal a mucosal mass lesion. Diffuse trigonal involvement often denotes transitional cell carcinoma (Fig. 26-4). Polypoid lesions away from the trigone have a higher likelihood of being benign (Fig. 26-5). An intravenous urogram to evaluate the bladder lumen may be done if a urethral catheter cannot be passed or if ureteral obstruction is suspected. Hydronephrosis or hydroureter associated with bladder tumors is a poor prognostic sign since involvement of the trigone is likely. Sublumbar lymph nodes and the lumbar vertebrae should be examined radiographically for metastasis. Thoracic radiographs are generally performed but are only occasionally positive at the time of initial diagnosis.[34]

Bladders may be biopsied by means of cystoscopy[35,36] or, more commonly, at laparotomy.

TREATMENT

Before opening the bladder, the abdomen should be carefully inspected for metastatic disease. Particular attention should be paid to the sublumbar lymph nodes and any palpable nodes removed or biopsied for staging purposes. The ureters should also be inspected for increased size and tumor invasion. The bladder is then carefully palpated and a cystotomy incision made at least 1 cm away from suspect tumor. Transitional cell carcinoma is usually red and friable (Fig. 26-6). Benign lesions (usually small, well circumscribed, and pedunculated) can be excised with a conservative, full-thickness bladder wall removal (Fig. 26-7). Malignant lesions pose a greater surgical problem. Most patients have advanced-stage disease in a critical location. The ureters and trigone are frequently involved, making resection and reconstruction of a continent lower urinary tract difficult, if not impossible. Transposition of ureters to the body of the bladder is possible but unlikely to be curative. If the cancer is in the apex of the bladder, a very wide full-thickness partial cystectomy

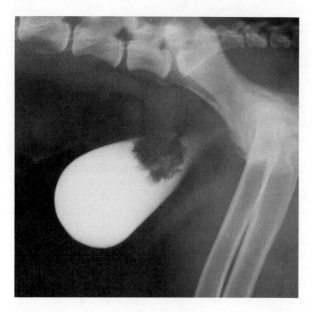

Figure 26-4. Positive contrast cystogram of an 8-year-old male dog with a large filling defect in the area of the trigone. A diagnosis of transitional cell carcinoma was confirmed by excisional biopsy. A partial cystectomy with transplantation of one ureter resulted in cessation of signs for 5 months, at which time local recurrence and metastasis to regional lymph nodes were evident.

may be attempted. Over 80% of the bladder may be removed with eventual return to normal or near-normal capacity.

Attempts at complete cystectomy with rerouting of urine into the bowel have yielded only short-term success and must be considered experimental in animals. In a series of 10 dogs who underwent complete cystectomy (± prostatectomy or urethrectomy) and ureterocolostomy, mean survival was only 2.8 months.[37] Complications such as pyelonephritis, ureteral obstruction, and hyperchloremic acidosis were common (Fig. 26-8). Metastasis to regional or distant sites occurred in 5 cases. The morbidity of the procedure coupled with a high metastatic rate makes this procedure less than ideal.[37a] Ureterostomy to the skin, or to bowel and then skin, has been rarely reported in the dog,[38] although it is commonly performed in humans. Maintaining attachment of collection bags to the skin and excoriation of surrounding skin have been major problems when this was attempted in the dog.

Intraoperative irradiation (delivery of large doses of radiation [15–30 Gy] during operative exposure) followed by fractionated external beam

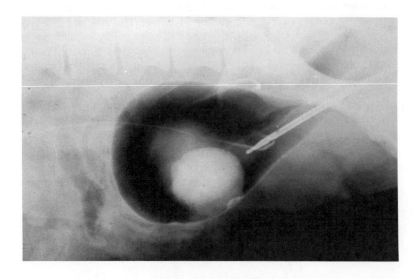

Figure 26-5. Double contrast cystogram of an 11-year-old dog with a circular mass visible on the floor of the bladder. This was a fibroma.

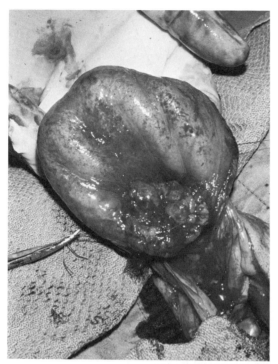

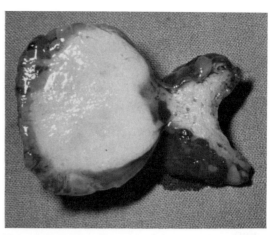

Figure 26-7. Cross-section of tumor and section of removed bladder wall depicted in Fig. 26-5. Note homogeneous white density and narrow stalk compatible with a benign lesion. Recovery was uneventful and the patient is free of disease 3 years postoperatively.

Figure 26-6. Typical appearance of a friable and hemorrhagic transitional cell carcinoma of the trigone of the bladder. Tumor infiltrated both ureters and was not resectable.

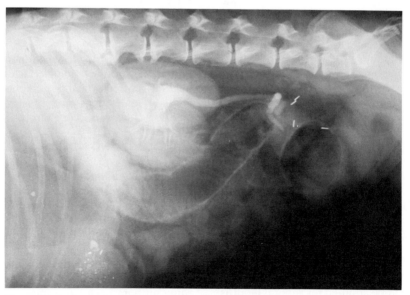

Figure 26-8. Intravenous urogram of a dog 4 months after complete cystectomy and urethrectomy followed by ureterocolonic anastomosis for transitional cell carcinoma. Metal clips note sites where ureters enter the colon. Ureteral and renal pelvis dilation is evident. Contrast material can be noted in terminal colon, which now acts as a reservoir for feces and urine. Although this patient did well clinically, she was euthanatized for bone and lung metastasis 9 months postoperatively.

irradiation (30 Gy) resulted in poor local control and serious bladder fibrosis with resultant incontinence in a series of 12 dogs treated.[39] In another paper utilizing intraoperative irradiation to treat canine bladder cancer, the one-year survival was 61%, and the two-year survival 15%. Most dogs died or were euthanized for metastasis, local recurrence, or side effects of treatment.[39a] Fractionated external beam irradiation is generally not recommended owing to the high dosages required to eradicate advanced cancer and subsequent serious risk of bowel injury.

Systemic chemotherapy is infrequently reported and does not look encouraging at this time. Cisplatin was used to treat 8 dogs with urinary tract transitional cell carcinoma. In spite of one partial response and stabilization of disease in 4 dogs, most survivals were less than 6 months.[39b] Local infusion of chemotherapy is an attractive idea,[40] but drugs usually do not penetrate beyond the submucosa; unfortunately, most animal tumors have infiltrated to muscularis or serosa. Hyperthermic chemotherapy infusions or infusions of immunotherapy are being investigated in humans.[41]

Attempts at using intralesional BCG cell wall preparations at the time of partial excision have yielded variable results. Two of seven dogs treated this way seemed to benefit from the intralesional therapy, but two dogs developed severe granulomatous reactions that resulted in a complete obstruction.*

Appropriate combinations of surgery, chemotherapy, and radiation need further investigation for treatment of bladder cancer in the dog and cat.[42]

PROGNOSIS

The prognosis for malignant cancer of the urinary bladder (especially transitional cell carcinoma) is poor owing to the usually advanced stage at diagnosis. Even if resection is possible, most patients suffer local recurrence or metastasis within 1 year.[43] However, palliation of symptoms with surgery can be attained for several months.

Benign lesions may be cured with surgical resection.

* MacEwen EG, Matus R: Personal communication, the Animal Medical Center, New York, NY, 1983

COMPARATIVE ASPECTS[18]

Numerous chemical carcinogens, often associated with industrial exposure, have been implicated in the development of human bladder cancer. Naturally occurring substances in urine may also be growth-promoting factors (urea and glycoprotein).

Ninety percent of epithelial cancers are transitional cell carcinoma. Multicentric tumors are common, presumably owing to diffuse exposure and alteration of the bladder mucosa to carcinogens (probably true in animals as well).

Carcinoma in situ may be treated with transurethral resection while more advanced stages are often treated with complete cystectomy and urinary diversion. Radiation may be employed curatively or adjuvantly. Chemotherapy may be systemic (cis-platinum) or through intravesicular routes (thiotepa, doxorubicin, and so forth). Intravesicular chemotherapy is usually reserved for superficial lesions.

Tumor size, stage, and histologic grade are important prognostic variables.

URETHRAL TUMORS

INCIDENCE AND RISK FACTORS

Urethral tumors are less common than bladder tumors. The same etiologic factors that induce bladder tumors probably influence the urethra. Older female dogs are most commonly affected.[44,45] Cats are very rarely affected.

PATHOLOGY AND NORMAL BEHAVIOR

The most common histologic types of cancer are transitional cell carcinoma and squamous cell carcinoma. Theoretically, the proximal one-third of the urethra should develop transitional cell carcinomas, and the distal two-thirds squamous cell carcinoma. Since most of these tumors involve the entire length of the urethra and biologic differences have not been identified, some authors prefer the more general term of urethral carcinoma.[46] Benign tumors are very rare, but granulomatous urethritis (resembling cancer) has been reported.

Metastasis is to regional lymph nodes and further in over half the cases evaluated.[44–47]

HISTORY AND CLINICAL SIGNS

The history and signs such as stranguria and hematuria are essentially the same as for bladder tumors.

DIAGNOSTIC TECHNIQUES AND WORK-UP

The approach is similar to that for bladder tumors. In male dogs, the most common site is the prostatic urethra, which may be palpated as a firm, irregular prostate by digital rectal examination and may mimic prostatic adenocarcinoma. Females often have a small mass palpable near the urethral papilla on the floor of the vagina. A vaginal smear may reveal transitional cells suggestive of neoplasia.[46]

A contrast urethrogram usually reveals an irregular and narrowed urethral lumen (Fig. 26-9). If the urethra cannot be catheterized, an intravenous pyelogram or direct injection cystogram may be performed to evaluate the bladder neck. In the male dog the proximal prostatic urethra and trigone are often involved, whereas in females the entire length of the urethra including the trigone may be involved (Fig. 26-10).[48]

A confirmation biopsy may be obtained through a vaginoscope in the female or by open abdominal biopsy of lymph nodes and urethra in the male or female.

TREATMENT

Treatment is generally ineffective owing to extensive involvement of the urethra and almost uniform proximity to the trigone, ureters, and blood supply to the bladder. As with bladder cancer, complete urethrectomy, cystectomy, and urinary diversion must be considered experimental.

Trigonal colonic anastomosis or antepubic urethrostomy (in females), after partial urethrectomy, has been suggested but is rarely if ever possible owing to the frequent involvement of the trigone.[44-50] A permanent cystostomy can be attempted palliatively for relief of bladder obstruction, but it is associated with skin scalding from urine and is usually rapidly followed by ureteral obstruction.

Intraoperative radiation therapy has been unsuccessful in controlling this disease in my experience.[39] Chemotherapy using *cis*-platinum has been recommended, but conclusive proof of efficacy is lacking.[39b]

PROGNOSIS

The prognosis for cure or significant palliation of malignant urethral cancer is very poor. Untreated animals have lived as long as 6 months after diagnosis but have experienced a gradual progression of symptoms ending in complete occlusion of the urethra or metastatic symptoms.

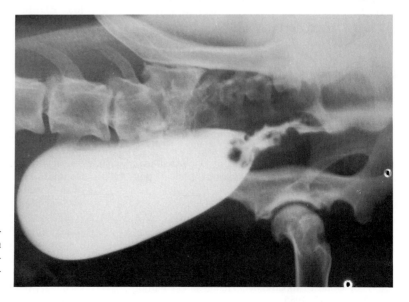

Figure 26-9. Urethrogram revealing filling defects in urethra and trigone which were confirmed as transitional cell carcinoma.

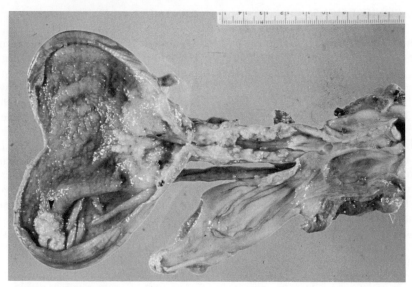

Figure 26-10. Bladder, urethra, and vagina from a dog with transitional cell carcinoma of the trigone and entire length of urethra. Note separate bladder lesion in lower left corner (arrow).

COMPARATIVE ASPECTS[18]

Urethral cancer in humans is rare. It is often preceded by a history of chronic urethritis. The disease is twice as common in women as in men. Proximal lesions are more likely to be transitional cell carcinoma, and distal lesions squamous cell carcinoma. Adenocarcinoma has also been reported. Surgery with or without radiation therapy is the treatment of choice.

REFERENCES

1. Klein MK, Cockerell GL, Harris CK, et al: Canine primary renal neoplasms: A retrospective review of 54 cases. J Am Anim Hosp Assoc 24:443–452, 1988

2. Hayes HM, Fraumeni JF: Epidemiological features of canine renal neoplasms. Cancer Res 37:2553–2556, 1977

3. Suter M, Lott–Stolz G, Wild P: Generalized nodular dermatofibrosis in six Alsatians. Vet Pathol 20:632–634, 1983

4. Lium B, Moe L: Hereditary multifocal renal cystadenocarcinomas and nodular dermatofibrosis in the German shepherd dog: Macroscopic and histopathologic changes. Vet Pathol 22:447–455, 1985

5. Caywood DD, Osborne CA: Oncology section: Urinary system. In Slatter DH (ed): Textbook of Small Animal Surgery, pp. 2561–2574. Philadelphia, W.B. Saunders, 1985

6. Weller RE, Stann SE: Renal lymphosarcoma in the cat. J Am Anim Hosp Assoc 19:363–367, 1983

7. Cadwallader JA, Goulden BE, Wyburn RS, Jolly RD: Renal hemangioma in a dog. New Z Vet J 21:48–51, 1973

8. Nafe LA, Herron AJ, Burk RL: Hypertrophic osteopathy in a cat associated with renal papillary adenoma. J Am Anim Hosp Assoc 17:659–662, 1981

9. Caywood DD, Osborne CA, Stevens JB, Jessen CR, O'Leary TP: Hypertrophic osteoarthropathy associated with an atypical nephroblastoma in a dog. J Am Anim Hosp Assoc 16:855–865, 1980

10. Konde LJ, Park RD, Wrigley RH, Lebel JL: Comparison of radiography and ultrasonography in the evaluation of renal lesions in the dog. J Am Vet Med Assoc 188:1420–1425, 1986

11. Peterson ME, Zanjani ED: Inappropriate erythropoietin production from a renal carcinoma in a dog with polycythemia. J Am Vet Med Assoc 179:995–996, 1981

12. Scott RC, Patnaik AK: Renal carcinoma with secondary polycythemia in the dog. J Am Anim Hosp Assoc 8:275–283, 1972

12a. Gorse MJ: Polycythemia associated with renal fibrosarcoma in a dog. J Am Vet Med Assoc 192:793–794, 1988

12b. Lappin MR, Latimer KS: Hematuria and extreme neutrophilic leukocytosis in a dog with renal tubular carcinoma. J Am Vet Med Assoc 192:1289–1292, 1988

13. Jeraj K, Osborne CA, Stevens JB: Evaluation of renal biopsy in 197 dogs and cats. J Am Vet Med Assoc 181:367–369, 1982

14. Mooney SC, Hayes AA, Matus RE, et al: Renal lymphoma in cats: 28 cases (1977–1984). J Am Vet Med Assoc 191:1473–1477, 1987

15. Lucke VM, Kelly DF: Renal carcinoma in the dog. Vet Pathol 13:264–276, 1976

16. Baskin GB, DePaoli A: Primary renal neoplasms of the dog. Vet Pathol 14:591–605, 1977

17. Burger GT, Moe JB, White JD, Whitney GD: Renal carcinoma in a dog. J Am Vet Med Assoc 171:282–283, 1977

18. Paulson DF, Perez CA, Anderson T: Genitourinary malignancies. In DeVita VT et al (eds): Cancer: Principles and Practice of Oncology, pp. 732–742. Philadelphia, J.B. Lippincott, 1982

19. Liska WD, Patnaik AK: Leiomyoma of the ureter of a dog. J Am Anim Hosp Assoc 13:83–84, 1977

20. Berzon JL: Primary leiomyosarcoma of the ureter in a dog: Clinical reports. J Am Vet Med Assoc 175(4):374–376, 1979

21. Hattel AL, Diters RW, Snavely DA: Ureteral fibropapilloma in a dog. J Am Vet Med Assoc 188(8):873, 1986

22. Hanika C, Rebar AH: Ureteral transitional cell carcinoma in the dog. Vet Pathol 17:643–646, 1980

23. Okajima E, Hiramatsu T, Hirao K, Ijuin M, et al: Urinary bladder tumors induced by n-butyl-n-(4-hydroxybutyl)nitrosamine in dogs. Cancer Res 41:1958–1966, 1981

24. Macy DW, Withrow SJ, Hoopes J: Transitional cell carcinoma of the bladder associated with cyclophosphamide administration. J Am Anim Hosp Assoc 19:965–969, 1983

25. Weller RE, Wolf AM, Oyejide A: Transitional cell carcinoma of the bladder associated with cyclophosphamide therapy in a dog. J Am Anim Hosp Assoc 15:733–736, 1979

26. Osborne CA, Low DG, et al: Neoplasms of the canine and feline urinary bladder: Incidence, etiologic factors, occurrence and pathologic features. Am J Vet Res 29:2041, 1968

27. Schwarz PD, Greene RW, Patnaik AK: Urinary bladder tumors in the cat: A review of 27 cases. J Am Anim Hosp Assoc 21:237–245, 1985

28. Crow SE: Urinary tract neoplasms in dogs and cats. Comp Cont Educ 7:607–618, 1985

29. Caywood DD, Osborne CA, Johnston GR: Neoplasms of the canine and feline urinary tracts. In Kirk RW (ed): Current Vet Therapy VII, pp. 1203–1212, 1980

30. Halliwell WH, Ackerman N: Botryoid rhabdomyosarcoma of the urinary bladder and hypertrophic osteoarthropathy in a young dog. J Am Vet Med Assoc 165:911–913, 1974

30a. Esplin DG: Urinary bladder fibromas in dogs: 51 cases (1981–1985). J Am Vet Med Assoc 190:440–444, 1987

31. Johnston SD, Osborne CA, Stevens JB: Canine polypoid cystitis. J Am Vet Med Assoc 166:1155–1160, 1975

32. Stone EA: Urogenital tumors. Vet Clin North Am 15:597–608, 1985

33. Brodey RS, Riser WH, Allen H: Hypertrophic pulmonary osteoarthropathy in a dog with carcinoma of the urinary bladder. J Am Vet Med Assoc 162:474–477, 1971

34. Walter PA, Haynes JS, Feeney DA, Johnston GR: Radiographic appearance of pulmonary metastases from transitional cell carcinoma of the bladder and urethra of the dog. J Am Vet Med Assoc 185:411–418, 1984

35. McCarthy TC, McDermaid SL: Prepubic percutaneous cystoscopy in the dog and cat. J Am Anim Hosp Assoc 22:213–219, 1986

36. Cooper JE, Milroy JG, Turton JA, Wedderburn N, Hicks RM: Cystoscopic examination of male and female dogs. Vet Rec 115:571–574, 1984

37. Stone EA, Withrow SJ, Page RL: Ureterocolonic anastomosis in ten dogs with transitional cell carcinoma. Vet Surg 17:147–153, 1988

37a. Montgomery RD, Hankes GH: Ureterocolonic anastamosis in a dog with transitional cell carcinoma of the bladder. J Am Vet Med Assoc 190:1427–1432, 1987

38. Bjorling DE, Mahaffey MB, Crowell WA: Bilateral ureteroileostomy and perineal urinary diversion in dogs. Vet Surg 14:204–212, 1985

39. Withrow SJ, Gillette EL, Hoopes PJ, et al: Intraoperative irradiation of 16 spontaneously occurring canine neoplasms. Vet Surg 18:7–11, 1989

39a. Walker M, Breider M: Intraoperative radiotherapy of canine bladder cancer. Vet Rad 28:200–204, 1987

39b. Shapiro W, Kitchell BE, Fossum TW, et al: Cisplatin for treatment of transitional cell and squamous cell carcinomas in dogs. J Am Vet Med Assoc 193:1530–1533, 1988

40. Blumenreich MS, Needles B, Yagoda A, Sogani

P, Grabstald H, Whitmore WF: Intravesical cisplatin for superficial bladder tumors. Cancer 50:863–865, 1982

41. Kubota Y, Shuin T, Miura T, Nishimura R, et al: Treatment of bladder cancer with a combination of hyperthermia, radiation and bleomycin. Cancer 53:199–202, 1984

42. Smith JA, Bata M, Grabstald H, Sogani PC, et al: Preoperative irradiation and cystectomy for bladder cancer. Cancer 49:869–873, 1982

43. Burnie AG, Weaver AD: Urinary bladder neoplasia in the dog: A review of seventy cases. J Small Anim Pract 24:129–143, 1983

44. Tarvin G, Patnaik A, Greene R: Primary urethral tumors in dogs. J Am Vet Med Assoc 172:931–933, 1978

45. Wilson GP, Hayes HM, Casey HW: Canine urethral cancer. J Am Anim Hosp Assoc 15:741–744, 1979

46. Magne ML, Hoopes PJ, Kainer RA, et al: Urinary tract carcinomas involving the canine vagina and vestibule. J Am Anim Hosp Assoc 21:767–772, 1985

47. Szymanski C, Boyce R, Wyman M: Transitional cell carcinoma of the urethra metastatic to the eyes in a dog. J Am Vet Med Assoc 185:1003–1006, 1984

48. Ticer JW, Spencer CP, Ackerman N: Transitional cell carcinoma of the urethra in four female dogs: its urethrographic appearance. Vet Radiol 21:12–17, 1980

49. Yoshioka MM, Carb A: Antepubic urethrostomy in the dog. J Am Anim Hosp Assoc 18:290–294, 1982

50. Bovee KC, Pass MA, Wardley R, et al: Trigonal-colonic anastamosis: A urinary diversion procedure in dogs. J Am Vet Med Assoc 178:184–191, 1979

27

TUMORS OF THE NERVOUS SYSTEM

Richard A. LeCouteur

INTRACRANIAL NEOPLASIA

INCIDENCE AND RISK FACTORS

Intracranial neoplasia appears to be more common in dogs than in other domestic species.[1–3] Vandevelde has suggested an incidence of brain tumors in dogs of approximately 14.5 per 100,000 of the population at risk.[3] The same author suggests an incidence in cats of approximately 3.5 per 100,000 population.[3]

Historically, gliomas (astrocytomas and oligodendrogliomas) have been reported to be the most frequently occurring primary brain tumors of dogs.[1,4] More recently, however, meningiomas have been shown to be the most commonly recognized intracranial neoplasms of dogs.[1,2,5,6] This apparent alteration in incidence may be due to use of advanced diagnostic modalities and longer life expectancy of dogs. Primary brain tumors other than meningiomas or gliomas occur infrequently in dogs.[1] While canine brain tumors are usually solitary, multiple primary brain tumors have been seen in dogs and cats. Multiple meningiomas have been reported in cats[7] and dogs,[8,9] and cerebrospinal fluid (CSF) metastases of choroid plexus carcinoma[10] and medulloblastoma[1] have been reported in dogs. Extracranial metastasis of primary brain meningioma has been seen in dogs. Of secondary tumors, local extension of nasal adenocarcinoma, metastases from mammary adenocarcinoma, and extension of pituitary adenoma or carcinoma are seen most commonly.[1] Skull tumors that affect brain by local extension include osteosarcoma and multilobular osteochondrosarcoma.[10a]

Brain tumors occur most frequently in dogs more than 5 years old, with greatest incidence between 6 and 11 years of age, although they may occur at any age.[1,3,9] Tumors of congenital maldevelopment (e.g., craniopharyngioma, teratoma, epidermoid cysts) are seen most frequently in young dogs,[1] and a high incidence of medulloblastomas or ventricular tumors may be seen in young dogs.[1,10b] In one study of 215 brain tumors of dogs, 135 occurred in males and

80 in females; in the same study, females were affected by meningiomas almost twice as often as male dogs (64 females, 39 males).[9] Glial cell tumors and pituitary tumors occur commonly in brachycephalic breeds, whereas meningiomas occur most frequently in dolichocephalic breeds.[1,3,8] Reticulosis or histiocytic lymphoma is seen most frequently in terriers or poodles and other toy breeds.[1]

Brain neoplasms occur less commonly in cats than in dogs. Zaki and Hurvitz reported 87 central nervous system (CNS) neoplasms in 75 of 3915 cats necropsied over a 12-year period.[11] Meningioma was the most frequently reported tumor in this series. Older male cats appear to be most susceptible to meningiomas.[7] There is a high incidence of multiple meningiomas in cats.[7] An unusually high incidence of meningiomas has been reported in cats with mucopolysaccharidosis.[12] Vandevelde reviewed 216 primary brain tumors in cats and found 10 neuroectodermal tumors (including 3 astrocytomas and 3 oligodendrogliomas) and 148 mesenchymal tumors (including 117 meningiomas).[3] It appears that primary brain tumors other than meningiomas are comparatively rare in cats.[11] Ependymoma,[13] astrocytoma,[14,14a] pituitary adenoma,[15,15a] oligodendroglioma,[16,16a] and lymphoma have been reported to occur in the brain of cats.[11] Lymphoma may be primary or secondary, or it may be one aspect of multicentric lymphoma. Metastatic carcinoma has been reported in the brain of cats.[16] There does not appear to be a breed predisposition for the development of intracranial tumors in cats.[17]

PATHOLOGY

Brain tumor classification in dogs and cats has been attempted by numerous authors.[18] A classification based on that of Escourolle and Poirier[19] is often used (Fig. 27-1), but 15% to 20% of animal neuroectodermal tumors (especially gliomas) remain unclassified.[18]

Brain neoplasms may be classified as primary or secondary.[19,20] Primary brain tumors originate from cells normally found within the brain and meninges, including neuroepithelium,[21] lymphoid tissues,[22,22a] germ cells,[23,23a] endothelial cells and malformed tissues. Gliomas include astrocytomas, oligodendrogliomas, choroid plexus papillomas, and ependymomas. Meningiomas are usually benign; however malignant forms

(meningeal sarcoma, malignant meningioma), occasionally with extracranial metastases, have been reported.[8,24] Intracranial lymphoid tumors of dogs generally have been classified under the heading of reticulosis or granulomatous meningoencephalitis (GME) (Fig. 27-2); however some lesions previously classified as reticulosis or GME may in fact be lymphoma.[18,22,25,26] Neoplastic angiotheliomatosis is a rare brain disorder of dogs that appears to be a B-cell lymphoma.[27,27a]

Secondary brain tumors may reach the brain by hematogenous metastasis from distant sites or by local extension from adjacent tissues such as bone or pituitary gland.[19,20] Most pituitary tumors involve the pars distalis; therefore, dorsal growth is generally favored, resulting in diencephalic encroachment and hypothalamic dysfunction.[2]

HISTORY AND CLINICAL SIGNS

The nature and course of neurologic signs resulting from a brain tumor depend on tumor location and extent, and on the rate of growth of the tumor.[18] The typically slow growth of brain tumors permits CNS compensation.[5] Clinical signs may be extremely subtle until such time as decompensation occurs, or until tumor growth leads to secondary effects such as hemorrhage, edema, or herniation.[28] Rapidly growing tumors are usually associated with acute onset of neurologic dysfunction.

The most frequently observed clinical sign associated with a brain neoplasm in a dog or cat is seizures.[18] Other signs are behavioral changes, circling, head pressing, altered states of consciousness, or associated locomotion disturbances.[5] Olfactory lobe tumors of dogs may grow to a large size before causing clinical signs[28a] (Fig. 27-3). Should a neoplasm involve the brain stem, cranial nerve signs may be seen.[28b]

DIAGNOSTIC TECHNIQUES AND WORK-UP

Following complete physical and neurologic examinations, a hemogram, serum chemistry panel, and urinalysis should be done.[18] Further serum biochemical tests may be indicated by the results of these initial studies. For example, should pituitary-dependent hyperadrenocorticism be suspected, an ACTH stimulation test, or dexamethasone suppression test, may be required. Survey radiographs of thorax and abdomen may

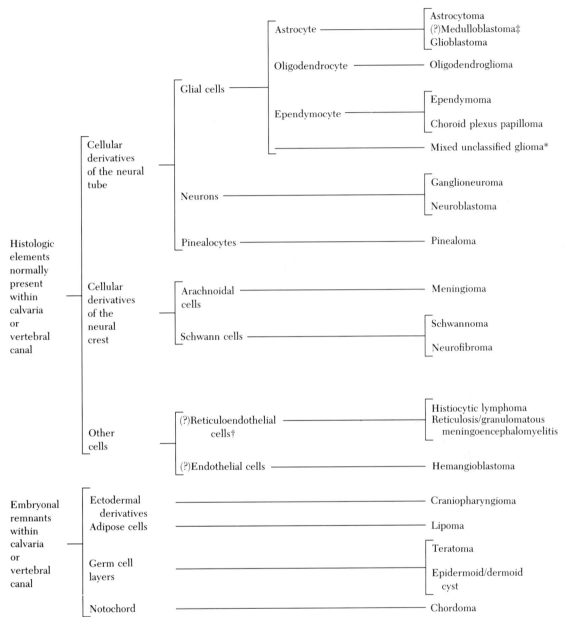

* Up to 20% of all canine glial tumors are composed of variable amounts of astrocytic, oligodendroglial, or ependymal differentiation often with mixtures of poorly differentiated glial cells.[18,21]

† The cells of origin of primary histiocytic lymphoma and reticulosis of the brain are unknown. A resident mononuclear phagocyte population is present in the normal canine brain, and it is suspected that neoplastic transformation of these cells may give rise to a histiocytic tumor or reticulosis.[22]

‡ The neuroglial precursor cell of origin of the medulloblastoma is unknown. Likely candidates are the cells that populate the external granule cell layer of the fetal neonatal cerebellum and the cells of the medullary vela.[1,20,98a]

Fig 27-1. Simplified histologic classification of primary central nervous system tumors of dogs and cats. (Modified from Escourolle R, Poirier J: Manual of Basic Neuropathology, 2nd ed, p 21. Philadelphia, WB Saunders, 1978.[19])

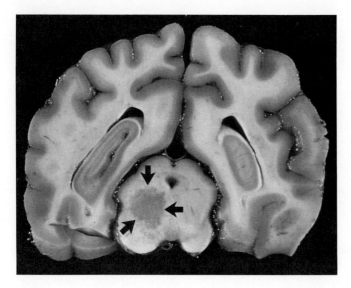

Fig 27-2. Transverse section of the brain of an 8-year-old spayed Airedale terrier at the level of the midbrain. The dog had a 2-month history of progressive loss of balance and a tendency to circle toward the left side. Skull radiographs and CT images of the brain were normal. There is a well-circumscribed space-occupying lesion on the left side of the midbrain and medulla (arrows). The histologic diagnosis was reticulosis.

help to rule out a primary malignancy elsewhere in the body.

Plain skull radiographs are of limited value in the diagnosis of a primary brain neoplasm. Occasionally, lysis or hyperostosis of the skull may accompany a primary brain tumor (e.g., meningioma), or there may be radiographically visible calcification within a neoplasm (Fig. 27-4).[2,5,29] Skull radiographs may be helpful in the detection of primary tumors of the skull or nasal tumors that have invaded the calvaria.

Cerebrospinal fluid collection and analysis are essential for differentiation of neoplastic from non-neoplastic brain diseases.[18] This technique is easily completed while the dog is under anesthesia for other diagnostic studies. Care must be used where increased intracranial pressure is suspected. Pressure measurements are of limited usefulness and are affected by such phenomena as anesthetic agent used and patient positioning. In general, increased CSF pressure and protein content in association with a normal to slightly increased white blood cell count has been considered "typical" of CNS neoplasia.[30,30a] In one study, only 39.6% of dogs with primary brain tumors had "typical" CSF alterations, while 10% had normal CSF protein content, and white blood cell count.[30] The remaining 50.4% of dogs had a variety of CSF alterations.[30] Cerebrospinal fluid from dogs with a meningioma often has a high white blood cell count (>50 cells/µl) with more than 50% being polymorphonuclear cells.[30] Neoplastic cells may be

found in CSF cells, particularly when sedimentation techniques are used in analysis. Little information is available regarding the CSF findings in association with feline brain tumors.[30a] It is assumed that results would be similar to those reported for dogs.

Numerous brain-imaging techniques, such as ventriculography, cerebral angiography, cavernous sinus venography, optic thecography/basal cisternography[31] and scintigraphy, are available for use in dogs and cats.[32,33] Each of these techniques has advantages in specific instances (e.g., optic thecography for diagnosis of a large pituitary neoplasm); however, each has pronounced limitations. The major disadvantage of these techniques is that while they may confirm the presence of a space-occupying lesion, they fail in most instances to define exactly the location and extent of a neoplasm and its relationship to surrounding normal structures. This information is essential for precise treatment planning of surgery or radiotherapy. Computed tomography (CT)[10,16,34,35] and magnetic resonance imaging (MRI)[1] permit precise localization of intracranial neoplasia in dogs and cats and have largely replaced the other techniques. Preliminary data suggest MRI may have some advantages over CT in imaging of the caudal fossa of dogs.[1,36]

While the major tumor types in dogs are reported to have characteristic CT features,[37] it must be remembered that non-neoplastic space-occupying lesions may mimic the CT appear-

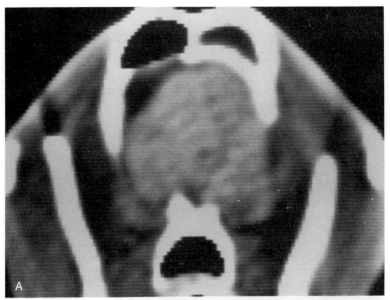

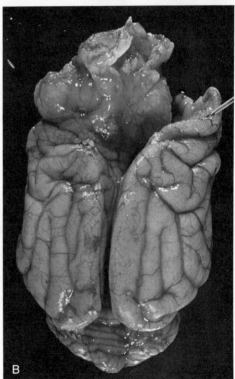

Fig 27-3. (*A*) Transverse postcontrast CT image of the head of a 9-year-old spayed Shetland sheepdog with a history of six seizures that had occurred during the previous 4 months. The image is at the level of the frontal sinuses. There is a large space-occupying lesion that obliterates the frontal lobes of the cerebrum and extends laterally to erode the frontal bone of the skull. The histologic diagnosis was malignant meningioma. (*B*) Dorsal view of the brain of the dog in *A*. A large malignant meningioma is seen arising from the left frontal lobe of the cerebrum. Although this tumor has grown to a large size in this location, clinical signs were mild.

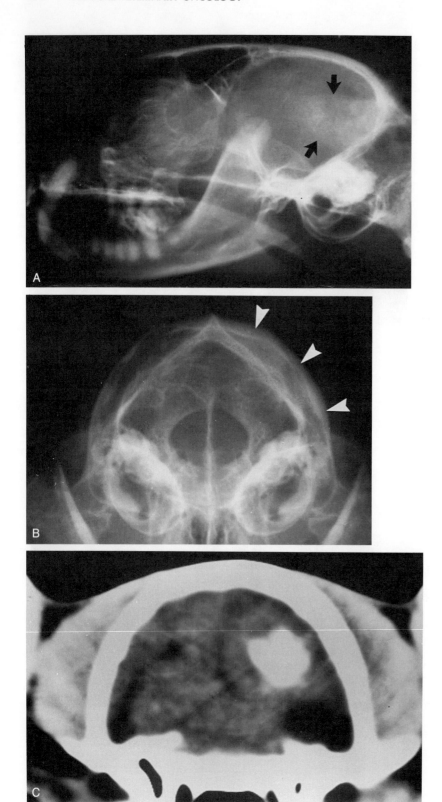

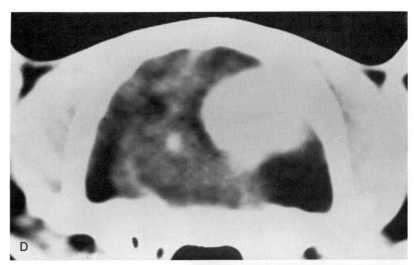

Fig 27-4. (*A*) Lateral radiograph of the skull of an 8-year-old castrated domestic shorthair cat. The cat had a 2-month history of abnormal behavior that consisted of vocalizing and hiding from its owner. The cat had a tendency to circle toward its left side. Note the region of mineralization within the cranial vault (arrows). (*B*) Rostrocaudal projection of the cranial vault of the cat in *A*. Note the mineralized opacity in the region of the left parietal bone and the increased thickness of the left parietal bone. (*C*) Transverse precontrast CT image of the head of the cat in *A*. Note the focal area of calcification within the left occipital lobe of the cerebrum. (*D*) Transverse postcontrast CT image of the head of the cat in *A* at a similar level to the CT image in *C*. There is a well-demarcated region of uniform contrast uptake in the region of the focal area of calcification that was seen in the precontrast image. In addition, there are areas of lucency around the periphery of the enhanced region that are consistent with peritumoral edema. The contrast enhancement pattern is typical of that seen with meningioma. (*E*) Dorsal view of the brain of the cat in *A*. There is a large space-occupying lesion in the left occipital lobe of the cerebrum. The histologic diagnosis was meningioma. (Photographs courtesy of Dr. Allen F. Sisson.)

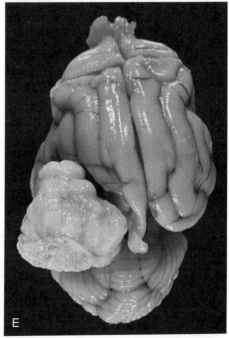

ance of a neoplasm (Fig. 27-5) and that occasionally a metastasis may have a similar CT appearance to a primary brain tumor (Fig. 27-6). Therefore, biopsy is necessary for definitive diagnosis of intracranial neoplasia; ideally, intracranial lesions should be biopsied prior to therapy.[32,38]

THERAPY

The major goals of therapy for a brain tumor are to control secondary tumor effects such as edema or elevated intracranial pressure, and to eradicate the tumor or to decrease its size.[32] Beyond general efforts to maintain homeostasis, palliative therapy of dogs or cats with a brain tumor consists of corticosteroids for reduction of peritumoral edema and, in some cases, tumor growth. Certain animals may show dramatic improvement for several weeks or months with only corticosteroid therapy. Dexamethasone may be administered intravenously during acute episodes of decompensation. Prednisone or prednisolone may be given orally over a prolonged

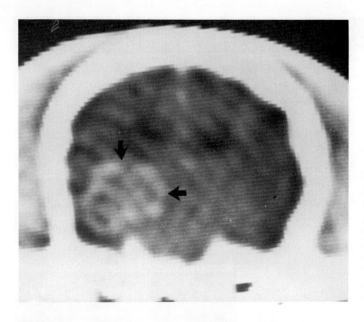

Fig 27-5. Transverse postcontrast CT image of the head of a 6-year-old cocker spaniel dog at the level of the thalamus. Note the well-circumscribed space-occupying lesion to the left of the thalamus (arrows). This lesion has many of the characteristics of a primary brain tumor; however, it was confirmed to be an encapsulated hematoma following surgical removal.

time period. Corticosteroid therapy may be combined with anticonvulsant medications should seizures be a problem. Phenobarbital is the drug best suited for control of seizures.

Eradication or reduction in size of a neoplasm is the primary consideration for the long-term survival of an animal with a brain tumor.[32] There are four major treatment methods, used either alone or in combination, for this purpose: surgery, radiation therapy, chemotherapy, and im-munotherapy (or biologic response modification). At this time, only surgery and radiation therapy have been used extensively in dogs or cats with an intracranial neoplasm.

Surgery

Before the widespread use of CT, only superficial meningiomas or bony lesions that compressed the brain were removed by surgery. With the precise information regarding location and ex-

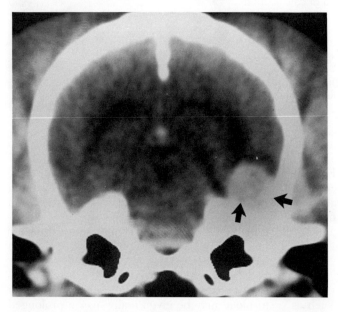

Fig 27-6. Transverse postcontrast CT image of the head of a 12-year-old spayed miniature schnauzer dog. The image is at the level of the tympanic cavities The dog had a history of seizures. There is a well-circumscribed, uniformly enhancing space-occupying lesion located superficially in the right temporal lobe of the cerebrum (arrows). The lesion has a broad meningeal attachment and has all the CT characteristics of a meningioma. The tumor was removed surgically and the histologic diagnosis was metastatic chemodectoma. The dog died 7 months following surgery at which time chemodectoma and hemangiosarcoma metastases were found in all organs examined except the brain, which was free of tumor.

tent of a neoplasm available by means of CT, and the development of advanced neurosurgical and anesthetic techniques, surgical therapy has been more widely used. Neurosurgical intervention is currently an essential consideration in the management of intracranial neoplasia, whether for complete excision, partial removal (debulking or cytoreduction), or biopsy (Fig. 27-7).[32] It must be remembered, however, that the small brain size of dogs and cats, combined with the limited access of veterinary neurosurgeons to advanced equipment, such as an operating microscope, intraoperative ultrasound, ultrasonic aspirator, and carbon dioxide laser, make such techniques difficult in these species.

The possibility of complete removal of a brain tumor is limited by the location and invasiveness of the lesion. Meningiomas, particularly those located over the cerebral convexities or in the frontal lobes of the cerebrum, often may be completely and uneventfully removed with surgery,[16,29] whereas surgical removal of a meningioma located in the caudal fossa may be accompanied by significant morbidity. Partial removal of a brain tumor may relieve signs associated with the tumor and decrease tumor size before other modes of therapy are attempted. Cytoreduction must, however, be approached with caution because "seeding" of a tumor through CSF pathways may result. Malignant brain tumors often are located deep within the brain

and seldom can be completely excised (Fig. 27-8). In such cases, surgical biopsy may precede other therapies, such as irradiation. Although surgical biopsy of a brain tumor is recommended prior to radiation therapy or other treatment modalities, practical considerations such as cost and morbidity may preclude it. The development of CT-guided stereotactic biopsy procedures for use in dogs and cats in the future may allow pretreatment biopsy to be done with little risk to the animal.[39]

Radiation Therapy

Irradiation is indicated for therapy of most primary brain tumors of dogs and cats.[32,40–42] It is used either alone or following surgical intervention (Fig. 27-9).[43] Radiation therapy is also indicated for secondary brain tumors. Both metastases and pituitary macroadenomas and carcinomas have been successfully managed by means of irradiation.[43a] Lymphoma and reticulosis of the brain may also be sensitive to radiation therapy.

External beam, megavoltage irradiation is currently being used for treatment of brain tumors in dogs and cats.[32,40–42] At this time few data exist regarding optimal total dose and number of fractions that should be given and time over which radiation therapy should extend.[32] The total dose currently used at Colorado State University is 45 Gy given in 15 equal

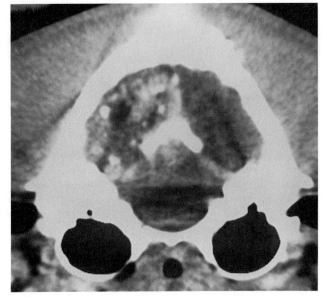

Fig 27-7. Transverse postcontrast CT image of the head of a 9-year-old castrated black Labrador retriever dog. The image is at the level of the tympanic cavities. The dog had a history of generalized seizures, blindness in the right eye, and mild right-sided postural reaction deficits. Note the irregularly enhancing space-occupying lesion in the left occipital lobe of the cerebrum. There are areas of calcification within the lesion. The tumor was partially excised surgically by means of lateral craniotomy. Surgery was followed by irradiation of the brain (45 Gy in 15 fractions over 3 weeks). The dog is alive 1 year following completion of therapy, and clinical signs other than infrequent seizures have resolved. The histologic diagnosis was chondrosarcoma.

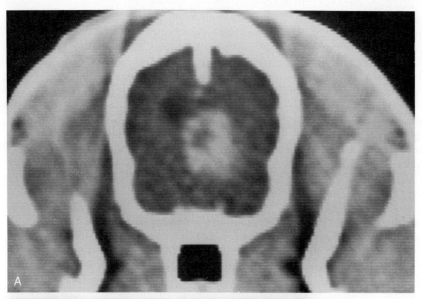

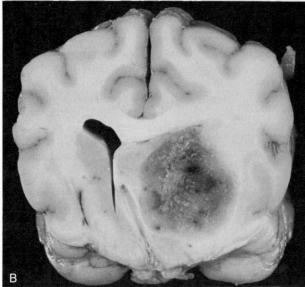

Fig 27-8. (A) Transverse postcontrast CT image of the head of a 12-year-old spayed boxer dog. The dog had a 3-week history of depression and anorexia. The image is at the level of the rostral thalamus. Note the enhancing space-occupying lesion to the right of the midline in the region of the thalamus. The mass is obliterating the right lateral ventricle. Histololgic diagnosis was glio-blastoma multiforme. (B) Transverse section of the brain of the dog in A at a level similar to that of the CT image. Note the malignant glioma that has expanded to displace the midline toward the left side.

fractions over 3 weeks. Interstitial radiation therapy also has been attempted in dogs; however, insufficient data exist to determine the role of this type of therapy.[1]

Chemotherapy

Factors that must be considered in the use of chemotherapeutic agents for treatment of a brain tumor include the possibility that the blood–brain barrier may prevent exposure of a tumor to a drug injected parenterally, and tumor cell heterogeneity, which means that only certain cells are sensitive to a given agent.[44,45] Several chemotherapeutic agents have been used in treating malignant gliomas of people.[44,45] As single agents, BCNU, CCNU (a lipid-soluble nitrosurea), and procarbazine (a monoamine oxidase inhibitor) have been shown to modestly increase patient survival in randomized clinical trials in people. BCNU is currently under in-

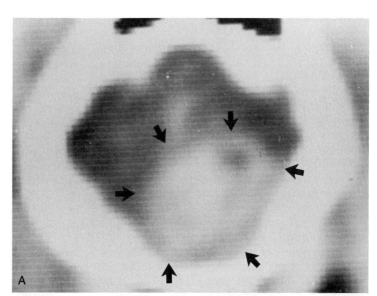

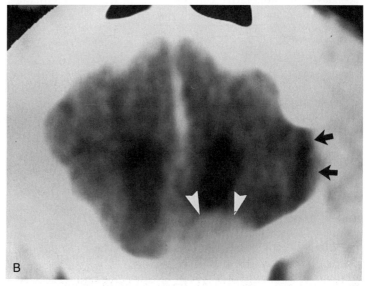

Fig 27-9. (*A*) Transverse postcontrast CT image of the head of a 13-year-old spayed miniature poodle dog at the level of the frontal lobes of the cerebrum. The dog had a history of seizures. There is a large space-occupying lesion to the right of midline (arrows). (*B*) Transverse postcontrast CT image of the head of the dog in *A* completed 436 days after partial surgical removal of the space-occupying lesion and post-surgical irradiation (4000 Gy in 10 fractions over 22 days). The diagnosis was meningioma. Note the craniotomy site in the right frontal bone (black arrows). There is apparent recurrence of the tumor on the floor of the calvaria (white arrows). The dog was reoperated and meningioma was removed from this site. The dog was free of signs 2 years after the second surgery.

vestigation for use in dogs with cerebral neoplasia. As a treatment modality for brain tumors, chemotherapy should be considered palliative only.[44,45]

Immunotherapy

Immunotherapy involves modification of the immune response of a patient so that a tumor may be eliminated immunologically.[46,47] Numerous immunotherapy approaches have been attempted in people with malignant gliomas; however, to date these studies have failed to

show increased survival in treated patients compared to a control group.[46,47]

Recently attempts have been made in dogs with a malignant glioma to mobilize cell-mediated immunity against a tumor by culturing autologous lymphocytes to increase their numbers and cytotoxic effectiveness and then returning these cells to the tumor bed after tumor cytoreduction.[48] In the future, immunotherapy, either alone or as an adjunct to other treatments, may improve survival of dogs and cats with a brain tumor.

PROGNOSIS

Few data exist concerning survival times of dogs or cats with a brain tumor that have received only palliative therapy. Results of one study indicate a mean and median survival time of 81 days and 56 days, respectively, following CT diagnosis of a brain tumor in each of eight dogs.[41] Six of the eight dogs died within 64 days of brain tumor diagnosis.[41] However, the range of survival times in this group of dogs was 10 to 307 days, indicating that occasionally a dog may survive for many months in the absence of specific antitumor therapy.[41]

There are several reports of successful surgical removal of a primary brain tumor in dogs.[43,49] A recent report of four dogs with an olfactory lobe meningioma that was surgically removed indicated postoperative survival times of 63 to 203 days.[49] Postoperative complications in this group of dogs included seizures, infection, and bronchopneumonia.[49]

Survival data for cats that have received only palliative therapy for an intracranial neoplasm do not exist. It does appear, however, that solitary superficial meningiomas in cats are amenable to surgical removal and that many cats so treated may be expected to survive for several years.[29,50,50a]

Radiation therapy has been used in both dogs and cats, either alone or in combination with surgery, for treatment of primary brain tumors.[40–43] Preliminary results suggest that the prognosis for dogs or cats with a brain tumor can be greatly improved by radiation therapy following surgical removal of a tumor, or by radiation therapy alone. In one study, mean survival time for 16 dogs that received only irradiation for a meningioma was 233 days, and for 10 dogs with a glioma, was 176 days.[42] In another study, 5 dogs that received radiation therapy alone survived from 159 to 751 days following completion of therapy.[40] Effects of radiation on a brain tumor include decrease in tumor size and better definition of tumor margins.[40,41] Adverse effects of radiation therapy for a brain tumor occur infrequently in dogs and cats.[40]

COMPARATIVE ASPECTS

The average annual incidence of primary intracranial tumors in humans is 9.2 per 100,000 adult human beings.[51] Incidence increases with age. The incidence of brain tumors is bimodal, with an early peak in childhood, and a later and broader peak covering the fifth, sixth, and seventh decades. Males are more often affected than females.[51] Almost half of the intracranial tumors in adults are gliomas; glioblastomas, representing 25%, are the most common type of tumor.[51] In children, cerebellar astrocytomas and ventricular ependymomas predominate.[51]

Morbidity and mortality associated with brain tumors in humans vary with histologic type. Only 10% of patients with malignant astrocytoma or glioblastoma multiforme are alive 18 to 24 months following therapy, regardless of the type of therapy used.[51] Some combination of surgery and irradiation is required to achieve 50% to 70% 5-year survival rates in virtually all adult cases of low-grade astrocytoma, oligodendroglioma, or ependymoma.[51] Approximately 80% of patients are free of recurrence at 5 years after excision of a meningioma, and 50% are free of tumor at 20 years after operation.[52] The only factor significantly associated with recurrence-free survival following resection of a meningioma is the completeness of surgical excision.[51] Radiation therapy is successful in improving survival of patients that have had incomplete surgical excision of a meningioma.[53,54]

SPINAL CORD NEOPLASIA

INCIDENCE AND RISK FACTORS

Tumors affecting the spinal cord may be considered as extradural, intradural-extramedullary, or intramedullary.[2] Extradural neoplasms comprise approximately 50% of all spinal neoplasms, while intradural-extramedullary tumors and intramedullary tumors comprise 35% and 15%, respectively.[2] Reported series are not large enough to yield reliable data concerning age, breed, or sex predilections.[55] In one study 8 of 29 dogs or cats (27.6%) were 3 years of age or less, and 90% of tumors occurred in large breeds of dogs.[20,56] It appears, however, that primary spinal cord neoplasms occur infrequently in dogs. Meningiomas appear to be the most frequently diagnosed primary spinal neoplasm of dogs.[55] Such tumors appear to have a high incidence in the cervical spinal cord.[55] A primary spinal cord neoplasm with a high incidence in young dogs (6 months to 3 years of age) is neuroepithelioma.[57,57a,58,58a] With the exception of lymphoma, spinal cord neoplasms rarely have been reported in cats.[20]

Etiologic factors of spinal tumors are poorly defined in cats and dogs. In cats, feline leukemia virus is frequently associated with lymphoma and therefore must be considered a risk factor in the development of spinal lymphoma.[59] However, a cat with spinal lymphoma may test negative for the feline leukemia virus.[59]

PATHOLOGY

Histologic classification of spinal cord neoplasms is similar to that used for brain neoplasms (Fig. 27-1).[56,60] In dogs, the most frequently reported extradural tumors are primary bone tumors.[56,60] The most frequently reported primary vertebral neoplasm is osteosarcoma (Fig. 27-10); however, chondrosarcoma, hemangiosarcoma, fibrosarcoma, and multiple myeloma also have been seen.[61] There are reports of secondary vertebral tumors causing spinal cord compression in dogs.[56,60] The most frequently reported secondary tumor in one series was metastatic carcinoma.[61] Extradural lymphoma and lipomas of dogs have also been described.[1]

Meningiomas and peripheral nerve sheath tumors are the most commonly occurring intra-dural-extramedullary neoplasms of dogs.[55] These tumors are reported to occur most frequently in older dogs of either sex.[55] A less common intradural-extramedullary spinal cord neoplasm is neuroepithelioma, also classified by several authors as ependymoma, nephroblastoma, and medullary epithelioma.[57,57a,58,58a] This neoplasm occurs in young dogs, usually between T10 and L2 spinal cord segments.[57,58]

Intramedullary spinal tumors of dogs occur rarely.[1] They are predominantly of glial cell origin, and astrocytoma, lymphoma, and ependymoma have been reported.[1]

Primary spinal cord neoplasms other than lymphoma are extremely rare in cats.[1,62] Lymphoma, however, occurs commonly in cats, most frequently in an extradural location.[59] Occasionally, lymphoma may invade the spinal cord parenchyma.

HISTORY AND CLINICAL SIGNS

Extramedullary spinal neoplasms typically are slow growing and result in gradual spinal cord compression. Signs of spinal cord dysfunction usually worsen over weeks or months. Occasionally, an acute onset of signs may accompany hemorrhage or ischemia associated with a neoplasm. Intramedullary tumors may grow more

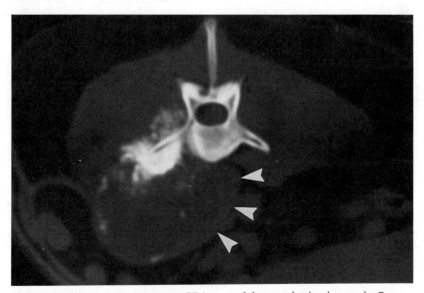

Fig 27-10. Transverse precontrast CT image of the vertebral column of a 7-year-old spayed Australian shepherd dog at the level of the L4 vertebra. There is a large tumor arising from the right transverse process of the L4 vertebra. The tumor involves the body of this vertebra. Note the soft tissue mass crossing the midline ventrally (arrows). The histologic diagnosis was osteosarcoma.

rapidly and are characterized by a higher incidence of ischemia, necrosis, and hemorrhage.

Clinical signs seen in association with a spinal cord tumor usually reflect the location of the neoplasm and are often indistinguishable from signs caused by other transverse myelopathies at the same location.[60] The presence of certain signs should cause suspicion of a spinal cord neoplasm. Extradural tumors may involve meninges, spinal nerves, or nerve roots, resulting in discomfort that may progress to extreme spinal hyperesthesia.[60] Neurologic deficits (e.g., paresis) may not be seen initially and, when present, may be intermittent (i.e., worsen with exercise). There is usually a progressive worsening of neurologic function caudal to the lesion. Intradural-extramedullary tumors may also result in prolonged, intermittent expression of clinical signs and hyperesthesia; however, the signs may be alleviated by exercise.[55] Brachial or lumbar intumescence involvement may be evidenced by lameness, holding up of a limb, neurogenic muscular atrophy, and depressed spinal reflexes. Rarely unilateral spinal cord compression may cause deficits in the contralateral limb. In contrast, intramedullary spinal cord tumors usually cause rapid progression of neurologic dysfunction.[56] Hyperesthesia is rarely associated with such tumors.[63]

DIAGNOSTIC TECHNIQUES AND WORK-UP

Diagnosis of a neoplasm affecting the spinal cord requires a systematic approach. The procedure is based on collection and interpretation of a minimum data base that includes appropriate serologic tests (hemogram, biochemical profile) and thoracic radiographs for primary or metastatic neoplasia.[18] Following this, survey spinal radiographs, CSF collection and analysis, and myelography may be completed during a single period of anesthesia.[18]

General anesthesia permits accurate positioning of a dog or cat for survey radiographs of the vertebral column and allows stressed or oblique views to be done.[18] Either primary or secondary vertebral tumors may produce bone lysis or new bone production or both.[2] The vertebral body and arch are more frequently involved than the dorsal spinous process or transverse processes. Plain radiographic abnormalities are uncommon with primary nervous system neoplasms.[2,55] Expansion of a spinal tumor may result in enlarge-

ment of an intervertebral foramen, widening of the vertebral canal, or thinning of surrounding bone (Fig. 27-11).[2]

Cerebrospinal fluid collection and analysis are indicated when plain radiographs do not provide a complete diagnosis. A lumbar puncture is recommended for CSF collection, and the needle may be left in place for myelography, pending results of cytologic examination of CSF. Alterations in CSF caused by spinal tumors should be interpreted according to the same criteria discussed for brain tumor diagnosis;[30] however, it must be remembered that the protein content of CSF collected from a lumbar location is normally higher than that of CSF collected from the cerebellomedullary cistern.[64] Lymphosarcoma affecting the spinal cord often results in a high white cell count, predominantly abnormal lymphocytes.

Myelography is essential for the accurate determination of location and extent of a spinal cord neoplasm.[18] Tumors may be classified as extradural (Fig. 27-12), intradural-extramedullary (Fig. 27-13) or intramedullary (Fig. 27-14) on the basis of myelography results, although this distinction cannot always be made. For example, occasionally it is not possible to distinguish between an intramedullary and an intradural-extramedullary lesion on the basis of myelographic findings.[55] In such cases, CT or MRI may provide more exact localizing information.

TREATMENT

A limited number of therapeutic options exist for a dog or cat with a spinal cord neoplasm.[65] Appropriate therapy depends on tumor location, extent, and histologic type. An immediate goal of therapy is to relieve the deleterious effects of sustained spinal cord compression. This may be achieved medically (e.g., glucocorticoids) or surgically. Surgical management may permit complete removal or cytoreduction and biopsy of a neoplasm.[55] In cases where complete removal is not possible, recurrence is to be expected, and adjunctive therapy such as irradiation is recommended. Currently, intramedullary neoplasms are not resectable.[65]

Accurate biopsy diagnosis of lymphoma is essential because lymphoma of the spinal cord may be treated successfully with irradiation alone or with intrathecal chemotherapy and craniospinal irradiation in combination.[66] In cer-

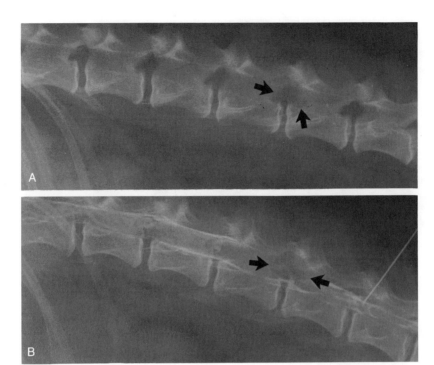

Fig 27-11. (A) Lateral radiograph of the lumbar vertebral column of a 10-year-old spayed Australian shepherd dog with a 3-week history of progressive lameness in the left pelvic limb. Severe atrophy of the left quadriceps muscle was seen in association with an absent left patellar reflex. A diagnosis of left femoral neuropathy was made. Note the lysis surrounding the L4–5 intervertebral foramen (arrows). (B) Myelogram of the lumbar vertebral column of the dog in A. There is a filling defect at the level of the L4–5 intervertebral foramen consistent with a space-occupying lesion (arrows). The histologic diagnosis was schwannoma. Note the positioning of the spinal needle for CSF collection and injection of contrast material.

tain cases, radiation therapy may be done prior to chemotherapy in order to effect a rapid reduction in tumor mass.[66]

PROGNOSIS

Few cases with long-term follow-up exist in the veterinary literature.[65] The prognosis depends on resectability, histologic type, location, and severity of clinical signs. Generally, dogs or cats with an extradural metastatic neoplasm or vertebral neoplasm have a poor prognosis, and palliative therapy only is attempted.[65] Occasionally, intradural-extramedullary tumors may be completely resected, and in such cases the prognosis must be considered good. In one study, 5 of 13 dogs survived for longer than 6 months following surgical resection of a meningioma.[55] One of the 5 dogs that survived was

alive 5 years after surgery.[55] Few data exist regarding irradiation or chemotherapy of spinal cord neoplasms; however, such therapies should be considered.

COMPARATIVE ASPECTS

Intradural spinal cord tumors are uncommon in humans; their incidence is from 3 to 10 per 100,000 population.[67] The ratio of intradural to extradural tumors is approximately 3 to 2. These tumors occur predominantly in the middle decades of life, and except for an unusually high incidence of meningiomas in females, the sex incidence is about equal. Of the intradural-extramedullary tumors, peripheral nerve sheath neoplasms comprise about 30%, and meningiomas comprise about 25%. Astrocytoma and ependymoma, each with a similar incidence, are

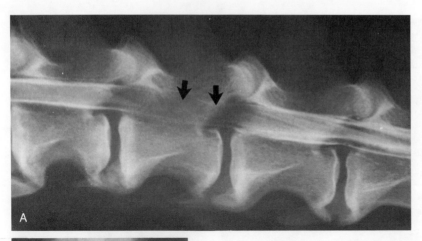

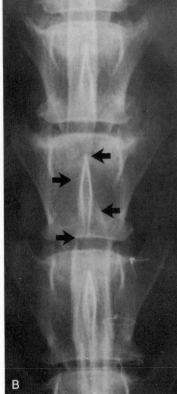

Fig 27-12. Lateral (*A*) and ventrodorsal (*B*) myelogram of the midlumbar region of the vertebral column of a 12-year-old spayed Bouvier des Flandres dog with progressive paraparesis that had started 72 hours previously. Noncontrast vertebral radiographs were normal. There is a severe extradural spinal cord compression centered over the body of L4 vertebra. The spinal cord is severely compressed from the dorsal direction and from the left and right sides (arrows). The histologic diagnosis was metastatic thyroid carcinoma within the L4 vertebra.

the most common intramedullary tumors. A high percentage (approximately 90%) of all intradural spinal cord tumors in humans are benign and potentially resectable.[67] Therefore, in contrast to animals, humans have an excellent outlook following surgical therapy.

In humans, the majority of extradural spinal cord tumors are metastases.[67] Approximately 5%

of cancer patients develop spinal epidural tumors, although not all of these become clinically evident. Primary CNS tumors such as neurofibromas or meningiomas occasionally may be limited to the extradural space. The prognosis for humans with extradural spinal neoplasms depends on the histologic type, rate of onset, and severity of symptoms. A correlation between

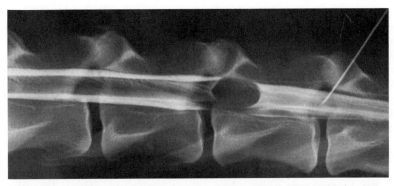

Fig 27-13. Lateral myelogram of the lumbar region of the vertebral column of a 10-year-old spayed Labrador retriever dog. The dog had progressive paraparesis of several months' duration. Noncontrast vertebral radiographs were normal. Note the well-defined intradural-extramedullary lesion at the level of L5–6 vertebrae. The mass was removed surgically and the histologic diagnosis was meningioma. The dog made a complete recovery and was normal 6 months following surgery.

pretreatment motor status and functional outcome emphasizes the value of early diagnosis and treatment of such neoplasms. In humans, palliation is the goal in the management of patients with spinal metastasis. Radiation therapy and surgical decompression individually or in combination may be used for this purpose.[67]

TUMORS OF PERIPHERAL NERVES

INCIDENCE AND RISK FACTORS

Primary neoplasms of peripheral nerves occur relatively infrequently in domestic animals, al-though they have been reported in dogs, cats, cattle, horses, goats, sheep, and pigs.[68,69] Primary tumors of cranial and spinal nerves and nerve roots are common in dogs. Peripheral nerve sheath tumors represented 26.6% of canine nervous system tumors in one report.[4] Neurofibromatosis has been reported in dogs.[70] Of 60 schwannomas of dogs of 23 breeds reported in one study, 4 involved cranial, 39 involved spinal, and 17 involved peripheral nerves.[9] The age distribution was from 2 to 17 years, with 43 tumors occurring between 5 and 12 years of age.[9] Forty-two dogs were males and 18 were females.[9] In the same study, 4 dogs with intraparenchymal schwannomas (1 brain, 3 spinal

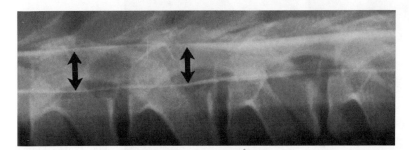

Fig 27-14. Lateral myelogram of the thoracic vertebral column of a 3-year-old spayed Labrador retriever dog with progressive paraparesis of 6 months' duration. Plain radiographs of this region were normal. The lateral myelogram outlined an expansile intramedullary lesion at the level of T5–6 vertebrae (arrows). The dog's signs continued to worsen, and 2 months following this study, the dog was euthanatized. An astrocytoma of the spinal cord was confirmed at the level of the T5–6 vertebrae.

cord) were reported.[9] Primary nerve sheath neoplasms appear to be extremely rare in cats. A solitary nerve sheath tumor has been described in the skin of a cat and a thoracic vertebra of a cat.[11] Neurofibromatosis has not been reported in cats.

Neuronal or nerve cell tumors arise most frequently from the sympathetic and paraganglionic components of the autonomic nervous system. Those arising from the sympathoblasts of the sympathetic system are neuroblastomas, while the paraganglionic system gives rise to paragangliomas, the best known being pheochromocytoma and chemodectoma.[71] Such tumors occur infrequently in dogs and cats.

Of secondary tumors that involve the cranial and spinal nerves and nerve roots of dogs or cats, lymphoma is the most common. It has been reported frequently in cats (Fig. 27-15).[11,22,72–74]

PATHOLOGY AND NATURAL BEHAVIOR

Primary peripheral nerve tumors may affect cranial nerves, peripheral nerves, sympathetic nerves and ganglia, and adrenal gland nerves. Most tumors of peripheral nerves, excluding those of the sympathetic nervous system, result from neoplastic transformation (usually benign) of periaxonal Schwann cells (Fig. 27-1). Such

tumors are called schwannomas.[75] They have also been called neurinomas or neurilemmomas because they arise in a nerve or nerve sheath. The terms neurofibroma or neurofibrosarcoma have been used to describe tumors thought to be derived from endo- or epineurally located fibroblasts within the nerve sheath. Peripheral nerve sheath tumors have also been called perineural fibroblastomas based on a theory that they arise from perineural fibroblasts.[75] Other less frequently used terms include Schwann cell tumor, lemmoma, and lemnocytoma.[76]

Classification of neural sheath tumors has been widely disputed.[18,20,77,78] A controversy concerning nomenclature hinges on whether such tumors arise from Schwann cells, which produce myelin, or the fibroblasts that are responsible for producing the endo-, peri-, and epineurium. The most reliable classification is based on a combination of ultrastructural features and immunocytochemical demonstration of cell-specific marker proteins.[76] On this basis, evidence has not been found for an endo-, peri-, or epineural derivation of nerve sheath tumors;[76] therefore it is recommended that peripheral nerve tumors be called schwannomas[79] or nerve sheath tumors[80] and that other terms be discarded. Results of tissue culture studies of nerve sheath tumors also accord with the notion that nerve sheath tumors are derived from Schwann

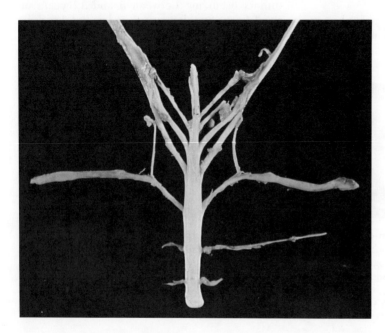

Fig. 27-15. Dorsal view of the lumbosacral plexus of a 7-year-old spayed domestic shorthair cat with a chronic history of progressive paraparesis. Note thickening of multiple nerve roots and peripheral nerves that has resulted from infiltration by lymphoma.

cells.[81] It has been suggested that the term neurofibroma be retained to describe a schwannoma without a capsule;[68] however, this classification may cause confusion if it is used for animals.

For each benign form of peripheral nerve tumor, there is a corresponding rare but distinct malignant form in which the cells of origin become anaplastic and on occasion may invade neighboring structures or metastasize.[80] Invasion and metastases are most common in tumors of the sympathetic nervous system.[80] Malignant neural sheath tumors, which are infrequent, are characterized by mitosis, cellularity, anaplasia, and rarely metastases to lymph nodes or lungs.[79]

Peripheral nerve sheath tumors of dogs most frequently occur in the brachial plexus nerves (C6–T2), although other nerves are occasionally affected.[20] Secondary extension by means of nerve roots into the spinal canal may result in spinal cord compression.[20] These tumors also commonly affect cranial nerves;[5,78] the vestibulocochlear nerve is frequently affected.[82] Occasionally the trigeminal nerve, oculomotor nerve, or other cranial nerves may be affected. Schwannomas occur as nodular or varicose thickenings of large nerves and usually are firm, white to gray in color, and well circumscribed (Fig. 27-16).

The granular cell myoblastoma has been described in peripheral nerves as a growth of Schwann cells.[18,83] It is not clear whether this tumor is a true neoplasm or a lipid disturbance of Schwann cells. Such tumors have been reported to occur in the tongue of dogs; they may also occur within the CNS as primary tumors.[18]

HISTORY AND CLINICAL SIGNS

Signs of peripheral nerve neoplasia reflect the location of the neoplasm, which may involve a single cranial or peripheral nerve, spinal nerve or nerve root, several cranial or peripheral nerves, a plexus, or multiple spinal nerves or nerve roots. Peripheral nerve neoplasms are slow growing, and signs usually progress over weeks to months. Occasionally, signs may develop rapidly.

The brachial plexus, or C6 through T2 spinal nerves and nerve roots, are the most common sites for peripheral nerve sheath tumors.[84] This tumor always should be suspected in adult dogs with unilateral thoracic limb lameness of obscure cause.[18] With progression of the neoplasm, paresis of the affected limb and atrophy of muscles innervated by the involved nerves may develop. An animal may hold the limb off the ground. Passive movement of the limb or neck may cause apparent pain to the animal, and a pain response may be elicited by deep palpation cranial to the first rib. Occasionally, a palpable enlargement of a nerve or plexus is apparent. Ipsilateral *Horner's* syndrome, either partial (miosis only) or complete (miosis, ptosis, enophthalmos, third eyelid prolapse), may occur where the T1 or T2 nerve roots are involved.[85] Ipsilateral loss of the

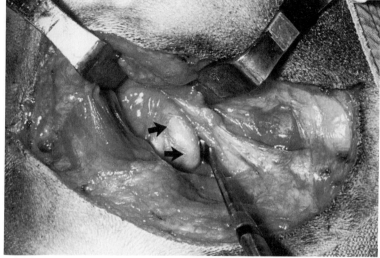

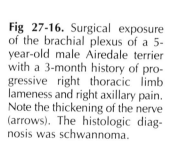

Fig 27-16. Surgical exposure of the brachial plexus of a 5-year-old male Airedale terrier with a 3-month history of progressive right thoracic limb lameness and right axillary pain. Note the thickening of the nerve (arrows). The histologic diagnosis was schwannoma.

panniculus reflex may also be detected. Occasionally, a brachial plexus schwannoma may extend proximally through an intervertebral foramen to compress the spinal cord.[68,86] Signs of spinal cord involvement usually follow a chronic period of forelimb lameness and progressive muscle atrophy, although occasionally they may precede or occur concurrently with forelimb lameness or atrophy.[18] The myelopathy usually results in asymmetric pelvic limb paresis. The contralateral forelimb may or may not be affected.

Schwannomas of the lumbosacral plexus most often cause progressive lameness of a single pelvic limb.[18] Progression of signs is similar to that described for a schwannoma of the brachial plexus; however, apparent pain is less consistently seen in association with lumbosacral plexus nerve sheath neoplasms. Urinary or fecal incontinence may be present in those cases where a schwannoma invades the spinal canal. Contralateral limb involvement may also be seen late in the course of the disease.

Involvement by a schwannoma of a solitary nerve root, spinal nerve, or cranial nerve results in neurologic deficits that reflect the nervous system structure involved. Should a schwannoma of a nerve root or spinal nerve extend proximally to involve the spinal cord, then myelopathy may be the only sign.

Lymphoma affecting the peripheral nervous system may be indistinguishable from schwannoma on the basis of clinical signs.

DIAGNOSTIC TECHNIQUES AND WORK-UP

A neoplasm affecting a peripheral nerve should be suspected when a complete physical and neurologic examination reveals the signs described in the previous section.[18] Single limb paresis and muscle atrophy in association with apparent pain on manipulation of the affected limb are the most commonly recognized signs of plexus neoplasms.

Electrophysiologic testing may define the location and extent of peripheral nerve involvement.[18] Electromyography (EMG) may distinguish between atrophy resulting from disuse or denervation, or may confirm involvement of muscles not yet atrophied. EMG of the entire animal may be completed to detect more widespread neuromuscular involvement. Determinations of motor and sensory nerve conduction velocity may also provide information regarding nerve involvement. Evoked spinal cord potentials in combination with these determinations may be used to provide functional evidence of sensory nerve fiber connections with the spinal cord.[85,87]

Mapping of atrophied muscles and regions of decreased cutaneous sensation of an affected limb may help to localize a peripheral nerve sheath neoplasm to a specific sensory or motor nerve, to a plexus, or to a group of spinal nerves or nerve roots.[85]

Plain radiographs of the vertebral column, CSF analysis, and myelography are essential in cases where secondary spinal cord involvement is suspected. The most frequently observed plain radiographic abnormality seen with a schwannoma is widening of an intervertebral foramen due to bone remodeling around an enlarged nerve root (Fig. 27-11),[68] although plain radiographs are frequently normal.[84] Lymphoma does not result in alterations visible on plain spinal radiographs. Myelography is essential in cases where neoplasia of spinal nerves or nerve roots is suspected in order to detect invasion of the vertebral canal that may not be clinically apparent. At the time a myelogram is done, CSF collection and analysis may be completed; however, CSF analysis rarely aids in more definitive diagnosis. The most commonly observed CSF alteration is an elevation in protein content in the absence of a cellular response.

Surgical exploration for biopsy of a cranial or peripheral nerve, nerve root, or plexus is essential for diagnosis. In some cases, this may be the only way to confirm the presence of a neoplasm.

THERAPY

Presently, treatment of peripheral neural sheath tumors is limited to surgical excision. Early detection and diagnosis of such tumors allow complete excision in only a few, unusual cases. In the majority of cases complete excision is impossible owing to proximal extension of the tumor into the spinal canal or spinal cord.[88] Because a schwannoma generally involves several spinal nerves or nerve roots, excision of spinal nerves as far proximally as possible, either at the level of the intervertebral foramen or at the level of the spinal cord following laminectomy, is most commonly accompanied by amputation of a limb.

Irradiation of schwannomas may be attempted, but it has not yet been adequately investigated. Irradiation of peripheral nerves or plexus is complicated by the proximity of other structures (e.g., the spinal cord). In the future, irradiation may be combined with surgical removal of nerve sheath tumors.

Chemotherapy for schwannomas may be of palliative benefit. A combination of vincristine, doxorubicin, and cyclophosphamide has been recommended.[18] Lymphoma of the peripheral nervous system is treated the same way it is treated elsewhere in the body.

PROGNOSIS

Survival following surgical excision of schwannomas has been reported to range from 2 months to 2 years.[68] Recurrence is common.[68] Postsurgical metastases to lungs have been reported. The high rate of local recurrence following surgical excision of a peripheral nerve sheath neoplasm may reflect proximal extension of a tumor within a nerve trunk. Grossly visible margins of a tumor at the time of operative resection may not accurately demarcate the extent of tumor invasion. Radical excision must be considered to offer the best prognosis, and nerve roots should be excised as far proximally as possible. This may include a laminectomy for transection of nerve roots where they enter the spinal cord parenchyma. The effect on prognosis of adjunctive radiation therapy following surgery has yet to be determined.

COMPARATIVE ASPECTS

It appears that types of peripheral nerve sheath tumors of dogs and cats are very similar to those occurring in humans. The controversy concerning classification of peripheral nerve sheath tumors in humans is similar to that described for animals.[89] The goals of treatment for a benign peripheral nerve sheath tumor in humans are tumor resection and preservation of nerve function. Most benign schwannomas in humans can be totally enucleated without nerve damage, and recurrences are quite rare.[89] Malignant nerve sheath tumors in humans have a high

tendency to recur following local excision. A recurrence rate of over 40% following local excision has been reported.[89] Radical excision, often in combination with amputation, is therefore recommended for treatment of malignant nerve sheath tumors. Although the benefit of postoperative irradiation has not been proven, it has been recommended in humans.

Multiple cutaneous and peripheral neurofibromas are the hallmark of von Recklinghausen's neurofibromatosis.[89] The peripheral nerve tumors associated with this disease may be benign or malignant in behavior, although a tendency exists toward malignant transformation. The similarity between this human disease and neurofibromatosis in cattle and dogs has been noted; however, the disease as it occurs in humans has not been confirmed in dogs at this time.[70]

NEUROLOGIC COMPLICATIONS OF SYSTEMIC CANCER

The incidence of neurologic complications of systemic cancer in dogs and cats is unknown; however, direct and indirect effects on the nervous system of cancer originating outside the nervous system are known to occur.[90-94]

Over 20% of humans with systemic cancer develop neurologic symptoms either as direct or indirect effects of their underlying disease.[95,96] These are summarized in Table 27-1. Metastasis to the brain is the most common complication of systemic cancer. Autopsy studies confirm that 25% of patients who die from cancer have intracranial metastases at the time of death. Metastasis to the spinal cord and nerve roots is the second most common neurologic complica-

Table 27-1. Neurologic complications
of systemic cancer

METASTASIS TO THE NERVOUS SYSTEM
Intracranial neoplasia
Spinal neoplasia
Leptomeningeal neoplasia
Cranial/peripheral nerve neoplasia
NONMETASTATIC NEUROLOGIC COMPLICATIONS
Metabolic encephalopathy
Central nervous system infections
Cerebrovascular disorders
Adverse effects of treatment
Paraneoplastic effects

tion of systemic cancer; it occurs in 5% to 10% of human patients with cancer.[95]

Nonmetastatic nervous system complications of systemic cancer in humans occur less commonly than metastatic disease.[95] Frequently nonmetastatic complications develop acutely. They are often fully reversible, but they may be fatal if they are not recognized and treated.

Metabolic encephalopathy is a common nonmetastatic complication. It is a behavioral change that results from failure of cerebral metabolism due to a systemic illness such as electrolyte imbalance, hepatic and renal failure, hypoxia, or sepsis.[95]

Cancer patients may be susceptible to CNS infections due to altered immune mechanisms or to neutropenia. Neutropenia is common in patients with hematologic malignancies, in those with bone marrow depletion by a metastatic tumor, and in those receiving chemotherapy.[95]

A high incidence of thrombocytopenia or coagulation deficits results in increased risk of cerebrovascular complications. Embolic infarction may occur secondary to endocarditis or sepsis.

Neurologic complications may also result from cancer treatment.[95] Although permanent damage to the nervous system from radiation therapy is rare, it is known to occur. Several chemotherapeutic agents (*e.g.*, methotrexate, cisplatin, vinca alkaloids, fluorouracil) may produce neurotoxicity in the central or peripheral nervous system either directly or indirectly by toxicity to other organs such as liver or kidney.[97]

Paraneoplastic syndromes or "remote effects" are nervous system abnormalities that occur in patients with malignant systemic tumors but that are not caused by metastatic invasion of the nervous system or by any identifiable effect of cancer on the nervous system, such as infection or chemotherapy.[96,98,98a] In about 50% of cases nervous system symptoms precede the diagnosis of cancer. The cause and pathogenesis of paraneoplastic syndromes are not known, although possible mechanisms include autoimmune reactions, viral infections, toxins secreted by a tumor, and nutritional deprivation. Commonly recognized paraneoplastic effects are sensorimotor polyneuropathy, myasthenia gravis (associated with thymoma), and polymyositis.

REFERENCES

1. Kornegay JN: Central nervous system neoplasia. In Kornegay JN (ed): Neurologic Disorders: Contemporary Issues in Small Animal Practice, Vol 5, pp. 78–108. New York, Churchill-Livingstone, 1986
2. Prata RG, Carillo JM: Nervous system. In Slatter DH (ed): Textbook of Small Animal Surgery, pp. 2499–2522. Philadelphia, W.B. Saunders, 1985
3. Vandevelde M: Brain tumors in domestic animals: An overview. Proceedings, Conference on Brain Tumors in Man and Animals, Research Triangle Park, North Carolina, September 5–6, 1984
4. Hayes HM, Priester WA, Pendergrass TW: Occurrence of nervous-tissue tumors in cattle, horses, cats and dogs. Int J Cancer 15:39–47, 1975
5. Braund KG, Ribas JL: Central nervous system meningiomas. Comp Cont Educ Pract Vet 8:241–248, 1986
6. Stunzi H, Hauser B, Isler D: Tumoren des Ruckenmarkes beim Hund. Schweiz Arch Tierheilkd 118:225–232, 1976
7. Nafe LA: Meningiomas in cats: A retrospective clinical study of 36 cases. J Am Vet Med Assoc 174:1224–1227, 1979
8. Patnaik AK, Kay WJ, Hurvitz AI: Intracranial meningioma: A comparative pathologic study of 28 dogs. Vet Pathol 23:369–373, 1986
9. McGrath JT: Morphology and classification of brain tumors in domestic animals. Proceedings, Conference on Brain Tumors in Man and Animals, Research Triangle Park, North Carolina, September 5–6, 1984
10. LeCouteur RA, Fike JR, Cann CE, et al: Computed tomography of brain tumors in the caudal fossa of the dog. Vet Radiol 22:244–251, 1981
10a. Straw RC, LeCouteur, RA, Powers BE, et al: Multilobular osteochondrosarcoma of the canine skull: Sixteen cases (1978–1988). J Am Vet Med Assoc (in press)
10b. Ribas JL, Mena H, Braund KG, et al: A histologic and immunocytochemical study of choroid plexus tumors of the dog. Vet Pathol 26:55–64, 1989
11. Zaki FA, Hurvitz AI: Spontaneous neoplasms of the central nervous system of the cat. J Small Anim Pract 17:773–782, 1976
12. Haskins ME, McGrath JT: Meningiomas in young cats with mucopolysaccharidosis. J Neuropathol Exp Neurol 42:664–670, 1983

13. Fox JG, Snyder SB, Reed C, et al: Malignant ependymoma in a cat. J Small Anim Pract 14:23–26, 1973

14. Komarnisky MD: Astrocytoma in a cat. Can Vet J 26:237–240, 1985

14a. Sarfaty D, Carrillo JM, Patnaik AK: Cerebral astrocytoma in four cats: Clinical and pathologic findings. J Am Vet Med Assoc 191:976–978, 1987

15. Lichtensteiger CA, Wortman JA, Eigenmann JE: Functional pituitary acidophil adenoma in a cat with diabetes mellitus and acromegalic features. Vet Pathol 23:518–521, 1986

15a. Nelson RW, Feldman EC, Smith MC: Hyperadrenocorticism in cats: Seven cases (1978–1987). J Am Vet Med Assoc 193:245–250, 1988

16. LeCouteur RA, Fike JR, Cann CE, et al: X-ray computed tomography of brain tumors in cats. J Am Vet Med Assoc 183:301–305, 1983

16a. Smith DA, Honhold N: Clinical and pathological features of a cerebellar oligodendroglioma in a cat. J Small Anim Pract 29:269–274, 1988

17. Kornegay JN: Intracranial neoplasia of dogs and cats. Proc 3rd Ann Medical Forum, Am Coll Vet Int Med, pp. 60–63. San Diego, California, 1985

18. Holliday TA, Higgins RJ, Turrel JM: Tumors of the nervous system. In Theilen GH, Madewell BR (eds): Veterinary Cancer Medicine, 2nd ed, pp. 601–617. Philadelphia, Lea & Febiger, 1987

19. Escourolle R, Poirier J: Manual of Basic Neuropathology, 2nd ed, p. 21. Philadelphia, W.B. Saunders, 1978

20. Braund KG: Neoplasia of the nervous system. Comp Cont Educ Pract Vet 6:717–722, 1984

21. Vandevelde M, Fankhauser R, Luginbuhl H: Immunocytochemical studies in canine neuroectodermal brain tumors. Acta Neuropathol 66:111–116, 1985

22. Vandevelde M: Morphological and histochemical characteristics of GME and reticulosis: one disease or two? The Bern perspective. Proc 4th Ann Medical Forum, Am Coll Vet Int Med, pp. 11/81–11/83. Washington, DC, 1986

22a. Britt JO, Simpson JG, Howard EB: Malignant lymphoma of the meninges in two dogs. J Compar Pathol 94:45–53, 1984

23. Cordy DR: Intracranial germinoma in a dog. Vet Pathol 21:357–358, 1984

23a. Valentine BA, Summers BA, de Lahunta A, et al: Suprasellar germ cell tumors in the dog: A report of five cases and review of the literature. Acta Neuropathol 76:94–100, 1988

24. Andrews EJ: Clinicopathologic characteristics of meningiomas in dogs. J Am Vet Med Assoc 163:151–157, 1973

25. Fankhauser R, Fatzer R, Luginbuhl H, et al: Reticulosis of the central nervous system in dogs. Adv Vet Sci Comp Sci 16:35–71, 1972

26. Vandevelde M, Fatzer R, Fankhauser R: Immunohistological studies on primary reticulosis of the canine brain. Vet Pathol 18:577–588, 1981

27. Summers BA, deLahunta A: Cerebral angioendotheliomatosis in a dog. Acta Neuropathol 68:10–14, 1985

27a. Dargent FJ, Fox LE, Anderson WI: Neoplastic angioendotheliomatosis in a dog: An angiotropic lymphoma. Cornell Vet 78:253–262, 1988

28. Kornegay JN: Pathogenesis of disease of the central nervous system. In Slatter DH (ed): Textbook of Small Animal Surgery, pp. 1266–1284. Philadelphia, W.B. Saunders, 1985

28a. Foster ES, Carrillo JM, Patnaik AK: Clinical signs of tumors affecting the rostral cerebrum in 43 dogs. J Vet Int Med 2:71–74, 1988

28b. Sarfaty D, Carrillo JM, Peterson ME: Neurologic, endocrinologic, and pathologic findings associated with large pituitary tumors in dogs: Eight cases (1976–1984). J Am Vet Med Assoc 193:854–856, 1988

29. Lawson DC, Burk RL, Prata RG: Cerebral meningioma in the cat: Diagnosis and surgical treatment of ten cases. J Am Anim Hosp Assoc 20:333–342, 1984

30. Bailey CS, Higgins RJ: Characteristics of cisternal cerebrospinal fluid associated with primary brain tumors in the dog: a retrospective study. J Am Vet Med Assoc 188:414–417, 1986

30a. Vandevelde M, Fankhauser RR: Liquoruntersuchungen bei neurologisch kranken Hunden und Katzen. Schweiz Arch Tierheilk 129:443–456, 1987

31. LeCouteur RA, Scagliotti RH, Beck KA, et al: Indirect imaging of the canine optic nerve using metrizamide (optic thecography). Am J Vet Res 43:1424–1428, 1982

32. LeCouteur RA, Turrel JM: Brain tumors in dogs and cats. In Kirk RW (ed): Current Veterinary Therapy. IX. Small Animal Practice, pp. 820–825. Philadelphia, W.B. Saunders, 1986

33. Barber DL, Oliver JE, Mayhew IG: Neuroradiography. In Oliver JE, Hoerlein BF, Mayhew IG (eds): Veterinary Neurology, pp. 65–110. Philadelphia, W.B. Saunders, 1987

34. LeCouteur RA, Cann CE, Fike JR: Computed tomography. In Gourley IG, Vasseur PB (eds): Textbook of Small Animal Soft Tissue Surgery,

pp. 989–1002. Philadelphia, J.B. Lippincott, 1985

35. Fike JR, LeCouteur RA, Cann CE, et al: Computerized tomography of brain tumors of the rostral and middle fossas in the dog. Am J Vet Res 42:275–281, 1981

36. Panciera DL, Duncan ID, Messing A, et al: Magnetic resonance imaging in two dogs with central nervous system disease. J Small Anim Pract 28:587–596, 1987

37. Turrel JM, Fike JR, LeCouteur RA, et al: Computed tomographic characteristics of primary brain tumors in 50 dogs. J Am Vet Med Assoc 188:851–856, 1986

38. Silverman JF, Timmons RL, Leonard JR: Cytologic results of fine-needle aspiration biopsies of the central nervous system. Cancer 58:1117–1121, 1986

39. Broggi G, Franzini A, Migliavacca F, et al: Stereotactic biopsy of deep brain tumors in infancy and childhood. Child's Brain 10:92–98, 1983

40. LeCouteur RA, Gillette EL, Dow SW, et al: Radiation response of autochthonous canine brain tumors. Int J Radiat Oncol Biol Phys 13:166, 1987

41. Turrel JM, Fike JR, LeCouteur RA, et al: Radiotherapy of brain tumors in dogs. J Am Vet Med Assoc 184:82–86, 1981

42. Turrel JM, Higgins RJ, Child G: Prognostic factors associated with irradiation of canine brain tumors. Vet Cancer Soc, 6th Ann Conference, West Lafayette, Indiana, 1986

43. LeCouteur RA, Sisson AF, Dow SW, et al: Combined surgical debulking and irradiation for the treatment of a large frontal meningioma in 8 dogs. Vet Cancer Soc, 7th Ann Conference, Madison, Wisconsin, 1987

43a. Dow SW, LeCouteur RA, Rosychuk RAW, et al: Radiotherapy of functional canine pituitary tumors. Vet Cancer Soc 7th Ann Conference, Madison, Wisconsin, 1987

44. Levin VA: Chemotherapy of primary brain tumors. Neurol Clin 3:855–866, 1985

45. Wilson CB, Levin V, Hoshino T: Chemotherapy of brain tumors. In Youmans JR: Neurological Surgery, Vol 5, 2nd ed, pp. 3065–3095. Philadelphia, W.B. Saunders, 1982

46. Lee Y, Bigner DD: Aspects of immunobiology and immunotherapy and uses of monoclonal antibodies and biologic immune modifiers in human gliomas. Neurol Clin 3:901–917, 1985

47. Mahaley MS, Gillespie GY: Immunotherapy of patients with glioma: Fact, fancy and future. Prog Exp Tumor Res 28:118–135, 1984

48. Shelden CH, Ingram M, Jacques S, et al: Apparent destruction of spontaneous glioblastoma in a dog by autologous lymphocytes. Pulse; So Calif Vet Med Assoc, December 1984, pp. 13–14

49. Kostolich M, Dulisch ML: A surgical approach to the canine olfactory bulb for meningioma removal. Vet Surg 16:273–277, 1987

50. Shell L, Colter SB, Blass CE: Surgical removal of a meningioma in a cat after detection by computerized axial tomography. J Am Anim Hosp Assoc 21:439–442, 1985

50a. Fingeroth JM, Hansen B, Myer CW: Diagnosis and successful removal of a brain tumor in a cat. Companion Anim Pract 2:6–15, 1988

51. Salcman M: The morbidity and mortality of brain tumors: A perspective on recent advances in therapy. Neurol Clin 3:229–257, 1985

52. Adegbite AB, Khan MI, Paine KWE, et al: The recurrence of intracranial meningiomas after surgical treatment. J Neurosurg 58:51–56, 1983

53. Carella RJ, Ransohoff J, Newall J: Role of radiation therapy in the management of meningioma. Neurosurgery 10:332–339, 1982

54. Solan MJ, Kramer S: The role of radiation therapy in the management of intracranial meningiomas. Int J Radiat Oncol Biol Phys 11:675–677, 1985

55. Fingeroth JM, Prata RG, Patnaik AK: Spinal meningiomas in dogs: 13 cases (1972–1987). J Am Vet Med Assoc 191:720–726, 1987

56. Luttgen PJ, Braund KG, Brauner WR, et al: A retrospective study of twenty-nine spinal tumors in the dog and cat. J Small Anim Pract 21:213–226, 1980

57. Summers BA, deLahunta A: Unusual intradural extramedullary spinal cord tumors in twelve dogs. J Neuropathol Exp Neurol 45:322, 1986

57a. Summers BA, deLahunta A, McEntee M, et al: A novel intradural extramedullary spinal cord tumor in young dogs. Acta Neuropathol 75:402–410, 1988

58. Tamke PG, Foley GL: Neuroepithelioma in a dog. Can Vet J 28:606–608, 1987

58a. Blass CE, Kirby BM, Kreege JM, et al: Teratomatous medulloepithelioma in the spinal cord of a dog. J Am Anim Hosp Assoc 24:51–54, 1988

59. Kornegay JN: Feline neurology. Comp Cont Educ Pract Vet 3:203–213, 1981

60. Wright JA, Bell DA, Clayton–Jones DG: The clinical and radiological features associated with spinal tumors in thirty dogs. J Small Anim Pract 20:461–472, 1979

61. Morgan JP, Ackerman N, Bailey CS, et al: Vertebral tumors in the dog: A clinical, radio-

logic, and pathologic study of 61 primary and secondary lesions. Vet Radiol 21:197–212, 1980

62. Haynes JS, Leininger JR: A glioma in the spinal cord of a cat. Vet Pathol 19:713–715, 1982

63. Neer TM, Kreeger JM: Cervical spinal cord astrocytoma in a dog. J Am Vet Med Assoc 191:84–86, 1987

64. Bailey CS, Higgins RJ: Comparison of total white blood cell count and total protein content of lumbar and cisternal cerebrospinal fluid of healthy dogs. Am J Vet Res 46:1162–1165, 1985

65. Gilmore DR: Neoplasia of the cervical spinal cord and vertebrae in the dog. J Am Anim Hosp Assoc 19:1009–1014, 1983

66. Couto CG, Cullen J, Pedroia V, et al: Central nervous system lymphosarcoma in the dog. J Am Vet Med Assoc 184:809–813, 1984

67. Wara WM, Sheline GE: Radiation therapy of tumors of the spinal cord. In Youmans JR (ed): Neurological Surgery, Vol 5, 2nd ed, pp. 3222–3226. Philadelphia, W.B. Saunders, 1982

68. Bradley RL, Withrow SJ, Snyder SP: Nerve sheath tumors in the dog. J Am Anim Hosp Assoc 18:915–921, 1982

69. Innes JRH, Saunders LZ. Neoplastic diseases. In Innes JRH, Saunders LZ (eds): Comparative Neuropathology, pp. 721–752. New York, Academic Press, 1962

70. Goedegebuure SA: A case of neurofibromatosis in the dog. J Small Anim Pract 16:329–335, 1975

71. Lewis JC, Reardon MJ, Montgomery A Jr: Paraganglioma involving the spinal cord of a dog. J Am Vet Med Assoc 168:864–865, 1976

72. Allen JG, Amis T: Lymphosarcoma involving cranial nerves in a cat. Aust Vet J 51:155–158, 1975

73. Luginbuhl H, Fankhauser R, McGrath JT: Spontaneous neoplasms of the nervous system in animals. Progr Neurol Surg 2:85–164, 1968

74. Schaer M, Zaki FA, Harvey HJ, et al: Laryngeal hemiplegia due to neoplasia of the vagus nerve in a cat. J Am Vet Med Assoc 174:513–515, 1979

75. Russel DS, Rubinstein LJ: Pathology of tumors of the nervous system, 4th ed, pp. 372–436. Baltimore, Williams & Wilkins, 1977

76. Dahme E, Bilzer T, Stavrou D: Classification of canine PNS-tumors based on EM- and PAP-techniques. Proc Joint Meeting, The World Association of Veterinary Pathologists, Utrecht, The Netherlands, 1984

77. Lusk MD, Kline DG, Garcia CA: Tumors of the brachial plexus. Neurosurgery 21:439–453, 1987

78. Zachary JF, O'Brien DP, Ingles BW, et al: Multicentric nerve sheath fibrosarcomas of multiple cranial nerve roots in two dogs. J Am Vet Med Assoc 188:723–726, 1986

79. Cordy DR: Tumors of the nervous system and eye. In Moulton JE (ed): Tumors of Domestic Animals, 2nd ed, pp. 430–455. Berkeley: University of California Press, 1978

80. Cravioto H: Neoplasms of peripheral nerves. In Wilkins RH, Rengachary SS (eds): Neurosurgery, pp. 1894–1899. New York, McGraw-Hill, 1985

81. Cravioto H, Lockwood R: The behavior of acoustic neuroma in tissue culture. Acta Neuropathol 12:141–157, 1969

82. deLahunta A: Veterinary Neuroanatomy and Clinical Neurology, 2nd ed., pp. 249–251. Philadelphia, W.B. Saunders, 1983

83. Budzilovich GN: Granular cell "myoblastoma" of vagus nerve. Acta Neuropathol 10:162–165, 1968

84. Carmichael S, Griffiths IR: Tumors involving the brachial plexus in seven dogs. Vet Rec 108:435–437, 1981

85. Bailey CS: Patterns of cutaneous anesthesia associated with brachial plexus avulsions in the dog. J Am Vet Med Assoc 185:889–899, 1984

86. Boring JG, Swaim SF: Malignant schwannoma (neurilemmoma): An extramedullary-intradural tumor causing cervical cord compression in a dog. J Am Anim Hosp Assoc 9:342–345, 1973

87. Holliday TA, Weldon NE, Ealand BG: Percutaneous recording of evoked spinal cord potentials of dogs. Am J Vet Res 40:326–333, 1979

88. Bradney IW, Forsyth WM: A schwannoma causing cervical spinal cord compression in a dog. Aust Vet J 63:374–375, 1986

89. Youmans JR, Ishida WY: Tumors of peripheral and sympathetic nerves. In Youmans JR (ed): Neurological Surgery, pp. 3299–3315. Philadelphia, W.B. Saunders, 1982

90. Braund KG, McGuire JA, Amling KA, et al: Peripheral neuropathy associated with malignant neoplasms in dogs. Vet Pathol 24:16–21, 1987

91. Braund KG, Steiss JE, Amling KA, et al: Insulinoma and subclinical peripheral neuropathy in two dogs. J Vet Int Med 1:86–90, 1987

92. Griffiths IR, Duncan ID, Swallow JS: Peripheral polyneuropathies in dogs: A study of five cases. J Small Anim Pract 18:101–116, 1977

93. Presthus J, Teige J Jr: Peripheral neuropathy associated with lymphosarcoma in a dog. J Small Anim Pract 27:463–469, 1986

94. Sorjonen DC, Braund KG, Hoff EJ: Paraplegia and subclinical neuromyopathy associated with a primary lung tumor in a dog. J Am Vet Med Assoc 180:1209–1211, 1982

95. Patchell RA, Posner JB: Neurologic complications of systemic cancer. Neurol Clin 3:729–750, 1985

96. Silverstein SR, Marx JA: Neurologic emergencies in patients with cancer. Top Emerg Med 8:1–10, 1986

97. Kaplan RS, Wernik PH: Neurotoxicity of anti-tumor agents. In Perry MC, Yarbro J (eds): Toxicity of Chemotherapy. New York, Grune & Stratton, 1984

98. Posner JB: Neurological complications of systemic cancer. Med Clin North Am 63:783–800, 1979

98a. Kornblith PL, Walker MD, Cassady JR: Neurologic Oncology, pp. 38–39. Philadelphia, J.B. Lippincott, 1987

28

OCULAR TUMORS

James F. Swanson
Richard R. Dubielzig

Tumors of the eye, adnexa, and orbit comprise a small but significant niche in clinical veterinary oncology. The delicate nature of the visual system and its close proximity to the central nervous system make it susceptible to severe dysfunction and visual loss following invasion by tumors that otherwise exhibit benign histologic or biologic characteristics.

The following are examples of the more commonly seen ocular neoplastic conditions in small animals.

TUMORS OF THE EYELIDS

Incidence and Risk Factors

Tumors of the eyelid are the most commonly diagnosed ocular neoplasms in small animals. The dog is more frequently affected than the cat. Squamous papillomas are found more often in dogs less than 1 year of age, and sebaceous adenomas and adenocarcinomas are found with increasing frequency in aging dogs. Other commonly noted canine eyelid tumors include histiocytomas, mast cell tumors, melanomas, and basal cell carcinomas. Eyelid tumors in cats tend to be malignant and include squamous cell carcinomas (SCC), sebaceous adenomas/adenocarcinomas, basal cell carcinomas, fibroma/fibrosarcoma, and mast cell tumors. SCC is the most common eyelid tumor in the feline and is usually found in white cats with poorly pigmented eyelids.[1] Increased exposure to solar radiation is felt to be a factor in the development of SCC in cats. In a report of four dogs affected with eyelid SCC, two of the dogs had nonpigmented eyelids and two had normal pigmentation.[2]

Pathology and Natural Behavior

In dogs, the majority of lid tumors are benign. One survey of canine lid tumor biopsies noted that only 24.7% of the tumors were malignant.[3] A more recent survey indicated an even lower (8.2%) incidence of malignancy.[4]

Squamous papillomas are an infectious, self-limiting neoplastic process of young dogs caused by a papovavirus. These growths are most commonly found on the inner surface of the lips but may also affect the skin and mucocutaneous junctions of the eyelids. The tumors are well demarcated and show no tendency to invade the underlying dermis.[3]

Sebaceous tumors often arise from the meibomian glands and are the most common eyelid tumor of the dog. These tumors tend to occur in older dogs and range histologically from largely inflammatory lesions to those exhibiting characteristics of malignancy. Malignant sebaceous tumors tend to be more infiltrative but do not metastasize and often do not appear significantly different clinically from more benign tumors. Grossly, these tumors may be seen on the inner aspect of the lid and extend above the lid margin to appear as pink to gray well-delineated masses.

Squamous cell carcinoma is the most common ocular adnexal tumor of the cat. It frequently develops from a preinvasive actinic plaque at the eyelid margin as an intraepithelial epithelioma or carcinoma *in situ*.[1] The tumor may subsequently invade the conjunctiva, nictitating membrane, and orbit. We have noted regional extension along the optic nerves in rare cases.

History and Clinical Signs

Eyelid tumors may produce no clinical signs other than an obvious mass lesion. Tumors touching the bulbar conjunctiva or globe surface typically cause signs of frictional irritation including lacrimation and blepharospasm. Secondary ulcerative keratitis may also be noted. Neoplasms infiltrating and blocking the nasolacrimal system may produce epiphora. Extensive growth causes lid deformation and dysfunction.

Squamous papillomas typically appear as multiple pedunculated, irregularly serrated masses along the lid margins, periocular skin, or other ocular structures (Fig. 28-1).

Older dogs affected with sebaceous adenomas are usually presented for evaluation of slow-growing, well-defined, pigmented masses of the eyelid margins.

Squamous cell carcinomas may present as small lumps on the lid margins or periocular skin. More commonly, the patient is presented for evaluation of an ulcerated, thickened, and misshapen lid margin that is unresponsive to symptomatic therapy. The globe or other adnexal structures may be secondarily involved.

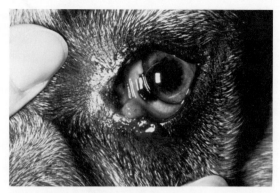

Figure 28-1. Typical appearance of squamous papilloma in a young dog. Masses may be multiple and are typically pedunculated.

Diagnostic Techniques and Work-Up

The diagnosis of eyelid tumors is by observation of a mass or ulcerative lesion. The clinical appearance may suggest the type of tumor. However, biopsy and histopathology remain the most accurate methods for determination of tumor type. Extensive tumor invasion may indicate local, regional, or distant metastasis.

Tumors must be differentiated from parasitic infestation, chronic blepharitis with nodule formation or ulceration, chalazia, eyelid pyogranulomas, and traumatic lid disease. Careful inspection, cytologic evaluation, and biopsy are helpful diagnostic aids.

Therapy

Tumors whose appearance or behavior suggest malignancy, or tumors causing secondary disease of the globe or adnexa should be biopsied as soon as the general physical condition of the patient allows. Small tumors should be completely removed. In cases of larger, more aggressive masses, an initial biopsy may be indicated because knowledge of specific tumor type is necessary in planning further resection and alternative therapeutic strategies. Resection methods including wedge, four-sided, and sliding or rotating skin-grafting techniques have been described.[5,6] In general, tumors involving one-fourth of the lid margin or less, depending on breed, may be excised without additional plastic surgical techniques.

Additional or alternate treatment modalities for eyelid tumors include cryosurgery, radiation therapy, and hyperthermia. Cryosurgery following partial debulking has been effective in treating canine eyelid tumors including papilloma, sebaceous adenoma, and sebaceous adenocarcinoma that are too large for primary resection. (See Chapter 12.)[7] The tumor is stabilized with a chalazion clamp and frozen twice. The iceball should extend 3–5 mm beyond visible tumor. Care should be taken to prevent contact of the cryogen with other structures. Nitrous oxide may be used as a cryogen but is effective only for small tumors. Swelling and sloughing of tumor for 10–14 days is common and temporary lid margin depigmentation and permanent leukotrichia can be expected.[4]

Prognosis

In the dog, lid tumors rarely recur following surgical removal. Incompletely treated benign or malignant tumors can be expected to recur with local extension. Additional primary tumors often arise and may be confused with local recurrence. Metastasis of eyelid tumors other than mast cell tumor is rare in the dog. Squamous cell carcinoma in the cat may exhibit extensive local invasion that precludes complete removal.

TUMORS OF THE CONJUNCTIVA AND MEMBRANA NICTITANS

Incidence and Risk Factors

The incidence of primary neoplasia of the conjunctiva and membrana nictitans is unknown but appears to be low in the dog and cat. Reported tumors include squamous papilloma, squamous cell carcinoma, hemangioma and hemangiosarcoma, adenoma and adenocarcinoma, fibrosarcoma, and melanoma. Most arise from the bulbar conjunctiva, although the membrana nictitans and palpebral conjunctiva are also affected.

Papillomas can affect palpebral and bulbar conjunctiva and encroach on the cornea. Although the precise relationship between oral and ocular papillomatosis remains unclear, viral particles compatible with the papillomavirus group have been demonstrated in one reported case.[8] As with oral and eyelid papillomas, young dogs are primarily affected.

Squamous cell carcinoma is reported in both the dog and the cat and affects the mucosa of the membrana nictitans and the perilimbal bulbar conjunctiva (Fig. 28-2). Eyelid SCC may

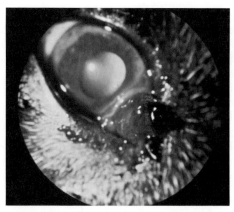

Figure 28-2. Squamous cell carcinoma may affect the mucosa of the membrana nictitans and the perilimbal bulbar conjunctiva.

invade the palpebral conjunctiva in extensive tumors. Hemangiomas and hemangiosarcomas have been described on the bulbar conjunctiva and third eyelid but are uncommon.[9]

Pathology and Natural Behavior

Squamous papillomas and SCC exhibit similar pathologic and behavioral characteristics to those described for eyelid tumors. Papillomas adjacent to the limbus may also involve the cornea. The natural history of conjunctival papillomas is unknown. Similarly, little is reported on the natural progression of untreated conjunctival SCC, although continued infiltration of adjacent tissue can be expected.

Hemangiomas of the subjacent conjunctival stroma have been reported.[9] These tumors exhibit variable growth, tend to recur following incomplete excision, but appear to remain confined to the subepithelial stroma. The propensity for metastasis is unknown. Hemangiosarcomas exhibit a more aggressive course, and it is important to determine whether the observed lesion is a primary or metastatic site. The natural behavior of adenocarcinomas of the gland of the third eyelid is unknown in small animals. We have observed regional lymph node metastasis 8 months after removal of a similar tumor in a horse.

History and Clinical Signs

Papillomas occur in young dogs and appear as elevated, papillary, roughened growths with surface clefts. Squamous cell carcinomas may present as a focally thickened or roughened lesion on the perilimbal conjunctiva or third eyelid. SCC may also have a similar appearance to papillomas and should be considered in older dogs exhibiting papillomatous growths.

Hemangiomas and hemangiosarcomas are usually focal, raised, dark-red masses on the bulbar conjunctiva or third eyelid that may hemorrhage if manipulated.

In most cases, signs of ocular discomfort are minimal unless tumor growth is extensive enough to cause frictional irritation or lagophthalmia.

Diagnostic Techniques and Work-up

Because of the mobility of the bulbar conjunctiva, small tumors may be easily excised for histopathologic examination with fine scissors following application of topical anesthestic. General anesthesia and more extensive biopsy procedures including superficial keratectomy or third-eyelid gland removal should be considered for invasive tumors.

Biopsy and histopathologic examination are necessary to differentiate neoplastic conditions from inflammatory conditions of the episclera and membrana nictitans, including fibrous histiocytoma and nodular fasciitis.[10] Although ocular squamous papilloma and adenomatous hyperplasia of the gland of the third eyelid ("cherry eye") are relatively common in young dogs, biopsy of similar appearing lesions in older animals should be considered to rule out potentially malignant neoplastic conditions.

Additional diagnostic techniques may be indicated in extensive disease and include orbital, skull, and thoracic radiography, orbital angiography, orbital ultrasonography, and regional lymph node cytology/biopsy.

Therapy

Squamous papillomas in young dogs are best left untreated because the condition is usually self-limiting. Exceptions include papillomas causing secondary ocular disease and those cases in which SCC is considered likely. Smaller tumors of the conjunctiva are easily removed and respond well to surgery.

Complete removal of larger or fixed tumors may not be possible without extensive resection, including excision of the third eyelid, enucleation, or orbital exenteration. Alternative therapy including cryosurgery, radiation, or hyperthermia should be considered in attempts to save

vital structures or if clinical or histopathologic assessment indicates incomplete excision. In these cases, additional preoperative work-up is imperative to determine whether regional or distant metastatic disease is present.

Prognosis

Published reports of conjunctival and third-eyelid tumors indicate that metastasis is unlikely in small animals following complete removal. However, long-term follow-up studies of significant numbers of cases are not available for any tumor of the conjunctiva or membrana nictitans.

PRIMARY OCULAR TUMORS

CANINE OCULAR MELANOMA

Incidence and Risk Factors

Among primary canine ocular neoplasms, tumors of melanocytic origin are the most common and important. Melanocytic tumors of the globe can be roughly subdivided into two categories: those occurring within the globe, and those occurring in the sclera near the limbus. Melanocytic tumors of the limbic sclera occur more frequently in German shepherd dogs than in other breeds.

No breed or sex predilection has been demonstrated for intraocular melanoma. Causes or risk factors associated with melanocytic tumors of the globe are not known.

Pathology and Natural Behavior

Melanocytic tumors of the canine globe can be subdivided according to anatomic location. Melanomas of the perilimbal sclera (epibulbar melanoma) are slow-growing, heavily pigmented tumors that are first evidenced as black, well-delineated, raised masses apparent beneath the conjunctival surface and near the limbus.[11] Epibulbar melanomas have never been demonstrated to metastasize.

Canine intraocular melanoma is almost always a disease of the anterior uveal tract.[12,13] Small numbers of discretely localized, pigmented masses of the iris which do not appear to grow by local infiltration have been reported in young dogs. These tumors are considered benign and probably distinct from the more common invasive melanomas of the anterior uveal tract in adult animals. Invasive anterior uveal melanomas can be subdivided into benign and malignant categories based on morphologic indicators of cellular anaplasia. Although a number of different criteria could be used, most reports would indicate that mitotic index is most useful to distinguish between benign and malignant anterior uveal melanomas.[13]

Both categories of anterior uveal melanomas are destructive and invasive within the ocular tissues. Recent reports indicate that metastatic disease is uncommon.[13] However, all cases of demonstrated distant metastasis have occurred in dogs with primary ocular tumors exhibiting cytologic features of malignancy.

Small numbers of primary tumors of the choroid have been reported in dogs, and these tumors appear as sharply delineated, dark, raised subretinal masses.[14] Some of these tumors have been followed funduscopically for many years and show either no growth or gradual expansion with no tendency to invade the sclera. Metastasis has never been demonstrated.

Diagnostic Techniques and Work-Up

Intraocular melanomas are usually detected when the tumor mass extends to the anterior chamber either by invasion through the iris root or extension beyond the pupillary margin (Fig. 28-3). Melanocytic tumors of the limbus can be observed as focal, flat to raised, dark masses beneath the bulbar conjunctiva or extending into the peripheral cornea. Gonioscopy may be useful in determining the extent of tumor invasion of the filtration angle. In cases of ocular media opacity caused by glaucoma or of intraocular hemorrhage or inflammation, ocular ultrasonography is often useful in delineating mass lesions.

The use of intraocular fine-needle aspiration to obtain tumor for cytologic evaluation is controversial but is described in both veterinary and human medicine.[15,16] Potential complications of fine-needle aspiration include laceration of the iris or lens, intraocular hemorrhage, retinal detachment, and local tumor dissemination. Excisional or incisional biopsy and histopathologic examination is the most efficient method for definitive diagnosis of epibulbar tumors.

Therapy

Although canine ocular melanomas are the most frequent primary ocular tumor, they occur rarely and little is known about the comparative values and risks of differing therapeutic modalities. Because metastatic disease is a rare consequence of most primary intraocular melanomas, debate has continued whether enucleation or any treatment at all is necessary for small tumors unassociated with secondary disease. Attempts to remove intraocular tumor and retain globe function have been largely unsuccessful. In more advanced cases, enucleation without adjuvant therapy has been considered a satisfactory treatment in all but the most invasive tumors. Large tumors with extrascleral extension must be completely removed by orbital exenteration. Frequently, in exenterations of heavily pigmented tumors, it is impossible to remove all the pigmented material from the orbit, and densely pigmented, graphitelike material remains. Histologically, this material is composed of large, round, heavily pigmented cells that are not thought to be capable of participating in continued neoplastic growth and invasion. However, in these circumstances, the surgeon is left with the dilemma of not knowing definitively whether potentially malignant tissue remains. For this reason, radiation or chemotherapy may be indicated following excision of large orbital melanomas with scleral penetration. More experience is needed to determine the value of these additional treatments.

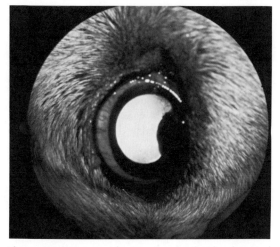

Figure 28-3. Intraocular tumors may first be detected after extension into the anterior chamber by invasion through the iris root or proliferation beyond the pupillary margin.

Small epibulbar tumors can be removed successfully by careful dissection. Full-thickness corneal and scleral resection or enucleation may be necessary for larger, more destructive masses. Cryosurgery may also be considered, but little information is available to indicate its effectiveness against epibulbar tumors.

Prognosis

The metastatic potential of intraocular melanoma, regardless of histologic category, is low. Localized pigmented tumors of the iris in young dogs and well-delineated pigmented masses of the choroid not associated with secondary complication should be treated conservatively because the risk of complications is minimal. The prognosis may be considered less favorable in cases of extrascleral extension and with tumors exhibiting high mitotic indices.

FELINE OCULAR MELANOMA

Incidence and Risk Factors

Although primary ocular melanoma in cats is even less common than in dogs, it is the most frequent primary ocular neoplasm in the feline. Its most frequent form is the diffuse iris melanoma.[17] The age, breed, and sex predilection for ocular melanoma in the feline is unknown.

Pathology and Natural Behavior

Diffuse iris melanoma begins with proliferation and anterior redistribution of melanocytes in the iris. These accumulate on the anterior iris surface, and the first indication of clinical disease is often a change in coloration of the iris. As the disease progresses, the tumor becomes invasive, causing irregular swelling of the entire iris. Proliferating tumor cells exfoliate into the anterior chamber and filtration angle. Glaucoma secondary to entrapment of tumor cells in the filtration angle is a consequence of diffuse tumor proliferation. Continued tumor growth will lead to scleral penetration and disfigurement. Although limited numbers of cases have been followed, ocular melanoma in cats appears to warrant a worse prognosis than its counterpart in dogs. Metastatic disease was seen in 12 of 18 cases with minimum follow-up of 16 weeks or longer.[18] Metastasis to the abdomen, particularly the liver, is most common.[18] The prognostic significance of histologic variations is unknown.

History and Clinical Signs

The earliest indication of clinical disease is the recognition of iridal pigment changes (Fig. 28-4). Localized pigmentary changes are commonly seen in aging cats, and their significance as a precancerous change is unknown. Thus, recommendations based' on clinically observable, focally increased iris pigmentation alone cannot be made without further study. Secondary consequences of diffuse iris melanoma in cats may occur rapidly because of tumor invasion of the filtration angle. The coexistence of increased iris pigmentation, irregular thickening of the iris, and glaucoma should be considered evidence of diffuse iris melanoma.

Therapy

Enucleation is the treatment of choice and should be performed as soon as possible following diagnosis. The authors have no experience with other therapeutic modalities.

Prognosis

There is some evidence indicating that prognosis is better following enucleation of small tumors than in instances where considerable ocular disfigurement has occurred.[18] The latency period between enucleation and clinical metastatic disease is variable but can be several years.[18]

TUMORS OF CILIARY BODY EPITHELIAL ORIGIN IN DOGS AND CATS

Incidence and Risk Factors

Ciliary body epithelial tumors are seen only sporadically. Breed or sex predilection has not been well defined. A review of ciliary body epithelial tumors in dogs and cats indicated ages ranging from 1½ to 14 years in affected animals, but most tumors occurred in middle-aged to older dogs.[15]

Pathology and Natural Behavior

Ciliary body epithelial tumors are rare, and little is known about the significance of morphologic variations. These tumors usually arise locally within the pars plicata of the ciliary body. Although local infiltration within the eye is common, these tumors usually remain fairly well-delineated and ocular destruction or scleral penetration is unusual. Metastasis of ciliary body

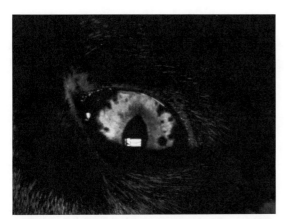

Figure 28-4. Diffuse iris melanomas may first appear clinically as multifocal to diffuse iridal pigment changes as seen in this cat.

epithelial tumors has been documented but appears to be uncommon in the dog and cat.[15]

Tumors are classified as adenoma or adenocarcinoma on the basis of standard morphologic features of malignancy. The tendency to cause secondary ocular disease cannot be correlated with morphology.

Care must be taken to differentiate epithelial tumors of the ciliary body from metastatic foci of malignant tumors originating in other organs.

History and Clinical Signs

Clinical disease occurs when the tumor extends into the anterior chamber at the iris root or when protrusion occurs at the pupillary margin. Tumors may be either pigmented or nonpigmented and therefore vary in clinical appearance. Ciliary epithelial tumors are usually well-delineated, soft, multinodular masses and often occur without secondary clinical ocular disease. However, the presence of ciliary body epithelial tumors should be considered when otherwise unexplained ocular pain, glaucoma, or intraocular hemorrhage are present. The occurrence of intraocular neoplasia in animals exhibiting non-specific ocular signs underscores the importance of histologic examination of all excised ocular structures.

Therapy

Intraocular tumors associated with secondary ocular disease should be treated by enucleation as soon as possible. Whether small ocular tumors unassociated with secondary ocular disease should be enucleated is controversial.[13] Techniques are described for resection of small tumors leaving the globe and vision intact, but the difficulty of completely removing the tumor and the propensity of the canine and feline eye to become phthisical following the severe inflammation that accompanies this invasive surgery limit this option to very selected cases.

Prognosis

Distant metastasis for ciliary body epithelial tumors is rare but has been reported in both the dog and the cat. The prognosis is guarded, especially if there is extensive and rapid tumor growth in the presence of secondary ocular disease.[15]

FELINE POST-TRAUMATIC SARCOMA

Incidence and Risk Factors

Post-traumatic sarcoma (P-TS) is a rare but interesting tumor of cat eyes.[19,20] P-TS is probably second only to melanoma in frequency as a primary ocular tumor of cats. It occurs in eyes that have previously suffered serious injury. Although the nature of the initial ocular damage is not always discernible, trauma seems to be the most common antecedent event. Lens perforation has been a feature of ocular disease associated with sarcoma in all cases studied to date.[19,20]

Pathology and Natural Behavior

The latency period between ocular damage and tumor development is between 1 and 10 years, with an average of more than 5 years. Post-traumatic sarcomas have a tendency to line the internal aspects of the globe circumferentially; early destruction of the retina and colonization of the subretinal space occur. Subsequently, there is invasion of the choroid, followed by extension of the tumor into the limbic sclera and cornea. P-TS has been shown to invade the central nervous system through the optic nerve.[19,20]

Several histologically distinct sarcoma types have been seen in previously traumatized cat eyes. Fibrosarcoma is the most common tumor type; however, osteosarcoma and anaplastic sarcoma have also been seen.[20]

History and Clinical Signs

Objective signs of P-TS may be nonspecific, but the following clinical signs are suggestive. The cornea of the affected eye may be opaque and may exhibit a white to pinkish coloration. The globe is often firm, enlarged, and distorted. Consequences occurring as a result of optic nerve and chiasm involvement include unilateral to bilateral loss of vision. Further extension to the central nervous system is associated with additional neurologic signs.

Diagnostic Techniques and Therapy

Post-traumatic sarcoma should be suspected in cats with a history of ocular trauma who develop ocular opacity, firmness, buphthalmia, exophthalmia, or infrequently, pain. Excisional biopsy is the most effective method of diagnosis and treatment. Care should be taken to remove as much of the optic nerve as possible with the globe. There have been no reports on the potential benefit of radiation treatment or chemotherapeutic agents.

Prognosis

The entire excised optic nerve should be examined histologically for evidence of tumor, as the prognosis is largely dependent on whether the process has extended beyond the surgical site. Eight cats with follow-up histories were euthanized owing to problems resulting from the tumors. Six cats developed blindness and CNS disorders owing to optic nerve invasions and extension to the brain. Only one cat had distant metastasis.[20]

TUMORS OF THE OPTIC NERVE AND ORBIT

Incidence and Risk Factors

Neoplasms represent an uncommon but serious cause of orbital disease in the dog and cat. Primary tumors from neoplastic transformation of orbital bone, vascular tissue, connective tissue, and epithelial elements have been documented. Secondary orbital tumors also occur from extension of primary tumors from other ocular structures, the oral or nasal cavities, or cranial vault. With the exception of lymphoma, orbital metastasis from distant primary tumor sites is rare.

A retrospective study of orbital neoplasms in 23 dogs indicated no breed or sex predilection.[21] The study results also suggest that orbital neoplasia is a disease of older dogs and that most orbital tumors are malignant.

Numerous types of primary and secondary tumors have been reported in the dog, including osteosarcoma, mast cell tumor, meningioma, reticulum cell sarcoma, glioma, schwannoma, reticulosis, chrondroma rodens, nasal and lacrimal adenocarcinoma, squamous cell carcinoma, plasma cell tumor, and lymphoma. With the exception of lymphoma, orbital neoplasia is less frequently reported in the cat. Documented feline orbital tumors include undifferentiated sarcoma, osteosarcoma, rhabdomyosarcoma, extension of conjunctival SCC, and ocular malignant melanoma.

Pathology and Natural Behavior

Many types of orbital neoplasms exhibit locally aggressive behavior with invasion or displacement of adjacent orbital structures. Direct invasion of the globe is unusual but has occurred in squamous cell carcinoma, nasal adenocarcinoma, and meningioma. Invasion and destruction of periorbital structures including the oral and nasal cavities, cranial vault, and frontal and maxillary sinuses is common in extensive lesions. With the exception of lymphoproliferative tumors, widespread metastasis is less likely than invasion of regional lymph nodes by means of lymphatics.

Primary orbital meningiomas arise from the arachnoid cells of the meninges of the optic nerve. Meningiomas may also invade the orbit as an extension of an intracranial tumor. Large or aggressive tumors may cause distortion of the globe or invade it directly, and pulmonary metastasis, although rare, has been reported.

Although considered uncommon as a primary orbital tumor in the dog, osteosarcoma comprised approximately 25% of orbital tumors in one retrospective study.[21] Unlike osteosarcoma of the appendicular skeleton, osteosarcoma of the skull more frequently affects older dogs of smaller breeds. Osteosarcoma may arise from any of the orbital bones and is first recognized as a firm bony enlargement.

Adenocarcinomas of the lacrimal gland or any malignancy within the nasal sinuses may involve the orbit by extension from the primary site.

History and Clinical Signs

Dogs and cats with space-occupying orbital disease typically present with a history of progressive, nonpainful exophthalmia and protrusion of the membrana nictitans (Fig. 28-5). Retropulsion and normal motility of the globe are reduced to absent. Pronounced exophthalmia may inhibit lid closure and produce secondary exposure keratitis. Distortion of the globe and retinal detachment may occur. Tumor necrosis and inflammation may produce signs of orbital cellulitis. Invasion into or from the nasal sinuses may result in ipsilateral epiphora or sanguino-purulent nasal discharge. Extension along the optic nerve or other cranial nerves may cause blindness or ophthalmoplegia.

Diagnostic Techniques and Work-Up

Thorough examination of the head is essential and should include the oral cavity and external nares. A complete ophthalmologic examination is necessary including palpation of both orbits, neuro-ophthalmologic and funduscopic examinations.

Additional diagnostic techniques to be considered are fine-needle aspiration and cytology or biopsy of palpable masses, orbital radiography with or without contrast studies (orbital angiography/venography, dacryocystorhinography, positive contrast orbitography, sialography, optic thecography), orbital ultrasonography, and computed tomography.[21a–21c]

Orbital neoplasms must be differentiated from orbital cysts, foreign bodies, cellulitis, and fractures of the orbital bones.

Therapy

Surgery remains the major mode of therapy. Limited and extensive exploration of the orbit have been described. These techniques should be considered when localized or well-circumscribed neoplasms are excised.[22] Unfortunately, the limits of many orbital neoplasms are poorly defined or the tumor has invaded the orbit enough by the time of diagnosis to require more radical surgery. In many cases, removal by exenteration of as much of the orbital contents as possible is the method of choice. Techniques for orbital exenteration are described elsewhere.[22]

Complete resection of extensive orbital tumors is often impossible. Additional treatment modalities to consider include radiation therapy and chemotherapy.

Prognosis

In most cases, the prognosis for elimination of orbital neoplasms is unfavorable. Many such tumors are malignant, and because the time interval from initial clinical signs to diagnosis and treatment is often prolonged, cure by complete surgical excision is unlikely. Recurrence of tumor at the primary site is common, and local and regional metastasis occurs with frustrating regularity. Early diagnosis, aggressive surgical management when possible, and follow-up ancillary treatment procedures are necessary to deal effectively with orbital cancer.

COMPARATIVE ASPECTS

Retinoblastoma is the most common primary tumor of the eye in children. There are approximately 11 new cases of retinoblastoma per 1 million children under the age of 5 years.[23] These tumors may be congenital, inherited, or acquired; and tumors can undergo spontaneous regression. More than 85% of the children with retinoblastoma survive, and the vast majority have both local tumor control and preservation of vision following surgery or irradiation.[24]

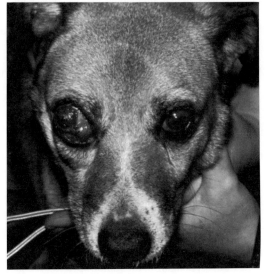

Figure 28-5. Animals with orbital neoplasia usually exhibit nonpainful exophthalmia and nictitans protrusion. Retropulsion of the globe is inhibited.

In adults, malignant melanoma of the eye is the most common primary tumor of that organ. The choroid within the uveal tract is the most common site of origin, whereas melanoma of the iris accounts for 8% of melanomas of the eye.[25] Intraocular melanomas occur most commonly in white, middle-aged women.

Clinical features predicting malignant behavior of uveal melanoma include large tumor, multiple patches of orange pigment in tumor, retinal detachment, and blood vessels within tumor.[25] Uveal melanomas metastasize to the liver through hematogenous routes without regional lymph node metastases. Six- to ten-year mortality rates vary from 15% to 25% and 35% to 36%, respectively. The treatment of these tumors has been enucleation.[26] Recent data suggest significantly longer survival when radiotherapy is applied to the orbit after enucleation.[25]

Melanoma of the iris has a better prognosis than melanomas of the choroid. Treatment consists of complete excision without enucleation. Death due to metastases from melanoma of the iris is rare.[25]

REFERENCES

1. Peiffer RL: Feline ophthalmology. In Gelatt KN (ed): Veterinary Ophthalmology, pp. 521–568. Philadelphia, Lea & Febiger, 1981
2. Barrie KP, Gelatt KN, Parshall CP: Eyelid squamous cell carcinoma in four dogs. J Am Anim Hosp Assoc 18:123–127, 1982
3. Krehbiel JD, Langham RF: Eyelid neoplasms of dogs. Am J Vet Res 36:115–119, 1975
4. Roberts SM, Severin GA, Lavach JD: Prevalence and treatment of palpebral neoplasms in the dog: 200 cases (1975–1983). J Am Vet Med Assoc 189:1355–1359, 1986
5. Brightman AH II: Lids. In Slatter DH (ed): Textbook of Small Animal Surgery, pp. 1448–1468. Philadelphia, W.B. Saunders, 1985
6. Peiffer RL, Gelatt KN, Karpinski LG: The canine eyelids. In Gelatt KN (ed): Veterinary Ophthalmology, pp. 296–305. Philadelphia, Lea & Febiger, 1981
7. Vestre WA: Cryosurgical techniques in veterinary ophthalmology. Comp Cont Educ 6:481–490, 1984
8. Bonney CH, Koch SA, Confer AW, Dice PF: A case report: A conjunctivocorneal papilloma

with evidence of a viral etiology. J Small Anim Pract 21:183–188, 1980
9. Peiffer RL: Episcleral hemangioma in a dog. J Am Vet Med Assoc 173:1338–1340, 1978
10. Cook CS: Inflammatory disease of the canine sclera and episclera. Schering Veterinary Clinical Classroom I, pp. 1–8. Princeton Junction, NJ, Veterinary Learning Systems, 1984
11. Martin CL: Canine epibular melanomas and their management. J Am Anim Hosp Assoc 17:83–90, 1981
12. Diters RW, Dubielzig RR, Aguirre GD, Acland GM: Primary ocular melanoma in dogs. Vet Pathol 20:379–395, 1983
13. Wilcock BP, Peiffer RL: Morphology and behavior of primary ocular melanomas in 91 dogs. Vet Pathol 23:418–424, 1986
14. Aguirre GD, Brown G, Shields JA, Dubielzig RR: Melanoma of the choroid in a dog. J Am Anim Hosp Assoc 20:471–476, 1984
15. Peiffer RL: Ciliary body epithelial tumours in the dog and cat; a report of thirteen cases. J Small Anim Pract 24:347–370, 1983
16. Augsburger JJ, Shields JA, Folberg R, et al: Fine needle aspiration biopsy in the diagnosis of intraocular cancer. Ophthalmology 92:39–48, 1985
17. Acland GM, McLean IW, Aguirre GD, Trucksa R: Diffuse iris melanoma in cats. J Am Vet Med Assoc 176:52–56, 1980
18. Dubielzig RR, Everitt J, Shadduck JA, Albert DM: Morphological and clinical features of primary ocular melanoma in cats. Vet Pathol, in press.
19. Dubielzig RR: Ocular sarcoma following trauma in three cats. J Am Vet Med Assoc 184:578–581, 1984
20. Dubielzig RR, Everitt J, Shadduck JA, Albert DM: Clinical and morphological features of post-traumatic ocular sarcomas in cats. Vet Pathol, in press
21. Kern TJ: Orbital neoplasia in 23 dogs. J Am Vet Med Assoc 186:489–491, 1985
21a. Fike JR, LeCouteur RA, Carr CE: Anatomy of the canine orbital region: Multiplanar imaging by CT. Vet Radiol 25:32–36, 1984
21b. LeCouteur RA, Fike JR, Scagliotti RH et al: Computed tomography of orbital tumors in the dog. J Am Vet Med Assoc 180:910–913, 1982
21c. LeCouteur RA, Scagliotti RH, Beck KA et al: Indirect imaging of the canine optic nerve, using metrizamide (optic thecography). Am J Vet Res 43:1424–1428, 1982

22. Slatter DH, Chambers ED: Orbit. In Slatter DH (ed): Textbook of Small Animal Surgery, pp. 1549–1569. Philadelphia, W.B. Saunders, 1985

23. Pendergrass TW, Davis S: Incidence of retinoblastoma in the United States. Arch Ophthalmol 90:1204–1210, 1980

24. Pizzo PA, Cassady JR, Miser JS et al: Solid tumors of childhood. In DeVita VT Jr, Hellman S, Rosenberg SA (eds): Cancer: Principles and Practice of Oncology, 2nd ed, pp. 1536–1540. Philadelphia, JB Lippincott, 1985

25. Sinkovics JG: Tumors of pigment cells. In Medical Oncology, vol I, pp. 425–426. New York, Marcel Dekker, 1988

26. Weiss JS, Albert DM: Intraocular melanoma. In DeVita VT Jr, Hellman S, Rosenberg SA (eds): Cancer: Principles and Practice of Oncology, 2nd ed, pp. 1423–1435. Philadelphia, JB Lippincott, 1985

29

HEMATOPOIETIC TUMORS

Feline Retroviruses

William D. Hardy, Jr.
E. Gregory MacEwen

At present the only known oncogenic viruses of pet animals exist in cats. Despite numerous studies, no oncogenic viruses have been isolated from dogs with lymphosarcoma or mammary adenocarcinomas. In cats, oncogenic retroviruses are numerous, but oncogenic herpes viruses have not been found.

Retroviruses are an ever-expanding family of RNA-containing viruses of animals and humans characterized by the ability to copy their single-stranded viral RNA into double-stranded DNA (reverse transcription) by means of a unique enzyme known as the reverse transcriptase. The DNA copy of the viral genome becomes integrated into the infected cell's chromosomes. This process of "viral genetic engineering" takes only a few hours to change the cell's chromosomes forever.

There are three subfamilies of retroviruses: Oncovirinae, Lentivirinae, and Spumavirinae. Oncoviruses include the cancer-inducing leukemia, sarcoma, and carcinoma viruses such as the feline leukemia virus (FeLV), feline sarcoma viruses (FeSV), avian leukosis viruses (ALV), and murine leukemia viruses (MuLV). Lentiviruses, long ignored because they "only" caused rare diseases of farm animals in far-off lands, are now very important because the human AIDS viruses (human immunodeficiency viruses, HIV-1 and -2) have been shown to be members of this subfamily. In addition, and of importance to veterinarians, a new feline lentivirus that induces acquired immunodeficiency syndrome (AIDS) in cats has recently been discovered and has been named the feline immunodeficiency virus (FIV).[1] Spumaviruses, or foamy viruses, occur in many animals; they cause inapparent infections but are not known to cause any disease. Cats are infected with representatives of all three subfamilies of retroviruses, and there are now two feline retroviruses from different subfamilies that cause AIDS in cats, FeLV and FIV (Tables 29-1 and 29-2).

Table 29-1. Feline Retroviruses: Method of Transmission and Effects

RETROVIRUS	METHOD OF TRANSMISSION/EFFECTS
Subfamily Oncovirinae	
Endogenous viruses	Genetically transmitted
RD-114	Xenotropic—does not replicate in cats
	No known disease association
FeLV-related sequences	Full length and shorter sequences
	Cannot be induced to replicate
	Recombines with exogenous FeLV-A to form FeLV-B and FeLV-C
Exogenous viruses	Spread contagiously
FeLV	
Subgroup A	Ecotropic—found in all infected cats
Subgroup B	Amphotropic—found in 50% of infected cats
Subsgroup C	Amphotropic—found rarely (< 1%)
Defective FeLV-myc	Found in 14% of FeLV-infected thymic LSAs
	Recombinant proviruses
FeSV: 11 well-characterized isolates	Recombinants between FeLV and cellular oncogenes
Subfamily Lentivirinae	
FIV (feline immunodeficiency virus)	Induces AIDS syndrome
Subfamily Spumavirinae	
FeSFV (feline syncytium-forming virus	Causes no known disease

Xenotropic: Grows in heterologous (noncat) cells only.
Ecotropic: Grows in homologous (cat) cells only.
Amphotropic: Grows in homologous and heterologous cells, broad host range.

Table 29-2. Classification of Retroviruses by Subfamily

A. Oncovirinae
  1. Leukemia and sarcoma viruses
     a. Avian—ALV, ASV
     b. Murine—MuLV, MuSV
     c. Feline—FeLV, FeSV, RD-114
     d. Bovine—BLV
     e. Baboon—BaEV
     f. Wolly monkey—SSV
     g. Gibbon ape—GaLV
     h. Monkey—STLV-I
     i. Human—HTLV-I, HTLV-II
  2. Carcinoma viruses
     a. Murine—MMTV
     b. Monkey—MPMV
B. Lentivirinae
  1. Amemiagenic: Equine—EIAV
  2. Neurotropic: Ungulates—Visna & Maedi viruses
  3. Immunosuppressive
     a. Feline—FIV
     b. Bovine—BIV
     c. Monkey—SIV (STLV-III)
     d. Human—HIV-1, 2 (HTLV-III/LAV, HTLV-IV/LAV-2)
C. Spumavirinae: Foamy viruses
     a. Feline—FeSFV
     b. Many species
     c. Human—HuSFV

About 2% of the estimated 50 million pet cats, or almost 1 million cats, in the United States are infected with FeLV.[2] The virus was discovered in the 1960s in Scotland in a cat that lived with several cats that had developed lymphoma (LSA).[3] At that time is was thought that all retroviruses were endogenous viruses that were transmitted genetically (vertically) as a Mendelian trait.[4] However, from veterinarian's observations of pet cats living in natural household environments,[5,6] later confirmed in laboratory experiments,[7] it was found the FeLV is an exogenous retrovirus that is transmitted contagiously among cats. It is now known that all disease-inducing retroviruses of animals and humans, except those of inbred laboratory mice, are exogenous and are contagiously transmitted among members of a single species.[8,9]

FELINE LEUKEMIA VIRUS (FeLV)

VIROLOGY OF FeLV

There are two major groups of feline oncogenic retroviruses, the endogenous and exogenous viruses (Table 29-1). The RD-114 virus is an endogenous virus of domestic cats.[10,10a] Multiple complete copies of the RD-114 viral genomes (proviruses) are found in all cats' cells, but the virus does not replicate in cats. RD-114 is closely related to the baboon endogenous virus (BaEV).[11] It is likely that RD-114 and BaEV originated together and that the original virus occurred as a result of horizontal transmission from one species to the other or via horizontal transmission from a third species into ancestral cats and baboons at approximately the same time.[10] RD-114 is not associated with any known feline disease.

ENDOGENOUS FeLV-RELATED SEQUENCES

Cellular DNA of normal cats contains sequences partially homologous to the exogenous horizontally transmitted FeLV.[10,11] The endogenous FeLV sequences are arranged as multiple (8–12 copies), discrete copies in a nonrandom fashion in the chromosomes.

The exogenous infectious FeLVs probably originated from cross-species infection of an endogenous rat retrovirus into ancestors of the domestic cat.[10,11] Three subgroups of FeLV—FeLV-A, -B, and -C—are identified by their envelope gp70 molecules (Table 29-1).[12,13] FeLV-A is ecotropic; that is, it has a highly restricted host range and grows almost exclusively in cat cells. FeLV-A is found in all infected cats, either alone (50%) or in combination with FeLV-B (49%) or FeLV-C (1%).[14,15] FeLV-B is amphotropic; it has a wide host range and can replicate in cat, dog, mink, hamster, dog, pig, bovine, monkey, and human cells. FeLV-C is also amphotropic, but it has an intermediate range of hosts; it can replicate in cat, dog, mink, guinea pig, and human cells.[12,13] There is no clear association of any subgroup of FeLV with any specific naturally occurring disease. However, under experimental conditions the Rickard strain of FeLV-A induces mainly thymic LSA, a variant of FeLV-A causes the feline acquired immune deficiency snydrome (FAIDS), and several isolates of FeLV-C induce erythroid hypoplasia (aplastic anemia).[16–20] It is now known that FeLV-A gives rise to FeLV-B and FeLV-C viruses *de novo* by means of recombination of its genome with the endogenous FeLV-B or FeLV-C-related *env* sequences that are present in the DNA of all cats.[21–23]

FeLV Genome

FeLV is a replication-competent chronic leukemia virus that does not possess a transforming gene (oncogene). The FeLV genome consists of the 5'-*gag-pol-env*-3' genes flanked by two long terminal repeats (LTR). The *gag* gene encodes the p15, p12, p27, and p10 internal viral structural proteins, the *pol* gene encodes the viral reverse transcriptase, and the *env* gene encodes the gp70 and p15E envelope proteins (Fig. 29-1).[8,9]

The FeLV proteins are produced in great excess in the cytoplasm of infected cells, and most of these antigens are never packaged into viral particles.[24,25] Detection of FeLV antigens in the cytoplasm of peripheral blood leukocytes by an indirect immunofluorescent antibody (IFA) test, or as soluble antigens in the plasma by an enzyme-linked immunosorbent assay (ELISA), has been used in the study of the occurrence and control of FeLV in pet cats.[14,24,26–28] A positive IFA test indicates persistent, usually lifelong (in 97% of IFA-positive cats) viremia and shedding of the virus in the saliva.[2,24,29] In contrast, approximately 30% to 50% of ELISA-positive cats do not have infectious FeLV in their plasma, nor do they shed the virus in their saliva.[2,29–31] The most likely explanation for this discrepancy is erroneous, or "false positive," ELISA test results.

FeLV Replication

FeLV is composed of a nucleocapsid core covered by a lipid envelope. The nucleocapsid contains the RNA genome surrounded by proteins, and the envelope is a lipid bilayer membrane with protruding glycoproteins.[32] FeLV infects a cell by binding, by means of the major envelope glycoprotein (gp70), to a receptor on the surface of a target cell. After the virus has penetrated the target cell, the viral reverse transcriptase directs the transcription of the viral RNA genome into DNA.[33,34] The DNA copy of the viral genome is duplicated and a circularized form of the double-stranded DNA integrates into the host cell DNA. The integrated double-stranded DNA form of the virus, called a provirus, thus becomes part of the genome of the host cell (Fig. 29-2).

Pathogenesis of FeLV Infection

As many as 2×10^6 infectious FeLVs per ml occur in the saliva of infected cats. The virus is

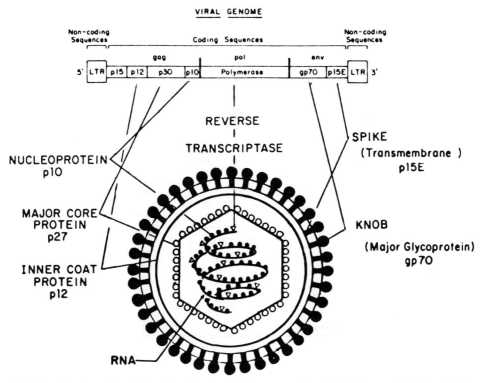

Fig 29-1. Structure of the feline leukemia virus and its genome. Reprinted with permission from Wolfe JH, Hardy WD, Jr: Immunogenetics of murine and feline retroviruses. In Litwin SD, Scott D, Flaherty L, Reisfeld R, Marcus D (eds): Human Immunogenetics: An Advanced Text. New York, Marcel Dekker, 1988.

transmitted through the saliva to the ocular, oral, and nasal membranes of uninfected cats.[29,35] After entering the cat's body, the virus replicates in lymphocytes of the local lymph nodes of the head and neck. Most exposed cats reject the virus at this early stage and become immune.[2,14,35] However, in cats that do not reject the virus, FeLV spreads to the bone marrow, where it replicates to high titers. Leukocytes and platelets released from the infected bone marrow, or free plasma virus, spread the infection throughout the cat's body. Ninety-seven percent of cats that have widespread replication of FeLV in their bone marrow remain persistently infected throughout life.[2] Within a few weeks the virus spreads to the salivary glands and respiratory epithelial cells, from which it is shed. FeLV can also be transmitted *in utero* to unborn fetuses and through the milk of infected queens.[2] Although the period of time from FeLV infection to disease development is highly var-

iable, 83% of infected healthy cats die within 3.5 years.[36]

Latent FeLV

FeLV can persist in a latent, unexpressed, nonreplicating state in a small number of mononuclear cells of the bone marrow of cats that have rejected the virus and become immune.[37] The virus can be activated from the bone marrow cells by treating such cats with very high doses of corticosteroids or by stimulating bone marrow cultures with corticosteroids or *Staphylococcus aureus* Cowan I.[37] Activation of latent virus has not been shown to occur often, if at all, in immune pet cats living in natural household environments. Although a small percentage of latently infected cats are intermittently positive by ELISA testing, most express no circulating viral antigen. The prognosis for the latently infected cat is not clear. As long as the animal remains aviremic, it is probably not at high risk

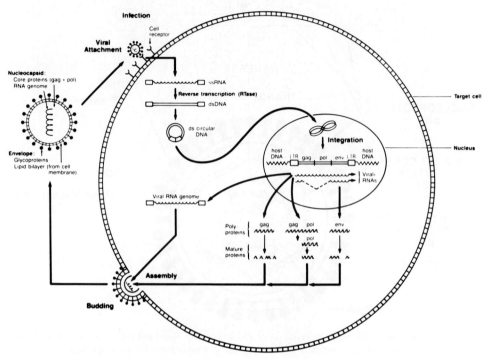

Fig 29-2. Replication of the feline leukemia virus. FeLV attaches by its envelope gp70 to the gp70 receptors on the cell membrane, enters the cell, and is uncoated, releasing the viral RNA genome. The viral RNA genome is copied into double-stranded DNA by the viral reverse transcriptase and cat cellular enzymes. The double-stranded DNA circularizes and is integrated into the cell's chromosomes, and the integrated DNA (provirus) is then transcribed into viral messenger RNA. New viral RNA, proteins, and reverse transcriptase are synthesized and assembled into a complete virus particle, which buds from the cell membrane as infectious FeLV. (Reprinted with permission from Wolfe JH, Hardy WD Jr: Immunogenetics of murine and feline retroviruses. In Litwin SD, Scott D, Flaherty L, Reisfeld R, Marcus D (eds): Human Immunogenetics: An Advanced Text. New York, Marcel Dekker, 1988).

of manifesting most FeLV-related diseases. However, FeLV-negative lymphoid tumors may develop if feline oncornavirus-associated cell membrane antigen antibody (FOCMA) titers decline. Latently infected cats have not been shown to spread the virus to uninfected contacts. Latently infected queens, though they have been reported to bear FeLV-infected offspring, are unlikely to do so. Glucocorticoid activation of latent infection may be of little significance because of the relatively short duration of the latent phase and the infrequency of experimental reactivation in cats carrying most strains of FeLV. However, no serologic test is available to identify latent FeLV infections, and tech-

niques for marrow cultures are expensive and not widely available. Cats at risk for latent infection are those known to have been transiently infected (particularly within the previous 6–12 months), as well as recently acquired FeLV-exposed cats. To reduce the risks of activating viremia in potential carriers, the following precautions are suggested:

1. Screen all suspects with a reliable ELISA or IFA assay; consider repeat testing 12 weeks after the exposure period.
2. Avoid steroid administration, pregnancy, and other stresses.
3. Consider FeLV immunization.

Table 29-3.   Consequences of Exposure to FeLV

FeLV EXPOSURE	PERMANENT FeLV STATUS	FeLV IMMUNE RESPONSE	PERCENTAGE OF CATS
Not exposed	Not infected	Not immune	30
Exposed	Not infected	Immune	42*
Exposed	Infected	Not immune	28

* Transiently infected

Consequences of FeLV Exposure

The immunologic response of cats to FeLV exposure determines their fate, and exposure to FeLV does not invariably result in persistent infection and development of LSA. Only about 10% to 20% of persistently infected pet cats develop LSA, whereas far more die of the immunosuppressive effects of the virus.[2,14,29,36,38–40] Forty-two percent of cats exposed to FeLV become immune to the virus, 28% become persistently infected, and the remaining 30% become neither immune nor infected (Table 29-3).[2,14] An adequate antibody response to the viral envelope constituents, the gp70 and p15E, will result in neutralization of the virus and clearance from the body. An inappropriate antibody response in some cats against the FeLV *gag* antigens p15, p12, p27, and p10 is not beneficial and in persistently infected cats may lead to the formation of immune complexes, immunosuppression, and the development of immune complex glomerulonephritis.[2,41,42]

EPIDEMIOLOGY OF FeLV

Occurrence of FeLV

During the 1960s, many veterinarians observed the clustering of cases of LSA in unrelated cats living in the same households which suggested that contagious transmission of FeLV was occurring in these environments.[29,43,44] In 1973 we devised a simple and accurate IFA test for FeLV[24] that enabled large epidemiologic surveys of the occurrence of FeLV to be done in the United States and Europe.[2,14,15,24,27,29–31,35–37] Infected cats were mainly found in exposure households, such as multiple-cat households where other cats with FeLV infection or LSA had lived. We found that 28% of healthy FeLV-exposed cats were persistently infected, whereas only 1% to 2% of household cats with no known exposure were infected.[2,14,29] Less than 1% of stray cats and 2% of shelter cats that we tested were infected with FeLV.

FeLV Testing Methods

In 1973 a specific sensitive and rapid immunofluorescent antibody (IFA) test for detection of FeLV antigens in leukocytes in the peripheral blood of cats was introduced into veterinary medicine.[24] A positive IFA test indicates FeLV infection but is not diagnostic of any FeLV disease. FeLV can be isolated from the blood of 97.5% of IFA-positive cats (Table 29-4), and an IFA-positive cat sheds the virus in its saliva.[24,29,45] Ninety-seven percent of IFA-positive cats remain positive for life, whereas 3% are able to reject the virus and become immune.

Table 29-4.   Correlation of IFA Test for Detection of FeLV with Tissue Culture Isolation Test and ELISA Test

IFA TEST RESULTS*	ELISA TEST RESULTS†	NO. CATS TESTED	NO. CATS FeLV ISOLATED IN TISSUE CULTURE‡	NO. CATS IFA POSITIVE	AGREEMENT (%)
Negative		153	3	ND**	98
Positive		121	118	ND	97.5
	Negative	661	ND	88	86.7
	Positive	7819	ND	3193	40.8

* FeLV IFA tests performed by the National Veterinary Laboratory.
† ELISA tests performed by practitioners or veterinary laboratories. ELISA test kits produced by Pitman Moore, TechAmerica, Symbiotics, Norden, and Idexx.
‡ Tissue culture isolation performed by WDH at Memorial Sloan Kettering Cancer Center.
**ND = not done.

FeLV cannot be isolated from 98% of IFA-negative cats. Thus there is excellent correlation between the IFA test result for FeLV and the ability to isolate the virus from the blood.

In the past several years in-hospital enzyme-linked immunosorbent assay (ELISA) tests for FeLV have been introduced into veterinary medicine, and comparative studies of the IFA and ELISA tests have been performed (Table 29-4). In general there is fairly good correlation between ELISA negative tests and the IFA test results. We have found an 86% agreement with negative ELISA tests; this indicates, however, that more than 13% of ELISA negative tests performed by practicing veterinarians are incorrect. More important, we have found only a 40.8% agreement between ELISA positive tests and the IFA test. Other workers have reported around a 70% agreement between ELISA positive and IFA positive tests.[30,46] We strongly recommend that all positive ELISA tests be confirmed with an accurate FeLV IFA test.

IMMUNE RESPONSE TO FeLV

Feline Oncornavirus-Associated Cell Membrane Antigen (FOCMA)

FOCMA was initially detected on cell membranes of cultured feline LSA cells.[47,48] Cats with high titers of FOCMA antibody are resistant to FeLV-induced LSA.[14] FOCMA antibody and FeLV-neutralizing (VN) antibody are not always present together in the same cat, suggesting that FOCMA is not an FeLV structural antigen, at least not an FeLV-A or -B structural antigen.[14,49] In addition, FOCMA is found on the cell membranes of all feline T- and B-LSA cells, irrespective of their FeLV status, on FeSV-induced fibrosarcoma cells, and on FeLV-infected erythroid and myeloid leukemic cells.[45,50–52] In contrast, FOCMA is not found on normal feline lymphocytes, even those productively infected with FeLV-A and -B. The finding of FOCMA on FeLV-negative LSA cells indicates that FOCMA is a marker of FeLV leukemogenesis, i.e., a tumor-specific antigen.[45,50,51] FOCMA isolated from FeLV-positive and FeLV-negative LSA cells was found to be a protein of 70,000 daltons (p70) molecular weight, which was found to be different from the gp70 molecules of FeLV-A and -B.[49,51,52] It is now known that FOCMA is related to, but is serologically distinguishable from, FeLV-C gp70 and is biologically a marker

of FeLV and FeSV neoplasia (tumor-specific antigen).[45,51]

Immune Response to Virus-Neutralizing Antibody

The fate of an FeLV-exposed cat depends mainly on its humoral immune response to the viral gp70, the virus-neutralizing (VN) antibody, and the FeLV-induced tumor-specific antigen, FOCMA. However, a high antibody titer to the FeLV gp70 alone is sufficient to protect the cat against both FeLV infection and FeLV-induced diseases, except FeLV-negative LSA. Cats with protective titers of VN antibody (1:10 or greater) have rejected the virus and are resistant to subsequent viral infection. Cats with protective titers of FOCMA antibody (1:16 or greater), in the absence of protective titers of VN antibody, are resistant to the development of LSA or other FeLV-induced tumors but are not resistant to the development of FeLV infection and non-neoplastic FeLV diseases.[14,39,47]

Seroepidemiologic studies have shown that unexposed pet cats do not have VN antibodies to FeLV subgroups A and B, whereas about 42% of exposed cats have FeLV-A and -B neutralizing antibodies.[2,53] No FeLV-infected cats have protective VN antibody to FeLV-A and -B.[2,53] However, there is an unexplained high prevalence of VN antibodies to FeLV-C in all populations of cats, especially in FeLV-A and -B infected cats (45%), most of whom (98%) have no VN antibodies to FeLV-A and -B.[2,53]

Immune Response to FOCMA

FOCMA antibody protects cats from developing FeLV-induced LSA, but does not protect them from FeLV infection or from developing FeLV-induced non-neoplastic diseases.[47] FOCMA antibody is found mainly in cats exposed to FeLV (38.4%), only rarely in unexposed cats, and never in specific pathogen free (SPF) cats.[2,14] Twenty-five percent of FeLV-infected cats have protected titers of FOCMA antibody. FOCMA antibody has even been used therapeutically to induce remission of LSA in pet cats.[54]

PREVENTION OF THE SPREAD OF FeLV

An IFA test and removal program has been used successfully in veterinary medicine for the past 16 years.[2,26,27,55] In this program, all cats are tested for FeLV and any infected cats are removed from the household. After the infected cats have been removed, the uninfected cats are quarantined in the household and are retested 3 months later. The 3-month retest is needed because the incubation period of FeLV infection can be as long as 3 months. If any of the initially uninfected cats are found to be FeLV positive in the second FeLV test, they are removed and a third test is done 3 months later. When all cats test negative in two consecutive tests done 3 months apart, the cats in the household are declared free of FeLV infection. With this program we were able to reduce the spread of FeLV 40-fold over households that did not remove infected cats from contact with uninfected cats.[27] It must be stressed that, owing to the poor correlation between ELISA and IFA positive tests, FeLV in all ELISA-positive cats must be confirmed with an accurate IFA test before the cats are removed or euthanatized.

FeLV VACCINE

The first retrovirus vaccine was developed in veterinary medicine and is now available for potential protection of cats against FeLV infection.[56,57] The vaccine preparation is inactivated to ensure that there is no infectious FeLV in the product. Clinical trials of the efficacy of the vaccine performed by the manufacturer demonstrated an 80% protection against virus challenge.[58] However, another study of the immunogenicity and efficacy of the vaccine reported poorer protection.[59] Only 50% of vaccinated cats developed good antibody to FeLV gp70-related antigens, and the response to virus challenge was disappointing.

One of us (WDH) has observed numerous vaccine "breaks" while testing cats for FeLV. Because these observations were not made in rigorous, controlled studies we cannot conclude that they were more than the expected 20% of cats that the producer of the vaccine claims may not be protected by vaccination. We recommend that cats be vaccinated with the current FeLV vaccine until a more efficient one is developed. However, it must be stressed that the vaccine does not reverse FeLV infection in a viremic cat. In addition, cats should be tested for FeLV at the time of the first dose of vaccine, and those infected should be removed from the household or strictly isolated and should not receive subsequent vaccinations. Employing the FeLV test

and removal program along with vaccination should markedly reduce the spread of FeLV among pet cats.

Recently a second FeLV vaccine has been marketed, but efficiency studies have not yet been performed.

FeLV DISEASES

FeLV replicates most efficiently in rapidly dividing lymphoid and myeloid cells and can induce proliferative (neoplastic) and degenerative (blastopenic) diseases in these cells (Table 29-5). FeLV-induced diseases are collectively the leading cause of death among pet cats.[2,40,60,61,62] At present it is not known if the vaccine has significantly lowered the occurrence of FeLV diseases.

Lymphoma (LSA) is the proliferative lymphocyte disease caused by FeLV, whereas thymic atrophy and general lymphoid depletion are the degenerative diseases of lymphocytes.[17,40,63] FeLV-induced proliferative diseases of erythrocyte precursors are erythremic myelosis and erythroleukemia, whereas the degenerative erythrocyte disease, erythroblastopenia, occurs far more often in pet cats than the proliferative diseases.[16,61,64] Severe immunosuppression induced by the virus, which results in the development of secondary opportunistic infections and death, is the most frequent clinical manifestation of FeLV infection.[40,60] This syndrome is called the FeLV-induced feline acquired immune deficiency syndrome, or FeLV-FAIDS.[65]

Lymphoma

Pet cats have the highest incidence of naturally occurring LSA of any animal, with 200 cases occurring per 100,000 cats at risk.[2,60] One-third of all cat tumors are hematopoietic tumors, and 90% of these are LSA.[66] The multicentric form, in which the tumor localizes in internal organs and lymph nodes, is the most common anatomic form of LSA in cats. About 30% of cats with LSA have leukemic blood profiles, and these cats are classified as having multicentric LSA.[60,61] Thymic LSA is the second most common form, followed by alimentary LSA, which localizes in the gastrointestinal tract and usually is FeLV-negative.[50,61]

The majority of feline LSAs are T cell tumors, although B cell LSAs occur frequently in the

Table 29-5.   FeLV Diseases by Cell Type

CELL TYPE	PROLIFERATIVE DISEASES (NEOPLASTIC)	DEGENERATIVE DISEASES (BLASTOPENIC)
Lymphocytes	Lymphosarcoma	Thymic atrophy Lymphopenias Feline acquired immune deficiency syndrome (FAIDS)
Bone Marrow Cells		
Primitive mesenchymal cell	Reticuloendotheliosis	
Erythroblast	Erythremic myelosis	Erythroblastosis
	Erythroleukemia	Erythroblastopenia Pancytopenia
Myeloblast	Granulocytic leukemia	Myeloblastopenia
Megakaryocyte	Megakaryocytic leukemia	Thrombocytopenia
Fibroblast	Myelofibrosis	
Osteoblast	Medullary osteosclerosis Osteochondromatosis	
Kidney	—	FeLV immune complex glomerulo-nephritis
Uterus	—	Abortions and resorptions
Fibroblasts, skin	FeSV-induced multicentric fibrosarcomas	—

gastrointestinal tract.[45,50] About two-thirds of cats with LSA have nonregenerative anemias.[61]

Thirty percent of cats with LSA are FeLV negative.[45] In these cases, no FeLV antigens are detected, nor can infectious FeLV be isolated from any tissue.[45,50] However, the FeLV-induced FOCMA is present on the membranes of both FeLV-positive and -negative LSA cells.[45,50] Cats with FeLV-positive LSA are usually less than 7 years old and have T cell multicentric or thymic LSA, whereas cats with FeLV-negative LSA are usually over 7 years of age and have alimentary B cell LSA.[45,50,67]

FeLV-negative cases of LSA occur frequently in households where FeLV-infected cats live.[2,14,24,43] A large epidemiologic study found that cats who developed FeLV-negative LSA were exposed to FeLV as often as cats who developed FeLV-positive LSA.[45,50] No FeLV proviral sequences, above the level of endogenous FeLV sequences present in all uninfected cat cells, can be found in the FeLV-negative LSA tumor tissues; this suggests an indirect mechanism of leukemogenesis in these cases.[68] However, additional FeLV sequences can be found in non-LSA tissues, most often bone marrow cells, in 60% of these cats, indicating that cats with FeLV-negative LSA were previously infected with FeLV and that integrated exogenous FeLV sequences exist in some non-LSA tissues. This finding and the observation that in healthy cats with FOCMA antibody the titers remain high for many years suggest that there is continual FeLV stimulation. Latent FeLV can be reactivated from the bone marrow of healthy FeLV-immune cats and from the bone marrow (but not from the lymphoma cells) of cats with FeLV-negative LSA.[37] Thus, it is apparent that FeLV induces both FeLV-positive and FeLV-negative LSA in cats. FeLV can also induce FeLV-negative LSA in puppies.[69] Puppies inoculated with FeLV during the first day of life developed FeLV-negative LSA, whereas those inoculated in utero developed FeLV-positive LSA.

Feline lymphoma can be treated with combination chemotherapy.[70–73] The most commonly used protocols include vincristine, cyclophosphamide, prednisone, cytosine arabinoside, methotrexate, and L-asparaginase (Table 29-6, Protocol A). In a recent study,[70] a complete response (100% regression of disease) was obtained in 64 of 103 (62%) cats treated. The cats with a complete response had a median survival time of 7 months; 30% (19 of 64 cats) survived a year or longer. Twenty-one cats had a partial response (>50% regression of disease) with a median survival time of 2.5 months. Cats with a less than 50% regression had a median survival time of 1.5 months. FeLV-negative cats with less advanced disease (Stages I or II) had median survival times of 17–18 months. Median survival time for FeLV-positive cats was 4.2 months, as compared to 9 months for FeLV-negative cats.

Table 29-6.   Feline Lymphoma Protocols

PROTOCOL A

Induction of remission

Week 1: 0.5 to 0.7 mg/m² vincristine IV; 400 i.u./kg L-asparaginase IP, IM; 2 mg/kg prednisone daily, divided twice a day, orally

Week 2: 200 mg/m² cyclophosphamide IV

Week 3: 0.5 to 0.7 mg/m² vincristine IV

Week 4: 0.8 mg/kg methotrexate IV*

Repeat treatments on weekly basis for another 4 treatments (except for L-asparaginase).

Maintenance of Remission

Continue same treatments (except for L-asparaginase) on an every 2-week basis

PROTOCOL B: RENAL LYMPHOSARCOMA

Induction of Remission

2 cycles (8 weeks) of Protocol A

Maintenance of remission

Every 2 weeks:

   1st drug: 0.5 to 0.7 mg/m² vincristine IV

   2nd drug: 30 mg/kg or 600 mg/m² cytosine arabinoside SQ divided into 4 doses at 12-hour intervals over 48 hours

   3rd drug: 0.5 to 0.7 mg/m² vincristine IV

   4th drug: 0.8 mg/kg methotrexate IV*

* Adriamycin (doxorubicin) can be substituted for methotrexate at a dose of 25 mg/m² IV (maximum dose 200 mg/m²). Wait 14 days before giving the next vincristine treatment.

Renal lymphoma can be treated with a somewhat altered chemotherapy protocol (Table 29-6, Protocol B). In a recent study[73] of 28 cats treated, the median survival time was 5.5 months for cats achieving a complete remission. Cats that were FeLV negative had a median survival time of 8.5 months, as opposed to 4 months for FeLV-positive cats.

We have seen cats presented with prominent generalized lymphadenopathy[74] with histologic features resembling lymphoma. All cats were FeLV negative and the cause of the lymphadenopathy was unknown. In five of the six cats reported, the lymph nodes regressed spontaneously without any therapy. Four of the six cats were recovering from either upper respiratory tract or urinary tract infections. Therefore, all cats with suspected lymphoma should undergo a thorough physical examination, including a history of previous or concurrent viral infection or exposure, thoracic and abdominal radiography, FeLV testing, and bone marrow and lymph node biopsy to determine a diagnosis.

Lymphoblastic leukemia is characterized by a predominance of immature cells (lymphoblasts) in the bone marrow. Response to treatment is not as good for leukemias as it is for lymphomas. These can be treated with combination chemotherapy (Table 29-6). Combination chemotherapy using cyclophosphamide, vincristine, and prednisone has been used, and in one study a complete remission was achieved in 27% of cats with lymphoblastic leukemia.[71]

Degenerative Lymphoid Diseases and FeLV-Induced Feline Acquired Immune Deficiency Syndrome (FeLV-FAIDS)

FeLV replicates to high titers in feline lymphoid cells and often induces severe depletion or dysfunction of these cells (Table 29-7).

Thymic Atrophy. Thymic atrophy is a degenerative lymphoid disease of T-lymphocytes of the thymus gland of FeLV-infected young cats.[40,63] Depletion of thymic lymphocytes occurs, probably as a result of viral lysis, and results in a

Table 29-7.   Parameters of the FeLV-induced Feline Acquired Immune Deficiency Syndrome (FeLV-FAIDS)

I. Immune cell deficiencies

   A. Lymphoid depletions

      1. Thymic atrophy—kittens

      2. General lymphoid depletion—adults

   B. Myeloid depletion: Neutropenias—myeloblastopenia syndrome

II. Immune cell dysfunctions

   A. Deficient cell-mediated immune response: Cutaneous anergy—decreased allograph rejection

   B. Deficient antibody-mediated immune response to threshold antigen stimulation

III. Pathogenic antibody immune-mediated disease: Immune complex glomerulonephritis

IV. Complement deficiency

deficient cell-mediated immune response. In-fected kittens are susceptible to opportunistic infectious microorganisms. Many kittens with thymic atrophy develop bronchopneumonia or enteritis and usually die of these diseases in the first 3 months of life.

Lymphoid Atrophy. Lymphoid hyperplasia occurs early in most FeLV-infected cats but usually progresses to lymphoid atrophy, lymphopenia, and death from opportunistic infections.[40]

Secondary Diseases FeLV-FAIDS. More pet cats die from FeLV-FAIDS than from neoplastic diseases.[40,75] About half of cats with feline infectious peritonitis (feline coronavirus), one-third of cats with chronic abscesses or nonhealing lesions of the skin, half of cats with chronic upper-respiratory disease and pneumonia, half of cats with chronic generalized infections (septicemias and pyothorax), and 87% of kittens with thymic atrophy are infected with FeLV.[40,63,75] In order to diagnose this common disorder, the veterinarian must diagnose the chronic secondary disease in an FeLV-positive cat.

Mechanisms of FeLV Immunosuppression. Two feline retroviruses, FeLV and FIV, are now known to induce feline AIDS.[1] In FeLV-FAIDS, FeLV replicates in lymphoid and myeloid cells of the immune system and often causes degenerative blastopenic diseases (lymphopenias and neutropenias) involving these cells.[2,24,40,60,75] FeLV-infected cats often develop immune-cell deficiencies characterized by drastic reductions in lymphocytes and neutrophils[2,40] and immune-cell dysfunctions consisting of cutaneous anergy,[76] reduced T cell blastogenic responsiveness,[5,76–78] and impaired antibody production, particularly to T cell-dependent antigens (Table 29-7).[40,79]

In addition to T cell dysfunctions, B cell dysfunctions also occur in FeLV-infected cats.[40,79] FeLV-infected cats are less able (4-fold) to produce antibody to threshold doses of antigens than are uninfected cats. This deficiency may have very significant consequences under natural conditions of exposure to pathogens.[40,79]

FeLV may induce immunosuppression by one of the following mechanisms:

1. By the process of viral replication and budding from the cell membranes FeLV may cause lysis or may sensitize cells to cell-mediated immune destruction. The thymus-dependent T cell appears to be the primary target of FeLV.

2. FeLV-soluble circulating antigens may cause immunosuppression. In this regard, purified p15E has been reported to decrease *in vitro* blast transformation by 45% to 92%.[77–80] In addition, Orosz et al.[81,82] reported that inactivated FeLV and the p15E envelope antigen interfered with the production and function of murine IL-2. Furthermore, a recent study has shown that FeLV-infected cats have a T-helper cell suppression as evidenced by failure to produce IL-2.[82a]

3. Circulating immune complexes (CIC) are immunosuppressive, and CIC composed of whole infectious FeLV, FeLV gp70, p27, p15, and p15E occur in FeLV-infected pet cats.[40–42] In addition, when CICs were therapeutically removed by *ex vivo* immunosorption on *Staphylococcus aureus* Cowans I columns, several FAIDS cats and cats with leukemia-lymphoma showed marked clinical improvement.[83,84,84a]

The complement system is also affected in cats infected with FeLV. In one study all FeLV-infected cats with LSA, and 50% of FeLV-infected healthy cats, were hypocomplementemic.[85] The hypocomplementemia observed in FeLV-infected cats probably contributes to the generalized immunosuppression.

There are numerous similarities between human AIDS and FeLV-FAIDS in pet cats.[65,86] In both species, the syndromes are characterized by lymphopenias, reduced lymphocyte blastogenesis, cutaneous anergy, reduced numbers of T cells, impaired antibody response, and the occurrence of secondary infectious diseases.[65,87]

Bacterial infections are the most common problem associated with FAIDS. Broad-spectrum, bactericidal antibiotics should be used in cats with known bacterial infection. Wound care and bacterial cultures may also be indicated. Other concurrent infections, such as fungal infections, may develop. Cryptococcus can be diagnosed with cytology or antigen titers. Treatment for fungal infections includes the use of ketoconazole (10 mg/kg daily PO 4–8 weeks) and combination therapy with 5-fluorocytosine and amphotericin B. Toxoplasmosis can be diagnosed by means of serology and can be treated with sulfonamide (30 mg/kg BID) and pyrimethamine (0.5–1.0 mg/kg daily); this is considered more successful than sulfonamide-trimethoprim combinations alone (30 mg/kg BID 14–21 days).

Methods to abrogate the immune suppression with immunomodulators or immunorestorative procedures have been studied in the cat.[87a,87b] The agents used to treat immunosuppression fall under the category of biologic response modifiers (BRM). A review of BRM in the management of viral infections has been published.[87c] Antiviral therapy is undergoing intense study for treating AIDS in humans.[87d] Many of the agents used will be available for study in cats. A review of antiviral therapy in animals has recently been published.[88]

Erythroid Diseases

FeLV replicates in all nucleated erythroid cells in the bone marrow and can induce neoplastic or blastopenic diseases.[24,60,75]

Erythroid Neoplastic Diseases. FeLV rarely induces erythremic myelosis and erythroleukemia in infected cats. Feline erythroid neoplasms are similar to those that occur in chickens and mice infected with their oncogene-containing acute transforming retroviruses.[89,90]

Erythroid Blastopenic Diseases

Erythroid blastopenic diseases occur far more often in FeLV-infected pet cats than do erythroid neoplastic diseases.[60,61,75] There are three types of FeLV-induced anemias: erythroblastosis (regenerative anemia), erythroblastopenia (nonregenerative anemia), and pancytopenia.[18,60,74] FeLV-A has been shown to induce nonfatal transient erythroblastosis experimentally, whereas several FeLV-C isolates have induced fatal erythroblastopenias.[18,20] The most common types of erythroid blastopenic conditions seen are nonregenerative anemias and pancytopenias. Affected cats tend to have a very poor prognosis.

Treatment for these two conditions includes whole-blood transfusions, anabolic steroids, corticosteroids, and hematinics. In one study, 100 cats with nonregenerative anemia were treated with whole-blood transfusions—49 were euthanized before 2 weeks had elapsed because they had responded poorly to the initial transfusion.[91] The median survival time of the cats treated for longer than 2 weeks was 4 months; however, 8 cats had remission of their anemia. Some cats remained in remission for as long as 7 years.[91]

In general therapy for FeLV-anemias is unsuccessful.

Myeloid Diseases

FeLV replicates in all precursors and differentiated myeloid cells in the bone marrow.[24,75]

Myeloid Neoplastic (Myeloproliferative) Diseases. FeLV has been found in most naturally occurring myeloproliferative diseases of cats.[61,64] These diseases include reticuloendotheliosis, neutrophilic leukemia, myelofibrosis, and medullary osteosclerosis; they occur only rarely in pet cats. Myelofibrosis is characterized by replacement of the marrow by fibrous connective tissue resulting in aplastic anemia. Splenomegaly is present with severe extramedullary hematopoiesis (myeloid metaplasia). A marrow biopsy is needed to confirm the diagnosis. Medullary osteosclerosis has been seen in FeLV-positive cats with radiographically detectable thickening of the cortices of long bones with decreased medullary space.[90a]

Myeloproliferative diseases generally respond very poorly to treatment. The bone marrow is usually heavily infiltrated with malignant cells, which displace the normal marrow precursor cells. Anemia, leukopenia, and sepsis are common before and during therapy. Combination chemotherapy can be tried, but the overall prognosis is very poor. Drugs used include cyclophosphamide (200–300 mg/m² IV), vincristine (0.5–0.7 mg/m² IV), cytosine arabinoside (600 mg/m² IV slowly over a 48-hour period *or* divided SQ every 12 hours for 4 treatments), and prednisone (2 mg/kg PO daily). The approach to therapy consists of marrow ablation of leukemic cells using chemotherapy, followed by repopulation of marrow with normal precursor cells. Anemia, sepsis, and hemorrhage are common sequelae from the treatment as well as the disease. Anemia can be controlled with blood transfusions, but bleeding and sepsis are often fatal. Owing to the poor results with treatment, chemotherapy is rarely advised for cats with myeloproliferative diseases.

Myeloid Blastopenic Diseases. Blastopenic myeloid diseases occur more commonly in infected pet cats than do myeloproliferative diseases. FeLV-myeloblastopenia, a panleukopenia-like syndrome, is characterized by severe dysentery and panleukopenia. Erosion of the epithelium of the tips of the small intestinal villi permits opportunistic infections to enter, resulting in septicemia and death.[60,75] FeLV antigens and replicating virus are present in the intestinal epithelial cells and lymphocytes in the lamina propria.[60,75]

Cyclic neutropenia has been reported in FeLV-infected cats.[91a] FeLV-infected cats will have neutropenic episodes every 10 to 20 days, lasting 3 to 5 days. Treatment consists of supportive care, such as antibiotics and high-dose prednisone therapy (2.2 mg/kg PO every 12–24 hours). Special care must be given to cats during the neutropenic period. Maintenance doses of prednisone (1.1 mg/kg PO once daily) should be used if a remission develops.[91a]

Other FeLV Diseases

Abortions and Resorption Syndromes. FeLV can cause fetal abortions or resorptions late in gestation. The virus has been detected in two-thirds of cats with a history of abortions or fetal resorptions and has been shown experimentally to induce these disorders.[60,75]

FeLV Neurologic Syndrome. A neurologic syndrome similar to the neurologic syndrome observed in MuLV-infected wild mice occurs in FeLV-infected pet cats and is characterized by posterior paresis, paralysis, or tetraplegia.[60,75,92] However, FeLV has not yet been proven to cause this syndrome under experimental conditions. A similar neurologic syndrome characterized by paralysis occurs in humans infected with the human T cell leukemia virus (HTLV-I).[93]

FeLV Immune Complex Glomerulonephritis. Persistently FeLV-infected pet cats have a life-long viremia that is ideal for the formation of immune complexes and the induction of glomerulonephritis.[40–42,60,94] FeLV antigens, antibody (IgG), and complement deposited in the glomeruli have been found in 25% of the healthy FeLV-infected cats studied, but none of these cats had clinical glomerulonephritis.[40] Although there are many chronically viremic pet cats, clinical glomerulonephritis is not a frequent outcome of FeLV infection.

FELINE SARCOMA VIRUS (FeSV)

Feline sarcoma viruses (FeSV) are replication-defective acute transforming viruses that possess transforming genes, viral oncogenes (v-oncs), acquired through recombination of the FeLV genome with single-copy cellular c-onc (proto-oncogenes) genes.[95,96] Each FeSV is generated de novo in individual infected cats and does not appear to be transmitted contagiously.[95] FeSV induces neoplasms with a short latent period in animals and transforms tissue culture cells of various species, including human cells.[95–97] The transforming properties of FeSV are determined by the v-onc sequences.

Pet cats are an excellent source of viral oncogene-containing acute transforming viruses because approximately 1 million pet cats are chronically viremic with the replication-competent chronic leukemia virus FeLV. To date 11 naturally occurring FeSVs with 7 different oncogenes have been isolated from pet cats. The study of oncogenes appears to offer great promise to our understanding of the cause of cancer. However, only the oncogenes transduced into acute transforming viruses have been shown to be capable of transforming normal cells or inducing tumors in animals. The expression of cellular proto-oncogenes in normal and proliferating non-neoplastic cells has cast some doubt on the specificity of oncogene expression and cancer. The increasing number of viral-transduced oncogenes, presently about 30, that are shared by viruses isolated from the same species, as well as by those isolated in viruses from different species, implies that the number of oncogenes may be limited.

FeSV-INDUCED TUMORS OF PET CATS

Fibrosarcomas account for between 6% and 12% of all cat tumors.[42,46] FeSV induces multicentric fibrosarcomas of young (average age 3 years) pet cats, whereas the more common single fibrosarcomas that occur in older cats (average age 10 years) are not associated with FeSV.[97,98] FeSV-induced fibrosarcomas are usually poorly differentiated, multicentric, and more invasive than the non-FeSV-induced fibrosarcomas. We do not recommend treatment for FeSV-induced fibrosarcoma.

FELINE IMMUNODEFICIENCY VIRUS (FIV)

Retroviruses are an ever-expanding family of RNA-containing viruses of animals and humans.

A new feline lentivirus that induces AIDS in cats has recently been discovered and has been named the feline immunodeficiency virus (FIV).[1,1a] Thus, cats are infected with representatives of all 3 subfamilies of retroviruses, and there are now two feline retroviruses from different subfamilies that cause AIDS in cats: FeLV, an oncovirus and FIV, a lentivirus. FIV was recently discovered in a cattery in Northern California that was free of FeLV but had an outbreak of FAIDS in several cats living together in the same pen. As can be seen in Table 29-8, FeLV- and FIV-FAIDS are almost identical. Morphologically, FIV differs from FeLV in that it has a rod-shaped instead of an oval nucleoid. Unlike FeLV, which replicates in all nucleated cells of the lymphoid and myeloid series, FIV is highly T-lymphotropic; that is, it replicates almost exclusively in T-lymphocytes. However, like all retroviruses, FIV results in a persistent lifelong infection in cats who do not mount an appropriate immune response and clear the virus after exposure.

The clinical signs of FIV-FAIDS include generalized lymphadenopathy, fever, leukopenia, conjunctivitis, gingivitis, periodontitis, stomatitis rhinitis, emaciation, diarrhea, and pustular dermatitis. Cats infected can be categorized into two major phases.[1a] Phase I usually occurs approximately 4 to 6 weeks after exposure and is characterized by generalized lymphadenopathy, neutropenia, and fever. Some cats die owing to sepsis during this phase of the disease. The second phase is usually associated with cats chronically infected. These cats tend to be older (5–7 years of age) and free roaming; male cats

Table 29-8. Comparison of FeLV and FIV

FeLV	FIV
Subfamily: Oncovirinae	Subfamily: Lentivirinae
Pancytotropic—bone marrow and lymphoid cells	Highly T-lymphocyte tropic
Causes FAIDS, anemia, cancer, neurologic disorders	Causes FAIDS, anemia, neurologic disorders
Morphology: oval nucleoid	Morphology: rod-shaped nucleoid
Mg^{++}-dependent reverse transcriptase	Mn^{++}-dependent reverse transcriptase
Does not coexist with antibody	Coexists with antibody
Spreads via saliva—licking	Spreads via saliva—biting
Moderately contagious	Poorly contagious
Detected by presence of viral antigens	Detected by presence of viral antibodies

predominate. This phase of the disease is characterized by chronic oral infections (50% to 60%), upper respiratory infections (34%), chronic diarrhea (20%) and chronic conjunctivitis (11%). These cats may live several years with the disease.[99,100] A recent study of 580 serum samples from a diverse population of cats found that 2.4% were positive for FIV and frequently were coinfected (57%) with *Toxoplasma gondii*.[101] These findings suggested that FIV-associated immunosuppression may be a factor in active *Toxoplasma* infection in adult cats.

As with people infected with the AIDS viruses and cows with the bovine leukemia virus, cats infected with FIV produce antibodies to the viral proteins that coexist with the virus. The antibody immune response against FIV is not sufficient to clear the virus from the cat's body, and a persistent infection develops. FIV antibody can be detected by a fluorescent antibody test using FIV-infected cat T-lymphocytes as a target and by an ELISA test.[1] This method of detection differs from those used to detect FeLV infection, in which a fluorescent antibody test or an ELISA test detects the viral antigens in the absence of antibody to FeLV. Thus, in order to diagnose FIV-FAIDS, the clinician must diagnose the secondary disease syndrome in an FeLV test-negative cat who is positive for FIV antibody. It has been reported that between 12% and 16% of the cats will be coinfected with FIV and FeLV.[1a,99]

FIV, like FeLV, appears to be transmitted mainly by means of saliva. Transmission is slow, and the major mode of transmission appears to be through bite wounds. Cats with oral lesions have higher concentrations of virus in the saliva.[1a] There is a suggestion that free-roaming (outdoor/indoor, stray, feral) cats are at a higher risk, and bringing these cats together from such environments may lead to localized epizootics.[1,1a] FIV may be a recently introduced virus in cats; as was found for the human AIDS virus, it probably originated from another species.

Since only about 50% of pet cats with chronic immunosuppressive syndromes (FAIDS) are infected with FeLV, FIV may be responsible for some or most of the non-FeLV-caused immunosuppression observed in pet cats. Thus, FIV may represent a major new naturally occurring feline pathogen, and veterinarians should be aware of this possibility and be prepared to institute control measures to prevent the spread of this virus. Until an FIV vaccine can be developed, such control measures will include FIV testing programs. At present FIV-infected cats should be kept indoors, away from uninfected cats and should never be allowed to roam free outdoors. Since FIV does not replicate in human cells and since many FIV-infected cats can remain healthy for long periods, we do not recommend removal of these cats by euthanasia.

REFERENCES

1. Pederson NC, Ho EW, Brown ML, Yamamoto JK: Isolation of a T-lymphotropic virus from domestic cats with an immunodeficiency-like syndrome. Science 235:790–793, 1987

1a. Yamamoto JK, Hansen H, Ho WE, et al: Epidemiologic and clinical aspects of feline immunodeficiency virus infection in cats from continental United States and Canada and possible mode of transmission. J Am Vet Med Assoc 194:213–220, 1989

2. Hardy WD Jr: The feline leukemia virus. J Am Anim Hosp Assoc 17:951–980, 1981

3. Jarrett WFH, Crawford EM, Martin WB, Davie F: A virus-like particle associated with leukemia (lymphosarcoma). Nature 202:567–569, 1964

4. Huebner RJ, Todaro GJ: Oncogenesis of RNA tumor viruses as determinants of cancer. Proc Natl Acad Sci 64:1087–1094, 1969

5. Essex M, Cotter SM, Sliski AH, et al: Horizontal transmission of feline leukemia virus under natural conditions in a feline leukemia cluster household. Int J Cancer 19:90–96, 1977

6. Hardy WD Jr, Geering G, Old LJ, et al: Feline leukemia virus: Occurrence of viral antigen in the tissues of cats with lymphosarcoma and other diseases. Science 166:1019–1021, 1969

7. Jarrett WFH, Jarrett O, Mackey L, Laird H, Hardy WD Jr, Essex M: Horizontal transmission of leukemia virus and leukemia in the cat. J Natl Cancer Inst 51:833–841, 1973

8. Hardy WD Jr: Naturally occurring retroviruses (RNA tumor viruses). I. Cancer Invest 1:67–83, 1983

9. Hardy WD Jr: Naturally occurring retroviruses (RNA tumor viruses). II. Cancer Invest 1:163–174, 1983

10. Benveniste RE, Sherr CJ, Todaro GJ: Evolution of type C viral genes: Origin of feline leukemia virus. Science 190:886–888, 1975

10a. Livingston DM, Todaro GJ: Endogenous type-C virus from a cat cell clone with properties distinct from previously-described feline viruses. Virology 53:142–147, 1973

11. Todaro GJ: Interspecies transmission of mammalian retroviruses. In Klein G (ed): Viral Oncology, pp 291–309. New York, Raven Press, 1980

12. Jarrett O, Laird HM, Hay D: Determinants of the host range of feline leukaemia viruses. J Gen Virol 20:169–175, 1973

13. Sarma PS, Log T: Subgroup classification of feline leukemia and sarcoma viruses by viral interference and neutralization tests. Virology 54:160–169, 1973

14. Hardy WD Jr, Hess PW, MacEwen EG, McClelland AJ, Zuckerman EE, Essex M, Cotter SM, Jarrett O: Biology of feline leukemia virus in the natural environment. Cancer Res 36:582–588, 1976

15. Jarrett O, Hardy WD Jr, Golder MC, Hay D: The frequency of occurrence of feline leukemia virus subgroups in cats. Int J Cancer 21:334–337, 1978

16. Hoover EA, Kociba GJ, Hardy WD Jr, Yohn DS: Erythroid hypoplasia in cats inoculated with feline leukemia virus. J Natl Cancer Inst 53:1271–1276, 1974

17. Hoover EA, Olsen RG, Hardy WD Jr, Schaller JP, Mathes LE: Feline leukemia virus infection: Age related variation in response of cats to experimental infection. J Natl Cancer Inst 57:365–369, 1976

18. Mackey LJ, Jarrett W, Jarrett O, Laird H: Anemia associated with feline leukemia virus infection in cats. J Natl Cancer Inst 54:209–217, 1975

19. Mullins JT, Chen CS, Hoover EA: Disease-specific and tissue-specific production of unintegrated feline leukemia virus variant DNA in feline AIDS. Nature 319:333–336, 1986

20. Onions D, Jarrett O, Testa N, Frassoni F, Toth S: Selective effect of feline leukaemia virus on early erythroid precursors. Nature 296:156–158, 1982

21. Elder JH, Mullins JT: Nucleotide sequence of the envelope gene of Gardner-Arnstein feline leukemia virus B reveals unique sequence homologies with a murine mink cell focus-forming virus. J Virol 46:871–880, 1983

22. Soe LH, Devi BC, Mullins JL, Roy–Burman P: Molecular cloning and characterization of endogenous feline leukemia virus sequences from a cat genomic library. J Virol 46:829–840, 1983

23. Soe LH, Shimizu RW, Landolph JR, Roy–Burman P: Molecular analysis of several classes of endogenous feline leukemia virus elements. J Virol 56:701–710, 1985

24. Hardy WD Jr, Hirshaut Y, Hess P: Detection of the feline leukemia virus and other mam-

malian oncornaviruses by immunofluorescence. In Dutcher RM, Chieco–Bianchi L (eds): Unifying Concepts of Leukemia, pp 778–799. Basel, Karger, 1973

25. Yoshiki T, Mellors RC, Hardy WD Jr, Fleissner E: Common cell surface antigen associated with mammalian C-type RNA viruses. J Exp Med 139:925–942, 1974

26. Hardy WD Jr, McClelland AJ, Hess PW, MacEwen EG: Veterinarians and the control of feline leukemia virus. J Am Anim Hosp Assoc 10:367, 1974

27. Hardy WD Jr, McClelland AJ, Zuckerman EE, Hess PW, Essex M, Cotter SM, MacEwen EG, Hayes AA: Prevention of the contagious spread of feline leukaemia virus and the development of leukaemia in pet cats. Nature 263:326–328, 1976

28. Kahn DE, Mia AS, Tierney MM: Field evaluation of Leukassay F, an FeLV detection test kit. Feline Pract 10:41, 1980

29. Francis DP, Essex M, Hardy WD Jr: Excretion of feline leukemia virus by naturally infected pet cats. Nature 269:252–254, 1977

30. Jarrett O, Golder MC, Weijer K: A comparision of three methods of feline leukaemia virus diagnosis. Vet Rec 110:325, 1982

31. Lutz H, Pederson NC, Harris CW, Higgins BS, Theilein GH: Detection of feline leukemia virus infection. Feline Pract 10:13, 1980

32. Bolognesi DP, Montelaro RC, Frank H, Schafer W: Assembly of type C oncornaviruses: A model. Science 199:183–186, 1978

33. Baltimore D: Viral RNA-dependent DNA polymerase in virions of RNA tumor viruses. Nature 226:1209–1211, 1970

34. Teich N: Taxonomy of retroviruses. In Weiss R, Teich N, Varmus H, Coffin J (eds): RNA Tumor Viruses, p 25. New York, Cold Spring Harbor Laboratory, 1982

35. Rojko JL, Hoover EA, Mathes LE, Olsen RG, Schaller JP: Pathogenesis of experimental feline leukemia virus infection. J Natl Cancer Inst 63:759–768, 1979

36. McClelland AJ, Hardy WD Jr, Zuckerman EE: Prognosis of healthy feline leukemia virus infected cats. In Hardy WD Jr, Essex M, McClelland AJ (eds): Feline Leukemia Virus, p 121. New York, Elsevier, 1980

37. Rojko JL, Hoover EA, Quakenbush SL, Olsen RG: Reactivation of latent feline leukaemia virus infection. Nature 298:385–388, 1982

38. Cotter SM, Hardy WD Jr, Essex M: The association of feline leukemia virus with lymphosarcoma and other disorders in the cat. J Am Vet Med Assoc 166:449–454, 1975

39. Essex M, Sliski A, Cotter SM, Jakowski RM, Hardy WD Jr: Immunosurveillance of naturally occurring feline leukemia. Science 190:790, 1975

40. Hardy WD Jr: Immunopathology induced by the feline leukemia virus. In Klein G (ed): Springer Seminar on Immunopathology, p 75. New York, Springer-Verlag, 1982

41. Day NK, O'Reilly–Felice C, Hardy WD Jr, Good RA, Witken SS: Circulating immune complexes associated with naturally occurring lymphosarcoma in pet cats. J Immunol 126:2363–2366, 1980

42. Snyder HW Jr, Jones FR, Day NK, Hardy WD Jr: Isolation and characterization of circulating feline leukemia virus-immune complexes from plasma of persistently infected pet cats removed by ex vivo immunosorption. J Immunol 128:2726–2730, 1982

43. Brodey RS, McDonough S, Frye FL, Hardy WD Jr: Epidemiology of feline leukemia. In Dutcher RM (ed): Comparative Leukemia Research, p 333. Basel, Karger, 1970

44. Schneider R, Frye FL, Taylor DON, Dorn CR: A household cluster of feline malignant lymphoma. Cancer Res 27:1316–1322, 1967

45. Hardy WD Jr, McClelland AJ, Zuckerman EE, Snyder HW Jr, MacEwen EG, Francis D, Essex M: Development of virus non-producer lymphosarcomas in pet cats exposed to FeLV. Nature 288:90, 1980

46. Lutz H, Pederson NC, Theilen GH: Course of feline leukemia virus infection and its detection by enzyme-linked immunosorbent assay and monoclonal antibodies. Am J Vet Res 44:2054–2059, 1983

47. Essex M, Klein G, Snyder SP, Harrold JB: Correlation between humoral antibody and regression of tumors induced by feline sarcoma virus. Nature 233:195–196, 1971

48. Thelien GH, Kawakami TG, Rush JD, Munn RJ: Replication of cat leukaemia virus in cell suspension cultures. Nature 22:589–590, 1969

49. Snyder HW Jr, Hardy WD Jr, Zuckerman EE, Fleissner E: Characterization of a tumor-specific antigen on the surface of feline lymphosarcoma cells. Nature 275:656–658, 1978

50. Hardy WD Jr, Zuckerman EE, MacEwen EG, Hayes AA, Essex M: A feline leukaemia virus- and sarcoma virus-induced tumour-specific antigen. Nature 270:249–251, 1977

51. Snyder HW Jr, Singhal MC, Zuckerman EE, Jones FR, Hardy WD Jr: The feline oncornavirus-associated cell membrane antigen (FOCMA) is related to, but distinguishable from, FeLV-C gp70. Virology 131:315–327, 1983

52. Stephenson JR, Essex M, Hino S, Hardy WD Jr, Aaronson SA: Feline oncornavirus-associated cell-membrane antigen (FOCMA): Distinction between FOCMA and the major virion glycoprotein. Proc Natl Acad Sci 74:1219–1223, 1977

53. Russell PH, Jarrett O: The occurrence of feline leukemia virus neutralizing antibodies in cats. Int J Cancer 22:351–357, 1978

54. Hardy WD Jr, MacEwen EG, Hayes AA, Zuckerman EE: FOCMA antibody as specific immunotherapy for lymphosarcoma of pet cats. In Hardy WD Jr, Essex M, McClelland AJ (eds): Feline Leukemia Virus, p 227. New York, Elsevier, 1980

55. Weijer K, Uijtdehaag F, Osterhaus A: The control of feline leukaemia virus infection by a removal programme. Vet Rec 119:555–556, 1986

56. Olsen RG, Hoover EA, Mathes LE, Heding LD, Schaller JP: Immunization against feline oncornavirus disease using a killed tumor cell vaccine. Cancer Res 36:3642–3646, 1976

57. Olsen RG, Lewis M, Mathes LE, Hause W: Feline leukemia vaccine: Efficacy testing in a large multicat household. Feline Pract 10:13, 1980

58. Mastro JM, Lewis M, Mathes LE, Sharpee R, Tarr MJ, Olsen RG: Feline leukemia vaccine: Efficacy, contents and probable mechanism. Vet Immunol Immunopathol 11:205–213, 1986

59. Pedersen NC, Ott RL: Evaluation of a commercial feline leukemia virus vaccine for immunogenicity and efficacy. Feline Pract 15:7, 1985

60. Hardy WD Jr: Feline leukemia virus diseases. In Hardy WD Jr, Essex M, McClelland AJ (eds): Feline Leukemia Virus, p 3. New York, Elsevier, 1980

61. Hardy WD Jr: Hematopoietic tumors of cats. J Am Anim Hosp Assoc 17:921–940, 1981

62. Essex M: Feline leukemia and sarcoma viruses. In Klein G (ed): Viral Oncology, p 205. New York, Raven Press, 1980

63. Anderson LJ, Jarrett WFJ, Jarrett O, Laird HM: Feline leukemia-virus infection of kittens: Mortality associated with atrophy of the thymus and lymphoid depletion. J Natl Cancer Inst 47:807–817, 1971

64. Herz A, Theilen GH, Schalm OW: C-type virus in bone marrow cells of cats with myeloproliferative disorders. J Natl Cancer Inst 44:339, 1970

65. Hardy WD Jr, Essex M: FeLV-induced feline acquired immune deficiency syndrome (FAIDS): A model for human AIDS. In Klein E (ed): Acquired Immune Deficiency Syndrome. Progr Allergy 37:353–376, 1986

66. Dorn CR, Taylor DON, Schneider R, Hibbard HH, Klauber MR: Survey of animal neoplasms in Alameda and Contra Costa Counties, California. II. Cancer morbidity in dogs and cats from Alameda County. J Natl Cancer Inst 40:307–318, 1968

67. Francis DP, Cotter SM, Hardy WD Jr, Essex M: Comparison of virus-positive and virus-negative cases of feline leukemia and lymphoma. Cancer Res 39:3866–3870, 1979

68. Koshy R, Wong–Stall F, Gallo RC, Hardy WD Jr, Essex M: Distribution of feline leukemia virus DNA sequences in tissues of normal and leukemic domestic cats. Virology 99:135–144, 1979

69. Rickard CG, Post JE, Noronha F, Barr LM: Interspecies infection by feline leukemia virus: Serial cell-free transmission in dogs of malignant lymphomas induced by feline leukemia virus. In Dutcher RM, Chieco–Bianchi L (eds): Unifying Concepts of Leukemia, p 102. Basel, Karger, 1973

70. Mooney SC, Hayes AA, MacEwen EG, et al: Treatment and prognostic factors in feline lymphoma: 103 cases (1977–1981). J Am Vet Med Assoc 194:696–702, 1989

71. Cotter SM: Treatment of lymphoma and leukemia with cyclophosphamide, vincristine, and prednisone. II. Treatment of cats. J Am Anim Hosp Assoc 19:166–172, 1983

72. Jeglum KA, Whereat A, Young K: Chemotherapy of lymphoma in 75 cats. J Am Vet Med Assoc 190:174–178, 1987

73. Mooney SC, Hayes AA, Matus RE, et al: Renal lymphoma in cats: 28 cases (1977–1984). J Am Vet Med Assoc 191:1473–1477, 1987

74. Mooney SC, Patnaik AR, Hayes AA, et al: Generalized lymphadenopathy resembling lymphoma in cats: Six cases (1972–1976). J Am Vet Med Assoc 190:897–900, 1987

75. Hardy WD Jr: Feline leukemia virus non-neoplastic diseases. J Am Anim Hosp Assoc 17:941–949, 1981

76. Perryman LE, Hoover EA, Yohn DS: Immunologic reactivity of the cat: Immunosuppression in experimental feline leukemia. J Natl Cancer Inst 49:1357–1365, 1972

77. Cockerell GL, Hoover EA: Inhibition of normal lymphocyte mitogenic reactivity by serum from feline leukemia virus-infected cats. Cancer Res 37:3985–3989, 1977

78. Cockerell GL, Hoover EZ, Krakowka S, Olsen RG, Yohn DS: Lymphocyte mitogen reactivity and enumeration of circulating B- and T-cells

during feline leukemia virus infection in the cat. J Natl Cancer Inst 57:1095–1099, 1976

79. Trainin Z, Wernicke D, Ungar–Waron H, Essex M: Suppression of the humoral antibody response in natural retrovirus infections. Science 220:858–859, 1983

80. Mathes LE, Olsen RG, Hebebrand LC, Hoover EA, Schaller JP: Abrogation of lymphocyte blastogenesis by a feline leukemia virus protein. Nature 274:687–689, 1978

81. Orosz CG, Zinn NE, Olsen RG, et al: Retrovirus-mediated immunosuppression I FeLV-UV and specific FeLV proteins alter T lymphocyte behavior by inducing hyporesponsiveness to lymphokines. J Immunol 134:3396–3403, 1985

82. Orosz CG, Zinn NE, Olsen RG, et al: Retrovirus-mediated immunosuppression II FeLV-UV alters in vitro murine T-lymphocyte behavior by reversibly impairing lymphocyte secretion. J Immunol 135:583–590, 1985

82a. Tompkins MB, Ogilvie GK, Gast AM, et al: Interleukin–2 suppression in cats naturally infected with feline leukemia virus. J Biol Resp Modif 8:86–96, 1989

83. Jones FR, Yoshida LH, Ladiges WC, Kenny MA: Treatment of feline leukemia and reversal of FeLV by ex vivo removal of IgG. Cancer 46:675–684, 1980

84. Snyder HW Jr, Singhal MC, Hardy WD Jr, Jones FR: Clearance of feline leukemia virus from persistently infected pet cats treated by extracorporeal immunoadsorption is correlated with an enhanced antibody response to FeLV gp70. J Immunol 132:1538–1543, 1984

84a. Engelman RW, Tyler RD, Trang LQ, et al: Clinicopathologic responses in cats with feline leukemia–virus–associated leukemia–lymphoma treated with staphylococcal Protein A. Am J Pathol 118:367–378, 1985

85. Kobilinsky L, Hardy WD Jr, Day NK: Hypocomplementemia associated with naturally occurring lymphosarcoma in pet cats. J Immunol 122:2139–2142, 1979

86. Hardy WD Jr: Feline leukemia virus as an animal retrovirus model for the human T-cell leukemia virus. In Gallo RC, Essex M, Gross G (eds): Human T-cell Leukemia/Lymphoma Viruses, pp 35–43. New York, Cold Spring Harbor Laboratory, 1984

87. Masur H, Michelis MA, Green JB, Onorato I, Vande Stouwe RA, Holzman RS, Wormser G, Brettman L, Lange M, Murray HW, Cunningham–Rundles S: An outbreak of community-acquired pneumocystis carinii pneumonia. Initial manifestation of cellular immune dysfunction. N Engl J Med 305:1431–1438, 1981

87a. Weiss RC: Immunotherapy for feline leukemia, using staphylococcal protein A or heterologous interferons: Immunopharmacologic actions and potential use. J Am Vet Med Assoc 192:681–684, 1988

87b. Cummins JM, Tompkins MB, Olsen RG, et al: Oral use of human alpha interferon in cats. J Biol Resp Modif 7:513–523, 1988

87c. Ford RB: Biological response modifiers in the management of viral infection. Vet Clin North Am 16:1191–1204, 1986

87d. Fischl MA, Richman DD, Grieco MH, et al: The efficacy of azidothymidine (AZT) in the treatment of patients with AIDS and AIDS–related complex. New Engl J Med 317:185–191, 1987

88. Gustafson DP: Antiviral therapy. Vet Clin North Am 16:1181–1189, 1986

89. Roussel M, Saule S, Lagrou C, Rommens C, Bug H, Graf T, Stehelin D: Three new types of viral oncogenes of cellular origin specific for haematopoietic cell transformation. Nature 281:452–455, 1979

90. Scolnick EM: Hyperplastic and neoplastic erythroproliferative diseases induced by oncogenic murine retroviruses. Biochem Biophys Acta 651:273–283, 1982

90a. Hoover EA, Kociba GJ: Bone lesions in cats with anemia induced by feline leukemia virus. J Nat Cancer Inst 53:1277–1284, 1974

91. Cotter SM: Anemia associated with feline leukemia virus infection. J Am Vet Med Assoc 175:1191–1194, 1979

91a. Swenson CL, Kociba GJ, O'Keefe DA, et al: Cyclic hematopoeisis associated with feline leukemia virus infection in two cats. J Am Vet Med Assoc 191:93–96, 1987

92. Gardner MB, Henderson BE, Officer JE, Rongey RW, Parker JC, Oliver C, Estes JD, Huebner RJ: A spontaneous lower motor neuron disease apparently caused by indigenous type C RNA virus in wild mice. J Natl Cancer Inst 51:1243–1254, 1973

93. Osame M, Usuku K, Izumo S, Ijichi N, Amitani H, Igata A, Matsumoto M, Tara M: HTLV-I associated myelopathy: A new clinical entity. Lancet I:1031, 1986

94. Jakowski RM, Essex M, Hardy WD Jr, Stephenson JR, Cotter SM: Membranous glomerulonephritis in a household of cats persistently viremic with feline leukemia virus. In Hardy WD Jr, Essex M, McClelland AJ (eds): Feline Leukemia Virus, p 141. New York, Elsevier, 1980

95. Besmer P: Acute transforming feline retroviruses. Curr Top Microbiol Immunol 107:1–27, 1983

96. Frankel AE, Gilbert JH, Porzif FJ, Scolnick EM, Aaronson SA: Nature and distribution of feline sarcoma virus nucleotide sequences. J Virol 30:821–827, 1979

97. Hardy WD Jr: The feline sarcoma viruses. J Am Anim Hosp Assoc 17:981–997, 1981

98. Hardy WD Jr: The biology and virology of the feline sarcoma viruses. In Hardy WD Jr, Essex M, McClelland AJ (eds): Feline Leukemia Virus, p 79. New York, Elsevier, 1980

99. Ishida T, Tsukimi W, Kazushige T, et al: Feline immunodeficiency virus infection in cats of Japan. J Am Vet Med Assoc 194:221–225, 1989

100. Grindem CB, Corbett WT, Ammerman BE, et al: Seroepidemiologic survey of feline immunodeficiency virus in cats of Wake County, North Carolina. J Am Vet Med Assoc 194:226–228, 1989

101. Witt CJ, Moench TR, Gittelsohn Am, et al: Epidemiologic observations on feline immunodeficiency virus and Toxoplasma gondii coinfection in cats in Baltimore, Md. 194:229–233, 1989

Canine Lymphoma and Lymphoid Leukemias

E. Gregory MacEwen
Karen M. Young

INCIDENCE AND RISK FACTORS

Malignant lymphoma is one of the most common neoplasms seen in the dog. The annual incidence has been estimated to be 30 per 100,000 dogs at risk.[1] This is approximately twice the human incidence and two-thirds the incidence seen in the cat. Breeds of dogs reported to have a higher incidence include boxers, basset hounds, St. Bernards, Scottish terriers, Airedales, and bulldogs. Breeds at low risk for lymphoma include dachshunds and Pomeranians.[2] Some studies have reported a higher incidence of lymphoma in males than in females, although the reports are inconclusive. The average age at diagnosis is 6–7 years, with a range of 6 months to more than 15 years.

Lymphocytic leukemia is more common than nonlymphocytic leukemia and other myeloproliferative disorders (MPD). The true incidence is unknown. In a series of 30 cases of acute lymphoblastic leukemia (ALL), the median age was 5.5 years with a range of 1–12 years. Eight dogs were less than 4 years old. German shepherd dogs accounted for 27% of the cases seen. The male:female (M:F) ratio was 3:2.[3] Well-differentiated or chronic lymphocytic leukemia (CLL) is seen less commonly than ALL but more frequently than MPD. The median age is 11 years, and in one study of 20 dogs the M:F ratio was 2:1.[4]

Although the exact etiology of canine lymphoma and lymphoid leukemia is unknown, retroviruses have been implicated in the development of lymphoma and leukemia in diverse animal species such as fish, snakes, birds, rodents, rats, cats, cattle, and nonhuman primates; and there is now evidence that a retrovirus (HTLV—human T cell leukemia/lymphoma virus) is the causative agent of a form of cutaneous T cell leukemia and lymphoma in humans.[5] Earlier studies reported some evidence of retroviral particles seen by electron microscopy of canine tissue. In addition, viral particles were identified in beagle dogs following cellular transmission of the disease.[6,7] A canine lymphoma B cell line containing a retrovirus has also been established.[8] In 1980, reverse transcriptase activity was recognized in 3 of 14 short-term lymphoma cultures and in 2 of 11 crude preparations of canine tumor tissue.[9] More recently, analysis of tissues from 43 dogs with lymphoma as well as tissue from 40 clinically normal dogs revealed that reverse transcriptase levels were higher in the lymphoma supernates than in tissue from normal dogs.[10] High molecular weight (60–70S) RNA was detected in canine lymphoma cells and shown to be in association with this particular reverse transcriptase activity, while no such RNA was detected in culture supernates from normal canine lymphoid cells.[11] Although this evidence is not conclusive, it is highly suggestive that a viral etiology may exist.

Genetic predisposition is a potential etiologic factor, as some breeds of dogs are considered to have a higher risk of developing hematopoietic tumors than others. The development of lymphoma in a family of bull mastiffs has strengthened arguments for either a viral or genetic cause.[12]

Immune deficiencies and defects in immunologic recognition have also been proposed as a cause of cancer, particularly the lymphoproliferative tumors. Dogs with lymphoma and lymphoid leukemia have been shown to have decreased primary and secondary humoral and cellular immune reactivity and possible impairment of monocyte-macrophage function.[13] This suppression may be due to the disease itself and not necessarily to an underlying immune suppression. Lymphocyte reactivity has been shown to be suppressed in dogs with advanced disease and to return to normal following successful chemotherapeutic control of the disease. Evidence shows that immunologic incompetence is associated with lymphoma and leukemia, but it cannot be established as the cause or the effect of the disease.[14]

PATHOLOGY AND NATURAL BEHAVIOR

The classification of malignant lymphoma in dogs can be correlated with anatomic location and histologic criteria. The most common anatomic forms of lymphoma include the multicentric, cranial mediastinal, gastrointestinal, and cutaneous forms. Primary extranodal forms such as ocular and central nervous system are less commonly observed.

Eighty percent of dogs with lymphoma are presented with superficial lymphadenopathy. Lymph node enlargement is usually painless, rubbery, and discrete and may initially include only submandibular and prescapular involvement. Many animals are asymptomatic, but approximately 40% have a history of weight loss, lethargy, anorexia, and febrile episodes.

Approximately 20% of animals affected have thoracic involvement; mediastinal and hilar lymphadenopathy is the most common presenting feature. Pulmonary infiltration can also be seen, and in one report, this occurred in 27% of animals seen with multicentric lymphoma.[15]

Hepatosplenomegaly is the most common manifestation of abdominal involvement and is usually associated with an advanced stage of multicentric disease. Primary alimentary involvement is less common and represents less than 10% of cases seen. Dogs with infiltrative disease of the intestinal tract have weight loss,

anorexia, and evidence of malabsorption. Pathologically these neoplasms resemble plasma cell tumors, and aberrant production of immunoglobulins may occur. We have seen IgA-secreting tumors with hyperviscosity syndrome (see "Plasma Cell Neoplasms," this chapter).

Lymphoma can result in acute spinal cord compression, testicular masses, and ocular masses. This tumor can occur in almost any location in the body.

In acute lymphoblastic leukemia (ALL) the blast cells always infiltrate the bone marrow, resulting in variable degrees of anemia, thrombocytopenia, and neutropenia. Infiltration of the spleen and liver are common, and extramedullary sites, such as the nervous system, bone, and gastrointestinal tract, may be involved as well. Some animals may have lymph node involvement and develop generalized lymphadenopathy.

In chronic lymphocytic leukemia (CLL) the marrow is infiltrated with small, well-differentiated lymphocytes. The extent of marrow infiltration is less than that seen with ALL or MPD. Dogs tend to have a mild anemia, and the granulocytes and platelets are also only mildly reduced. Splenomegaly is common, and lymph nodes can be minimally enlarged. Despite the well-differentiated appearance of the lymphocytes in CLL, these cells function abnormally. Some animals with CLL have an accompanying monoclonal gammopathy.[16] This immunoglobulin spike in the serum is associated with production of immunoglobulins by the leukemic cells (B cells). The immunoglobulin is usually IgM, and the term macrogammaglobulinemia is used (see "Plasma Cell Neoplasms," this chapter) to describe this gammopathy.

Hypercalcemia is commonly associated with lymphoma and has a profound effect on the kidney. Hypercalcemic nephropathy with resultant renal failure is a common complication of untreated hypercalcemia. The central nervous system and gastrointestinal tract are also affected. Possible mechanisms for hypercalcemia include direct tumor osteolysis, osteolysis by prostaglandins of the E series, ectopic production of a parathyroidlike hormone, and production of a bone-resorbing substance similar to osteoclast-activating factor (OAF). In canine lymphoma, hypercalcemia is most likely associated with an OAF-like substance.[17] (See Chapter 5.)

HISTOLOGIC CLASSIFICATION

The classification systems applied to canine malignant lymphoma have been predominantly based upon Rappaport's older classification of non-Hodgkin's lymphoma in humans.[18] These systems categorize tumors by general architectural pattern as either diffuse or nodular (also termed follicular), and by cell type as lymphocytic well-differentiated, lymphocytic poorly differentiated, histiocytic, and undifferentiated.[19–21] The description of cell type is based solely on morphologic appearance without consideration of immunologic or functional criteria. For example, histiocytic tumors have cells that morphologically resemble tissue histiocytes or macrophages, but these cells have been shown to be lymphoid in origin by more sophisticated immunologic techniques.[22] The frequency of various cell types and architectural patterns of canine lymphomas reported has varied widely,[22–25] and although these systems are simple and convenient, they have provided little or no useful information about survival or response to therapy.[23,25,26]

Recently, attempts have been made to employ more relevant classification systems with the following aims:

1. To adopt a system currently used to classify human lymphomas, taking advantage of the more sophisticated systems that incorporate both histopathologic and clinical features and permitting comparisons to be made between canine and human lymphomas. Obviously, successful adaptation of such a system would depend upon its applicability to canine tumors.
2. To utilize the histologic classification to predict response to therapy and survival, identifying animals that might benefit from the application of various therapeutic regimens.
3. To classify tumors by histologic, functional, and immunologic criteria in order to determine prognoses.

Several human classifications[27–29] have recently been applied to canine lymphomas[30,31] with some success. For example, 289 cases of lymphoma in dogs[31] were classified by the Lukes and Collins system, a frequently used classification in human medicine that accounts for architectural, histocytologic, and immunologic

features. Although it appears that, from the standpoint of histopathology, canine tumors can be feasibly classified according to these systems, no data are available yet on the capacity of these systems to predict survival and therapeutic response.

In 1982, the National Cancer Institute published the results of a study it sponsored on the classification of non-Hodgkin's lymphoma in humans. The study resulted in the development of the Working Formulation for Clinical Usage.[32] This formulation was not intended to be a separate classification system or to replace other systems; rather, it was to provide a common ground for communication among the existing systems, allowing comparison of various clinical studies. Due to the prognostic significance of the subgroups in the Working Formulation (WF), however, oncologists for humans have readily adopted it as a classification system. Based primarily on architecture (diffuse or follicular) and cell type (for example, small, large, cleaved, noncleaved), tumors are placed into low-, intermediate-, or high-grade categories with 10 subgroups (Table 29-9). Low-grade tumors are associated with the best survival times because of a slower progression of disease, whereas intermediate- and high-grade categories are associated with poorer prognoses without chemotherapy, but they respond to chemotherapy much better than the low-grade lymphomas.

Two groups have used the WF to classify canine lymphomas, and the histologic criteria established for architecture, mitotic index, and nuclear and nucleolar morphology have been found to be applicable to canine tumors with few modifications.[30,33] While reporting different

Table 29-9. Working Formulation for Non-Hodgkin's Lymphoma (Simplified)*

Low Grade	Small lymphocytic, diffuse
	Small cleaved cell, follicular
	Mixed small cleaved and large cell, follicular
Intermediate Grade	Large cell, follicular
	Small cleaved cell, diffuse
	Mixed small and large cell, diffuse
	Large cell, diffuse
High Grade	Immunoblastic
	Lymphoblastic
	Small noncleaved cell

* Adapted.[32,33]

distributions of cell types, both groups agree that most canine tumors have a diffuse architectural pattern and that the percentages of high- and intermediate-grade tumors are higher in dogs than in humans. This may reflect different biologic behavior or later detection of lymphoma in canine patients.

The major disadvantage of the WF is its failure to take into account the immunologic classification of tumor cells. For example, it treats immunoblastic tumors as one category, although B and T cell immunoblastic lymphomas may respond differently to therapy.[34] Studies of surface markers on canine lymphoma cells indicate that the majority are B cells, but some phenotypic heterogeneity exists within most lymphomas.[22,30] Interestingly, cells expressing a lymphocyte differentiation marker were less responsive to therapy than cells that lacked the marker.[30] Presumably the negative cells were less differentiated and therefore more responsive to therapy. The use of a relevant classification system coupled with identification of immunologic markers will facilitate selection of candidates for therapeutic protocols. The capacity to directly compare canine and human tumors may provide diagnostic and therapeutic advances to veterinary clinicians and models for the study of human lymphoma.

HISTORY AND CLINICAL SIGNS

Multicentric lymphoma, usually characterized by generalized lymphadenopathy with or without hepatosplenomegaly and bone marrow involvement,[35] is the most frequently encountered lymphoma in the dog. Generalized lymphadenopathy may be associated with weight loss and a decrease in appetite and activity. Cranial mediastinal lymphoma may result in respiratory compromise caused by a space-occupying mass and pleural effusion. The intestinal form of lymphoma may result in weight loss and cachexia associated with malabsorption, especially with the infiltrative form. Vomiting or diarrhea may be present in animals with the nodular form of lymphoma in the gastrointestinal tract. Colonic lymphomas are usually single or multiple discrete nodules resulting in straining to defecate and hematochezia. Dogs with less common forms of lymphoma may have an ocular mass, dementia or seizures associated with cerebral involve-

ment, or pain, paresis, and paralysis associated with extradural spinal cord compression.

The differential diagnosis of lymphadenopathy will depend on the dog's age and the size, shape, feel, and location of the lymph nodes involved. Other causes of lymphadenopathy to consider are bacterial and viral infections, parasites (*Toxoplasma* sp., *Leishmania* sp.), *Neorickettsia* (Salmon poisoning, *Ehrlichia* sp.), and fungal agents (*Coccidiodes* sp., *Histoplasma* sp.). Discrete, hard lymph nodes, particularly if fixed, may indicate metastatic tumor such as a mast cell sarcoma or carcinoma. Immune-mediated diseases such as systemic lupus erythematosis may also be associated with lymphadenopathy.

Mediastinal involvement must be differentiated from a primary thymoma (see Chapter 30) and metastatic thyroid adenocarcinoma. Pulmonary infiltrate and other lymphadenopathy in the thoracic cavity must be differentiated from fungal infection (histoplasmosis and blastomycosis). Primary or metastatic tumor of the lung must also be considered.

Canine lymphoma may also be associated with various paraneoplastic syndromes. Anemia is probably the most common lymphoma-related paraneoplastic syndrome.[36] The most frequently described anemia is nonregenerative anemia of chronic disease. Hypercalcemia is characterized by anorexia, weight loss, muscular weakness, lethargy, polyuria and polydipsia, and rarely central nervous system depression and coma. Other paraneoplastic disease syndromes include immune-mediated anemias, monoclonal gammopathies, cachexia, and hypoglycemia.[37-39] (See Chapter 5.)

Dogs with acute lymphoblastic leukemia usually have a history of anorexia, weight loss, and lethargy. Splenomegaly is common, and other physical abnormalities may include hemorrhages, lymphadenopathy, and hepatomegaly. Some animals have gastrointestinal disturbances. Anemia, thrombocytopenia, and an elevated white blood cell (WBC) count are common. The anemia may be severe and is usually characterized as normocytic and normochromic. WBC counts are usually elevated owing to an increased number of circulating immature lymphocytes ($>14,000$ cells/μl); some dogs, however, may be leukopenic. Infiltration of bone marrow by neoplastic lymphoblasts is extensive with resultant depression of normal hematopoietic elements.

In chronic lymphocytic leukemia, mild lymphadenopathy and splenomegaly may be present. Most dogs tend to be anemic and mildly thrombocytopenic (130,000 to 190,000 platelets/µl). The WBC count is usually greater than 30,000 cells/µl, but it can vary from normal to greater than 100,000 cells/µl owing to an increase in circulating mature lymphocytes. Granulocytes are usually present in normal numbers.

Cutaneous lymphoma is an uncommon manifestation of the spectrum of disease conditions associated with lymphoproliferative tumors in the dog.[40] The disease may be a primary cutaneous manifestation (primary cutaneous lymphoma or mycosis fungoides) or part of the spectrum of multicentric lymphoma. Primary cutaneous lymphoma has (or is associated with) a variety of clinical forms. The lesions associated with lymphoma include nodules, plaques, ulcers, erythroderma, and exfoliative dermatitis. Histologically, the lesions of primary cutaneous lymphoma are characterized by a diffuse dermal and subcutaneous infiltration by malignant lymphocytes. One study indicates that these cells may be of B cell origin.[22] The dog may initially be free of any systemic clinical signs, but as the disease progresses the lymph nodes may become involved and start to enlarge.[35,41]

HISTOLOGIC CLASSIFICATION OF PRIMARY CUTANEOUS LYMPHOMA

Mycoses fungoides is a T cell lymphoma characterized histologically by hyperkeratosis, acanthosis, epidermatropism, and Pautrier micro-abscesses.[42,43] The neoplastic cells are pleomorphic and are seen in association with neutrophils and plasma cells. It is suspected that these neoplastic cells are of the T cell lineage, although this has not been firmly established.[43] Mycosis fungoides in the dog often begins as a generalized, pruritic exfoliative dermatitis or erythroderma and slowly, over many months, progresses to firm, enlarged nodular growths. Dogs presented in the exfoliative stage are often misdiagnosed as having severe seborrhea.[35,41]

DIAGNOSTIC TECHNIQUES AND WORK-UP

For most animals with suspected lymphoma the diagnostic work-up should include a complete blood count (CBC) with a differential cell count,

platelet count, a serum chemistry profile with particular interest in evaluating serum calcium, renal function, and liver enzymes, bone marrow aspiration or biopsy, and lymph node biopsy or fine-needle aspiration. To permit accurate histopathologic evaluation of lymphomas, specimen preparation should be optimal. Practical considerations include the method of collection, timely and proper fixation, and previous cytotoxic therapy. While Tru-cut® biopsies may be prepared satisfactorily, they are best avoided owing to crush artifact and inadequate sample size.[33] Most pathologists prefer whole-node biopsies because they provide the maximum amount of information. Therefore, when a lymph node biopsy is performed, the entire lymph node should be removed, leaving the capsule intact to maintain the architecture. Autolysis of tissue obviously precludes adequate evaluation. Finally, cytotoxic drugs may result in changes in cell type or may obscure the histologic evaluation. Tissue should, therefore, be obtained prior to therapy. Care should be taken to avoid lymph nodes from reactive areas, such as submandibular lymph nodes; the prescapular or popliteal lymph nodes are preferable. Impression smears can be made from a carefully cut lymph node to help establish a diagnosis.

Thoracic and abdominal radiographs may be important in determining the extent of internal involvement. Ultrasonography has been useful to help determine liver and splenic involvement.[43a,43b] Cytologic examination of cerebrospinal fluid, pleural effusion, or a fine-needle aspirate from an intracavitary mass is indicated when appropriate. In animals with anemia or evidence of bleeding, a reticulocyte count, a platelet count, and coagulation studies may also be indicated. Dogs with a high total protein or evidence of an increased globulin fraction should be evaluated by serum electrophoresis. Monoclonal gammopathies have been reported to occur in 6% of dogs with lymphoma.[44]

Infiltration of bone marrow is the hallmark of both ALL and CLL, and examination of peripheral blood and bone marrow is essential in establishing a diagnosis of lymphocytic leukemia. If bone marrow cannot be adequately obtained by aspiration, a bone marrow biopsy should be performed. In ALL, lymphoblasts predominate in the bone marrow and are also present in peripheral blood. In most cases, these cells can be easily distinguished from blast cells of other hematopoietic lineages without the use of special cytochemical or immunologic markers. Perhaps the most distinguishing feature of lymphoblasts is the nuclear chromatin pattern, which is more condensed than the chromatin in myeloblasts. Lymphoblasts are larger than neutrophils; they have a high nuclear-cytoplasmic ratio and blue cytoplasm, which in some cases can be quite basophilic. Nucleoli, although present, are less prominent in lymphoblasts than in myeloblasts. The infiltration of bone marrow by lymphoblasts is accompanied by a concomitant decrease in the myeloid, erythroid, and megakaryocytic cell lines. The lymphocytes in CLL are small, mature cells that occur in excessive numbers in bone marrow early in the disease. Infiltration becomes more extensive as the disease slowly progresses, and eventually the neoplastic cells replace normal marrow.

After the diagnosis has been established, the extent of disease should be determined and correlated to the clinical stage of disease. The WHO staging system is routinely used to stage dogs with lymphoma (Table 29-10). Most animals are presented in an advanced stage of disease, either Stage III, IV, or V.

THERAPY

The vast majority of canine malignant lymphomas are best managed by combination chemotherapy. However, lymphoma of one site (es- pecially an extranodal site) may be treated with local radiation therapy (see Chapter 10). Single-agent chemotherapy has a limited role in the management of most of the clinical stages of lymphoma. Many protocols have been used; to date, not one of them has been shown to be superior. The most effective drugs are prednisone, vincristine, cyclophosphamide, L-asparaginase, and doxorubicin. Other drugs that have been included in protocols but are considered less effective are chlorambucil, methotrexate, dacarbazine (DTIC), and cytosine arabinoside. The most commonly used protocols are listed in Table 29-11.

The fund amentals of treatment are to induce a remission, maintain a remission, and reinduce a remission (rescue) after a relapse. Maintaining a first remission is much easier than inducing a second remission. Most of the presently used protocols result in 75% to 80% complete remission rate and median survival times of 8–14 months.[45–49a,66]

The response to therapy has been reported to depend on the extent of disease, stage, histologic grade, presence of concurrent medical problems such as hypercalcemia, and possibly gender.[39,45,46,48,49] Most dogs tolerate these protocols very well, and the results achieved provide the dog with a good quality of life. The cost depends on the number and frequency of the drugs given and the tests needed to monitor their toxic effects.

Table 29-10. Clinical Stages of Lymphosarcoma and Lymphoid Leukemia in Domestic Mammals* (Including Lymphosarcoma of the Skin)

ANATOMIC TYPE
  Generalized
  Alimentary
  Thymic
  Skin
  Leukemia (true)**
  Others (including solitary renal)

STAGE GROUPING (to include anatomic type)
  I   Involvement limited to a single node or lymphoid tissue in a single organ***
  II Involvement of many lymph nodes in a regional area (± tonsils)
  III Generalized lymph node involvement
  IV Liver and/or spleen involvement (± Stage III)
  V   Manifestation in the blood and involvement of bone marrow and/or other organ systems (± Stages I–IV)
Each stage is subclassified into:
  a) without systemic signs, or (b) with systemic signs

  * Excluding myeloma
 ** Only blood and bone marrow involved
*** Excluding bone marrow
(Owen L: WHO Clinical Staging. Geneva, World Health Organization, 1980. Extracted from document VPH/CMO/80, 20, p. 47, by permission of The World Health Organization, which retains the copyright)

Table 29-11. Protocols for Canine Lymphoma

PROTOCOL	NO. CASES	COMPLETE REMISSION RATE (%)	MEDIAN REMISSION TIME (DAYS)	MEDIAN SURVIVAL (DAYS)	REF
1. VCR* 0.7 mg/m² IV day 1, 14 L-Asparaginase† 400 IU/kg IP or IM day 1 CTX‡ 200–250 mg/m² IV day 7 MTX§ 0.6–0.8 mg/kg IV day 7 Repeat procedure above, except use L-asparaginase for rescue only; substitute chlorambucil[a] (1.4 mg/kg) PO for CTX if dog is in remission	147	77	140	265	MacEwen[15,37,45]
2. CTX 300 mg/m² PO every 3 wk VCR 0.75 mg/m²/wk IV × 4 wk, then every 3 wk Pred 1 mg/kg/day PO × 21 days, then every 48 hr	77	75	180	N.R.	Cotter[46,49]
3. CTX 50 mg/m² PO daily × 4 days/wk × 8 Ara-C# 100 mg/m² IV daily × 4 days VCR 0.5 mg/m²/wk IV × 8 Pred 40 mg/m² × 7 days, 20 mg/m² q 48 hr MAINTENANCE CTX 50 mg/m²w/day PO × 4 days/wk and Pred 10 mg/m² BID q 48 hrs *or* 6 MP** 50 mg/m²/day PO *or* MTX 2.5 mg/m² PO BID weekly	20	65	66	186	Madewell[47]
4. Doxorubicin†† 30 mg/m² IV of 21 days × 5 courses; rescue with CTX, VCR, Pred, L-asparaginase	37	59	131	230	Postorino[66]

* VCR, vincristine—Oncovin, Eli Lilly
† L-Asparaginase, Elspar, Merck Sharpe and Dohme
‡ CTX, cyclophosphamide, Cytoxan, Mead Johnson
§ MTX, methotrexate, Lederle
[a] Chlorambucil, Leukeran, Burroughs Wellcome
Ara C, cytosine arabinoside, Cytosar-U, Upjohn
** 6-MP, 6-mercaptopurine, Purinethol, Burroughs Wellcome
†† Doxorubicin, Adriamycin, Adria Laboratories

One of the authors (EGM) has considerable experience and survival data with Protocol 1 in Table 29-12. More than 200 dogs have been treated with this protocol, and the results have been recently published.[45] The results of Protocol 1 can be summarized as follows: A complete response was achieved in 113 dogs (77%), a partial response in 26 dogs (17.7%), and no response in 8 dogs (5.4%). The median survival time for the dogs with a complete response was 290 days; for those with a partial response, 152 days; and for those with no response, 26 days. The median survival time for dogs with a complete or partial response was 265 days. Approximately 15% of the dogs treated survived 2 years or longer. It has been our experience to stop chemotherapy after 3 years. Alternative protocols published or under evaluation use doxorubicin[66] (Table 29-11 and Table 29-12).

Doxorubicin is given at a dose of 30mg/m² I.V. every 3 weeks. The safe maximum cumulative dose is 175–225 mg/m². The maximum cumulative dosage is set to prevent lethal cardiac toxicity.

Once the protocol is chosen, it is the responsibility of the veterinarian and the client to work together to establish a successful treatment program. The veterinarian needs to understand the protocol and the associated toxicities. The veterinarian must establish a follow-up schedule to which the clients must adhere, and the veterinarian must make the client aware of the potential toxicities of the drugs and the clinical signs to watch for during the treatment phases. The exact follow-up procedure depends upon the protocol used. In general, a CBC should be repeated at each visit. If the neutrophil count falls below 3000 cells/μl, it may be necessary to

Table 29-12.   School of Veterinary Medicine, University of Wisconsin–Madison, Canine Lymphoma Protocol

	INDUCTION	DATE	DOSE GIVEN
Week 1	Vincristine 0.5–0.7 mg/m² IV	_____	_____
	400 IU/kg L-Asparaginase IM	_____	_____
	2 mg/kg Prednisone PO daily	_____	_____
Week 2	Cyclophosphamide 200–250 mg/m² IV or PO	_____	_____
	1.5 mg/Kg Prednisone PO daily	_____	_____
Week 3	Vincristine 0.5–0.7 mg/m² IV	_____	_____
	1 mg/kg Prednisone PO daily	_____	_____
Week 4	Doxorubicin 30 mg/m² IV	_____	_____
	0.5 mg/kg Prednisone PO daily	_____	_____
MAINTENANCE			
Week 6	Vincristine 0.5–0.7 mg/m² IV	_____	_____
	0.25 mg/kg Prednisone PO daily	_____	_____
Week 7	Chlorambucil 1.4 mg/kg PO (if in complete remission)	_____	_____
	Stop prednisone	_____	_____
Week 8	Vincristine 0.5–0.7 mg/m² IV	_____	_____
Week 9	Methotrexate 0.5–0.8 mg/kg IV	_____	_____
Week 10	Vincristine 0.5–0.7 mg/m² IV	_____	_____
Week 11	Chlorambucil 1.4 mg/kg PO	_____	_____
Week 12	Vincristine 0.5–0.7 mg/m² IV	_____	_____
Week 13	Doxorubicin 30 mg/m² IV	_____	_____

(1) Continue as above (week 6–13) treatments every 2 weeks, alternating methotrexate and doxorubicin. After week 28, treatments can be given every 3 weeks.

(2) Maximum dose of doxorubicin 175–225 mg/m². Then stop doxorubicin and continue methotrexate.

(3) Monitor weekly CBC for first 12 weeks, then periodically thereafter. Stop chemotherapy if WBC < 3,000 and administer prophylactic antibiotics.

administer bacteriacidal antibiotics to prevent infections during these leukopenic episodes. Chemotherapy should be withheld until the neutrophil count increases to greater than 3500/µl.

The platelet count should be monitored at periodic intervals and maintained above 100,000 cells/µl. If the count falls below this, therapy should be discontinued until the platelet count increases to an acceptable range. Repeated chemistry profiles are not absolutely necessary during chemotherapy, but it is advisable to repeat a chemistry profile at 3–4 month intervals to check for any potential toxicity or possible recurrence of disease.

Hypercalcemia is best managed by the use of intravenous administration of sterile 0.9% sodium chloride solution and furosemide, given at a dose of 5 mg/kg BW, and prednisone at a dose of 1–2 mg/kg BW divided and given twice daily. Furthermore, specific chemotherapy should be instituted once a diagnosis of lymphoma has been established.

REINDUCTION OF REMISSION (RESCUE)

Relapse can occur because the dose or frequency of drugs given is reduced too early, the tumor cells become resistant to the drugs used, or the tumor cells are resistant to all chemotherapeutic agents.

The following steps can be taken to try to reinduce remission:[37,49]

1. Start the remission induction protocol over again if relapse occurs when the animal is off drugs.

2. Substitute vinblastine (2.0 mg/m² IV) for vincristine.

3. Use L-asparaginase more frequently, *i.e.*, once weekly at 400 IU/kg intramuscularly.

4. Incorporate doxorubicin into the protocol at a dose of 30 mg/m² IV. We have found it best to substitute doxorubicin for methotrexate (when using Protocol 1). If treatment is begun with COP (when using Protocol 2), doxorubicin can be used as a single-agent rescue drug.

5. Administer cytosine arabinoside, 600 mg/m^2 IV over a 48-hour period. Repeat q 2–3 weeks or as needed to maintain a remission.
6. Administer dacarbazine (DTIC), 200 mg/m^2 IV once daily for 5 days. Repeat as needed.

In dogs with massive splenomegaly, chemotherapy should be used to reduce the size of the spleen. However, if the spleen remains enlarged, then splenectomy can be considered. Splenectomy can rapidly reverse clinical signs caused by massive splenomegaly and cytopenias secondary to hypersplenism. Splenectomy has been used in the management of dogs with lymphoma.[49b]

Tumor lysis syndrome (TLS) can occur in dogs undergoing chemotherapy and is associated with massive tumor destruction. TLS is characterized by hyperuricemia, hyperkalemia, hyperphosphatemia, and hypocalcemia. These changes lead to renal failure or sudden death due to calcium and electrolyte imbalances.[49c,49d] Treatment consists of administration of intravenous fluids containing calcium and bicarbonate. Allopurinal may help minimize the hyperuricemia.

TREATMENT APPROACHES USING IMMUNOLOGIC OR BIOLOGIC AGENTS

Results to date using immunologic procedures or biologic agents have been mixed. Studies using the chemical immunomodulator levamisole in combination with chemotherapy have proved to be unrewarding.[50] Studies using a mixed bacterial vaccine (*Serratia marcescens* and *Streptococcus pyogenes*) have improved remission time, but not survival time.[51]

Autogenous vaccines have been shown to have some positive effects in dogs when combined with chemotherapy. A tumor vaccine extract using lymphoma cells combined with Freund's adjuvant was administered to dogs after remission induction with combination chemotherapy. The median survival time was 336 days (11 dogs) for the vaccine-treated group as opposed to 196 days (9 dogs) for the chemotherapy alone group.[52] Unfortunately, a subsequent study by the same investigators reported that the prolonged survival was due to the Freund's adjuvant.[53]

Intralymphatic (IL) administration of tumor cell vaccine has been used in dogs placed in remission with a combination chemotherapy protocol. The median remission time for the

dogs given chemotherapy alone was 28 days as compared with 98 days for dogs given IL vaccine plus chemotherapy. Unfortunately, the survival times for the groups were not significantly different.[54]

Another approach to prolonging remission and survival times in dogs with malignant lymphoma is the addition of autologous bone marrow transplantation. This approach holds much promise for potential cure.[55,56] (See Chapter 15.)

TREATMENT OF ACUTE LYMPHOID LEUKEMIA (ALL)

The treatment for ALL is characteristically divided into two phases: The first is the initial or remission induction therapy, and the second is maintenance therapy. Table 29-12 gives a combination chemotherapy protocol that we have found useful for treating dogs with ALL. The cornerstone of remission induction is the combination of vincristine and prednisone. In one recently published paper on the use of this combination, 40% of the dogs responded, 20% with a complete remission and 20% with a partial remission.[3] As shown in Table 29-12, with the addition of doxorubicin and L-asparaginase, it is anticipated that response rates will increase over those reported for vincristine and prednisone alone.

The maintenance phase of treatment begins after the animal has achieved complete remission. Complete remission is defined as 100% regression of disease as based on bone marrow and peripheral blood evaluation. Chemotherapy treatments should be continued on a weekly basis except when doxorubicin is administered, and then a two-week rest period is indicated before the initiation of other drugs. This protocol has not been adequately evaluated in large numbers of animals with ALL, but on the basis of our experience this protocol is superior to vincristine and prednisone alone.

TREATMENT OF CHRONIC LYMPHOCYTIC LEUKEMIA (CLL)

Because of the indolent nature of CLL in many animals, it is controversial whether or not all dogs with the disease need to be treated.[57,58] The clinician may elect to observe the patient if the discovery of CLL is purely accidental and there are no accompanying physical or clinical signs and no significant hematologic abnormalities. If the animal is anemic and the white blood cell count is excessively high (>75,000/μl), therapy should be instituted. The most effective drug evaluated thus far is chlorambucil, which is given orally at a dose of 0.2 mg/kg once daily for 7–14 days. The dose can then be reduced to 0.1 mg/kg.

Corticosteroids are lymphocytolytic and have a major role in the systemic control of CLL. Studies in human beings have shown that the antitumor activity of chlorambucil combined with prednisone is better than that with chlorambucil alone. When the bone marrow is heavily infiltrated with CLL cells and neutropenia, thrombocytopenia, and anemia occur, more aggressive use of an alkalating agent, usually the platelet-sparing drug, cyclophosphamide, in combination with corticosteroids can be considered. The treatment of CLL is primarily palliative and complete remissions are rare, but owing to the indolent nature of this disease, survival times have been in the range of 2–3 years.[4,58]

TREATMENT OF CUTANEOUS LYMPHOMA AND LYMPHOMA-LIKE LESIONS

The clinical management of cutaneous lymphoma, with or without concurrent systemic involvement, has been generally unrewarding. Solitary lesions are best managed by complete surgical excision,[41] and dogs with solitary lesions may respond very well to surgery alone. Generalized cutaneous lymphoma has generally been considered poorly responsive to most combination chemotherapy protocols. The drugs that seem to be most effective in cutaneous lymphoma are vincristine, L-asparaginase, cyclophosphamide, and prednisone.[40,41] Recently, two dogs with solitary lymphoma were treated by radiation therapy alone. These dogs received 3000–4000 cGy and were free of disease for 3–6 years.[59]

Mycosis fungoides (MF) has been reported to respond to topical administration of nitrogen mustard.[43,60] Ten milligrams of nitrogen mustard is dissolved in 40 to 60 ml of water and applied directly to the entire skin surface after clipping. The mixture is applied 2–3 times/week initially and then once weekly or twice monthly as needed. Remissions have lasted for as long as 2 years in some dogs. Because nitrogen mustard

is a potent sensitizing agent in humans, rubber gloves should always be worn when applying the mixture.

Another agent that has been found to be beneficial in the treatment of MF is L-asparaginase. We have recently found that a polyethylene glycol (PEG) conjugate of asparaginase has been beneficial in dogs with multicentric and skin lymphoma.[61] We have documented 50% to 75% regressions of disease for up to 8 months with PEG-asparaginase alone. (See chapter 15.)

PEG-asparaginase has also been found to be very effective in treating another condition one of us (EGM) has recognized in dogs, termed granulomatous histiocytic dermatosis. This appears to be histologically benign, but dogs are presented with generalized nodular-type lesions, especially around the head and neck. Histologically this condition appears as granulomatous inflammation characterized by large epithelioid cells coexisting with plasma cells and lymphocytes.

PROGNOSIS

The prognosis of canine lymphoma is variable and dependent on a number of factors. Although it is not curable, complete remissions and good quality survival can be achieved. Factors that have been shown to influence the response to therapy and survival time include:

1. Clinical stage of disease
2. Anatomic location of tumor
3. Concurrent medical problems or paraneoplastic conditions, such as hypercalcemia, especially if renal failure is present
4. Sex of patient
5. Histologic grade of tumor

Clinical stage (based on extent of disease) has been shown to be of prognostic importance in three studies.[15,46,48] Dogs with localized disease, regional involvement, or multicentric involvement (without liver, spleen, or bone marrow involvement) seem to have a better prognosis.

The anatomic site of disease is also considered important. Primary cutaneous lymphoma (multiple sites), diffuse gastrointestinal lymphoma, and primary central nervous system involvement are associated with a poor response to therapy.

Hypercalcemia is a relatively common paraneoplastic condition in dogs with lymphoma and has been shown to influence survival adversely in dogs undergoing chemotherapy.[39] See Chapter 5 for the treatment of hypercalcemia.

Recently females have been shown to have a better prognosis than males.[45] In a study of 147 dogs with lymphoma treated with one chemotherapy protocol, females had a median survival time of 335 days versus 214 days for males.[45] Of the 12 dogs that survived 2 years or longer, 9 were females and 3 were males. The underlying reason for this difference is unknown.

Histologic classification has also been shown to be of prognostic importance. In a study of 41 dogs with lymphoma, an association was demonstrated between response to therapy and tumor cell type based on the Working Formulation.[48] Complete remission was achieved more frequently in animals with high-grade tumors, probably reflecting the presence of cells in active cycle that are responsive to the cytotoxic actions of chemotherapeutic drugs. Survival times were no different among dogs with low-, intermediate-, or high-grade tumors. The low-grade tumors probably have a slow, insidious course and are influenced very little by chemotherapy. Recently, further work using this classification system has demonstrated significant prognostic associations with specific cell types.*

In general, the prognosis of ALL in the dog is very poor. In a study of 21 dogs treated with vincristine and prednisone, among the 8 dogs achieving complete or partial remission the median survival time was 120 days, and few dogs survived longer than 8 months with that protocol.[3] In one case report, a dog with ALL was treated with infusion of fresh canine plasma and whole blood and a complete remission was maintained for 19 months without additional therapy.[62] This is a very unusual response and may indicate that normal blood contains some antileukemic factor. (See Chapter 11.)

We have seen several dogs with lymphocytic leukemia in which the lymphoblasts appear to be more well-differentiated than in most cases of ALL. Clinically, these dogs appear to have a better prognosis, and their disease may represent a subtype of canine ALL. Further studies are needed to define this subpopulation, if it exists at all.

* Carter RF: Personal communication, 1987

As stated before, CLL is a slowly progressive disease that does not always require therapy.[57] Overall, the prognosis is good, and those dogs undergoing therapy (chlorambucil and prednisone) have survival times of 18–30 months.

COMPARATIVE FEATURES[63–65]

The non-Hodgkin's lymphomas may present as "nodal" or "extranodal" disease. Approximately 64% of human patients present with peripheral lymphadenopathy, with the cervical nodes being the primary site in 60%. Most patients with non-Hodgkin's lymphoma tend to have disseminated disease.

Treatment must take into consideration such factors as histologic type, stage of disease, age, and "extranodal" involvement. For the older patient with a good prognosis histologically, the treatment may be palliative. This may involve low-dose radiation and single-agent chemotherapy (chlorambucil and prednisone). Patients with more aggressive histologic cell types may respond to radiation therapy and combination chemotherapy (cyclophosphamide, vincristine, doxorubicin, and prednisone).

The prognosis varies enormously with histology and clinical stage. For those with localized disease, survival rates of 60% to 80% are possible; for individuals with widespread disease treated with chemotherapy, the survival is about 30% to 40% at 5 years.

The treatment of ALL has seen major advances over the past 20 years. The first principle of management is to reduce the population of malignant cells to as near zero as possible by intensive combination chemotherapy. Remission is induced by a combination of cytotoxic agents (for example, prednisone, vincristine, daunorubicin, and L-asparaginase). Once remission is induced, consolidation and maintenance treatment with drugs such as 6-mercaptopurine, methotrexate, and cyclophosphamide is continued for up to 2 years or more. The central nervous system is treated with irradiation and intrathecal cytotoxic chemotherapy, usually methotrexate. The overall cure rate is greater than 80%.

The treatment of CLL in humans depends on the extent of disease and nature of the clinical symptoms. Treatment is usually initiated if anemia or thrombocytopenia is present. Radiotherapy may reduce the size of lymph nodes or spleen, but the usual treatment is continuous oral chlorambucil with or without prednisone. The prognosis of CLL is generally good despite the broad spectrum of the disorder. The median survival time is more than 5 years.

REFERENCES

1. Dorn CR, Taylor DON, Schneider R, et al: Survey of animal neoplasms in Alameda and Contra Costa Counties, California. II. Cancer morbidity in dogs and cats from Alameda County. Natl Cancer Inst 40:307–318, 1968

2. Priester WA: The occurrence of tumors in domestic animal. NCI Monogr 54:158, 1980

3. Matus RE, Leifer CE, MacEwen EG: Acute lymphoblastic leukemia in the dog: A review of 30 cases. J Am Vet Med Assoc 183:859–862, 1983

4. Leifer CE, Matus RE: Lymphoid leukemia in the dog. Vet Clin North Am (Small Anim Pract) 15:723–739, 1985

5. Gallo RC, Meyskens FL: Advances in viral etiology of leukemia and lymphoma. Semin Hematol 15:379–398, 1978

6. Kakuk TJ, Hinz RW, Langhan RF, et al: Experimental transmission of canine malignant lymphoma to a Beagle neonate. Cancer Res 28:716–723, 1968

7. Chapman NL, Bopp RRJ, Brightwell AS, et al: A preliminary report on virus-like particles in canine leukemia and derived cell cultures. Cancer Res 27:18–25, 1967

8. Strandstrom HV, Rimaila-Parnanenm E: Canine atypical malignant lymphoma. Am J Vet Res 40:1033–1034, 1979

9. Onions D: RNA dependent DNA polymerase activity in canine lymphosarcoma. Eur J Cancer 16:345–349, 1980

10. Armstrong SJ, Thomley FM, Nunes deSouza PA, et al: Reverse transcriptase activity associated with canine leukemia and lymphosarcoma. In Yohn DS, Blakeslee JR (eds): Advances in Comparative Leukemia Research, 1981, pp 411–412. New York, Elsevier, 1982

11. Tomley FN, Armstrong SJ, Nahy BWJ, et al: Reverse transcriptase activity and particles of retroviral density in cultured canine lymphosarcoma supernatants. Br J Cancer 47:277–284, 1983

12. Onions D: A prospective survey of familial canine lymphosarcoma. J Natl Cancer Inst 72:909–912, 1984

13. Weiden PL, Storb R, Korb HJ, et al: Immune reactivity in dogs with spontaneous malignancy. J Natl Cancer Inst 53:1049–1053, 1974

14. Kersay JH, Spector BD, Good RA: Immunodeficiency and cancer. Adv Cancer Res 18:211–230, 1973

15. MacEwen EG, Brown NO, Patnaik AK, et al: Cyclic combination chemotherapy of canine lymphosarcoma. JAMA 178:1178–1181, 1981

16. MacEwen EG, Hurvitz AJ, Hayes AA: Hyperviscosity syndrome associated with lymphocytic leukemia in three dogs. J Am Vet Med Assoc 170:1309–1312, 1977

17. Weller RE: Paraneoplastic disorders in dogs with Hematopoietic tumors. Vet Clin North Am (Small Amin Pract) 15:805–816, 1986

18. Rappaport H: Tumors of the hematopoietic system. In Atlas of Tumor Pathology, Sect 3, Fasc 8, pp 91–206. Washington, DC, US Armed Forces Institute of Pathology, 1966

19. Jarrett WFH, Mackey LJ: Neoplastic diseases of the haematopoietic and lymphoid tissues. Bull WHO 50:21–34, 1974

20. Moulton JE, Dungworth DL: Tumors of the lymphoid and hemopoietic tissues. In Moulton JE (ed): Tumors in Domestic Animals, ed 2, pp 150–204. Berkeley, University of California Press, 1978

21. Nielson SW: Classification of tumors in dogs and cats. J Am Anim Hosp Assoc 19:13–60, 1983

22. Holmberg CA, Manning JS, Osburn BI: Canine malignant lymphomas: Comparison of morphologic and immunologic parameters. J Natl Cancer Inst 56:125–135, 1976

23. Squire RA, Bush M, Melby EC, Neeley LM, Yarbrough B: Clinical and pathologic study of canine lymphoma: Clinical staging, cell classification, and therapy. J Natl Cancer Inst 51:565–574, 1973

24. Valli VE, McSherry BJ, Dunham BM, Jacobs RM, Lumsden JH: Histocytology of lymphoid tumors in the dog, cat and cow. Vet Pathol 18:494–512, 1981

25. Weller RE, Holmberg CA, Theilen GH, Madewell BR: Histologic classification as a prognostic criterion for canine lymphosarcoma. Am J Vet Res 41:1310–1314, 1980

26. Gray KN, Raulston GL, Gleiser CA, Jardine JH: Histologic classification as an indicator of therapeutic response in malignant lymphoma of dogs. J Am Vet Med Assoc 184:814–817, 1984

27. Lennert K, Mohri N, Stein H, Kaiserling E: The histopathology of malignant lymphoma. Br J Haematol (Suppl) 31:193–203, 1975

28. Lukes RJ, Collins RD: Immunologic character-

ization of human malignant lymphomas. Cancer 34:1488–1503, 1974

29. Rappaport H, Brylan RC: Changing concepts in the classification of malignant neoplasms of the hematopoietic system. In Rebuck JW, Berard CW, Abell MR (eds): The Reticuloendothelial System, pp 1–19. Baltimore, Williams and Wilkins, 1975

30. Appelbaum FR, Sale GR, Storb R, Charrier K, Deeg HJ, Graham T, Wulff JC: Phenotying of canine lymphoma with monoclonal antibodies directed at cell surface antigens: Classifications, morphology, clinical presentation and response to chemotherapy. Hematol Oncol 2:151–168, 1984

31. Gendron–Fitzpatrick AP: A functional classification of canine malignant lymphomas (abstr). 37th Annual Meeting American College of Veterinary Pathologists and 21st Annual Meeting American Society for Veterinary Clinical Pathologists, p 124, 1986

32. Non-Hodgkin's Lymphoma Pathologic Classification Project: National Cancer Institute sponsored study of classification of non-Hodgkin's lymphomas. Cancer 49:2112, 1982

33. Carter RF, Valli VEO, Lumsden JH: The cytology, histology and prevalence of cell types in canine lymphoma classified according to the National Cancer Institute Working Formulation. Can J Vet Res 50:154–164, 1986

34. Levine AM, Taylor CR, Schneider DR, Koehler SC, Forman SJ, Lichtenstein A, Lukes RL, Feinstein DI: Immunoblastic sarcoma of T-cell versus B-cell origin: I. Clinical features. Blood 58:52–61, 1981

35. MacEwen EG, Patnaik AK, Wilkins RJ: Diagnosis and treatment of canine hematopoietic neoplasms. Vet Clin North Am (Small Anim Pract) 7:105–118, 1977

36. Madewell BR, Feldman BF: Characterization of anemias associated with neoplasia in small animal. J Am Vet Med Assoc 176:419–425, 1980

37. Madewell BR: Canine lymphoma. Vet Clin North Am (Small Anim Pract) 15:709–722, 1985

38. MacEwen EG, Siegel SD: Hypercalcemia: A paraneoplastic disease. Vet Clin North Am (Small Anim Pract) 7:187–194, 1977

39. Weller RE, Theilen GH, Madewell BR: Chemotherapeutic responses in dogs with lymphosarcoma and hypercalcemia. J Am Vet Med Assoc 181:891–893, 1982

40. Brown NO, Nesbitt GH, Patnaik AK, et al: Cutaneous lymphosarcoma in the dog: A disease with variable clinical and histologic manifestations. J Am Anim Hosp Assoc 16:565–572, 1980

41. Goldschmidt MH, Bevier DE: Skin tumors in the dog. III. lymphohistiocytic and melanocytic tumors. Comp Cont Educ Pract Vet, 3:588, 1981

42. Shadduck JA, Reedy LN, Lawton G, et al: A canine cutaneous lymphoproliferative disease resembling mycosis fungoides in man. Vet Pathol 15:716, 1978

43. Kwochka KW: Clinical diagnosis and management of cutaneous neoplasia in the dog. In Gorman NT (ed): Oncology: Contemporary Issues in Small Animal Practice, pp 195–212. New York, Churchill-Livingstone, 1986

43a. Nyland TG: Ultrasonic patterns of canine hepatic lymphosarcoma. Vet Radiol 25:167–172, 1984

43b. Wrigley RH, Konde LJ, Park RD, et al: Ultrasonographic features of splenic lymphosarcoma in dogs: 12 cases (1980–1986). J Am Vet Med Assoc 193:1565–1568, 1988

44. MacEwen EG, Hurvitz AI: Diagnosis and management of monoclonal gammopathies. Vet Clin North Am (Small Anim Pract) 7:119–131, 1977

45. MacEwen EG, Hayes AA, Matus RE, et al: Evaluation of some prognostic factors for advanced multicentric lymphosarcoma in the dog: 147 cases 1978–1981. J Am Vet Med Assoc 190:564–568, 1987

46. Cotter SM: Treatment of lymphoma and leukemia with cyclophosphamide, vincristine, and prednisone. I: Treatment of dogs. J Am Anim Hosp Assoc 19:159–165, 1983

47. Madewell BR: Chemotherapy of canine lymphosarcoma. Am J Vet Res 36:1525–1528, 1975

48. Carter RF, Harris CK, Withrow SJ, et al: Chemotherapy of canine lymphoma with histopathologic correlation: Doxorubicin alone compared to COP as first treatment regimen. J Am Anim Hosp Assoc 23:587–596, 1987

49. Cotter SM: Clinical management of lymphoproliferative, myeloproliferative, and plasma cell neoplasia. In Gorman NT (ed): Oncology Contemporary Issues in Small Animal Practice, pp. 169–194. New York, Churchill-Livingstone, 1986

49a. Cotter SM, Goldstein MA: Comparison of two protocols for maintainance of remission in dogs with lymphoma. J Am Anim Hosp Assoc 23:495–499, 1987

49b. Brooks MB, Matus RE, Leifer CE, et al: Use of splenectomy in the management of lymphoma in dogs: 16 cases (1976–1985). J Am Vet Med Assoc 191:1008–1010, 1987

49c. Page RL: Acute tumor lysis syndrome. Vet Med Surg 1:58–60, 1980

49d. Laing EJ, Carter RF: Acute tumor lysis syndrome following treatment of canine lymphoma. J Am Anim Hosp Assoc 24:691–696, 1988

50. MacEwen EG, Hayes AA, Mooney S, et al: Levamisole as adjuvant to chemotherapy for canine lymphosarcoma. J Biol Response Mod 4:427–433, 1985

51. MacEwen EG, Hess PW, Hayes AA, et al: A clinical evaluation of the effectiveness of immunotherapy combined with chemotherapy for canine lymphosarcoma. In Bentvelzen J, Yohn DS (eds): 8th Symposium on Comparative Research on Leukemia and Related Disease, pp 395–399. Amsterdam, Elsevier/North Holland Biomedical Press, 1977

52. Crow SE, Theilen GH, Benjamin E, et al: Chemoimmunotherapy for canine lymphosarcoma. Cancer 40:2102–2108, 1977

53. Weller RE, Theilen GH, Madewell BR, et al: Chemoimmunotherapy for canine lymphosarcoma: A prospective evaluation of specific and nonspecific immunomodulation. Am J Vet Res 41:516–521, 1980

54. Jeglum KA, Young KM, Barnsley K, et al: Chemotherapy versus chemotherapy with intralymphatic tumor cell vaccine in canine lymphoma. Cancer 61:2042–2050, 1988

55. Weiden PL, Storb R, Deeg HJ, et al: Prolonged disease-free survival in dogs with lymphoma after total-body irradiation and autologous marrow transplantation consolidation of combination-chemotherapy-induced remission. Blood, 54:1039–1049, 1979

56. Appelbaum FR, Deeg HJ, Storb R, et al. Marrow transplant studies in dogs with malignant lymphoma. Transplantation 39:499–504, 1985

57. Harvey JW, Terrell TG, Hyde DM, et al: Well-differentiated lymphocytic leukemia in a dog: Long-term survival without therapy. Vet Pathol 18:37–47, 1981

58. Hodgkins EM, Zinkl JG, Madewell BR: Chronic lymphocytic leukemia in the dog. J Am Vet Med Assoc 117:704–707, 1980

59. Thrall DE, Dewhirst MH: Use of radiation and/or hyperthermia for treatment of mast cell tumors and lymphosarcoma in dogs. Vet Clin North Am (Small Anim Pract) 15:835, 1985

60. Miller WH: Canine cutaneous lymphomas. In Kirk RW (eds): Current Veterinary Therapy VII, p 493. Philadelphia, W.B. Saunders, 1980

61. MacEwen EG, Rosenthal R, Matus R, et al: An evaluation of asparaginase: Polyethylene glycol conjugate against canine lymphosarcoma. Cancer 59:2011–2015, 1987

62. MacEwen EG, Patnaik AK, Hayes AA, et al: Temporary plasma-induced remission of lymphoblastic leukemia in a dog. Am J Vet Res 42:1450–1452, 1981

63. DeVita VT, Jaffee ES, Hellman S: Hodgkin's disease and the non-Hodgkin's lymphoma. In DeVita VT, Hellman S, Rosenburg S (eds): Cancer: Principles and Practice of Oncology, ed 2, pp 1623–1710. Philadelphia, J.B. Lippincott, 1985

64. Wiernik PH: Acute leukemia of adults. In Devita VT, Hellman S, Rosenburg S (eds): Cancer: Principles and Practice of Oncology, ed 2, pp 1711–1738. Philadelphia, J.B. Lippincott, 1985

65. Canellos GP: Chronic leukemia. In DeVita VT, Hellman S, Rosenburg S (eds): Cancer: Principles and Practice of Oncology, ed 2, pp 1739–1752. Philadelphia, J.B. Lippincott, 1985

66. Postorino NC, Susaneck SJ, Withrow SJ, et al: Single agent therapy with adriamycin for canine lymphosarcoma. J Am Anim Hosp Assoc 25:221–225, 1989

Canine Myeloproliferative Disorders

Karen M. Young
E. Gregory MacEwen

INCIDENCE AND RISK FACTORS

Nonlymphocytic leukemias and myeloproliferative disorders (MPD) are uncommon in the dog; they occur 10 times less frequently than lymphoproliferative disorders.[1] The most frequently reported MPD are granulocytic and myelomonocytic leukemia. There is no known age, breed, or sex predisposition. The etiology of spontaneously occurring leukemia is unknown; genetic factors, environmental factors (including exposure to radiation, drugs, or toxic chemicals), and aberrant function of the immune system have all been implicated. Certain forms of leukemia have been produced experimentally following irradiation.[2–4] In contrast to MPD in cats, no causative viral agent has been demonstrated in dogs.

PATHOLOGY AND NATURAL BEHAVIOR

Before discussing the pathogenesis of MPD, a review of normal hematopoiesis will aid in understanding the various manifestations of MPD. Hematopoiesis is the process of proliferation, differentiation, and maturation of stem cells into terminally differentiated blood cells. A simplified scheme is presented in Fig. 29-3. Pluripotent stem cells differentiate into either lymphopoietic or hematopoietic stem cells. Under the influence of specific regulatory and microenvironmental factors, multipotent hematopoietic stem cells in bone marrow differentiate into progenitor cells committed to a specific hematopoietic cell line—for example, erythroid, granulocytic-monocytic, or megakaryocytic. Maturation results in the production of well-differentiated blood cells—erythrocytes, granulocytes, monoctyes, and platelets—which are delivered to the circulation. In some cases, as in the maturation of reticulocytes to erythrocytes, final development may occur in the spleen.

Proliferation and differentiation of hematopoietic cells is directed by a group of regulatory growth factors.[5] Of these, erythropoietin is the best characterized; it regulates erythroid proliferation and differentiation. The myeloid compartment is dependent on a group of factors, collectively referred to as colony-stimulating factors or activities (CSF or CSA), which direct the development of granulocytic, monocytic, and megakaryocytic cell lines. These factors act at the level of the committed progenitor cells. In some cases, multiple factors are required for normal development. Both megakaryocyte (Meg)-CSA and thrombopoietin, for example, are essential for normal megakaryocyte development *in vitro*. Interestingly, it is now known that some of these factors also influence the functional capabilities of mature cells. For example, granulocytic-monocytic (GM)-CSF increases the cytotoxic capacity of mature neutrophils.[6] Except for erythropoietin, which is produced in the kidney, the site of production of many of these factors is unknown. CSF are produced *in vitro* by a multitude of cell types, including monocytes, macrophages, lymphocytes, and endothelial cells. The *in vivo* site of production is unknown. While production of these factors is stimulated by hypoxia in the case of erythropoietin and endotoxin in the case of GM-CSF, exact regulatory mechanisms are largely unknown. Many of these factors have been well characterized in humans and mice, but less so in other species.

Myeloproliferative disorders result from defective proliferation of one or more of the hematopoietic cell lines. MPD are now known to be clonal disorders affecting hematopoiesis at the level of the stem cell or committed progenitor cell.[7] Since hematopoietic cells share a common stem cell, these disorders may be manifested by abnormalities in any or all the different cell lines. In addition, transformation from one MPD to another may occur. Clonal disorders of bone marrow include myeloaplasia (usually referred to as aplastic anemia), myelodysplasia, and myeloproliferation. A preleukemic syndrome, characterized by peripheral pancytopenia and bone marrow hyperplasia with maturation arrest, is more correctly termed hematopoietic dysplasia because the syndrome does not always progress to overt leukemia. This

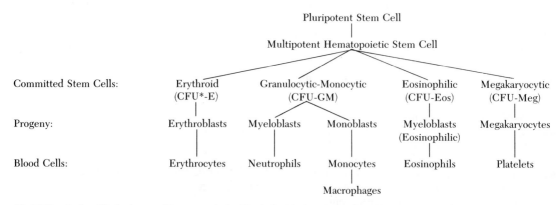

Fig 29-3. A simplified scheme of hematopoiesis. (Copied with permission from Young KM: Myeloproliferative disorders. Vet Clin North Am (Small Anim Pract) 15:770, 1985)

* CFU = colony forming units.

syndrome has been described in cats, usually in association with feline leukemia virus infection, but has only rarely been recognized in dogs.[8]

Several classification systems for MPD exist; one useful system distinguishes acute from chronic disorders. This classification is based on the degree of cellular differentiation, but it also correlates with presentation and clinical course. Disorders resulting from uncontrolled proliferation of cells that exhibit progressive maturation lead to accumulation of well-differentiated cells. These disorders are termed "chronic" myeloproliferative disorders and include polycythemia vera, chronic granulocytic leukemia, primary (essential) thrombocythemia, and primary (idiopathic) myelofibrosis. Disorders resulting from uncontrolled proliferation of cells incapable of progressive maturation lead to accumulation of poorly differentiated or "blast" cells. These disorders are termed "acute" myeloproliferative disorders or acute nonlymphocytic leukemias. In general, the acute disorders have a more sudden onset and are more aggressive. In both acute and chronic disorders, however, abnormalities in proliferation, maturation, and functional characteristics can occur in any hematopoietic cell line.[9] In addition, normal hematopoiesis is adversely affected. Owing to bone marrow infiltration and displacement of normal hematopoietic cells, animals with leukemia often have decreased numbers of circulating normal cells. Anemia is particularly common. Neutropenia and thrombocytopenia result in infection and hemorrhage, which may be more deleterious to the animal than the primary disease process. Despite the disseminated nature of the disease at the time of diagnosis, parenchymal organ dysfunction usually occurs only in very advanced cases of myeloproliferative disorders.

In the following section, each disease entity is considered separately. Chronic MPD will be considered first, followed by a discussion of the acute disorders.

CHRONIC MYELOPROLIFERATIVE DISORDERS

These disorders are characterized by excessive production of well-differentiated bone marrow cells, resulting in accumulation of erythrocytes (polycythemia vera), granulocytes (chronic granulocytic leukemia, basophilic leukemia), or platelets (primary thrombocythemia). Primary myelofibrosis, characterized by proliferation of fibroblasts with accumulation of collagen in bone marrow, is included in this group of diseases, but it may actually result from an abnormality in megakaryocyte production (see below).

Polycythemia Vera

Neoplastic proliferation of the erythroid series with terminal differentiation of red blood cells is termed *polycythemia vera*. The disease has been reported in dogs that tend to be middle-aged with no breed or sex predilection.[10–14] The disease is characterized by an increased red blood cell mass evidenced by an elevated packed cell volume (PCV), red blood cell count, and hemoglobin concentration. The bone marrow is hyperplastic, although the myeloid-erythroid ratio (M:E) tends to be normal. In contrast to the disease in humans, other cell lines do not appear to be involved, and transformation to other MPD has not been reported. The disease in dogs may be more appropriately termed primary erythrocytosis.

Chronic Granulocytic Leukemia (CGL)

Chronic granulocytic leukemia is a neoplastic proliferation of the neutrophilic series. Owing to the low incidence of CGL and the failure to distinguish between acute and chronic granulocytic leukemia in the literature, good epidemiologic information is not available. It appears, however, that CGL can occur in dogs of any age but may be more common in young dogs.[15] Neutrophils and neutrophilic precursors accumulate in bone marrow and peripheral blood and invade other organs. The peripheral white blood cell (WBC) count is usually, but not always, greater than $100,000/\mu l$. Both immature and mature neutrophils are present; mature forms are usually more numerous, but sometimes an "uneven" left shift is present. Eosinophils and basophils may also be increased. The bone marrow is characterized by granulocytic hyperplasia, and morphologic abnormalities may not be present. Erythroid and megakaryocytic lines may be affected, resulting in anemia, thrombocytopenia, or thrombocytosis. In humans, characteristic cytogenetic abnormalities are present in all bone marrow cells, signifying a lesion at the level of an early multipotent stem cell. Typically these individuals have a chromosomal translocation, resulting in the Philadelphia chromosome.[16] No consistent cytogenetic abnormalities have been demonstrated in spontaneously occurring CGL in dogs.

In addition to accumulating in bone marrow and peripheral blood, leukemic cells also invade the red pulp of the spleen, the periportal and sinusoidal areas of the liver, and sometimes lymph nodes. Other organs, such as kidney, heart, and lung, are less commonly affected. In addition, extramedullary hematopoiesis may be present in liver and spleen. Death is usually due to complications of infection or hemorrhage secondary to neutrophil dysfunction and thrombocytopenia. In some cases, CGL may terminate in "blast crisis," in which there is a transformation from a predominance of well-differentiated granulocytes to excessive numbers of poorly differentiated blast cells in peripheral blood and bone marrow. This phenomenon is well documented in the dog.[17,18]

Eosinophilic and Basophilic Leukemia

Eosinophilic and basophilic leukemia may be considered variants of chronic granulocytic leukemia. Eosinophilic leukemia has not been definitively reported in the dog. Disorders associated with eosinophilia, such as parasitism, skin diseases, or diseases of the respiratory and gastrointestinal tracts, should be considered first in an animal with eosinophilia owing to the rarity of the myeloproliferative disorder. Basophilic leukemia, although rare, has been reported in the dog and was characterized by an elevated WBC count with a high proportion of basophils in peripheral blood and bone marrow.[19] Hepatosplenomegaly, lymphadenopathy, anemia, and thrombocytosis were also present. This disorder should be distinguished from mastocytosis.

Primary Thrombocythemia

Primary or essential thrombocythemia has not been reported in dogs. In humans it is characterized by platelet counts of greater than 1 million/μl, marked megakaryocytic hyperplasia of the bone marrow, splenomegaly, and absence of a primary disorder associated with reactive thrombocytosis.[20] Thrombosis and bleeding are the most common sequelae. Attempts to recognize this disorder in dogs should account for these criteria. Differentials include causes of reactive thrombocytosis, such as iron-deficiency anemia, splenectomy, severe hemorrhage, and rebound from immune-mediated thrombocytopenia.

Primary Myelofibrosis

In humans, myelofibrosis is characterized by collagen deposition in bone marrow and increased numbers of megakaryocytes, many of which exhibit morphologic abnormalities. Focal osteosclerosis is sometimes present. Anemia, thrombocytopenia, splenomegaly, and myeloid metaplasia (production of hematopoietic cells outside the bone marrow) are consistent features. The extramedullary hematopoiesis is ineffective in maintaining or restoring normal peripheral blood counts.

Current thinking attributes the fibrosis to an accumulation in bone marrow of megakaryocytic cytoplasmic contents, which include several factors that promote fibroblast proliferation or inhibit collagen breakdown.[21] These factors are a normal component of megakaryocytes and are passed on to platelets, which deposit them at sites of vessel damage, thereby promoting wound repair. The accumulation of these factors in bone marrow may result from aberrant production and subsequent breakdown of megakaryocytes, or "ineffective megakaryocytopoiesis." Primary myelofibrosis may more correctly be a primary disorder of megakaryocytes with secondary fibrosis. Primary myelofibrosis is not well documented in the dog but has been reported secondary to megakaryocytic leukemia,[22] radiation damage,[23] and pyruvate kinase deficiency.[24]

ACUTE MYELOPROLIFERATIVE DISORDERS

These disorders are rare and are characterized by aberrant proliferation of a clone of cells without maturation. This results in accumulation of immature blast cells in bone marrow and peripheral blood. The WBC count is variable and ranges from leukopenia to counts greater than 500,000/μl. Spleen, liver, and lymph nodes are commonly involved, and other tissues, including tonsils, kidney, heart, and central nervous system (CNS), may be infiltrated as well. Young dogs may be more frequently affected.[15] The clinical course of these disorders tends to be rapid. Production of normal peripheral blood cells is usually diminished or absent, and anemia, neutropenia, and thrombocytopenia are common. Infection and hemorrhage are frequent sequelae. Occasionally, malignant blasts are present in bone marrow but not in peripheral blood. This is termed "aleukemic leukemia."

The neoplastic cells eventually accumulate in peripheral blood.

Acute myeloproliferative disorders are named for the lineage of the blast cells. Sometimes with standard Romanovsky stains the blast cells have distinguishing features; usually, however, the lineage must be determined with more sophisticated cytochemical techniques. In acute myelogenous leukemia (AML), the blasts are myeloid (or granulocytic) in origin. In some cases, the blast cells have features of both myeloid and monocytic cells; this disorder is referred to as acute myelomonocytic leukemia (AMML) and is probably the result of a lesion at the level of the committed progenitor cell that is shared by neutrophils and monocytes (see Fig. 29-3). AML and AMML are the most commonly reported acute MPD in the dog.[1,25–31] Other acute leukemias include monocytic leukemia, in which the cells may appear as undifferentiated blasts or well-differentiated monocytes;[1,32,33] megakaryocytic leukemia, with abnormal megakaryocytes and fibrosis in the bone marrow, dwarf megakaryocytes or blast cells in the peripheral blood, and low or high numbers of circulating platelets with morphologic abnormalities;[34] erythremic myelosis, in which erythroid precursors predominate; and erythroleukemia, in which blasts of both erythroid and myeloid cells are present. Spontaneously occurring erythremic myelosis and erythroleukemia have not been reported in the dog. Sometimes the lineage of the blasts cannot be determined with any of the currently available techniques. These leukemias are referred to as "undifferentiated." In general, acute leukemias behave similarly in terms of natural behavior and response to therapy, so sophisticated determinations of cell type may be academic. However, by acquiring this information, we may eventually be able to identify types of acute leukemias that respond to certain therapeutic regimens.

HISTORY AND CLINICAL SIGNS

Dogs with MPD have similar presentations regardless of the specific disease entity, although animals with acute MPD tend to have a more acute onset of illness and a more rapid clinical course. A history of lethargy, inappetence, and weight loss is common. Clinical signs include pallor, fever, hepatosplenomegaly, and less commonly lymphadenopathy and enlarged tonsils. Vomiting, diarrhea, and neurologic signs are variable features. Serum chemistries are frequently normal but may change if significant organ infiltration occurs. In polycythemia vera, dogs often have erythema of mucous membranes owing to the increase in red blood cell mass. In addition, neurologic signs, such as disorientation, ataxia, or seizures, may be present and are thought to be the result of hyperviscosity or hypervolemia.[14] Hepatosplenomegaly is usually absent.

Peripheral blood abnormalities are consistently found. In addition to the presence of neoplastic cells, other abnormalities, including a decrease in the numbers of normal cells of any or all hematopoietic cell lines and morphologic abnormalities, may be present. Nonregenerative anemia is a common laboratory finding. It is usually normocytic and normochromic, although macrocytic anemia is sometimes present. Pathogenic mechanisms include myelophthisis (crowding out of normal bone marrow cells by neoplastic cells), ineffective erythropoiesis, immune-mediated anemia secondary to neoplasia, and hemorrhage secondary to thrombocytopenia, platelet dysfunction, or disseminated intravascular coagulation. Anemia is most severe in acute MPD; it may be milder in animals with acute monocytic leukemia. In myelofibrosis, the anemia is characterized by anisocytosis and poikilocytosis with characteristic teardrop-shaped erythrocytes. In addition, pancytopenia and leukoerythroblastosis, in which immature erythroid and myeloid cells are in circulation, may be present. These phenomena probably result from replacement of marrow by fibrous tissue with resultant sheering of red cells and escape of immature cells normally confined to bone marrow. In polycythemia vera, the PCV is elevated, usually in the range of 65% to 80%. The bone marrow is hyperplastic, and the M:E is usually in the normal range.

DIAGNOSTIC TECHNIQUES AND WORK-UP

In all cases of MPD, the diagnosis depends upon examination of peripheral blood and bone marrow. Owing to the degree of differentiation of cells in chronic MPD, these disorders must be distinguished from non-neoplastic causes of increases in these cell types. In order to make a diagnosis of polycythemia vera, it must first be established that the polycythemia is absolute rather than relative. In absolute polycythemias, the red blood cell mass is increased. In relative polycythemias, there is no real increase in red blood cell mass, but owing to water loss, for example from dehydration, the PCV appears to be elevated. Absolute polycythemia should be suspected in an animal with an elevated RBC count, PCV, and hemoglobin concentration without dehydration. It can be confirmed by measuring the red blood cell mass by labeling cells with [51]chromium.[14] Following the establishment of the presence of absolute polycythemia, it must be determined if the polycythemia is primary or secondary. Primary polycythemia is a neoplastic myeloproliferative disorder in which serum erythropoietin levels are either normal or decreased. Secondary polycythemia results either from hypoxic conditions, for example cardiopulmonary disease, or from tumors which secrete erythropoietin.[35,36] In the former, blood gas analysis is helpful in distinguishing primary from secondary polycythemia. Unfortunately, measurement of serum erythropoietin is not widely available at this time.

In chronic granulocytic leukemia, pathognomonic findings do not exist, and other common causes for marked leukocytosis with a left shift ("leukemoid reaction") and granulocytic hyperplasia of bone marrow must be eliminated. These include infections, especially pyogenic ones, immune-mediated diseases, and other malignant neoplasms. In CGL maturation sometimes appears disorderly, and there may be variation in the size and shape of neutrophils at the same level of maturation. In addition, neoplastic leukocytes may disintegrate more rapidly and appear vacuolated.[15] Because of the invasive nature of CGL, biopsy of liver or spleen may also help to distinguish true leukemia from a leukemoid reaction, assuming the animal can tolerate the procedure. If characteristic cytogenetic abnormalities can be found in dogs with CGL, this analysis may be helpful.

Eosinophilic and basophilic leukemias are diagnosed on the basis of increased numbers of these cells in circulation and in bone marrow. Hypereosinophilic syndromes should be eliminated before a diagnosis of esoinophilic leukemia is made. Basophilic leukemia must be differentiated from mastocytosis based on the morphology of the cell type present. Basophils have a segmented nucleus, whereas mast cells have a round nucleus that may be partially or totally obscured by metachromatic-staining granules; however, it is usually possible to find cells with few enough granules to discern the morphology of the nucleus.

Myelofibrosis should be suspected in animals with cytopenias, morphologic abnormalities in erythrocytes, especially teardrop-shaped cells, and leukoerythroblastosis. Bone marrow aspiration is usually unsuccessful, resulting in a "dry tap." This necessitates a bone marrow biopsy taken with a Jamshidi needle. The specimen is processed for routine histopathologic examination, and if necessary, special stains for fibrous tissue can be used. Since myelofibrosis can occur secondary to other diseases, such as other MPD[22] or pyruvate kinase deficiency,[24] the clinician should look for a primary disease process.

Acute MPD are diagnosed on the basis of finding blast cells in peripheral blood and bone marrow. These cells may be present in low numbers in peripheral blood, and a careful search of the smear, especially at the feathered edge, should be made. Even if blasts are not present in peripheral blood, indications of bone marrow disease, such as pancytopenia or nonregenerative anemia, are usually present. Occasionally neoplastic cells can be found in cerebrospinal fluid in animals with invasion of the central nervous system.

Examination of blasts stained with standard Romanovsky stains may give clues as to the lineage of the cells. In AML, in addition to myeloblasts, some progranulocytes with their characteristic azurophilic granules may be present. In myelomonocytic leukemia, the blasts are usually very pleomorphic with round to lobulated nuclei. In some cells, the cytoplasm may contain large azurophilic granules or vacuoles. Blasts in megakaryocytic leukemia may contain vacuoles and have cytoplasmic blebs.

While these distinguishing morphologic features may suggest a definitive diagnosis, special stains are usually required to define the lineage of the blasts. Several investigators have reported modification of diagnoses following cytochemical staining.[37,38] Precise determination of cell type may be academic since acute nonlymphocytic leukemias behave in a similar manner and have a uniformly grave prognosis. It is important, however, to distinguish lymphocytic leukemia from nonlymphocytic leukemia because the prognosis and response to therapy are much better in the former. Lymphoblasts usually have a higher nuclear to cytoplasmic ratio and more condensed chromatin pattern, but the distinction cannot always be made with certainty on routinely stained smears. Moreover, with advances in therapy, it may eventually be important from a clinical standpoint to distinguish among the nonlymphocytic leukemias. In addition, if models for human disease are to be developed, precise identification of cell types is required.

Currently, the best way of distinguishing cell types is by performing a battery of special cytochemical stains on peripheral blood or bone marrow if blast cells are infrequent in peripheral blood. The most commonly used stains are Sudan black B (SBB), peroxidase, periodic acid-Schiff (PAS), chloracetate esterase (CAE), and α-naphthyl butyrate or acetate (nonspecific esterase, NSE) with and without fluoride inhibition. Procedures for performing these stains have been established for the dog.[39] Table 29-13 lists these stains along with their significance in interpreting the blast lineage. Another marker with potential use is acetylcholinesterase, which stains megakaryocytes.[40] It should be stressed that proper specimen handling, fixation, and staining procedures are critical to accurate interpretation of results. In addition, blasts must be in high enough frequency in peripheral blood or bone marrow to be distinguished from other cells.

Leukocyte alkaline phosphatase (LAP) is absent in neutrophils and their precursors in normal dogs.[39] However, several investigators have now reported its presence in leukemic blasts from dogs with AML and AMML.[27,37–39] In addition, LAP may be present in some neoplastic lymphoblasts in the dog.[38] In humans, by contrast, LAP activity is normally present in neutrophils, increased in leukocytosis due to infection or inflammation, and decreased in CGL. This enzyme marker may be useful in the differential diagnosis of leukemia in the dog.

Other techniques that are available to identify cell type are electron microscopy and flow cytometry. These require expensive instrumentation, experienced operators, and, in the case of flow cytometry, specific immunologic reagents. While these requirements appear formidable, many human hospitals and veterinary schools now have flow cytometers with trained operators; and if appropriate reagents can be developed, performance of these tests may facilitate that task of identifying cell types. Hematopoietic cells from people with leukemia often have abnormal chromosome patterns. Cytogenetic abnormalities have been found in leukemic cells from a small number of dogs.[41] While no consistent patterns could be correlated with the type of leukemia, cytogenetic analysis may eventually prove to be a valuable diagnostic and prognostic aid.

THERAPY

Two chemotherapeutic agents have been useful in treating chronic granulocytic leukemia and polycythemia vera. Hydroxyurea is the most

Table 29-13. Cytochemical Reactions in Blast Cells of Acute Leukemias

LEUKEMIA	SUDAN BLACK B	PEROXIDASE (LEUKOCYTE)	PAS	CAE	NSE	PEROXIDASE (PLATELET)
AML	+	+	+	+	−	
AMML	+	+/−	+/−	+	+	
AMoL	−	+/−	+/−	−	+*	
Erythroleuk	−	−	+	−	−	
Meg L			+			+
ALL	−	−	+†	−	+‡	
Undiff L	−	−	−	−	−	−

PAS, periodic acid-Schiff; CAE, chloracetate esterase; NSE, nonspecific esterase; AML, acute myelogenous leukemia; AMML, acute myelomonocytic leukemia; AMoL, acute monocytic leukemia; Erythroleuk, erythroleukemia; Meg L, acute megakaryocytic leukemia; ALL, acute lymphoblastic leukemia; Undiff L, undifferentiated leukemia. +, positive; −, negative; +/− weakly or occasionally positive.
* sodium fluoride-sensitive
† coarse blocks of PAS-positive material in cytoplasm
‡ focal positivity
(Copied with modification from Young KM: Myeloproliferative disorders. Vet Clin North AM [Small Anim Pract] 15:776, 1985)

effective agent and the drug studied most extensively. It can be given at a dosage of 40–50 mg/kg divided BID or 1 gm/m^2 PO until the desired effect is seen in the CBC.[14,19] Most animals tolerate this drug very well. One of the adverse side-effects of hydroxyurea is bone marrow suppression with the development of a megaloblastic anemia. One dog on long-term therapy developed changes in toenails and subsequently lost the nails. They grew back following cessation of hydroxyurea therapy. Another drug that has been used less frequently is busulphan, usually administered at a dosage of 0.1–0.2 mg/kg daily. In humans, busulphan therapy has been associated with the development of pulmonary fibrosis. This has not been described in dogs.

An important aspect of the therapy of chronic MPD is the monitoring of treatment. In treating polycythemia vera, therapy is aimed at reducing the red blood cell mass. It is most desirable to keep the PCV in the range of 50% to 60% during hydroxyurea administration. Periodically phlebotomy may be required to control the red cell mass. In treating CGL, hydroxyurea is initially administered over a 4- to 6-week period. A blood count should be monitored weekly, and treatment should be interrupted when the leukocyte count decreases to 10,000/µl. A safe approach to consider is to reduce the dosage by half when the leukocyte count is in the range of 10,000–12,000/µl or to alternate 7–10 days of therapy at the full dose with 7–10 days of no therapy. In most cases there is no urgent need to lower the blood counts, and this more gradual approach reduces the risk of severe myelosuppression. Once remission is achieved, monthly monitoring of the leukocyte count may be all that is necessary. Long-term complications of therapy are very rare.

In humans, blast crisis of CGL is considered a terminal event. This appears to be true for dogs as well. Effective therapy of blast crisis in the dog has not been achieved. If attempted, therapy is similar to the treatment of acute MPD (see below).

Treatment of acute myeloproliferative disorders with chemotherapy has been very discouraging. No dogs with acute MPD have been effectively placed in remission with current chemotherapeutic protocols. If therapy is to be attempted, it should begin as soon as possible owing to the rapidly progressive nature of these disorders. In Table 29-14 a protocol that could be attempted in dogs with acute MPD is presented.[42] The mainstay of treatment is provided by cytosine arabinoside, the thiopurines (6-thioguanine), and one of the anthracyclines (daunorubicin or doxorubicin). Significant bone marrow hypoplasia is required for normal bone marrow regeneration. For this reason, no matter what drugs are used initially, they must be administered intensively and for a time sufficient to induce clinically significant pancytopenia. Therefore, it is also necessary to support hemostasis and manage infection throughout the same period. Owing to the poor response, the major thrust of treatment at present is to provide palliative supportive therapy, including the treatment of anemia with blood transfusions and thrombocytopenia with transfusions of whole fresh blood or platelet-rich plasma. Neutropenia is common and renders animals extremely susceptible to infections; aggressive antibiotic therapy should be instituted immediately.

Treatment for myelodysplastic syndrome relies largely on the administration of blood components to combat cytopenias and antibiotics to counter infections. Both retinoic acid and cytosine arabinoside at low concentrations have been shown to induce differentiation of leukemia cells in tissue culture.[43,44] In humans with myelodysplastic syndromes, clinical trials using retinoic acid have shown some encouraging results.[45,46]

PROGNOSIS

The prognosis for polycythemia vera and chronic granulocytic leukemia is guarded, but significant remissions have been achieved with certain therapeutic regimes and careful monitoring. Animals commonly survive a year or more.[17,19] Development of blast crisis portends a grave prognosis. In general, the prognosis for animals with chronic MPD is better than for dogs with acute MPD, in which the prognosis is grave.

COMPARATIVE ASPECTS

The pathophysiology and therapy of nonlymphocytic leukemia in humans is being studied intensively. The myeloproliferative disorders have been demonstrated to be clonal with abnormalities evident in all hematopoietic cell

Table 29-14.   Protocol for the Treatment of Acute MPD[42]

DRUG	DOSAGE	ROUTE
REMISSION INDUCTION		
Cytosine arabinoside	100 mg/m²/day	IV for 3–4 days
6-Thioguanine	40 mg/m²	PO for 4 days
Doxorubicin	10–15 mg/m²	IV SID for 3 days
MAINTENANCE		
Cytosine arabinoside	100 mg/m²	SQ or IV once or twice weekly
6-Thioguanine	40 mg/m²	PO SID 2–4 days each week
Doxorubicin	30 mg/m²	IV every 3 weeks

lines. Cytogenetic abnormalities have been described in these disorders. Therapeutic modalities under investigation include combination chemotherapy, immunotherapy, and bone marrow transplantation. Still the prognosis is much poorer than for lymphocytic leukemias. The spontaneous canine diseases probably occur too infrequently to serve as useful models. MPD have been induced experimentally in the dog by irradiation and transplantation in an attempt to create models for study. Many similarities between human and canine MPD exist, and veterinary medicine may benefit from any therapeutic advances made in the human field.

REFERENCES

1. Nielsen SW: Myeloproliferative disorders in animals. In Clarke WJ, Howard EB, Hackett PL (eds): Myeloproliferative Disorders in Animals and Man, pp 297–313. Oak Ridge, TN, USAEC Division of Technical Information Extension, 1970
2. Anderson AC, Johnson RM: Erythroblastic malignancy in a beagle. J Am Vet Med Assoc 141:944–946, 1962
3. Seed TM, Tolle DV, Fritz TE, et al: Irradiation-induced erythroleukemia and myelogenous leukemia in the beagle dog: Hematology and ultrastructure. Blood 50:1061–1079, 1977
4. Tolle DV, Seed TM, Fritz TE, et al: Acute monocytic leukemia in an irradiated beagle. Vet Pathol 16:243–254, 1979
5. Metcalf D: The Hemopoietic Colony Stimulating Factors, pp 55–96. New York, Elsevier, 1984
6. Vadas MA, Nicola NA, Metcalf D: Activation of antibody-dependent cell-mediated cytotoxicity of human neutrophils and eosinophils by separate colony-stimulating factors. J Immunol 130:795–799, 1983
7. Lichtman MA: Classification of the hemopoietic stem cell disorders. In Williams WJ, Beutler

E, Erslev AJ, et al (eds): Hematology, ed 3, pp 144–150. New York, McGraw-Hill, 1983
8. Couto CG, Kallet AJ: Preleukemic syndrome in a dog. J Am Vet Med Assoc 184:1389–1392, 1984
9. Lichtman MA: Clinical manifestations of hemopoietic stem cell disorders. In Williams WJ, Beutler E, Erslev AJ, et al (eds): Hematology, ed 3, pp 54–58. New York, McGraw-Hill, 1983
10. Bush BM, Fankhauser R: Polycythaemia vera in a bitch. J Small Anim Pract 13:75–89, 1972
11. Carb AV: Polycythemia vera in a dog. J Am Vet Med Assoc 154:289–297, 1969
12. McGrath CJ: Polycythemia vera in dogs. J Am Vet Med Assoc 164:1117–1122, 1974
13. Miller RM: Polycythemia vera in a dog. Vet Med/Small Anim Clin 63:222–223, 1968
14. Peterson ME, Randolph JF: Diagnosis of canine primary polycythemia and management with hydroxyurea. J Am Vet Med Assoc 180:415–418, 1982
15. Jain NC: The leukemia complex. In Schalm's Veterinary Hematology, ed 4, pp 838–908. Philadelphia, Lea & Febiger, 1986
16. Rundles RW: Chronic myelogenous leukemia. In Williams WJ, Beutler E, Erslev AJ, et al (eds): Hematology, ed 3, pp 196–214. New York, McGraw-Hill, 1983
17. Leifer CE, Matus RE, Patnaik AK, et al: Chronic myelogenous leukemia in the dog. J Am Vet Med Assoc 183:686–689, 1983
18. Pollet L, Van Hove W, Matheeuws D: Blastic crisis in chronic myelogenous leukaemia in a dog. J Small Anim Pract 19:469–475, 1978
19. MacEwen EG, Drazner FH, McClelland AJ, et al: Treatment of basophilic leukemia in a dog. J Am Vet Med Assoc 166:376–380, 1975
20. Silverstein MN: Primary thrombocythemia. In Williams WJ, Beutler E, Erslev AJ, et al (eds): Hematology, ed 3, pp 218–221. New York, McGraw-Hill, 1983
21. Castro–Malaspina H: Pathogenesis of myelofibrosis: Role of ineffective megakaryopoiesis and megakaryocyte components. In Berk PD, Castro–Malaspina H, Wasserman LR (eds): Mye-

lofibrosis and the Biology of Connective Tissue, pp 427–454. New York, Alan R. Liss, 1984

22. Rudolph R, Huebner C: Megakaryozytenleukose beim hund. Kleintier-Praxis 17:9–13, 1972

23. Dungworth DL, Goldman M, Switzer JW, et al: Development of a myeloproliferative disorder in beagles continuously exposed to ^{90}Sr. Blood 34:610–632, 1969

24. Prasse KW, Crouser D, Beutler E, et al: Pyruvate kinase deficiency anemia with terminal myelofibrosis and osteosclerosis in a beagle. J Am Vet Med Assoc 166:1170–1175, 1975

25. Barthel CH: Acute myelomonocytic leukemia in a dog. Vet Pathol 11:79–86, 1974

26. Green RA, Barton CL: Acute myelomoncytic leukemia in a dog. J Am Anim Hosp Assoc 13:708–712, 1977

27. Jain NC, Madewell BR, Weller RE, et al: Clinical-pathological findings and cytochemical characterizations of myelomonocytic leukaemia in 5 dogs. J Comp Pathol 91:17–31, 1981

28. Linnabary RD, Holscher MA, Glick AD, et al: Acute myelomonocytic leukemia in a dog. J Am Anim Hosp Assoc 14:71–75, 1978

29. Moulton JE, Dungworth DL: Tumors of the lymphoid and hemopoietic tissues. In Moulton JE (ed): Tumors in Domestic Animals, ed 2, pp 150–204. Berkeley, University of California Press, 1978

30. Ragan HA, Hackett PL, Dagle GE: Acute myelomonocytic leukemia manifested as myelophthistic anemia in a dog. J Am Vet Med Assoc 169:421–425, 1976

31. Rohrig KE: Acute myelomonocytic leukemia in a dog. J Am Vet Med Assoc 182:137–141, 1983

32. Latimer KS, Dykstra MJ: Acute monocytic leukemia in a dog. J Am Vet Med Assoc 184:852–854, 1984

33. Mackey LJ, Jarrett WFH, Lauder IM: Monocytic leukaemia in the dog. Vet Rec 96:27–30, 1975

34. Holscher MA, Collins RD, Glick AD, et al: Megakaryocytic leukemia in a dog. Vet Pathol 15:562–565, 1978

35. Peterson ME, Zanjani ED: Inappropriate erythropoietin production from a renal carcinoma in a dog with polycythemia. J Am Vet Med Assoc 179:995–996, 1981

36. Scott RC, Patnaik AK: Renal carcinoma associated with secondary polycythemia in a dog. J Am Anim Hosp Assoc 8:275–283, 1972

37. Grindem CB, Stevens JB, Perman V: Cytochemical reactions in cells from leukemic dogs. Vet Pathol 23:103–109, 1986

38. Facklam NR, Kociba GJ: Cytochemical characterization of leukemic cells from 20 dogs. Vet Pathol 22:363–369, 1986

39. Jain NC: Cytochemistry of normal and leukemic leukocytes. In Schalm's Veterinary Hematology, ed 4, pp 909–939. Philadelphia, Lea & Febiger, 1986

40. Joshi BC, Jain NC: Experimental immunologic thrombocytopenia in dogs: A study of thrombocytopenia and megakaryocytopoiesis. Res Vet Sci 22:11–17, 1977

41. Grindem CB, Buoen LC: Cytogenetic analysis of leukaemic cells in the dog. A report of 10 cases and a review of the literature. J Comp Pathol 96:623–635, 1986

42. Theilen GH, Madewell BR, Gardner MB: Hematopoietic neoplasms, sarcomas and related conditions. In Theilen GH, Madewell BR (eds): Veterinary Cancer Medicine, ed 2, pp 392–407. Philadelphia, Lea & Febiger, 1987

43. Koeffler HP: Induction of differentiation of human acute myelogenous leukemia cells: Therapeutic implications. Blood 62:709–721, 1983

44. Kufe DW, Griffin JD, Spriggs DR: Cellular and clinical pharmacology of low-dose Ara-C. Semin Oncol 12:200–207, 1985

45. Clark RE, Lush CJ, Jacobs A, et al: Effect of 13-cis-retinoic acid on survival of patients with myelodysplastic syndrome. Lancet 1:763–765, 1987

46. Jacobs A: Treatment for the myelodysplastic syndromes. Hematologica 72:477–480, 1987

Plasma Cell Neoplasms

E. Gregory MacEwen

Plasma cell neoplasms arise when a cell of the B-lymphocyte lineage proliferates to form a large population of similar cells. This population is believed to be monoclonal—that is, derived from a single cell—because the cells produce homogeneous immunoglobulin. These malignant clonal expansions of B cells include multiple myeloma, primary (Waldenstrom's) macroglobulinemia, and lymphoma with monoclonal elaboration of IgG, IgA, and IgM immunoglobulin, and light-chain proteins.[1,2]

Monoclonal immunoglobulin (M component) spikes have also been reported to occur in association with certain non-neoplastic diseases and can include chronic infections and immune-mediated disorders. Monoclonal gammopathies have been associated with *Erhlichia canis* infection in the dog.[3] This section will deal with monoclonal immunoglobulin-producing tumors only.

INCIDENCE AND RISK FACTORS

Plasma cell tumors, including multiple myeloma and primary (Waldenstrom's) macroglobulinemia, in the dog have been reported infrequently. Their true incidence is unknown, but a rate of less than 1% of canine malignant tumors and approximately 8% of canine hematopoietic malignant tumors has been reported.[4] In the dog, plasma cell tumors account for 3.6% of all primary and secondary bone tumors diagnosed by biopsy.[5] Monoclonal immunoglobulin spikes are estimated to occur at a rate of 6 per 100 cases of lymphosarcoma and have been reported in several cases of chronic lymphocytic leukemia.[1,6,9] Macroglobulinemia without leukemia has been observed also.[2] Two cases of extramedullary plasmacytoma[7] and two cases of nonsecretory bone myeloma have also been described in the dog.[8] Cryoglobulinemia (monoclonal associated proteins that form preciptins at less than 37°C) has been found in association with both canine macroglobulinemia and multiple myeloma.[9,10,11] Light-chain disease (Bence Jones proteinuria) commonly occurs in association with multiple myeloma and rarely in macroglobulinemia and has been reported as a separate entity in only one dog.[12]

Plasma cell tumors are very rare in the cat and account for less than 1% of the hematopoietic tumors seen. Most affected cats are between the ages of 6 and 13 years. There appears to be a male to female ratio of one.[1,13]

The etiology of multiple myeloma is unknown. In humans multiple myeloma has been associated with chronic administration of antigens for desensitization of allergies.[14] In rodent models, chronic irritation and inflammation can be associated with monoclonal immunoglobulin spikes.[14]

PATHOLOGY AND NATURAL BEHAVIOR

Plasma cell tumors have a relatively uniform appearance on histologic sections and cytologic preparations. The plasma cell population often varies from small, mature cells, to larger cells with more cytoplasm, to more immature cells with a distinct nucleolus and multinucleated cells. In Wright-stained films, the plasma cell is round or oval with an eccentric nucleus composed of coarsely clumped chromatin, a densely basophilic cytoplasm, and a perinuclear clear zone containing the Golgi apparatus.

Plasma cells are produced mainly in hematopoietic bone marrow, lymph nodes, spleen, submucosa of the upper airway passages, and the gastrointestinal tract. Most plasma cell neoplasms form multiple tumors in bone and cause generalized increase in marrow plasma cells. These neoplasms rarely present as solid tumors in bone or in extramedullary sites. Extramedullary plasmacytomas have been reported in the gastrointestinal tract in two dogs,[7] and less commonly they have been seen in the spleen or lymph nodes and the skin.[7a] It is possible for them to occur in any site. Local amyloid deposits have been found in the biopsies of two dogs with extramedullary plasmacytomas.[7]

Solitary plasmacytomas of bone appear to be uncommon and may represent an early stage of multiple myeloma. With colleagues, I have recently published a report of two cases of solitary plasmacytoma that were nonsecretory (did not secrete immunoglobulin).[8]

Extramedullary plasmacytomas tend to stay localized to the regional area in which they are located, and they rarely metastasize to the bone.[2,7,7a] On the other hand, solitary bony plasma cell tumors tend to spread quite rapidly to other bones and become a more generalized disease seen in multiple myeloma.[2,8]

The disease manifestations of plasma cell neoplasms are exceedingly variable. These tumors can appear at almost any site, and the signs caused by the tumor must be added to those resulting from the myeloma protein produced by the neoplasm. Dogs may present with signs of bone pain or fracture when osteolytic lesions are present (Fig. 29-4).[1,15] Other classic features of this diseases include the hyperviscosity syndrome, hypercalcemia, and renal failure.[1,2,15]

Hypercalcemia is present at diagnosis in approximately 15% to 20% of animals presenting with plasma myeloma.[15] The serum calcium should be measured in any animal showing signs of polydipsia and polyuria. Hypercalcemia develops as a result of increased bone resorption stimulated by the release of an osteoclast-acti-

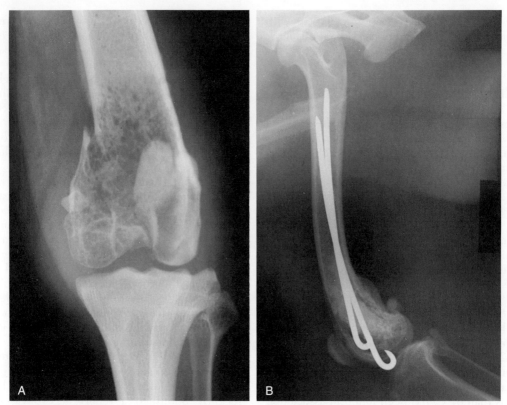

Fig 29-4. (*A*) Radiograph of a distal femur demonstrating severe osteolysis and a pathologic fracture. (*B*) Radiograph of the same pathologic fracture after surgical repair with Rush rods and bone cement. Local site was treated with adjuvant radiation. Dog was continued on chemotherapy for 2 more years and did well.[8]

vating factor (OFA) or other substances produced by the myeloma cells.[16]

Increased bone resorption leads to two major types of bony changes: generalized osteoporosis and more localized, purely osteolytic "punched-out lesions," with no evidence of osteoblastic bone repair at the margins.[1,2] Bone lesions are usually seen in about 50% of the dogs presenting for plasma cell myeloma.[15] The osteolytic lesions are more common than is diffuse osteoporosis. Most common sites are long bones, vertebral bodies, and pelvis.

Renal abnormalities will be seen in approximately one-third of patients with plasma cell myeloma.[15] Many factors contribute to the development of renal failure. In animals with hypercalcemia, excessive amounts of calcium may interfere with renal function. However, the important renal lesions specifically relate to plasma cell myeloma and myeloma cast forma-

tion and diffuse renal tissue precipitation of myeloma proteins.

Light chains are filtered and then reabsorbed and catabolized by renal tubular cells.[17] It is possible that renal tubular cells are injured during reabsorption and catabolism of light chains, either by the release of the lysosomal enzymes or by a direct nephrotoxic effect of the light chain. Renal tubular cell injury is manifest early by defects in the ability of the kidney to acidify and concentrate urine.[18] Cast formation appears to be an end stage of chronic progressive renal impairment. The glomerular filtration rate falls progressively if tumor growth continues unabated. The increased load of free light chains must be excreted by fewer nephrons, and an increased intratubular light-chain protein concentrations favors its precipitation and resultant cast formation. The distinctive dense casts are the hallmark of the "myeloma kidney."[19]

Dogs with myeloma who form tubular myeloma casts excrete many light chains in the urine, with albumin as a minor component. These light chains will not show up on routine urine dip stick examination. When the urine of these patients is concentrated and subjected to electrophoresis, a major protein spike resembling light chains is found in the beta and gamma region, usually along with a minor albumin component.

Although uncommon, amyloid may also be associated with renal dysfunction. Amyloid deposition is associated with specific light chains secreted by the myeloma cell. Amyloid in the kidney is usually deposited in the tubular basement membrane, the blood vessels, or the interstitium.

The hyperviscosity syndrome develops when the size, shape, and concentration of the serum myeloma protein causes a marked increase in serum viscosity.[1,2,14] Serum viscosity can be measured crudely by a simple laboratory procedure. Serum from the animal is drawn into a volumetric pipette (2 to 5 ml) and allowed to flow out of the pipette by gravity. The same procedure is done with an equal volume of water. If viscosity is normal the two values at room temperature will be similar, but in hyperviscosity syndrome severe enough to cause clinical signs the serum will take more than four times as long to flow from the pipette.[14a] The syndrome is seen most commonly in macroglobulinemia (IgM) and plasma myeloma due to IgA. The IgA may polymerize in the serum, thus producing a protein aggregate of very high molecular weight. IgG has also been shown to produce the hyperviscosity syndrome, although this is quite unusual.[20] The clinical features of the syndrome are essentially related to hypervolemia. The syndrome may manifest as either a bleeding diathesis, cerebral dysfunction, or congestive heart failure. Funduscopic abnormalities of characteristic retinal hemorrhage or detachment and venous dilation with sacculation and tortuosity are commonly apparent in the hyperviscosity syndrome. Blindness has also been reported associated with IgA myeloma.[20a] Approximately 20% of dogs with monoclonal gammopathies present with the hyperviscosity syndrome.[15]

In dogs with plasma cell myeloma, mild leukopenia and anemia are not uncommon findings and are due to bone marrow replacement. About 70% of affected dogs present with a nonregenerative anemia, and leukopenia has been seen in about 25%.[15] Severe thrombocytopenia is less common; it has been reported in about 16% of affected dogs.[15] Absolute thrombocytopenia is seen in about one-third of the dogs. Abnormal plasma cells circulating in the peripheral blood are quite uncommon; they are seen in about 10% of cases.[15]

Macroglobulinemia can be seen with lymphoplasmacytic neoplasms, and B-lymphocyte neoplasms such as chronic lymphocytic leukemia.[6,9] Animals with macroglobulinemia usually have hepatosplenomegaly and lymphadenopathy. It is extremely rare to see osteolytic bone lesions. Owing to the high molecular weight of IgM (900,000), it is more common to see the hyperviscosity syndrome. Cryoglobulinemia has also been reported in dogs with macroglobulinemia.[10,11]

Although rare, benign monoclonal gammapathies have been reported in the dog.[15a,15b] These are usually incidental findings on an electrophoresis and the bone marrow shows minimal plasma cell infiltration. These dogs are free of clinical signs associated with the monoclonal gammopathy. These dogs need to be followed for the development of signs, such as hyperviscosity syndrome, bone lesions, and bone marrow suppression.

HISTORY AND CLINICAL SIGNS

The clinical signs associated with plasma cell tumors can be attributed to organ infiltration by neoplastic cells or to their protein product (M component) or both. The most common clinical signs are bleeding diathesis, especially from the nasal cavity or mucous membranes, retinal hemorrhage, or dilated retinal vessels, and blindness. Severe dementia, depression, and rarely coma are seen. Congestive heart failure has been associated with the hyperviscosity syndrome.

Polydipsia and polyuria can be associated with hypercalcemia or renal dysfunction. Lameness and weakness can be seen with osteolytic or osteoporotic bone lesions. Other common signs seen in the dog are pale mucous membranes, fever, lethargy, and hepatosplenomegaly.

In the cat the most common clinical signs are anorexia, weight loss, listlessness, and fever. Polyuria and polydipsia may be present also.[13,21]

DIAGNOSIS AND STAGING

The diagnosis of a plasma cell neoplasm requires the demonstration of uncontrolled growth of a plasma cell clone. Evidence of uncontrolled growth is provided when plasma cells invade normal tissue and cause osteolytic bone lesions or plasmacytomas in extraskeletal sites. A progressive increase in the amount of serum myeloma protein or light-chain proteinuria provides additional evidence of uncontrolled growth. The criteria for diagnosis are as follows:

1. *Plasma cell myeloma.* The classical diagnostic triad for plasma cell myeloma is the association of bone marrow plasmacytosis, osteolytic bone lesions, and a serum or urine myeloma protein. In the absence of osteolytic lesions, the diagnosis is also established if marrow plasmacytosis is associated with a progressive increase in the M component as seen on repeated serum electrophoresis. For the diagnosis of plasma cell myeloma, plasma cells in excess of 20% (of 1,000 cells counted) or sheetlike growth of plasma cells in the marrow in addition to a monoclonal spike is necessary.

2. *Solitary osseous plasmacytoma.* A diagnosis of solitary osseous plasmacytoma is suspected when a solitary lytic lesion is discovered on a skeletal survey radiograph. The diagnosis is confirmed by a biopsy showing that the lytic lesion is composed of plasma cells. There may or may not be a monoclonal spike in the serum or light chains in the urine. A bone marrow aspiration from a radiographically normal site may or may not reveal an increased number of plasma cells.

3. *Extramedullary plasmacytoma.* Extramedullary plasmacytomas appear in the dog most commonly in the gastrointestinal tract and skin. Biopsy shows the tumors to be composed of plasma cells. Skeletal radiographs are usually normal, and marrow aspirations usually contain a normal number of plasma cells. The few cases that have been reported in the dog have been associated with very mild increases in the M component in the serum.[7,7a]

Specifically, each dog or cat suspected of having a plasma cell neoplasm should undergo the following evaluation:

1. Serum and urine electrophoresis to demonstrate a monoclonal immunoglobulin (in the serum) or light chains (in the urine)
2. A radiographic skeletal survey to demonstrate evidence of osteoporosis or osteolysis
3. Bone marrow aspirations to evaluate for an increase in number or clustering of plasma cells

A staging system for canine plasma cell myeloma[15] (see Table 29-15) has been adopted from the human staging system and to date has not been extensively studied to determine its full usefulness in the dog.

In addition, the clinical evaluation of an animal with suspected plasma cell tumor should also include a CBC, platelet count, urinalysis, and chemistry profile. Particular attention should be paid to renal function and calcium levels. Approximately one-third of affected dogs present with azotemia, and 15% to 20% present with hypercalcemia.[15] Additional tests that may be necessary include a coagulogram (aPTT, PTT, platelet count), particularly if the hyperviscosity syndrome is suspected. In dogs IgG and IgA tend to be equally represented as the class of immunoglobulin secreted.[15] In cats all myelomas reported have secreted IgG, except one that secreted IgA.[13]

It is relatively easy to differentiate the B-lymphocyte neoplasms associated with an IgM protein because affected animals have other features diagnostic of chronic lymphocytic leukemia or diffuse lymphocyte lymphomas (see section on Canine Lymphoma and Lymphoid Leukemias, this chapter).

TREATMENT

Animals with plasma cell tumors should be considered immunologic cripples. The mecha-

Table 29-15. Clinical Stages of Canine Multiple Myeloma

STAGE I—LOW TUMOR CELL MASS
PCV > 37%
Serum calcium < 11.5 mg/dl
No bony lesions
Total Immunoglobulin < 3 g/dl
STAGE II—INTERMEDIATE TUMOR CELL MASS
Fits neither Stage I nor Stage III values
STAGE III—HIGH TUMOR CELL MASS
PCV < 25%
Serum calcium > 11.5 mg/dl
Extensive bony lesions
Total immunoglobulin > 5 g/dl

nisms responsible for the failure of the primary immune response are complex and probably multifactorial. Defective neutrophil function may make patients with plasma cell neoplasms more susceptible to infections. Neutropenia is another inherent problem with myeloma patients. Human beings with myeloma have circulating suppressor factors thought to be suppressor macrophages, which have been shown to suppress lymphocyte function.[22] The infections seen in myeloma-infected animals are associated with bone marrow suppression and with immunosuppressive factors associated with the disease itself.[23] An important aspect in the treatment of myeloma is prompt and urgent investigation and treatment of any febrile episode. Appropriate bacterial cultures should be taken and their drug sensitivity determined, and serious infections should be treated with antibiotic therapy.

Renal function needs to be closely monitored and treated vigorously if abnormalities occur. Medical management should include establishment of hydration and renal perfusion with maintenance of adequate glomerular filtration. This may necessitate intravenous fluid support during initial treatment and during any hospitalization for infection or other illness. Owners should be instructed to make sure that animals have plenty of water at all times. If there is any evidence of illness or if the dog becomes anorexic or decreases its water intake, the dog's kidney function should be immediately evaluated.[1,2]

Another major concern that can require immediate treatment is hypercalcemia, which is not uncommon in canine multiple myeloma.[1,2,15] Calcium should be adjusted for the often decreased albumin concentration. The treatment of hypercalcemia should include the use of sodium chloride hydration in combination with furosemide, which causes a calcium diuresis. Prednisone therapy is indicated as an aid to decrease intestinal absorption of calcium and inhibits osteoclast activation. Other methods used to lower calcium can be diphosphanate therapy, although the results and benefits are not firmly established. In extreme cases, where the calcium cannot be lowered by conventional means, mithramycin therapy ($25\mu g/kg$ IV) can be used to lower serum calcium.[23a] In addition, chemotherapy should be initiated to control tumor cell progression.

Bony lysis and generalized osteoporosis may predispose an animal to a pathologic fracture.[1,2,8]

Attempts to repair pathologic fractures have been done in a limited number of cases, and have sometimes been quite successful clinically.[8] Repair generally requires usage of plates or rods supplemental with bone cement. If a pathologic fracture occurs around the vertebral bodies, localized radiation can be used. If severe paresis or paralysis due to spinal cord compression occurs, surgical decompression in addition to radiation therapy has been reported to be effective. Extreme caution should be used with surgical decompression because of the susceptibility of these patients to infection and a bleeding diathesis due to the monoclonal spike.[1,2] Whenever possible it is most desirable to treat bony lesions with either localized radiation therapy or combination chemotherapy.

Fortunately most animals do not require emergency intervention to treat the hyperviscosity syndrome. In some select cases, either because of severe neurologic impairment or hemorrhagic diathesis, plasmapheresis may be required to lower the serum viscosity.[24] However, the initiation of chemotherapy usually improves the viscosity in a matter of a few weeks.

The most effective way to manage plasma cell tumors is with chemotherapy.[1,2,15] Successful chemotherapy relieves bone pain, reduces myeloma cell mass, initiates skeletal healing, and lowers the level of serum immunoglobulin. It has also been shown to improve and lengthen survival time.[15] However, there is no evidence that neoplastic plasma cells can be completely eliminated by the chemotherapy currently available. Thus, the treatment of plasma cell neoplasms is largely palliative, being directed at controlling the disease during the chronic phase and preventing death from complications such as infections, hypercalcemia, hyperviscosity, renal failure, and so forth.

The agents that have received the most attention in treating multiple myeloma are the alkylating agents, which can be used in both dogs and cats.[1,2] The two alkylating agents that have been used to treat myeloma are melphalan and cyclophosphamide.[1,2,15] The addition of prednisone to alkylating agents increases their effectiveness. Although no optimal dosage schedule has been devised, melphalan has been used extensively in the dog at a dosage of 0.1 mg/kg of body weight, per os, SID for 10 days, then 0.05 mg/kg per os SID continuously. Cyclophosphamide can be used both as an intravenous bolus at 200–300 mg/m² IV once weekly, or given at a low dosage per os at 50 mg/m² per day for 4 days per week. Prednisone is usually administered at a dosage of 0.5 mg/kg SID per os for 10 days, then 0.5 mg/kg on alternate days for 60 days, then stopped. One side-effect of melphalan is bone marrow suppression, particularly platelet suppression. If this occurs, cyclophosphamide should be substituted for melphalan. Cyclophosphamide is less toxic to thrombopoiesis, and thrombocytopenic patients are usually able to tolerate it better than other alkylating agents.

Another combination therapy approach that has been used in the dog is cyclophosphamide, vincristine, melphalan, and prednisone.[8] This protocol is considered more aggressive, but it is tolerated quite well by most dogs. The dose of cyclophosphamide is 200 mg/m² q 14 days IV. Vincristine is given at 0.7 mg/m² q 14 days IV. Melphalan is given at 0.10 mg/kg SID per os × 10 days, then reduced to 0.05 mg/kg SID per os. Prednisone is given at 0.5 mg/kg SID per os. Chlorambucil is another alkylating agent that has been quite successful in treating macroglobulinemia.[1,6,10] The dosage is 0.2 mg/kg SID per os daily. Chlorambucil is a very safe alkylating agent that causes almost no clinical signs of toxicity at that dosage.

Animals with lymphoma and an associated monoclonal spike should be treated with a standard lymphoma protocol (see Canine Lymphoma and Lymphoid Leukemias).

PROGNOSIS

In a recent study of 37 dogs treated with melphalan, with or without cyclophosphamide and prednisone, the median survival time was 540 days (Fig. 29-5).[15] The median survival time of 12 dogs treated with prednisone alone was 220 days. In this study a complete response was noted in 43% (16 of 37 dogs) and a partial response in 48% (18 of 37 dogs). Only 8% (3 dogs) failed to respond to therapy. The clinical stage of disease did not seem to be a prognostic factor. Hypercalcemia, light chains of myeloma protein in the urine, and extensive bony lesions have been associated with poor prognosis (Fig. 29-6).[15] Sex, the type of monoclonal Ig class, serum viscosity, and presence of azotemia did not correlate significantly with prognosis, although a trend toward increased survival time was apparent in the nonazotemic group.

Although chemotherapy does not cure this disease, it significantly prolongs survival time. The vast majority of dogs tolerate the therapy very well with minimal side-effects. Treated dogs tend to improve clinically and to experience a good quality survival. If alkylating agents (at the standard dosage) and prednisone fail to control the disease, then attempt to induce

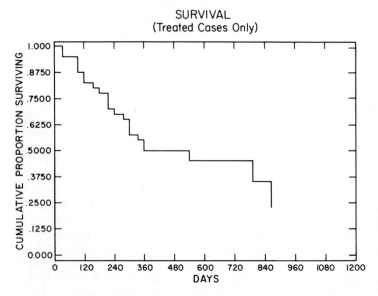

SURVIVAL
(Treated Cases Only)

Fig 29-5. Survival curve of 37 dogs with multiple myeloma treated with chemotherapy. The median survival time is 540 days. (Reprinted with permission from Matus RE, Leifer CE, MacEwen EG et al: Prognostic factors for multiple myeloma in the dog. J Am Vet Med Assoc 188:1288–1292, 1986)

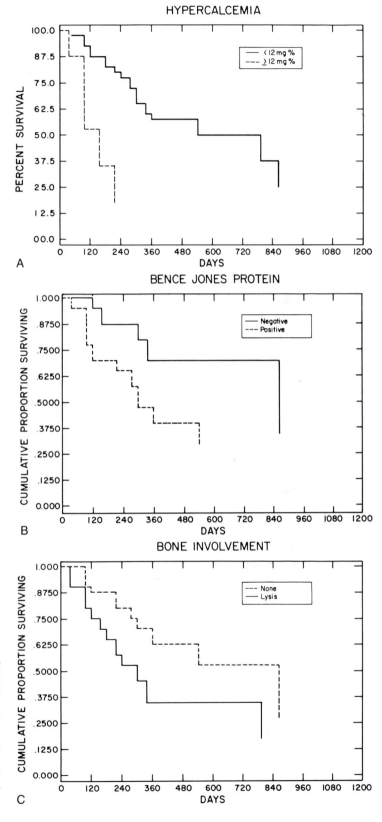

Fig 29-6. (A,B,C) Survival curves of 37 dogs with multiple myeloma treated with chemotherapy. The curves reveal that hypercalcemia, Bence Jones protein, and bony lysis are all associated with a poor prognosis ($p < 0.05$). (Reprinted with permission from Matus RE, Leifer CE, MacEwen EG et al: Prognostic factors for multiple myeloma in the dog. J Am Vet Med Assoc 188:1288–1292, 1986)

remission with vincristine (0.07 mg/m² IV weekly) and high dosages of cyclophosphamide (300 mg/m²). Doxorubicin can also be tried at 30 mg/m² IV every three weeks.

The response to therapy needs to be evaluated in terms of specific laboratory changes and radiographic findings. Monoclonal spikes usually decreases to less than 50% of the initial value within 8–12 weeks.[1,2] As therapy progresses, the immunoglobulin spike eventually disappears.

Although our experience with treating macroglobulinemia is not as large, the prognosis should be as good as that for animals with multiple myeloma.

COMPARATIVE FEATURES

In humans, plasma cell tumors occur slightly more frequently in males than in females. The incidence is about 30 per 100,000 persons over the age of 25 years.[25]

Most plasma cell neoplasms form multiple tumors in bone and cause a generalized increase in marrow plasma cells. The disorder rarely presents as a solitary tumor in bone or extramedullary sites. Plasma cell tumors originating in extramedullary sites usually develop in the upper airway passages. Less commonly they present in the spleen or lymph nodes, the skin, and the gastrointestinal tract.[14]

The treatment of multiple myeloma is very similar to the treatment used in the dog. In humans undergoing melphalan therapy alone the response varies from 25% to 40%, and the median survival time has been reported to be from 18 to 30 months.[26,27] With the addition of prednisone the response rate tends to go from 30% to 56%, and the median survival time to range from 19 to 39 months.[28,29]

Recently the effectiveness of many drug combinations has been tested in the treatment of plasma cell myeloma, but none is clearly more effective than melphalan and prednisone. Combinations of alkylating agents have been shown to induce higher percentages of response in high-risk human patients and may be associated with prolonged survival in patients with high tumor cell burden. The studies thus far have indicated that the response rate varies from 33% to 74%, and the median survival time seems to be between 30 and 40 months.[28,30,31] Combina-

tions of agents have usually included vincristine, melphalan, cyclophosphamide, doxorubicin, BCNU, prednisone.

In human patients undergoing therapy for multiple myeloma approximately 70% die from progressive disease. About 5% develop acute leukemia.[27] It has not been possible to determine whether treatment with leukemogenic agents (irradiation and alkylating agents) increases the risk of developing acute leukemia or whether the leukemia is due to an inherent defect in the stem cell which was associated with the original myeloma. Approximately 20% of patients die from causes not associated with multiple myeloma.[27] The two major causes of death for patients with multiple myeloma are renal failure and sepsis.[14]

REFERENCES

1. MacEwen EG, Hurvitz AI: Diagnosis and management of monoclonal gammopathies. Vet Clin North Am 7:119–131, 1977
2. Matus RE, Leifer CE: Immunoglobulin producing tumors. Vet Clin North Am 15:741–753, 1985
3. Breitschwerdt EB, Woody BJ, Zerbe CA, et al: Monoclonal gammopathy associated with naturally occurring canine ehrlichiosis. J Vet Int Med 1:2–9, 1987
4. Priester WA: The occurrence of tumors in domestic animals. NCI Monogr 54:36, 1980
5. Lui SK, Dorfman HD, Hurvitz AI, et al: Primary and secondary bone tumors in the dog. J Small Anim Pract 18:313–326, 1977
6. MacEwen EG, Hurvitz AI, Hayes AA: Hyperviscosity syndrome associated with lymphocytic leukemia in three dogs. J Am Vet Med Assoc 170:1309–1312, 1977
7. MacEwen EG, Patnaik AK, Johnson GF, et al: Extramedullary plasmacytoma of the gastrointestinal tract in two dogs. J Am Vet Med Assoc 184:1396–1398, 1984
7a. Lucke VM: Primary cutaneous plasmacytomas in the dog and cat. J Small An Pract 28:49–55, 1987
8. MacEwen EG, Patnaik AK, Hurvitz AI, et al: Non-secretory multiple myeloma in two dogs. J Am Vet Med Assoc 184:1283–1286, 1984
9. Braund KG, Everett RM, Albert RN, et al: Neurologic manifestations of monoclonal IgM gammopathy associated with lymphocytic leukemia in a dog. J Am Vet Med Assoc 172:1407–1410, 1978

10. Hurvitz AI, MacEwen EG, Middaugh CR, et al: Monoclonal cryoglobulinemia with macroglobulinemia in a dog. J Am Vet Med Assoc 170:511–513, 1977

11. Braund KG, Everett RM, Bartels JE, et al: Neurologic manisfestations of IgM multiple myeloma associated with cryoglobulinemia in a dog. J Am Vet Med Assoc 174:1321–1325, 1979

12. Hurvitz AI, Kehoe JM, Capra JD, et al: Bence-Jones proteinemia and proteinuria in the dog. J Am Vet Med Assoc 159:1112–1116, 1971

13. Drazner FH: Multiple myeloma in the cat. Comp Cont Educ 4:206–216, 1982

14. Bergsagel DE, Rider WD: Plasma cell neoplasms. In DeVita JR, Hellman S, Rosenberg SA (ed): Cancer: Principles and Practice of Oncology, ed 2, pp 1753–1795. Philadelphia, J.B. Lippincott, 1985

14a. Cotter SM: Clinical management of lymphoproliferative, myeloproliferative, and plasma cell neoplasia. In Gorman NT (ed): Oncology, vol 6, pp 169–194. London, Churchill Livingstone, 1986

15. Matus RE, Leifer CE, MacEwen EG, et al: Prognostic factors for multiple myeloma in the dog. J Am Vet Med Assoc 188:1288–1292, 1986

15a. Dewhirst MW, Stamp GI, Hurvitz AI: Ideopathic monoclonal IgA gammapathy in a dog. J Am Vet Med Assoc 170:1313–1316, 1977

15b. Hoenig M, O'Brien JA: A benign hypergammaglobulinemia mimicking plasma cell myeloma. J Am Anim Hosp Assoc 24:688–690, 1988

16. Mundy GR, Raisz LG, Cooper RA, et al: Evidence for the secretion of an osteoclast stimulating factor in myeloma. N Engl J Med 291(2):1041–1046, 1974

17. Solomon A, Waldmann TA, Fahey JL, et al: Metabolism of Bence-Jones proteins. J Clin Invest 43:103–117, 1964

18. DeFronzo RA, Kooke CR, Wright JR, et al: Renal function in patients with multiple myeloma. Medicine 57:151–166, 1978

19. Hill GS, Morel–Maroger L, Mery JP, et al: Renal lesions in multiple myeloma: Their relationship to associated protein abnormalities. Am J Kidney Dis 11:423–438, 1983

20. Thrall MA: Lymphoproliferative disorders. Vet Clin North Am (Small Anim Pract) 11:321–347, 1981

20a. Kirschner SE, Niyo Y, Hill BL, et al: Blindness in a dog with IgA-forming myeloma. J Am Vet Med Assoc 193:349–350, 1988

21. Carpenter JL, Andrews LK, Holzworth J: Tumors and tumor-like lesions. In Holzworth J (ed): Diseases of the Cat, pp 442–444. Philadelphia, W.B. Saunders, 1987

22. Krakauer RS, Strober W, Waldmann TA: Hypogammaglobulinemia in experimental myeloma: The role of suppressor factors from mononuclear phagocytes. J Immunol 118:1385–1390, 1970

23. Jacobson DR, Zolla–Pazner S: Immunosuppression and infection of multiple myeloma. Semin Oncol 13:282–290, 1986

23a. MacEwen EG, Siegel SD: Hypercalcemia: A paraneoplastic disease. In MacEwen EG (ed): Clinical Veterinary Oncology. Vet Clin of NA 7:187–194, 1977

24. Matus RE, Leifer CE, Gordon BR, et al: Plasma plasmapheresis and chemotherapy of hyperviscosity syndrome associated with monoclonal gammopathy in the dog. J Am Vet Med Assoc 183:215–218, 1983

25. Axelsson U, Bachman R, Hallen J: Frequency of pathological proteins (M-component) in 6995 sera from adult population: Acta Med Scand 179:235–247, 1966

26. Alexanian R, Bonnet J, Gehan E, et al: Combination chemotherapy for multiple myeloma. Cancer 30:382–389, 1972

27. Ahre A, Bjorkholm M, Mellstedt H, et al: Intermittent high-dose melphalan/prednisone versus continuous low-dose melphalan treatment in multiple myeloma. Eur J Cancer Clin Oncol 19:499–506, 1983

28. Abramson N, Lurie P, Mietlowski WL, et al: Phase III study of intermittent carmustine (BCNU) cyclophosphamide and prednisone versus intermittent melphalan and prednisone in myeloma. Cancer Treat Rep 66:1273–1277, 1982

29. Pavlovsky S, Saslavsky J, Tesamos PM, et al: A randomized trial of two vs five drug combination for untreated multiple myeloma. J Clin Oncol 2:832–836, 1984

30. Bergsagel DE, Bailey AJ, Laugley GR, et al: The chemotherapy of plasma-cell myeloma and the incidence of acute leukemia. N Engl J Med 301:743–748, 1979

31. Salmon SE, Haut A, Bonnet JD, et al: Alternating combination chemotherapy and levamisole improves survival in multiple myeloma. J Clin Oncol 1:453–461, 1983

30

MISCELLANEOUS TUMORS

Hemangiosarcoma

E. Gregory MacEwen

INCIDENCE AND RISK FACTORS

Hemangiosarcoma, also known as malignant hemangioendothelioma or angiosarcoma, is a malignant vascular neoplasm of endothelial origin. It occurs more frequently in the dog than any other species.[1,2] Hemangiosarcoma has been seen in 0.3% to 2% of recorded canine necropsies and represents about 5% of all nonskin primary malignant neoplasms in the dog.[3,4] Hemangiosarcomas are much less common in the cat. They have been reported to occur in 18 of 3145 cats examined at autopsy in one study.[5] In five combined surveys of cats, 20 of 1006 tumors were hemangiosarcomas.[6] The actual incidence in the cat varies from 0.1% to 1.5% of all nonhematopoietic neoplasms.

Dogs with hemangiosarcoma are usually older; the mean age varies between 8 and 10 years, although there are reports of dogs 1 year old or younger developing hemangiosarcoma.[4,7] In cats a mean age of 10 years has been reported.[5] Hemangiosarcoma can occur in any breed of dog or cat. In dogs the majority of reports find the German shepherd most commonly affected.[1,8] Other breeds reported are the boxer, Great Dane, English setter, golden retriever and pointers. Most reports do not cite a sex predisposition, but several indicate a higher incidence in males, as much as 3 times that in females.[4,8,9] In cats, males and females tend to be equally represented. Most hemangiosarcomas have been reported in the domestic short-haired cat. Although the etiology is unknown, reports in humans have been related to thorium dioxide, exposure to arsenicals, or exposure to vinyl chloride.[10,11] Local irradiation is also reported to be a contributory factor.[12] Methylnitrosamine is a carcinogen formed in fish meal and has been shown to cause hemangiosarcoma in mink.[4]

PATHOLOGY AND NATURAL BEHAVIOR

In the dog the site of primary involvement is usually the spleen, although the tumor has been reported in many locations. Other sites include the liver, heart, lungs, kidneys, skin, oral cavity, muscle, bone, and peritoneum. In the cat approximately 50% of hemangiosarcomas occur either in the liver, spleen, or mesentery; other sites reported are the subcutis, thoracic cavity, and nasal cavity.[6]

Hemangiosarcomas may be single or multiple in any organ. In an animal with multiple tumors, it may be difficult to determine which is the primary tumor site. The tumors are variable in size, pale gray to dark red, nodular, and soft. They may contain areas of hemorrhage and necrosis. They are poorly circumscribed, non-encapsulated, and often adhered to adjacent organs. Rupture and hemorrhage are frequently seen. On cut section the tumors may appear solid, or they may have irregular spaces formed by fragile trabeculae. The spaces may contain free or clotted blood or pink fluid that oozes from the cut surface. There are usually pale gray fibrous strands or foci and yellow to pink friable areas of necrosis. A large mass may vary greatly with regard to hemorrhage and neoplastic tissue, and multiple tissue samples may be required to establish a diagnosis.

Hemangiosarcomas tend to metastasize rapidly, and they may have widespread metastases. They tend to metastasize predominantly through the hematogenous routes, and the most frequently reported sites are liver and lungs. Other sites reported have been the kidney, muscle, peritoneum, omentum, lymph nodes, mesentery, adrenal glands, and diaphragm. In untreated cases death is usually due to metastases or rupture of the primary tumor.

Hemangiosarcoma in cats also tends to have a very high metastatic potential. In one recent report of 12 cats with hemangiosarcoma of the subcutis, all of them had recurrence or death due to disease within 1 month to 1 year after surgical removal.[6] In the cat visceral hemangiosarcomas are aggressive and metastasize readily. The liver appears to be the most common primary site followed by the omentum, diaphragm, pancreas, and lung. However, in cats, hemangiosarcomas of the liver may be less aggressive than those arising elsewhere in the

viscera. As opposed to the dog, hemangiosarcoma of the heart is very rare in the cat.

Overall, it can be stated that hemangiosarcomas are extremely malignant tumors, often multiple in number, that metastasize early in a wide distribution.

HISTORY AND CLINICAL SIGNS

The clinical signs vary depending upon the location and size of the primary tumor. The most dramatic presentation is sudden death from rupture of a tumor focus or acute blood loss. Clinical signs most commonly reported are weakness, distention of the abdomen, increased pulse and respiration, pale mucous membranes, and weight loss. The history may also reveal intermittent episodes of weakness or collapse, often with spontaneous recovery in 12–24 hours. Usually these incidents are associated with hemorrhage into a body cavity and subsequent blood resorption. Eventually, this trend becomes fatal; the majority of naturally occurring deaths in hemangiosarcoma are associated with hemorrhage from tumor rupture.

Other presenting signs can be related again to the specific organ of involvement and may include syncope, ataxia, or cardiac arrhythmias. Pericardial effusion or cardiac tamponade associated with right atrial hemangiosarcoma is also a common sequela in the dog.[13,14] Muffled heart sounds are detected with cardiac tamponade and the development of acute right heart failure.[15] The skin form most often presents as discrete subcutaneous masses, usually not ulcerative. Bone and muscle forms can be presented with localized swelling, lameness, and pain. Metastasis to the brain or vertebrae with spinal involvement can cause seizures, dementia, paresis, and other CNS signs.

In the cat signs of hemangiosarcoma depend on the location and extent of the primary and metastatic tumors. Cats with visceral tumors usually have a history of lethargy, anorexia, vomiting, dyspnea, or a distended abdomen. On physical examination, pallor, pleural or peritoneal fluid, and a palpable abdominal mass are often found. Bleeding, which is common because vascular channels in the tumor are friable, may be intermittent, causing episodic weakness, or acute, causing sudden collapse, sometimes in an apparently healthy cat. Most cats with visceral hemangiosarcoma are anemic. The anemia may be mild or severe, and it may have more than one cause.

In both dogs and cats recurrent hemorrhage may cause a regenerative anemia (normocytic, normochromic) characterized by polychromasia, anisocytosis, reticulocytosis, and nucleated red cells in the peripheral blood. Fragmentation of red cells, which occurs in humans and dogs with hemangiosarcoma, has not been documented in the cat.[16] Four causes have been proposed for this fragmentation seen in the dog[16]:

1. Local mechanical trauma to red cells traversing irregular vascular spaces of the tumor
2. Formation of spherocytes and destruction of older red blood cells with lower ATP when blood flow is sluggish and oxygen tension is low
3. Increased fragility of red blood cells made hypochromatic by blood loss and lower iron content
4. Altered cholesterol phospholipid ratios in red cells membranes due to altered hepatic lipoprotein metabolism, possibly accounting for acanthocytosis and fragmentation in dogs with hepatic hemangiosarcoma.

In dogs, anemia is the most common encountered hematologic abnormality.[2,4,8,17] In addition a neutrophilic leukocytosis may frequently be seen.

DIAGNOSTIC TECHNIQUES AND WORK-UP

The diagnosis of hemangiosarcoma in the dog and the cat is usually based on clinical history, physical examination, hematologic testing, radiographic findings, ultrasonic findings,[17a] and paracentesis, when indicated. Hemangiosarcoma effusions are serosanguinous (or frank blood if ruptured) and usually do not clot. Tumor cells are only rarely seen in these effusions. The ultimate diagnosis is based on histopathologic evaluation.

It is important to keep in mind that all canine splenic masses are not hemangiosarcomas. The majority of splenic masses will be hemangiosarcoma but other neoplasms to consider are lymphosarcoma and leiomyosarcoma. Benign conditions can include hematomas, hemangioma and splenic cysts. In a series of 100 dogs who underwent splenectomy for a splenic mass the following results were obtained: 1 benign neoplasia, 59 primary neoplasia, 6 metastatic neoplasia, and 34 non-neoplastic disease. Hemangiosarcoma (43 cases) was the most common splenic disease. Dogs with anemia or splenic rupture had a significantly greater chance of having splenic neoplasia.[17b]

The diagnosis of hemangiosarcoma is most reliably made by biopsy or removal of the primary or metastatic tumor. Cats with hemangiosarcoma often have pleural or peritoneal effusions. The fluid may be clear, milky, or bloody. In most cases it is blood tinged. Fusiform neoplastic cells are only rarely detected in cytologic examinations of fluids in both the dog and the cat.

In evaluating an animal with suspected hemangiosarcoma, particular attention should be directed toward evaluating for metastatic disease because the incidence of metastasis is extremely high (70% to 80%). All animals with suspected hemangiosarcoma should have radiographic evaluation of both the thoracic and abdominal cavity. Hematologic evaluation is important as discussed above. Echocardiography can be used to image cardiac masses, including hemangiosarcoma.[13,13a]

Radiographs of hemangiosarcoma of the bone show a typical primary bone neoplasm with a tendency to be more lytic than productive (Fig. 30-1).[18]

Another feature noted in dogs with hemangiosarcoma is the presence of nucleated red blood cells in the peripheral blood. This has been seen in about 25% of reported hemangiosarcoma cases, and the mean count is about 20 nucleated RBC/100 WBC. Table 30-1 demonstrates the typical hematologic findings in dogs with hemangiosarcoma. The physiological causes for nucleated RBC's in the peripheral blood may include bone marrow infiltration by malignant cells, extramedullary hematopoiesis, impairment of splenic function by tumor, and hypoxemia. Disseminated intravascular coagulation (DIC) can develop in dogs with hemangiosarcoma also. DIC is characterized by decreased platelets, increased prothrombin time, and decreased fibrinogen.

THERAPY

Surgery remains the treatment of choice for all dogs and cats with hemangiosarcoma. The sur-

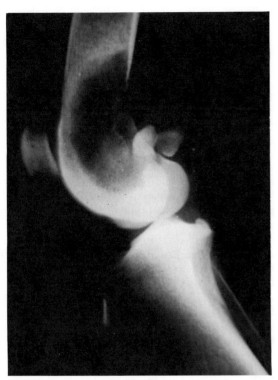

Figure 30-1. A primary hemangiosarcoma of the distal femur in a dog. Note the prominent lysis and minimal osteoblastic reaction.

gery should be as radical as possible, removing all affected tissue. In the case of hemangiosarcoma of the spleen, a complete splenectomy is necessary.[8] In dogs with hemangiosarcoma of the heart, particularly the right atrium, exploratory thoracotomy is indicated, not only as a diagnostic procedure, but as a treatment for the tumor.[14,19] Pericardiectomy alone for the relief of clinical signs due to cardiac tamponade is considered a palliative treatment for dogs with inoperable cardiac hemangiosarcoma. Perioperative ventricular and supraventricular arrhythmias are a common feature in dogs with primary cardiac hemangiosarcoma. Treatment of ventricular premature contractions and ventricular tachycardia may require the use of such agents as lidocaine and procainamide. Paroxysmal atrial tachycardia is seen less frequently and may require treatment with digoxin and propranolol hydrochloride.[14] It is essential that dogs with pericardial effusion be monitored electrocardiographically prior to, and following, pericardiocentesis.

In animals with primary bone hemangiosarcoma, a complete limb amputation is required.

Owing to the metastatic nature of this particular type of tumor and the overall poor prognosis, even with radical surgery, other forms of therapy need to be considered. Combination chemotherapy may offer the best chance of controlling this disease. Combination chemotherapy using cyclophosphamide, doxorubicin, and vincristine[13a,20] has shown potential in preliminary studies in the dog. Other combinations such as vincristine, cyclophosphamide, and methotrexate have also yielded minimal improvement in overall survival time.[8,17]

Table 30-1. Hematologic Abnormalities in Dogs with Hemangiosarcoma[17]

HEMATOLOGIC ABNORMALITIES	NORMAL VALUE	DOGS WITH HSA AT VARIABLE LOCATIONS (TOTAL: 98 DOGS)		DOGS WITH SPLENIC HSA (TOTAL: 60 DOGS)	
		Number of Dogs	Percent	Number of Dogs	PERCENT
Anemia	Hematocrit, 37–52% Hemoglobin, 12–18 g/dl Red blood cells, 5–8 × 10⁶	49	50	41	69
Neutrophilic leukocytosis	56–78% (3–10 × 10³)	49	50	40	67
Increase in band neutrophils	0–2%	55	56	42	70
Increased reticulocyte count	0–1% (<800 × 10³)	15	16	13	22
Thrombocytopenia	200–500 × 10³	35	36	31	51
Nucleated red blood cells	None seen	13	13	10	17

(Data from The Animal Medical Center, New York, July 1, 1980, to January 1, 1983 Brown NO: Vet Clin North Am 15:569–575, 1985)

Very few studies of biologic therapy have been done. One study using a mixed bacterial vaccine showed slight improvement in survival for dogs with splenic hemangiosarcoma.[8]

The same recommendations hold for cats with hemangiosarcoma. Chemotherapy protocols, in addition to surgery, should be considered. At this time the only potentially beneficial combination would be cyclophosphamide and doxorubicin.

Results of radiation therapy on hemangiosarcomas have not been published.

PROGNOSIS

Overall dogs and cats with hemangiosarcomas have a very poor prognosis regardless of the location of the primary tumor. In one small series of 7 dogs, the mean survival time was 3 months;[21] only 7 of 26 dogs in another series lived more than 1 year.[22] In a series of 19 dogs undergoing splenectomy for hemangiosarcoma the median survival was 8 weeks.[17b] In another study of 47 dogs treated by splenectomy, there was no difference in survival time according to stage of disease or therapy used.[8] Dogs were staged as outlined in Table 30-2. The results of treatment based on clinical stage are presented in Table 30-3. Eight dogs had Stage I disease (primary only), 15 had Stage II disease (rupture), and 24 dogs had Stage III disease (metastasis). Dogs were treated with surgery alone (21 dogs), surgery and immunotherapy (10 dogs), or surgery, immunotherapy, and chemotherapy (16 dogs). The immunotherapy consisted of the

Table 30-2.   Clinical Staging System of Canine Hemangiosarcoma

T, PRIMARY TUMOR
  T0—no evidence of tumor
  T1—tumor confined to spleen
  T2—tumor confined to spleen but ruptured
  T3—tumor invading adjacent structures

N, REGIONAL LYMPH NODES
  N0—no regional lymph node involvement
  N1—regional lymph node involvement
  N2—distant lymph node involvement

M, DISTANT METASTASIS
  M0—no evidence of distant metastasis
  M1—distant metastasis

STAGES
  I—T0 or T1, N0, M0
  II—T1 or T2, N0 or N1, M0
  III—T2 or T3, N1 or N2, M1

Table 30-3.   Splenic Hemangiosarcoma: Correlation of Survival Time to Stage Regardless of Treatment[8]

	STAGE I	STAGE II	STAGE III
Number of dogs	8	15	24
Median days	110	107	73
Mean days	79	156	96
Range days	14–211	35–476	5–533

administration of a mixed bacterial vaccine (*Serratia marcescens* and *Streptococcus pyogenes*). Chemotherapy consisted of vincristine, cyclophosphamide, and methotrexate. The median survival time for the 8 dogs in Stage I was 100 days; for the 15 dogs in Stage II, 107 days; and for the 24 dogs in Stage III, 73 days. Dogs treated by surgery alone had a median survival time of 70 days. Dogs treated by surgery plus mixed bacterial vaccines had a median survival time of 85 days, and dogs treated by combined surgery plus immunotherapy plus chemotherapy had a median survival time of 123 days. There was no significant difference between the three median survival times.

In another recent study of 38 dogs with primary cardiac hemangiosarcoma,[14] 16 dogs underwent an exploratory thoracotomy. Seven dogs (44%) were euthanatized at the time of surgery due to nonresectability of the primary tumor or to gross metastatic disease. In 9 dogs (56%) the tumor was resected by removing part of the right atrium. The mean survival time for these 9 dogs was 4 months, and the survival time ranged from 2 days to 8 months. In another study, right atrial appendage hemangiosarcomas were removed from four dogs, and all were dead within 3 to 5 months.[19]

In cats the prognosis for hemangiosarcoma is also very poor. Most cats die from recurrence of the primary lesion or metastasis within 6 months to 1 year after surgical removal.[6,23] Cats with nonabdominal sites survived slightly longer than cats with tumors of the abdominal organs.[23] The average time until recurrence is usually about 4–5 months.

In summary, surgery still offers the best approach to therapy. The value of adjuvant chemotherapy for the treatment of this neoplasm remains a point of considerable controversy. Too few studies have been done to truly evaluate the effectiveness of adjuvant chemotherapy or biologic therapy in conjunction with surgery.

More studies are needed to evaluate potential therapeutic modalities with this particular tumor.

COMPARATIVE ASPECTS

Hemangiosarcoma, angiosarcoma, and malignant hemangioendothelioma are malignant tumors that arise from the endothelial cells of the blood vessels. In man, they are almost uniformly high grade tumors and are considered uncommon and will only comprise approximately 2% of all soft tissue sarcomas.[24]

Hemangiosarcomas have an overall recurrence rate of 50%–54% with clinical metastases occurring in 12%–26%, and 34%–48% of patients die within 5 years.[24] Hemangiosarcoma of the heart occurs in adults. Right-sided congestive heart failure with hemorrhagic pericardial fluid may also develop, as is seen in the dog. Hematogenous metastases to liver, lungs, and elsewhere may occur. Hemangiosarcoma of the bone is treated by amputation or eu bloc resection and pulmonary metastases within two years are frequent.[24,25]

One type of hemangiosarcoma of the liver is a chemically induced tumor in man. Thorium dioxide, potassium arsenite (Fowler solution) ingestion, and exposure to vinyl chloride are etiologic factors. Splenic hemangiosarcoma is very rare. Splenic rupture and metastases to the liver may occur.[24]

Combination chemotherapy using cyclophosphamide, methotrexate, and doxorubicin have been used in primary hemangiosarcoma of the liver, with objective response in 3 of 4 patients treated.[24]

Overall, these tumors have a very poor prognosis in humans, as they do in the dog and cat.

REFERENCES

1. Priester WA, McKay FW: The occurrence of tumors in domestic animals. NCI Monogr 54: 1980
2. Madewell BR, Theilen GH: Skin tumors of mesenchymal origin. In Thielen GH, Madewell BR (eds): Veterinary Cancer Medicine, pp. 295–297. Philadelphia, Lea & Febiger, 1987
3. Moulton JE: Tumors in Domestic Animals, ed 2, pp. 35–36. Berkeley, University of California Press, 1978
4. Oksanen A: Hemangiosarcomas in dogs. J Comp Pathol 88:585–595, 1978
5. Patnaik AK, Liu SK: Angiosarcoma in cats. J Small Anim Pract 18:191–198, 1977
6. Carpenter JL, Andrews LK, Holzworth J: Tumors and tumor-like lesions. In Holzworth J (ed): Diseases of the Cat, Vol 1, pp. 480–483. Philadelphia, W.B. Saunders, 1987
7. Arp LH, Grier RL: Disseminated cutaneous hemangiosarcoma in a young dog. J Am Vet Med Assoc 185:671–673, 1984
8. Brown NO, Patnaik AR, MacEwen EG: Canine Hemangiosarcoma: Retrospective analysis of 104 cases. J Am Vet Med Assoc 186:56–58, 1985
9. Pearson GR, Head KW: Malignant hemangioendothelioma (angiosarcoma) in the dog. J Small Anim Pract 17:737–745, 1976
10. Adam YG, Huvos AG, Hajdu SI: Malignant vascular tumors in the liver. Ann Surg 175:375–383, 1972
11. Ludwig J, Hoffman HN: Hemangiosarcoma of the liver: Spectrum of morphologic changes and clinical findings. Mayo Clin Proc 50:255–263, 1970
12. Rebar A, Han FF, Halliwell WH, et al: Microangiopathic hemolytic anemia associated with radiation-induced hemangiosarcoma. Vet Pathol 17:443–454, 1980
13. Berg RJ, Wingfield W: Pericardial effusion in the dog: A review of 42 cases. J Am Anim Hosp Assoc 20:721–730, 1984
13a. deMadro E, Helfand SC, Stebbins KE: Use of chemotherapy for treatment of cardiac hemangiosarcoma in a dog. J Am Vet Med Assoc 190:887–891, 1987
14. Aronsohn M: Cardiac hemangiosarcoma in the dog: A review of 38 cases. J Am Vet Med Assoc 187:922–926, 1985
15. Kline LJ, Zook BC, Munson TO: Primary cardiac hemangiosarcoma in the dog. J Am Vet Med Assoc 157:326–337, 1970
16. Hirsch VM, Jacobsen J, Mills JHL: A retrospective study of canine hemangiosarcoma and its association with acanthocytosis. Can Vet J 22:152–155, 1981
17. Brown NO: Hemangiosarcoma. Vet Clin North Am (Small Anim Pract) 15:569–575, 1985
17a. Wrigley RH, Park RD, Konde LJ, et al: Ultrasonographic features of splenic hemangiosarcoma in dogs: 18 cases (1980–1986). J Am Vet Med Assoc 192:1113–1117, 1988
17b. Johnson KA, Powers BE, Withrow SJ, et al: Splenomegaly in dogs: Predictors of neoplasia and survival following splenectomy. J Vet Int Med, (in press)

18. Dueland R, Dahlin DC: Hemangioendotheli-oma of canine bone. J Am Anim Hosp Assoc 8:81–85, 1972

19. Wykes PM, Rouse GP, Orton EC: Removal of five canine cardiac tumors using a stapling instrument. Vet Surg 15:103–106, 1986

20. Couto CG, Helfand SC: VAC chemotherapy for metastatic and non-resectable soft tissue tumors in the dog. Proceedings of the Veterinary Cancer Society, 6th Annual Conference, Vol 6, April 28–30, 1986

21. Brodey RS: Vascular tumors of the canine spleen. Mod Vet Pract 45:39–43, 1964

22. Bartels P: Indications for splenectomy and post-operative survival rate. J Small Anim Pract 101:781–785, 1970

23. Scavelli TD, Patnaik AK, Mehlhaff CJ, et al: Hemangiosarcoma in the cat: Retrospective evaluation of 31 surgical cases. J Am Vet Med Assoc 187:817–819, 1985

24. Rosenberg SA, Suit HD, Baker LH: Sarcomas of soft tissue. In DeVita VT, Hellman S, Rosenberg SA (eds): Principles and Practice of Oncology, ed 2, p 1262. Philadelphia, J.B. Lippincott, 1985

25. Sinkovics JG: Soft tissue sarcomas. In Sinkovics JG (ed): Medical Oncology, Vol 1, pp 318–320. New York, Marcel Dekker, 1986

Thymoma

Stephen J. Withrow

INCIDENCE AND RISK FACTORS

Thymomas are rare in the dog and even more uncommon in the cat. Even though the normal thymus is larger and more active in puppies and kittens, the disease is generally diagnosed in the older animal. In dogs, the mean age is 9 years; in cats, 10 years. Although no consistent breed predilection is known, medium and large breed dogs may be over-represented.[1,2] One study demonstrated a female prevalence,[3] but most studies show no sex predilection.[1]

PATHOLOGY AND NATURAL BEHAVIOR

Thymomas originate from thymic epithelium but are variably and even predominantly infil-trated with mature lymphocytes. The epithelium is the neoplastic component. "Benign" thymo-mas are noninvasive and well encapsulated, whereas "malignant" thymomas invade adjacent structures (precava, rib cage, and pericardium) but rarely metastasize.[4] The terms "benign" and "malignant" are derived more from clinical features (resectability) of the tumors than from histologic features. Distant metastasis is rare but has been reported.[5]

Anterior mediastinal tumors include, in order of frequency of occurrence, lymphomas, thy-momas, branchial cysts, ectopic thyroid, che-modectoma, and a variety of rare neoplasms.[1,6]

HISTORY AND CLINICAL SIGNS

Most patients present with signs of respiratory distress (coughing, tachypnea, and dyspnea). Obstruction of venous and lymphatic drainage from the head, neck, and legs many cause precaval syndrome (facial, neck or front leg swelling). The paraneoplastic syndrome of myas-thenia gravis has also been documented in up to 40% of affected dogs; it is characterized by muscle weakness and megaesophagus.[1–3,7] In 20% to 40% of animals, nonthymic neoplasms, various autoimmune diseases, and polymyositis have also been associated with the presence of thymoma.[2,3,8]

DIAGNOSTIC TECHNIQUES AND WORK-UP

Physical examination may reveal painless, bilateral pitting edema of the head, neck, or front legs as a result of the precaval syndrome. Jugular veins may be enlarged and tortuous. Auscultation of the thoracic cavity may reveal decreased lung sounds over the anterior mediastinum (mass) or ventral lung fields (pleural effusion). The heart sounds may be heard more dorsally and caudally than normal as a result of cardiac displacement. In smaller dogs and cats, decreased compressibility of the anterior chest cavity may also be detected.

Routine hematologic and biochemistry tests are usually normal, although lymphocytosis has been reported.[5,9] Thoracic radiographs generally reveal a variable size mass in the anterior mediastinum, pleural effusion, and displacement of the cardiac silhouette caudally and dorsally (Fig. 30-2). Dilation of the esophagus caudal to the mass may be seen with myasthenia gravis.

Transthoracic fine-needle aspiration for cytologic preparations is a simple and safe procedure,

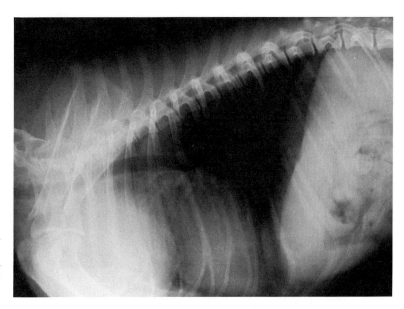

Figure 30-2. Anterior mediastinal mass (thymoma) is seen on lateral radiograph of a 13-year-old female mixed breed dog.

but it has been associated with unreliable results in my experience. Cytologic results usually reveal a preponderance of lymphocytes rather than the epithelial component of the tumor. Thymomas are commonly cystic and frequently yield nondiagnostic material (Fig. 30-3).[2] Since the major differential diagnosis is lymphoma, which is treated differently, the distinction between the two tumors is important. As opposed to thymoma, feline thymic lymphoma is usually seen in young cats (mean age 2 years) that are positive for feline leukemia virus (80%).[10] Canine thymic lymphoma is often associated with hypercalcemia (25% to 50%) or generalized lymphadenopathy.[11] Cytologic evaluation of pleural effusion in thymomas cases should yield mature lymphocytes as opposed to the lymphoblasts seen with lymphoma.[8]

Transthoracic needle-core biopsy can be diagnostic but often yields cystic and necrotic material with a preponderance of lymphocytes, making definitive diagnosis difficult.

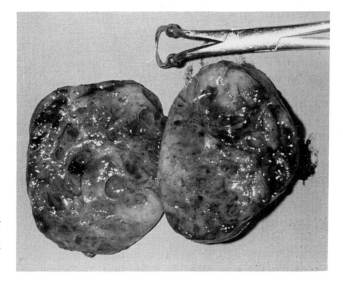

Figure 30-3. Cross-section of well-encapsulated thymoma surgically removed from patient in Fig. 30-2. Note cystic nature of lesion, which may complicate cytologic diagnosis. Patient was alive and free of disease more than 2 years postoperatively.

Angiography, ultrasound, and computed tomographic examinations of mediastinal masses are not sensitive means of differentiating thymoma from lymphoma.

A definitive presurgical diagnosis of thymoma is difficult. An attempt should be made, however, to rule out the more common diseases. Most thymic lymphoma cases respond rapidly and completely to aggressive chemotherapy. Thymoma should be suspected in patients with a partial remission or stable disease 10 to 14 days after chemotherapy administration for suspect lymphoma.

THERAPY

The definitive therapy for thymoma is surgical resection. Smaller masses may be approached by means of an intercostal thoracotomy, but the more common large masses should be approached by an anterior sternotomy. Once the mass is seen, the surgeon must make a clinical judgment of its resectability. Approximately 50% of thymomas are resectable, but nothing (including size) is uniformly predictive of resectability in the preoperative evaluation. Invasive and malignant thymomas adhere to surrounding tissues, especially major veins, making removal difficult or impossible.

Debulking of invasive thymomas can be attempted in hopes of alleviating symptoms of the physical mass or possibly enhancing potential chemotherapy treatment, but it is frequently associated with extensive morbidity.

If the mass is deemed unresectable, and if other treatments are to be pursued, large wedge biopsies should be taken at surgery, being careful not to contaminate the thoracic cavity and remembering that thymomas are cystic and not homogeneous.

Attempts at treatment with chemotherapy have been reported, but objective partial or complete remissions are very uncommon.[2,12] A combination of high-dosage cyclophosphamide and prednisone seems to be the most effective treatment and has resulted in at least a partial response in two cases. Radiation therapy has rarely been attempted, but either radiation alone[12a] or chemotherapy and radiation should decrease the lymphoid component of the mass.

Myasthenia gravis, if present, generally requires treatment with immunosuppression (prednisone) or anticholinesterase drugs.

PROGNOSIS

The prognosis for surgically resectable (benign) thymomas is good. Long-term remissions and cures can be expected.[5,7,12]

The outlook for patients with nonresectable thymomas remains poor until use of nonsurgical treatments (chemotherapy or radiation therapy) can be optimized.

Myasthenia gravis may improve with complete removal of the thymoma, but the improvement may require many months.[1] Two untreated thymoma patients, followed with thoracic radiographs only, lived 6 and 36 months, implying slow growth of some thymomas.[3]

COMPARATIVE ASPECTS[13]

Thymomas are very similar in animals and humans. Sixty-five percent are encapsulated and noninvasive, whereas 35% are invasive.

Multiple paraneoplastic syndromes have been associated with human thymomas (autoimmune, endocrine, infectious, and nonthymic cancer). Up to 50% of patients have symptoms of myasthenia gravis. Only 25% have improvement in muscle strength after removal of the thymoma.

Treatment is surgical removal, and at least 80% of treated patients are free of disease at 5 years. Radiation therapy is indicated for invasive thymomas, which are considered moderately sensitive to irradiation. Corticosteroids have caused regression of some thymomas. Other single agents with some efficacy include doxorubicin, cisplatin and alkylating agents.[13a]

REFERENCES

1. Stevenson S: Thymoma. In Slatter DE (ed): Textbook of Small Animal Surgery, pp 1235–1241. Philadelphia, W.B. Saunders, 1985
2. Aronsohn M: Canine thymoma. Vet Clin North Am 15:755–767, 1985
3. Aronsohn MG, Schunk KL, Carpenter JL, King NW: Clinical and pathologic features of thymoma in 15 dogs. J Am Vet Med Assoc 184:1355–1362, 1984
4. Robinson WC, Cantwell HD, Crawley RR, Weirich WE, Blevins WE: Invasive thymoma in a dog: A case report. J Am Anim Hosp Assoc 13:95–97, 1977

5. Bellah JR, Stiff ME, Russell RG: Thymoma in the dog: Two case reports and review of 20 additional cases. J Am Vet Med Assoc 183:306–311, 1983

6. Liu S-K, Patnaik AK, Burk RL: Thymic branchial cysts in the dog and cat. J Am Vet Med Assoc 182:1095–1098, 1983

7. Poffenbarger E, Klausner JS, Caywood DD: Acquired myasthenia gravis in a dog with thymoma: a case report. J Am Anim Hosp Assoc 21:119–124, 1985

8. Carpenter JL, Holzworth J: Thymoma in 11 cats. J Am Vet Med Assoc 181:248–251, 1982

9. Theilen GH, Madewell BR: Tumors of the respiratory tract and thorax. In Theilen GH, Madewell BR (eds): Veterinary Cancer Medicine, p 351. Philadelphia, Lea & Febiger, 1979

10. Hardy WD: Hematopoietic tumors of cats. J Am Anim Hosp Assoc 17:921–940, 1981

11. Theilen GS, Madewell BR: Leukemia-sarcoma disease complex. In Theilen GH, Madewell BR (eds), Veterinary Cancer Medicine, pp. 241–252. Philadelphia, Lea & Febiger, 1979

12. Willard MD, Tvedten H, Walshaw R, Aronson E: Thymoma in a cat. J Am Vet Med Assoc 176:451–453, 1980

12a. Hitt ME, Shaw DP, Hogan PM: Radiation treatment for thymoma in a dog. J Am Vet Med Assoc 190:1187–1190, 1987

13. Rosenberg JC: Neoplasms of the mediastinum. In DeVita VT et al (eds): Cancer: Principles and Practice of Oncology, p 486–492. Philadelphia, J.B. Lippincott, 1982

13a. Uematsu M, Kondo M: A proposal for treatment of invasive thymoma. Cancer 58:1979–1984, 1986

Canine Transmissible Venereal Tumor

E. Gregory MacEwen

INCIDENCE AND RISK FACTORS

Transmissible venereal tumor (TVT) is recognized only in dogs and is a naturally occurring tumor. It commonly affects the external genitalia and is usually transmitted at coitus. The development of the TVT as a coitally transmitted neoplasm in the dog is probably facilitated by some unique characteristic of sexual intercourse in this species that leads to injuries of the vaginal or penile mucosa which provide the bed for tumor transplantation. TVT are naturally transplanted tumors that are derived from a common origin; these tumors apparently have a cellular mode of transmission and have been maintained in the canine population for many generations.[1,2] The tumor has been reported to occur in most parts of the world but appears to be more prevalent in temperate climates. Studies have shown that the hospital prevalence of TVT is inversely correlated to geographic latitude and positively correlated to higher mean annual temperature and increased rainfall.[3,4] It is seen most often in young, roaming, sexually active dogs.

A viral etiology has been investigated but not verified.[5] Virus particles have been observed, but the tumor has not been transmitted by cell-free infiltrates.

PATHOLOGY AND NATURAL BEHAVIOR

The TVT consists of undifferentiated round cells that are loosely packed and regarded to be of reticuloendothelial origin. The TVT usually maintains a relatively consistent karyotype. Special staining and evaluation of TVT cell mitotic figures has demonstrated that most cells have a stem-line chromosome number of 59 (range 57–64).[6] Of these 59 chromosomes, 16 or 17 are metacentric and 43 or 42 are acrocentric. These constant and highly specific chromosome aberrations are regarded as suggesting a cellular mechanism of transmission. The normal dog karyotype is 78 chromosomes. It has also been shown that the same histocompatibility complex (DL-A) antigens are expressed on the surface of TVT cells that originate from different dogs in different locations.[7]

Overall, immunologic studies clearly demonstrate that the TVT tumor is antigenic in the dog and that the immune response against the tumor plays a major role in determining the course of disease. The TVT possesses tumor-associated antigens, as determined by both immunodiffusion and enzyme-linked immunosorbent assays (ELISA), and the immunologic response plays a major role in inhibiting the growth and spread of this neoplasm.[4] The anti-TVT immune response is mounted, at least in part, against DL-A. Regression of the tumor is followed by the development of immunity to subsequent reinfections. Passive transfer of post-regression sera if given before transplantation, can inhibit the growth of experimentally transplanted tumor and prevent development of the tumor.[4] Antibodies from regressor animals are cytotoxic to TVT cells in the presence of complement and may therefore destroy the tumor cells *in vivo* without the involvement of cellular effector mechanisms.[8] The demonstration that passive transfer of immune serum can induce tumor regression indicates that antibody-dependent mechanisms are involved in the induction of tumor regression. In addition, *in vitro* assays suggest that suppressive serum factors may facilitate tumor growth in the initial stages of disease.[8]

One interesting observation in animals heavily infected with large burdens of TVT is that they develop a polycythemia.[4] It has been suggested that TVT cells probably synthesize and secrete erythropoietin.

Once an animal becomes infected, the TVT may progress to a certain point or to a certain size and then regress if there is an appropriate antitumor immunologic response. This probably happens in most of the animals that are naturally infected with TVT. But the TVT may continue to grow and, rarely, even to metastasize. Metastasis has been seen in lymph nodes, skin, eye, liver, and brain.[2,8a] The TVT may also involve extragenital sites through autotransplantation (licking and sniffing). This may be the way in which TVT develops in the oral and nasal cavities.

HISTORY AND CLINICAL SIGNS

Most cases of naturally occurring TVT are confined to the external genitalia. In the vagina, TVT may range in size from 0.5 mm to more than 10 cm in diameter. They are usually cauliflowerlike in appearance, friable, and red to flesh-colored (Fig. 30-4). It is not uncommon to see areas of necrosis with superficial bacterial infection. Hemorrhage is a common problem, and many animals are presented because of persistent bleeding. In the male, a serosanguineous discharge from the prepuce is often the presenting clinical sign. TVT are frequently located around the gland of the penis and therefore require total extension of the penis for visualization (Fig. 30-5). Extremely large masses may preclude total extension of the penis. These tumors can also be multicentric along the penis. They tend to be very friable, and hemorrhage is common.

TVT can be seen in the oral cavity, the skin (Fig. 30-6), the sclera, and the anterior chamber. Intranasal TVT frequently cause epistaxis and sneezing.

TVT are usually diagnosed in dogs that are allowed to run free and have been exposed to an infected animal.

DIAGNOSTIC TECHNIQUES AND WORK-UP

The definitive diagnosis is based on either a histologic or cytologic evaluation of the tumor.

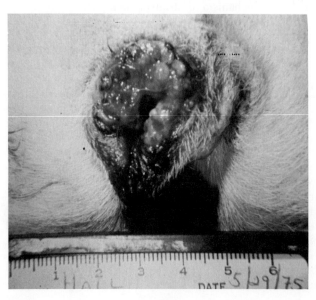

Figure 30-4. Vaginal TVT. Note the cauliflowerlike appearance.

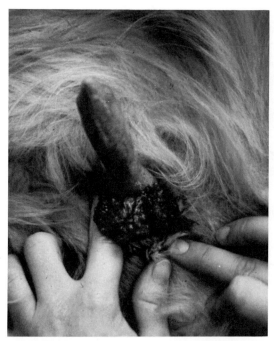

Figure 30-5. Proliferative TVT involving the base of the penis. The penis usually must be totally extended to visualize the tumor.

Cytologically, the TVT has a very distinct appearance. The cells appear round to oval, and mitotic figures are common (Fig. 30-7). Chromatin clumping and one or two prominent nuclei are obvious. Perhaps the most striking cytologic finding is the presence of multiple clear cytoplasmic vacuoles, frequently arranged in chains. The cytologic appearance of TVT is not readily confused with other neoplasms such as mast cell

tumors, histiocytoma, and malignant lymphomas. Some oral TVT have been misdiagnosed as amelanotic melanoma or poorly differentiated sarcoma. In some cases it is easier to make a definitive diagnosis with cytology than with histology. If a TVT is suspected, it is advisable to make impression smears of the tumor before or at the time of biopsy.

As previously mentioned, TVT have been associated with a relative polycythemia. A CBC should be performed during the evaluation of an animal with a TVT. Although metastasis is uncommon, regional lymph nodes should be evaluated thoroughly. If there is any evidence of regional lymphadenopathy, a fine-needle aspiration should be performed to rule out possible metastasis. Thoracic radiographs are invariably negative for metastasis.

THERAPY

Transmissible venereal tumors respond to many forms of therapy. Surgery can be effective for small, localized TVT. Usually the tumor is too extensive for an adequate surgical excision, and other therapies must be considered.[9] Another problem with surgical excision has been the high recurrence rate associated with it. Recurrence rates after surgery vary from 20% to 60%, depending on the location and extent of disease.[9]

Radiation therapy is also an effective method of treating TVT. Dosage recommendations range from 15 Gy (1500 rads) divided over 5 days to 45 Gy divided over 3 weeks. In a recent study, 18 TVT patients were treated with orthovoltage

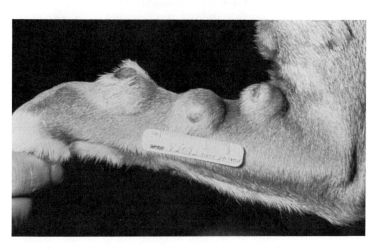

Figure 30-6. TVT nodules in the skin of a dog (photo courtesy of Dr. J. Broadhurst).

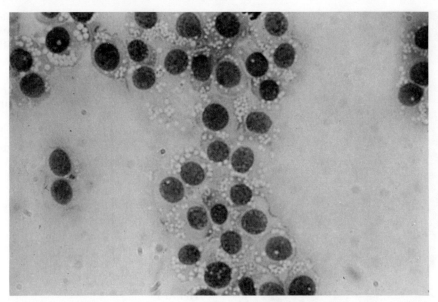

Figure 30-7. A characteristic cytologic preparation of a fine-needle aspirate from a TVT. Note the prominent nuclei and multiple clear cytoplasmic vacuoles.

radiotherapy, which induced complete regression of the tumor in all 18 dogs. No recurrence was observed within 1 year after treatment. A dose of 10 Gy was applied in each treatment, and in most cases, 3 treatments were required to induce complete remission.[10]

Chemotherapy offers the most effective and efficient treatment of TVT.[11] A number of agents have been used, including cyclophosphamide, vincristine, methotrexate, and doxorubicin. Vincristine has been reported to be one of the most effective agents in treating TVT.[12] It can be given at a dosage of 0.5–0.7 mg/m² IV once weekly. An average of 4–6 treatments are necessary to induce complete remission. Complete cure can be expected in more than 90% of cases treated. Doxorubicin has also been used quite effectively to treat TVT. The dosage commonly used is 30 mg/m² IV every 21 days. In my experience, two treatment courses are usually sufficient to induce complete and prolonged remissions.

Biologic response modifiers have also been used experimentally to treat TVT. Although responses have been noted with agents such as BCG, BCG cell walls, and Staphylococcus Protein A,[13,14] the results are inconsistent and recurrences frequent. To date, the use of biologic response modifiers must be considered investigative and not as effective as chemotherapy.

PROGNOSIS

With surgical excision alone, there tends to be a high recurrence rate, varying from 20% to 60% depending on the location and extent of disease.[15]

TVT is one neoplastic process that can be readily cured with chemotherapy. Most chemotherapy protocols effect cure in 90% to 95% of animals treated.[11,12] The two drugs that have been shown to be most effective are vincristine and doxorubicin.

REFERENCES

1. Stookey SL: Transmissible venereal tumors of dogs. NCI Monogr 32:315–320, 1969

2. Richardson RC: Canine transmissible venereal tumors. Comp Cont Educ 31:951–956, 1981

3. Higgins DA: Observations of the canine transmissible venereal tumor as seen in the Bahamas. Vet Rec 79:67–71, 1966

4. Cohen D: The canine transmissible venereal tumor: A unique result of tumor progression. Adv Cancer Res 43:75–112, 1985

5. Sapp WJ, Adams EW: C-type viral particles in canine venereal tumor cell cultures. Am J Vet Res 31:1321–1323, 1970

6. Murray M, James H, Martin WJ: A study of the cytology and karyotype of the canine trans-

missible venereal tumor. Res Vet Sci 10:565–568, 1969

7. Epstein RB, Bennett BT: Histocompatibility typing and course of canine venereal tumors transplanted into unmodified random dogs. Cancer Res 34:788–793, 1974

8. Bennett BT, Debelak–Fehir KM, Epstein RB: Tumor blocking and inhibiting serum factors in the clinical cause of canine venereal tumor. Cancer Res 35:2942–2947, 1975

8a. Yang TJ: Metastatic transmissible venereal sarcoma in a dog. J Am Vet Med Assoc 190:555–556, 1987

9. Brodey RS, Roszel JF: Neoplasms of the canine uterus, vagina, and vulva. A clinicopathologic survey of 90 cases. J Am Vet Med Assoc 151:1294–1307, 1967

10. Thrall DE: Orthovoltage radiotherapy of canine transmissible venereal tumors. Vet Radiol 23:217–219, 1982

11. Brown WO, Calvert C, MacEwen EG: Chemotherapeutic management of transmissible venereal tumors in 30 dogs. J Am Vet Med Assoc 176:983–986, 1980

12. Calvert CA, Leifer CE, MacEwen EG: Vincristine for treatment of transmissible venereal tumor. J Am Vet Med Assoc 181:163–164, 1982

13. Hess AD, Catchatourian R, et al: Intralesional Bacillus-Calmette-Guerin immunotherapy of canine venereal tumors. Cancer Res 37:3990–3994, 1977

14. Cohen D, Fer MF, Pearson, et al: Treatment of canine transmissible venereal tumor by intravenous administration of Protein A. J Biol Response Mod 3:271–277, 1984

15. Amber EI, Henderson RA: Canine transmissible venereal tumor: Evaluation of surgical excision of primary and metastatic lesions in Zaria-Nigera. J Am Anim Hosp Assoc 18:350–352, 1982

Mesothelioma

Richard R. Dubielzig
E. Gregory MacEwen

INCIDENCE AND RISK FACTORS

Mesothelioma is a rare neoplasm of dogs and cats affecting the lining epithelial cells of the various body cavities. In dogs, primary tumors affecting the thoracic cavity, abdominal cavity, pericardial sac, and vaginal tunic of the scrotum have been reported.[1,2] In cats, primary meso-theliomas have been reported in the pericardium, pleura, and peritoneum.[3,4] Exposure to asbestos may be an important contributing factor to development of mesothelioma in pet dog populations. Affected dogs frequently have owners with jobs or hobbies entailing exposure to asbestos.[5] The level of asbestos in lung tissues of affected dogs has been reported to be greater than that in controls.[5,6]

PATHOLOGY AND NATURAL BEHAVIOR

The normal mesothelium is a monolayer of squamous epithelial cells distinguished by the presence of microvilli and evidence of phagocytic potential. Disease conditions associated with inflammation or irritation of the lining of the body cavity commonly result in a marked physiological proliferation of the mesothelial cells. Fluid accumulation in the affected cavity promotes exfoliation and implantation, resulting in multiple tumor growths. Animals usually present with pleural or pericardial effusion characterized by nodules or pleural plaques or thickening of the lung bases or along fissures.

Mesothelial cells appear morphologically to be epithelial cells; however, their derivation is from mesoderm. Mesotheliomas may exhibit morphologic characteristics highly suggestive of epithelial neoplasms (carcinoma or adenocarcinoma), or they may show evidence primarily of mesenchymal proliferation (sclerosing mesothelioma).[1,7,8] The most useful criteria in establishing a diagnosis of mesothelioma is to demonstrate that the tumor is primarily a neoplasm of the coelomic cavity lining and that the principle method of tumor spread is by transcoelomic implantation. Mesothelioma should be considered when the bulk of the neoplastic tissue exists on the coelomic surface. Unfortunately there are no cellular markers that conclusively define the mesothelial cell. However, in cases where carcinoma or adenocarcinoma must be differentiated from mesothelioma, special stains can be helpful in making the distinction.[8,9] Little is known about the cellular markers useful in distinguishing mesothelioma from mesenchymal tumors.

HISTORY AND CLINICAL SIGNS

Classical mesotheliomas occur as a diffuse nodular mass covering the surfaces of the body cavity (Fig. 30-8). The most consistent clinical

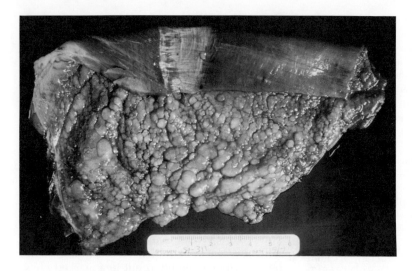

Figure 30-8. The diaphragm from a dog with abdominal mesothelioma is folded to show the affected side and the unaffected side.

feature is effusion and displacement of organs. Although malignant mesothelial cells easily exfoliate into the effusion fluid, they are difficult to distinguish cytologically from reactive hypertrophic mesothelial cells.

Sclerosing mesothelioma is a variation of mesothelial tumor seen primarily in male dogs, among which German shepherds are over-represented.[1] These tumors present as thick fibrous linings in the abdominal or pleural cavities (Fig. 30-9). The appearance of the body cavity at surgery is often interpreted as chronic inflammation. Since tumors of the abdomen are frequently located near the stomach or in the pelvic canal, vomition and urinary problems are often seen.

DIAGNOSTIC TECHNIQUES AND WORKUP

Mesothelioma should be suspected in adult dogs with evidence of chronic disease and fluid accumulation in any of the body cavities. Mesothelial cells can be expected to proliferate under any circumstance associated with fluid accumulation in the body cavity, making the distinction between physiological mesothelial proliferation and neoplasia difficult. Since phagocytic transformation normally occurs in hyperplastic

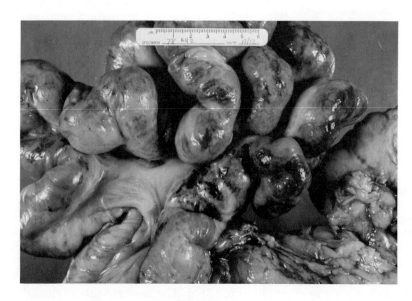

Figure 30-9. Loops of intestine from a dog with sclerosing mesothelioma. The thickening sclerosal surfaces must be distinguished from chronic inflammation.

mesothelial reactions, morphologic clues of malignancy may be difficult to assess.

The diagnosis is usually made at the time of exploratory surgery into the affected body cavity. The surgeon is cautioned to biopsy any body cavity lining when an obvious cause for fluid accumulation is not found. Sclerosing mesothelioma must be distinguished from chronic inflammatory disease of the body cavity, and histologic examination of biopsy material is essential to establish the diagnosis.

TREATMENT AND PROGNOSIS

No satisfactory treatment exists for mesothelioma. Radical excision may benefit some animals, but usually the tumors are too advanced and the tumor spreads within the body cavity early in the course of disease. Attempts at using intracavitary chemotherapeutic agents, such as Thio-Tepa, have been unrewarding. We have also tried intracavitary immunotherapy, using bacterial agents such as mixed bacterial vaccine (MBV) and *Corynebacterium parvum*, but have seen minimal response.

COMPARATIVE ASPECTS

In humans, mesothelioma is closely linked to exposure to aerosolized asbestos fibers.[10] A strong association is made between industrial exposure to asbestos crystals in asbestos-related occupations or avocations and mesothelioma. Occupations such as ship building, asbestos mining, auto mechanics, welding, and construction work are strong risk factors in the development of mesothelioma in humans.[10] Family members of industrial exposed populations are at risk owing to asbestos fiber exposure from the clothing. Affected individuals routinely have greatly increased counts of asbestos fibers in parenchymal lung tissue.[10]

Alterations in humoral and cellular immunity have been observed in patients with asbestos-related diseases and in asymptomatic asbestos-exposed individuals.[11,12] Suppression of cell-mediated immunity, especially depressed total T cells and T-helper cells has been found.[13,14] Thus, chronic immunosuppression may contribute to the development of the neoplasm.

Lung tissue from dogs with mesothelioma has been shown to contain high levels of asbestos.[5,6] In a case control epidemiologic survey of 18 histologically confirmed cases of mesothelioma in dogs, it was found that the owner's occupation or avocation in asbestos-related activities was a strongly positive risk factor for mesothelioma.[2] The epidemiologic association of mesothelioma in pet populations needs to be studied further in order to understand the degree of association with environmental risk factors. The latency period in pet animals between exposure and the development of environment-related diseases such as cancer would be expected to be considerably shorter than the similar latency period in humans. For this reason pet animals might be considered a sentinel population useful in predicting environmental hazards not yet manifest in the human population.

In humans the median survival from the time of diagnosis is approximately 12 months. Doxorubicin either alone or in combination with other chemotherapeutic agents has provoked some minimal responses. Radiation therapy can be used for palliation of pain.

REFERENCES

1. Dubielzig RR: Sclerosing mesothelioma in five dogs. J Am Anim Hosp Assoc 15:745–748, 1979
2. Thrall DE, Goldschmidt MM: Mesothelioma in the dog: Six case reports. J Am Vet Res Soc 19:107, 1978
3. Tilley LP, Owens JM, Wilkins RJ, et al: Pericardial mesothelioma with effusion in a cat. J Am Anim Hosp Assoc 11:60–65, 1978
4. Carpenter JL, Andrews LK, Holzworth J, et al: Tumors and tumor-like lesions. In Holzworth J (ed): Diseases of the Cat: Medicine and Surgery, pp. 583–585. Philadelphia, W.B. Saunders, 1987
5. Glickman LT, Domanski LM, Maguire TG, Dubielzig RR, Churg A: Mesothelioma in pet dogs associated with exposure of their owners to asbestos. Environ Res 32:305, 1983
6. Harbison ML, Godleski JJ: Malignant mesothelioma in urban dogs. Lab Invest 46:34A, 1982
7. Kannerstein M, Churg J: Desmoplastic diffuse malignant mesothelioma. Prog Surg Pathol 2:19–29, 1979
8. Whitaker D, Shilkin KB: Diagnosis of pleural malignant mesothelioma in life—A practical approach. J Pathol 143:147–175, 1984
9. Loosli M, Hurlimann J: Immunohistochemical study of malignant diffuse mesothelioma of the pleura. Histopathology 8:793, 1983

10. McDonald JC, McDonald AD: Epidemiology of mesothelioma from estimated incidence. Prov Mod 6:426, 1977

11. Kagan E, Solomon A, Cochran JC, et al: Immunological studies of patients with asbestosis. I. Studies of cell-mediated immunity. Clin Exp Immunol 28:261–267, 1977

12. Kagan E, Soloman A, Cochran JC, et al: Immunological studies of patients with asbestosis. II. Studies of circulating lymphoid cell numbers and humoral immunity. Clin Exp Immunol 28:268–274, 1977

13. Miller LG, Sparrow D, Ginns LC: Asbestos exposure correlates with alterations in circulating T-cell subsets. Clin Exp Immunol 51:110–116, 1983

14. Lew F, Tsang P, Holland JF, et al: High frequency of immune dysfunctions in asbestos workers and in patients with malignant mesothelioma. J Clin Immunol 6:225–233, 1986

31

DESIGNING CLINICAL CANCER TRIALS: BASIC CONSIDERATIONS

E. Gregory MacEwen

Studies designed to answer medical questions are called clinical trials. A study may deal with diagnostic, therapeutic, or surveillance issues. The environment in which the study is conducted may vary from a single clinic or hospital to a geographically dispersed consortium of institutions.

One of the most important contributions that veterinary medicine can make to clinical cancer research is the evaluation of new therapy approaches in well-designed and controlled clinical trials. The reasons for this are that veterinary hospitals are a unique source of animals with naturally occurring tumors, that the medicolegal considerations are less stringent than in human medicine, and that there are few accepted and effective treatments for many tumors that occur in pet animals. Thus, large numbers of animals can be obtained and new (experimental) therapies evaluated. An integrated program of clinical trials would not only improve the treatment of animals with cancer, but would also benefit research in the treatment of human cancer. At the present time, the primary objectives of clinical cancer trials in veterinary medicine are to accumulate data on the biologic behavior of different tumor types in animals and to evaluate new cancer therapy regimens. The purpose of this chapter is to describe the different types of clinical trials that are possible and the considerations that must be taken into account in designing them in order for them to provide useful data.

TYPES OF CLINICAL TRIALS[1,2]

There are three broad categories of clinical trials: Phase I, Phase II, and Phase III (Table 31-1). The information obtained in Phase I trials is used to plan Phase II trials, which in turn produces information used to help design Phase III trials. A short description of each type of trial follows.

Table 31-1.   Types of Clinical Trials

TRIAL	PURPOSE
Early trial (Phase I)	To determine dosage, toxicity, antitumor response
↓	
Preliminary trial (Phase II)	To evaluate response in one tumor type or stage of disease
↓	
Comparative trial (Phase III)	To determine if new therapy is better than the standard approach

PHASE I TRIAL

The purpose of a Phase I clinical trial is to determine the toxicity of the agent as well as whether a potential therapeutic agent has any antitumor activity and, if so, the best dosage and method of administration. These studies usually involve small numbers of animals and all types of tumors. Animals are usually assigned on the basis of histologic tumor type, extent of disease (clinical stage), general health status, and willingness of the owner to participate.

PHASE II TRIAL

The purpose of a Phase II clinical trial is to evaluate whether a therapy regimen or agent is effective against a variety of tumor types or stages of disease using the dosage and route determined in earlier Phase I trials.

PHASE III TRIAL

The purpose of a Phase III clinical trial is to determine whether a new therapy regimen or agent is better than the currently available forms of treatment. These trials, therefore, involve comparison of two or more treatments and require careful design in order to provide statistically meaningful results. The advice of a statistician is required regarding the number of patients needed, the randomization of animals, and stratification procedures. In some Phase III studies, new protocols may be compared with regimens previously reported in a scientific publication. However, the use of such historical controls is best avoided unless the biologic behavior of the tumor type being studied is very well known.

CONSIDERATIONS IN DESIGNING CLINICAL THERAPY PROTOCOLS

Careful planning is essential if a clinical trial is to provide useful data. The principles detailed below must be followed in order to design a meaningful clinical trial. The basic elements of a clinical protocol are presented in Table 31-2.

INITIAL STEPS

Before any clinical study is designed, the capabilities of the clinic in which the study is to be done must be realistically appraised. The caseload of the clinic and the tumor types seen are basic factors. The equipment available and the support (or lack of it) of other departments in the hospital must also be taken into consideration. If clinical trials have been done by the clinic in the past, they should be examined. Deficiencies in the experimental method should not be repeated in the new trial, and knowledge obtained in earlier studies can be used to help determine the objectives and methods of the proposed trial. A thorough review of previous work in the proposed field of study, as reported in the scientific press, is also important in this regard.

Table 31-2.   Elements of a Protocol

1. Introduction to scientific background for the study
2. Objectives of study
3. Design of study
4. Selection of patients
5. Treatment programs
6. Procedures in event of response, no response, or toxicity
7. Required clinical and laboratory data
8. Criteria for evaluating the effect of treatment
9. Statistical considerations
10. Informed consent, if needed
11. Record forms
12. Responsible investigator

If all the factors mentioned above are taken into consideration *before* a trial is designed and implemented, there is a good chance that the trial will produce useful results without requiring costly revisions at a later stage.

PURPOSE OF THE STUDY

The type of clinical trial that should be done depends on the current state of knowledge about the biology of the tumor type being treated and the type of protocol being evaluated. The trial should be designed to fulfill an objective that is realistic (in terms of being possible to achieve) and that will advance previous work.

Certain questions need to be addressed. Is the trial going to be a retrospective or prospective study? If it is prospective, then issues such as patient selection, patient allocation, type of controls, and criteria for evaluation need to be addressed.

PATIENT SELECTION

Another important consideration in designing a clinical trial is the type and number of patients that will be selected for the study. The factors taken into account will depend on the goals of the trial but will usually include:

1. Age
2. Previous therapy
3. Tumor type
4. Tumor site
5. Extent (stage) of disease
6. Other diseases, which may limit the patient's ability to participate fully in the trial
7. Prognostic factors
8. The availability of the patient for long-term follow-up studies, which may include a necropsy

The number of patients needed for any given trial depends on the purpose of the trial and the extent of the unavoidable variable factors that may be involved in achieving that purpose. The type of tumor selected for the study can have an important effect on the number of patients available. Whenever possible, the most common tumors should be selected so that a sufficient number of animals can be obtained in a reasonable length of time.

CLINICAL CONSIDERATIONS

The type of basic clinical information required in a study should be clearly stated in the overall design and should include the methods used to diagnose the disease, the number and frequency of hematologic examinations, the biochemical tests required, the radiographic procedures needed, and the criteria to be used for determining the clinical stage of a patient's disease.

CONTROLS

Occasionally a study is performed without controls because it can be argued that the course of the disease is so well known that no controls are necessary. Historical controls can be obtained from the literature or from previous studies by the same investigator. The best controls are concurrent nonrandomized or randomized controls.

PATIENT ALLOCATION PROCEDURES

Many clinical trials involve a comparison of the survival times of animals in two or more groups treated with different therapy regimens. It is, therefore, of critical importance that at the end of the study, the effectiveness of the treatment in the different groups of animals can be compared. The advice of a statistician must be obtained when designing a protocol as to whether there is a need to assign animals to different groups randomly or nonrandomly and, if randomization is to be used, the best method to be followed. The advantages of randomization include the elimination of bias, the balance of treatment groups with respect to prognosis, and a more valid statistical analysis that can assign significant levels to findings about the different groups under study.

Blinding can further eliminate bias by client responses regarding the effect of the treatment or the bias of the evaluating investigator. When treatment assignments are withheld from both the client (or patient) and the evaluating investigator, the study is said to be "double blind."

If a double-blind study is to be done, the methods of allocating patients to different therapy groups without the clinician's knowledge must be decided on *before* the study is begun.

Stratification tends to *balance* treatment groups according to the prognostic factors associated with the particular disease. The number of strata to be used in a particular clinical study should be roughly equivalent to the number of prognostic subgroups that can be distinguished in the study; for most studies, this number is between two and six. The more strata, the more patients need to be entered.

STANDARDIZATION

In an effort to reduce the number of unwanted variables in a study, all procedures and drugs used in a trial should be standardized. For instance, basic surgical procedures should be the same for different groups of animals (ideally, all surgery for a study should be done by the same surgeon), and chemotherapeutic or immunotherapeutic reagents should be from the same production batch. This is especially true for the biologic immunomodulators.

SAMPLE SIZE[3]

The most important factor related to the determination of sample size is the endpoint with respect to which the treatment is to be evaluated. Common endpoints in cancer clinical trials are objective response (tumor regression) and survival time. The question of sample size is closely related to how big the gain or difference can be expected for the treatment under evaluation. This question can be answered by ex-

amining the power of the statistical procedure. A powerful study is one with a high probability of detecting an important treatment difference. It has been proposed that if a study fails to reject the null hypothesis (no difference seen), then it is important to state the power of the study. Sample size (or power) calculations are relevant to study design, not analysis.[4]

In the design of studies to evaluate response rates, it is best to keep the standard error to 10% or less. Fig. 31-1 shows the relationship between a response rate and the standard error. For a given response rate, the standard error decreases as the sample size increases. From the figure a sample size of 25 patients corresponds to a standard error of 10% when the response rate is 50%. Because 10% error is generally regarded as adequate precision for an estimate in a Phase II study, 25 patients would be an adequate sample size.

In Phase III the sample size can be expected to be larger because the trial is comparative; that is, it involves two or more treatment groups. The typical objective of a Phase III study is to compare the effects of one treatment with another (usually to accepted or "standard" treatment) by comparing remission or survival duration, in addition to response rates. Table 31-3 can be used to determine the sample size in the comparison of a new treatment with a standard treatment.[3] For example, suppose you want to study a new treatment and you hope to reduce the recurrence rate of a tumor from 50% to 25% at 1 year. With an 80% power and a probability

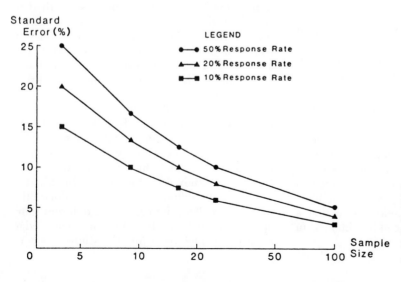

Figure 31-1. Relationship between response rate, standard error, and sample size (log scale). (Dixon DO: Sample size for clinical trials. Cancer Bull 32:207–213, 1980).

Table 31-3. Number of Patients Needed per Group to Compare Response Rates, for Given Level (One-Sided)* and Power for Specified Rates[3]

SMALLER RATE (%)	LARGER MINUS SMALLER RATE													
	5	10	15	20	25	30	35	40	45	50	55	60	65	70
5	330	105	55	40	33	24	20	17	13	12	10	9	9	8
	460	145	76	48	39	31	25	20	19	15	13	11	10	9
	850	270	140	89	63	37	41	34	21	25	22	18	16	14
10	540	155	76	47	37	30	23	19	16	13	11	11	9	8
	740	210	105	64	41	38	30	24	20	17	15	12	11	10
	1370	390	195	120	81	60	46	41	35	28	24	20	17	16
15	710	200	94	56	43	32	26	22	17	15	11	10	9	8
	990	270	130	77	52	43	34	26	23	19	16	12	11	10
	1820	500	240	145	96	69	52	41	37	30	24	22	18	16
20	860	230	110	63	42	36	27	23	17	15	12	10	9	8
	1190	320	150	88	58	46	36	29	23	18	16	12	11	10
	2190	590	280	160	105	76	57	44	39	30	27	22	18	16
25	980	260	120	69	45	37	31	23	17	15	12	10	9	—
	1360	360	165	96	63	46	38	30	23	18	16	12	11	—
	2510	660	300	175	115	81	60	46	40	33	27	22	17	—
30	1080	280	130	73	47	37	31	23	17	15	11	10	—	—
	1500	390	175	100	65	46	38	30	23	18	16	12	—	—
	2760	720	330	185	120	85	61	47	39	32	24	20	—	—
35	1160	300	135	75	48	37	31	23	17	15	11	—	—	—
	1600	410	185	105	67	46	38	30	23	18	15	—	—	—
	2960	750	340	190	125	85	61	46	39	30	24	—	—	—
40	1210	310	135	76	48	37	30	23	17	13	—	—	—	—
	1670	420	190	105	67	46	38	30	23	17	—	—	—	—
	3080	780	350	195	125	84	60	44	37	28	—	—	—	—
45	1230	310	135	75	47	36	26	22	16	—	—	—	—	—
	1710	430	190	105	65	44	36	26	20	—	—	—	—	—
	3140	790	350	190	120	81	57	41	34	—	—	—	—	—
50	1230	310	135	73	45	36	26	19	—	—	—	—	—	—
	1710	420	185	100	63	41	35	24	—	—	—	—	—	—
	3140	780	340	185	115	76	52	39	—	—	—	—	—	—

Upper figure, 5% level, 80% power; middle figure, 5% level, 90% power; and lower figure, 1% level, 90% power.
* One-sided—compares new treatment to standard treatment.
This table is organized to be used in planning clinical studies comparing a new treatment to an accepted or standard treatment. For example, suppose a surgical procedure is associated with a 50% recurrence rate at 6 months and a study is designed to incorporate a chemotherapeutic agent combined with surgery and this approach is expected to reduce the recurrence rate to 25% at 6 months. How many animals will be needed to address this in a clinical trial? Larger minus smaller rate (50 − 25 = 25) column headed 25 and smaller rate percent, headed 25. At the 80% power, 5% level (p = value) 45 animals will be needed in each arm of the study.

of 5% ($p = 0.05$), 45 animals would need to be studied in each arm of the study.

CRITERIA FOR EVALUATING THERAPY

The design of a clinical trial must include clear definitions of what is meant by remission time and survival time. Thus, the length of remission must be measured from an unequivocal starting point, such as the date when the animal is free of disease, to an unequivocal endpoint, such as the date of death or tumor recurrence. The methods used to measure the response to therapy must also be defined (*e.g.*, radiography, caliper measurement, biochemical assays, and so forth). The survival time is usually defined as the time between the date of histologic diagnosis and the time of death. In evaluating the effectiveness of a particular therapy, it is important to know whether the animals in the study die from natural causes or were euthanatized, and whether or not death was related to the tumor under study. A postmortem must therefore be done on *every* animal in a clinical study.

FOLLOW-UP PROCEDURES

An important aspect of every clinical trial is the frequency of follow-up examinations and the length of time that the patients who participated in the trial are followed after completing the therapy protocols. This information is of vital importance in the statistical evaluation of the results of the trial. Thus, the frequency of radiographic, hematologic, and other clinical examinations must be decided on in advance, as should the length of the follow-up period. For instance, a study may be continued until all animals that took part in it are dead, or for an arbitrary length of time such as 2 years or 5 years, depending on the purpose of the study.

It is often a mistake to plan a study for too long a period because the number of animals referred usually drops off after 3 to 4 years, new treatments are developed, and the clinic may not have sufficient resources to maintain the study.

STATISTICAL CONSIDERATIONS[5,6]

In a clinical trial, the analysis generally revolves around a time length measurement (*e.g.*, remission or survival). A number of statistical methods (survival curves) can be used to compare time intervals; these are the Kaplan–Meier methods, Log rank, the Breslow method, and the Savage method. Survival curves present results of the trial pictorially, helping avoid pitfalls that may result from reliance on numerical summaries only. An important consideration involving these types of survival or time length curves is how to account for study subjects who die of other causes or are lost or withdrawn from the study. These individuals are referred to as "censored" individuals.

An extensive review of the design and analysis of clinical trials points out that median survival times, though often used, are inefficient for comparing treatment groups, and average (mean) survival times are even worse. It is more accurate to analyze the survival difference by means of an appropriate statistical test to compare the differences between two survival curves.[4-6]

MISCELLANEOUS CONSIDERATIONS

The design of every clinical trial should include detailed instructions on the treatment of patients who fail the therapy, a written form of consent for experimental therapies (to be signed by the animal's owner), and the method of recording information on each patient.

COOPERATIVE CLINICAL TRIALS

Cooperative clinical trials—that is, trials done simultaneously at two or more institutions—have the advantage that a large number of animals and a wide range of tumor types can be obtained for the study in a shorter period of time than would be possible at any one institution. However, it is imperative that animals at the cooperating institutions be evaluated and treated *exactly* according to the therapy protocol. There are, therefore, certain requirements of institutions that cooperate in a clinical trial. The most important requirements are:

1. An established, reliable, retrievable medical records system
2. Clinical support facilities (*e.g.*, clinical pathology laboratory, radiographic equipment)
3. The ability to make accurate histologic diagnoses of tissues (histology slides must be available for pathology review)
4. Staff and methods for following up patients
5. A designated person to be responsible for the study on a day-to-day basis

Veterinary medicine has always been in a unique position to help advance knowledge of diseases. Veterinary oncology can and should assume a greater role in understanding cancer in humans, both its etiology and its control. Well-designed clinical cancer studies can offer significant advances in effective cancer therapy of animals and of humans. The most important aspects of a clinical trial are design, implementation, and data acquisition. No matter how much analysis is used, if the proper data are not collected uniformly on all patients, the full potential of the study will never be realized.

REFERENCES

1. Simon RM: Design and conduct of clinical trials. In DeVita VT, Hellman S, Rosenberg SA (eds): Cancer: Principles and Practice of Oncology, ed 2, pp. 329–350. Philadelphia, J.B. Lippincott, 1985
2. Carter SK: The design of clinical trials. In Theilen GH, Madewell BR (eds): Veterinary Cancer Medicine, ed 2, pp. 93–104. Philadelphia, Lea & Febiger, 1987

3. Dixon DO: Sample size for clinical trials. Cancer Bull 32:207–213, 1980
4. Matthews DE, Farewell VT: The question of sample size. In Using and Understanding Medical Statistics, pp. 184–195. Basel, S Karger, 1985
5. Peto R, Pike MC, Armitage P, et al: Design and analysis of randomized clinical trials requiring prolonged observations of each patient. I. Introduction and design. Br J Cancer 34:585–612, 1976
6. Peto R, Pike MC, Armitage P, et al: Design and analysis of randomized clinical trials requiring prolonged observations of each patient. II. Analysis and examples. Br J Cancer 35:1–39, 1977

32

THE VETERINARIAN'S ROLE IN PET LOSS: GRIEF EDUCATION, SUPPORT, AND FACILITATION

Laurel S. Lagoni
Suzanne Hetts
Stephen J. Withrow

A textbook devoted to the treatment of cancer in companion animals is evidence of the rapid and significant changes veterinary medicine has experienced during the past 10 years. Not only has the technical medicine aspect of the field changed but so have the roles veterinarians play in delivering health care to companion animals. Veterinarians' roles have changed because pets' roles in families have changed.

Families can be thought of as systems. Each family member fills a role in order to keep the system in a state of homeostasis or balance. Family structures have evolved from the traditional nuclear family to increasingly prevalent models such as never-married singles, childless dual-career couples, and widowed elderly women and men. Partially as a result of these life-style changes, companion animals have come to serve certain functions in balancing family systems. For many people pets are like children, parents, or friends;[1] they are significant members of the family. Many pets assume almost "people status" within the family system.[2]

Substantiating this statement is research showing that 56% of dog owners allow their dog to sleep on a bed with a family member, 64% give their dog tidbits from the table, and 54% celebrate their dog's birthday. Further evidence reports that 91% of cat owners carry pictures of their cat in their wallets or display them at home, and 91% believe that their cat understands their moods and emotions.[3] Today's veterinarians are treating important family members. In fact, clients most often compare their veterinarians to their pediatricians. Perhaps this is because both doctors care for the most dependent and vulnerable members of families.[4]

With pets playing such important roles in families, the illness or death of a companion animal can unbalance the family and trigger a grief response comparable to that caused by the loss of a human family member or friend. However, there is one significant difference between grief for humans and grief for pets. *Society does not generally support grief over the death of a pet and thus there are few available support systems for the bereaved pet owner.*[5]

Veterinarians who want to remain on the cutting edge of veterinary medicine will consider expanding the priorities of their practice in order to better respond to their human clients' beliefs and values about companion animals. Goals for these veterinarians may include:

1. Learning to deal better under stress and to feel more comfortable dealing with the emotions surrounding pet loss
2. Devising ways to educate their clients about normal grief responses
3. Supporting clients more effectively during times of crisis

In order to accomplish these goals, it is important to become knowledgeable about the nature of the human–companion animal bond and about the nature of grief.

ATTACHMENT AND LOSS

Perhaps more than any other disease or illness, the diagnosis of cancer or a malignancy instantly conjures up preconceived ideas. For many people, it predicts suffering and death. Regardless of the ultimate outcome, the diagnosis of cancer (or other serious illness) creates changes in the family system. For example, significant differences of opinion may exist among family members regarding the choice of treatment options. Caring for the sick animal, as well as making additional visits to the veterinarian, may require difficult changes in the family schedule. The cost of veterinary care may necessitate a restructuring of financial priorities, and this, plus the difficulties inherent in communicating about death and dying, can escalate tensions. Each family member may react to the pet's illness differently not only because each relationship with the pet is unique, but because individual members have different beliefs about the quality of the pet's life.

Experiencing any of these variables results in feelings of loss for each person connected to the pet. Loss associated with companion animals is experienced in many ways besides through death. Feelings of loss occur when a limb is amputated, when daily walks are suspended, and when exuberant greetings disappear. Especially significant is the loss of the naivete that allows pet owners to deny that their pets will die before they do.

People who choose to treat their pet's cancer invest significant amounts of time, money, and emotional energy in an attempt to do everything they can for their animal, even though the overall cure rate for all malignancies is only about 30%. Obviously, these clients have particularly strong attachments and commitments to their pets. Above-average attachments and commitments are formed for a variety of reasons. For example, pet owners may have lived with a pet during a significant or difficult time in their lives or they may currently live alone with their pet. In these circumstances, people often view their pets as their main sources of social support, reporting that their companion animals are always there for them. Because of these feelings, many strongly attached owners decide to do everything possible for their pet as they wish to reciprocate the support the pet has given them. Thus, the death of a pet who was relied on through "the rough times" can threaten the owner's well-being and sense of security. Sometimes the attachment between an owner and the companion animal grows stronger after the owner learns that the pet is ill. This frequently happens when the pet and a family member or close friend have both been diagnosed with cancer. Although there is no validating empirical research, clinical experience suggests that a certain percentage of clients have experienced the treatment or death of a parent, spouse, sibling, or child who had a cancer similar to that of their pet's. Sometimes, the clients themselves have undergone treatment for the same kind of cancer. This is not surprising in that current statistics predict that one in four U.S. citizens will develop cancer in his or her lifetime.

In these circumstances, the pet with cancer can become symbolic of many conflicting feelings and attitudes. Depending on the pet's response to treatment, it may come to represent hope, a "fighting spirit," the will to live, or the right to a peaceful, painless, and dignified death. The pet's situation may symbolize a parallel human situation and represent the range of options and outcomes that owners wish for themselves and their loved ones.

Companion animals can also be a symbolic link to a significant person no longer in a client's life. For instance, the pet may have been a gift from a friend or relative who has since died, or the pet may have been the special friend of an adult or a child now living far away. Often the pet is associated with a person who is alive but with whom the owner no longer has a relationship. Facing the possibility of the animal's death may trigger the unresolved feelings of loss still associated with that significant other.

GRIEF

Loss is pervasive in everyone's life, yet it often goes unrecognized. People find it difficult to acknowledge loss and even more difficult to permit themselves to experience the feelings of grief that naturally accompany a loss. Grief is a normal and healthy response to loss. At times, however, it seems unnatural because the nature and symptomatology of grief are unfamiliar to much of society.

One of the most important ways a veterinarian can assist grieving clients is to educate and reassure them that their feelings and behaviors are normal parts of the grief response. It may also be helpful to remind clients that pet loss is a socially negated loss. It is regarded as a trivial loss, and grieving pet owners may be characterized as "crazy," "hysterical," or "overly sensitive." As of yet, there are no socially sanctioned rituals such as funerals, wakes, or memorial services to help people draw closure to the loss of a pet. However, grief as a response to pet loss is not trivial, nor should it be reduced in concept to a "rehearsal" or preparation for the experience of human loss. It is a normal reaction to the loss of a significant part of a client's daily life.

Perhaps the most well-known theories pertaining to the grief response are those of Dr. Elizabeth Kubler–Ross. She outlined five "stages" of grief, including denial, anger, bargaining, depression, and acceptance.[6] Although these responses are usually part of normal grieving, grief is probably better described as a process rather than a series of sequential stages. Many other physical sensations, behaviors, and feelings are usually a part of normal grief, including appetite and sleep disturbances, inability to concentrate, restlessness, auditory or visual hallucinations, depression, "empty" feelings, tightness in the throat or chest, longing, loneliness, and a desire to be with or join the deceased. This last symptom represents a normal response to loss and is different from a suicidal reaction.

Grief is often referred to as "grief work," and alternative models to Kubler–Ross's describe tasks of mourning which theorists believe bereaved persons must accomplish in order to reconcile a loss. One such model was developed by Dr. J. William Worden of the Harvard Medical School and is especially pertinent here because of its relevance to pet loss. Dr. Worden states, "The well-being of the family and those close to a dying or recently deceased person is part of the health professionals' responsibility. Health care providers and the institutions they serve must understand the impact of grief and be sensitive to the needs of the bereaved by offering both support and information."[7]

The first task of mourning described by Dr. Worden is to accept the reality of the loss. Even in the case of a death from cancer where the family may have observed the deteriorating condition of the patient, there is a certain sense of unreality when the family learns that the patient is dead. Before people are able to face reality, veterinarians will see many examples of shock and denial and may feel that they are not "getting through" to their clients. By normalizing their grief and educating clients about the grief process, clinicians can support them through completion of this task.

Worden's second task of mourning is to experience the pain of the loss. Pain and grief are normally displayed outwardly through facial expressions, body postures, and emotions like crying or sobbing. Visible grief sometimes causes discomfort in people who are around the mourner who may then attempt to cut short this natural process. Veterinarians can facilitate this difficult task by accepting people's pain and giving them permission to show it. A very simple way to encourage clients to grieve openly is to have facial tissues available in exam rooms, in waiting rooms, and in private offices.

Adjusting to the loss is the third task of mourning. The ease of adjustment often depends on what the relationship was with the deceased and the role the pet played in the owner's life. Owners whose pets have played central roles in their lives can be expected to experience more difficult adjustments than owners whose pets have been on the peripheries of everyday routines.

Withdrawing emotional energy from the deceased and reinvesting energy in other relationships and activities is the fourth task in Worden's model. This is particularly relevant to pet loss. Bereaved owners are often encouraged to get another pet long before they are ready for one. Society's belief that pets are replaceable has trivialized pet loss and done much to thwart pet owners' movements through the natural grief process. Owners should be allowed to decide for themselves when they are ready for new pets. A new animal should probably not be obtained if the primary goal, wish, or expectation is to find one who is "just like" the deceased pet.[7]

EUTHANASIA

In spite of the fact that euthanasia is a difficult process for the owner and veterinarian alike, it is a privilege when conducted in an appropriate manner. Appropriate intervention to stop unmanageable pain and suffering is an act of kindness, not malice. Some pet owners seem to be able to decide, with a minimum of conflict, that euthanasia is the last humane and loving gift that they can give their dying companion animal. Others resist making the decision, reporting feeling as though they were deciding to kill their best friend. Feelings like these usually result in canceled appointments, stalled decisions, and guilt. Indecision and guilt are normal, yet frustrating for all involved. Guilt is especially difficult to cope with. Most pet owners have an intense awareness that their pet is totally dependent on them for care and for life itself. After the death of a pet, many owners are plagued with thoughts that they could have done more or that they in some way contributed to their pet's illness. Guilt serves to intensify and sometimes prolong or inhibit the normal grief process.

Clients deal more effectively with decision-making and the resulting feelings of grief when they realize that the grief process for most begins long before the actual death of a pet. Anticipatory grief is the reaction to the threat of loss and occurs quite often throughout the course of cancer treatment. Decision-making conflict and guilt feelings start at the time of diagnosis, when the client is encouraged to treat an often ultimately fatal disease. On one hand is the hope for remission or cure and on the other hand,

the realization that death from cancer waits ahead. As the animal's condition worsens, owners may begin to accept the reality of the impending death. However, if the animal improves, owners find themselves on an "emotional roller coaster" ranging from denial to hope to acceptance and back again. Recognizing that clients can and do grieve before the death of a pet can help in understanding the sense of alienation they sometimes feel toward their pet during the course of treatment. Alienation can be a defense mechanism and can be used to detach or dis-invest energy from ill pets. If a sense of alienation persists, owners may want to euthanize an animal before it is necessary, in an attempt to stop their own pain. An alert veterinarian can use this as a "teachable moment" and help people realize the extent of their grief. Then, even if the euthanasia takes place, the owner may be more able to allow the grief feelings to come and go naturally instead of suppressing them and denying that they exist.

THE VETERINARIAN'S ROLE IN PET LOSS

The diagnosis and treatment of a potentially life-threatening illness is a painful, upsetting, and stressful time for families and veterinarians alike. The death of a pet can be traumatic and even devastating. Men and women who have chosen careers in veterinary medicine find themselves in unique situations when faced with stressed or grieving families. Sensitive veterinarians work hard to create positive, caring environments and, consequently, gain the trust and respect of their clients. Because their knowledge, skills, and attitudes help people feel secure during their pet's healthy times, they are also relied on for emotional help during a pet's illness and death. This added role, however, can create problems for clients as well as for the veterinary team as, all too often, neither party knows quite what to expect from the other.

The shock, denial, and fear of ridicule people feel at the time of a pet's death may keep them from turning to their usual sources of support. Bereaved pet owners may shy away from confiding in friends or family, knowing that their grief may be ridiculed or misunderstood. Lacking other empathetic supports, clients often turn to the person who has shown consistent interest in their pet—their veterinarian.

During the treatment of a chronic disease like cancer, veterinarians fill the role of caregiver. Quite often, because they have spent time with families, they become "affiliate family members," privy to their human clients' private lives and to their deepest feelings of loss and grief. Because of this "affiliate family member" status, the boundaries between being a professional outsider and a family member sometimes become blurred. When this happens, some clients aren't satisfied to allow veterinarians to remain on the outside but rather insist that they become part of the family and take part in all aspects of their crisis.

What, then, is the veterinarian's role in pet loss? How much involvement is healthy both for clients and for their veterinarians? Since role ambiguity is correlated with job tension, job satisfaction, self-esteem, and depression these are important questions to explore.[8–10]

In terms of pet loss and the grief process, it might be easier to begin to define what the veterinarian's role is by first defining what it is not:

Veterinarians are not psychiatrists, psychologists, social workers, or family therapists. Most veterinarians are compassionate and want to help their human clients in any way they can. It's tempting for many to take advantage of their role as "affiliate family members" and step in to "fix" communication difficulties, relationship strains, or other problems that prevent the family from working together. Unfortunately, though, without therapeutic training, this "fixing" often takes the form of problem-solving, advice-giving, or rescuing, none of which are helpful or appropriate when dealing with another person's emotions.

The best way to avoid this dilemma is to learn to draw boundaries and set limits. Veterinarians should ask themselves how much they are really willing to do for their clients' recoveries. Once veterinarians learn to identify their own personal boundaries between support and over-commitment, they begin to feel more comfortable about referring clients to human service professionals. Clients who are having difficulties with any of the tasks of mourning can be gently and legitimately referred to a therapist or grief counselor. Suggesting to clients that they see a grief coun-

selor with whom the veterinarian is acquainted does not mean that they are being viewed as "crazy" or "over the edge." It simply means that the veterinarian has recognized that some clients have needs that veterinarians have not, as yet, been trained to meet.

Veterinarians are not members of the clergy. Clients sometimes begin to question their religious beliefs during the grieving process. They may feel that their God or higher power has betrayed them or let them down by "letting their pet die." Without this source of strength, they may turn to their veterinarian for emotional help. When veterinarians find themselves working very hard to reaffirm their clients' religious beliefs, they have probably crossed the boundary between offering support and "fixing" a problem. Referring clients to someone who can help sort out their religious beliefs about pet death can comfort them and help facilitate the grief process.

Veterinarians are not suicide prevention workers. Occasionally, a client hints at suicide or designates the end of his pet's life as the end of his own. While it is very important to take these threats seriously and to ask a client outright if they are considering suicide, the veterinarian's role in suicide prevention is limited. Veterinarians can listen openly to what a client has to say and assess the lethality of the situation. This is done by determining if the client has decided on a method and a plan for suicide, and if he has begun to act on that plan. If the client has taken such steps, the lethality of the situation is high; it may be appropriate to notify the police or county mental health facility. If the client does not articulate a specific method or plan, it is not appropriate, in most cases, to intervene in any way except to refer the client to a reputable mental health worker.

Every veterinarian should know what local professionals to contact in case a potential or attempted suicide needs to be reported. Suicide resource networks (hotlines, emergency clinics, therapists) should be researched and telephone numbers made available to everyone involved in the case. Actual suicides due to pet loss are rare, but in case a suicidal client does call a veterinarian for help, it's imperative to know what to do.

If veterinarians find themselves making pacts or contracts with suicidal clients (*i.e.*, "Promise to call me if you think you're going to hurt yourself") of if they attempt to make a rescue without professional help, they are in over their heads. Professional ethics dictate that veterinarians keep the boundaries between treating animals and treating humans clear.

Veterinarians are not members of their clients' families. It's normal for a sense of closeness and intimacy to develop between veterinarians and some of their clients, especially those for whom the clinician has provided long-term care. However, client requests that the veterinarian make the final decision regarding issues like euthanasia or surgery must be denied and given back to the family. Leaving decisions up to the family is healthier for both client and veterinarian— even if the outcome is different from what the veterinarian believed would be the best decision. When veterinarians find themselves caught up with family decisions or find they have angry, volatile feelings toward their clients, the boundaries between affiliate family member and professional may have been crossed.

Veterinarians are (in addition to their primary role of medical expert) educators, facilitators, and sources of support. They are also business people who share the need and desire to recruit new clients while maintaining their loyal ones. By learning to maintain the delicate balance between educating (talking), supporting (listening), and facilitating (acting), veterinarians will automatically enhance their skills at practice management.

THE ROLE OF EDUCATOR

Death education is a controversial subject. Opinions range from the belief that people should be educated formally about death to the belief that learning should take place during "teachable moments" only as part of the natural grief process.[11] In terms of veterinary medicine, where the death of a pet is a nearly inevitable part of pet ownership, a case for formalized education can be made. Veterinarians who recognize the impact of loss may take steps to educate themselves, their staffs, and their clients about the grief process. This is done in many ways. Perhaps two of the most important ways are by making books, pamphlets, videos, and grief counselors available to clients and by sponsoring educational workshops, trainings, or even support groups for colleagues and clients.

THE ROLE OF SUPPORT PERSON

Lending support means being available to listen to the nonmedical concerns of clients without taking action toward solving their problems. Lending support to a grieving client means normalizing their sense of loss, giving them permission to grieve, and listening to them as they remember the good times with their pet as well as struggle with its death. Listening is an overlooked skill in veterinary medicine. Veterinarians often deal with nonresponsive clients (who are in shock) by repeating themselves and saying too much. Grieving people often find just sitting with someone in understanding silence infinitely more comforting than talking.

Much of support is nonverbal. Veterinarians can show this by lightly touching a client's arm or by allowing tears of their own to fall when they participate in or learn of a pet's death. Nonverbal support during euthanasia is especially important and can be communicated in several ways. Scheduling euthanasias during a quiet time of the day and allowing clients to prepay are two of the best ways. Allowing them to be present at the euthanasia, to stay with the body afterwards, and to use an alternate way out of the office in order to avoid the waiting room are three others.

THE ROLE OF FACILITATOR

Facilitators ask, suggest, remind, and attempt to gain consensus on decisions. They try to stay neutral and provide just enough structure so that emotions and interpersonal issues don't interfere with the task at hand. Veterinarians spend a great deal of time facilitating decision-making processes and the resulting emotional responses of their clients.

Elizabeth Kubler-Ross calls death the final stage of growth. She advocates planning and preparing for it during healthy times so that last-minute decisions don't have to be made during a crisis. Facilitation of the grief process can begin the first time a veterinarian sees a client. By taking a life-span approach to health care, clinicians can help clients face the inevitability of their pet's death and help them to prepare and plan for it. A way to begin an open discussion of death and grief in a veterinary practice is to consistently say, "When your pet dies," as opposed to "If your pet dies." This can help clients face the inevitable reality of loss.

Veterinarians can also make information about cremation, burial memorials, and good-bye rituals available to their clients at all times, not just at the time of an illness or death. This will encourage them to think ahead and plan for their pet's death. Knowing ahead of time what will be most meaningful to all involved will make the decisions about treatment, euthanasia, and disposal of the body easier when it actually happens.

Because the procedure of euthanasia is somewhat unique to veterinary medicine, we will describe several concrete steps that can be taken to facilitate a client's bereavement at the time of euthanasia. These steps would be appropriate, however, no matter how the pet's death occurs.

When clients feel the time has come to euthanatize, encourage them to bring a friend or family member with them for support. Encouraging them to ask another person for help is very important because many people believe they shouldn't impose their burdens on anyone else. If whole families have been involved in the ongoing treatment of their pet, encourage all of them to be present at the euthanasia. This includes children. Most children are resilient and deal with death better when they are included in the grief process than when they are "protected" or left out. Even very young children intuitively know when a crisis has occurred. If they are not talked to about it, they may feel they did something wrong or even that they in some way were responsible for the death.

Before the euthanasia, procedures should be explained and clients should be told exactly what to expect. Everyone involved should be allowed to decide for themselves whether or not to be present during the euthanasia. Many clients have a desire to be with their pet as it dies, but don't feel they have the right to be in on a "medical procedure" unless the veterinarian has invited them. Most will be extremely grateful for the option. Good-byes should be said while the pet is still alive. Family members often need permission from the veterinarian to do this. A sentence or two can help families overcome the awkwardness of the situation and say and do what they need to in order to draw closure to the relationship with their pet.

After the euthanasia, allow the family to be with the body for as long as they desire. If some family members elected not to be present at the time of death, allow them to view the body afterwards. Viewing the body is important no matter what the mode of death. There is nothing like the confrontation with a beloved pet's body to bring home the reality of a loss. Viewing the body makes death real and tangible. It sets the stage for acceptance and recovery. "A program that encourages this and makes provision for it can make an important contribution to bereavement."[7]

Suggesting that clients determine an appropriate and meaningful way to say a final good-bye to their pet may be the final step in facilitating a euthanasia. Funerals, memorials, scrapbooks, or tree plantings are rituals that have been carried out by many bereaved pet owners. A ritualized good-bye helps validate the loss and can encourage conversation about the pet who has died. Talking about a pet and remembering the various episodes and phases of its life can help clients deal with the feelings of sadness, anger, guilt, relief, and anxiety that they may experience. As with any death, condolence letters should be sent to the owners immediately after the death with information about the grief process and grief counseling services enclosed.

CLIENT GRIEF AND PRACTICE MANAGEMENT

Pet owners elect to use veterinary services and select specific veterinarians for a variety of reasons. These factors include the type of bond that exists between people and their pets, the role of the pet in the family, their past experiences with veterinarians, and their beliefs about the outcomes of veterinary care.[4] In addition, a survey of owner attitudes revealed that 15% of former pet owners do not currently own a pet because the pain experienced when the pet died was too great.[12] In order for a veterinarian to maintain a healthy practice, new clients must be attracted and old ones must be retained. Because the death of a pet is such a traumatic and stressful event, the veterinarian's conduct during that time will most likely be remembered. If clients feel their veterinarians were distant, stoic, or calloused, they may never return to that practice. Instead, they will most likely choose veterinarians who are perceived as compassionate, caring, and sensitive to their and their pets' needs.

The December 1985 issue of *The Futurist* magazine predicted that a glut of veterinarians would persist in the United States during the 1980s. By 1990, the forecast said, there will be 40,000 veterinarians.[13] Although this is double the 1960 figure, job opportunities have not doubled correspondingly. Thus, from a pragmatic practice management perspective, learning how to better deal with pet loss, client grief, and the physical and emotional stresses inherent in the practice of veterinary medicine makes good business sense.

COMMON QUESTIONS AND ANSWERS

Colorado State University's Veterinary Teaching Hospital has established a grief education and support program called CHANGES: Support for People and Pets. CHANGES offers clients support during the emotionally difficult times of diagnosis, treatment, the euthanasia or death of a pet, and the days, weeks, months, and even years during which clients are actively grieving.

In the process of working with over 700 clients, the CHANGES program has identified several questions that veterinarians have asked repeatedly. These questions, and brief versions of their answers, are included here so that several issues not focused on in the text of this chapter may be addressed.

1. What mental health professionals are available should I decide to refer a client for additional emotional support? Many professional resources including hospice workers, crisis intervention teams, psychiatrists, psychologists, family therapists, social workers, members of the clergy, grief counselors, and numerous grief-oriented support groups may be accessible to members of your community. The most important consideration, though, is whether or not the professional is sensitive and understanding about pet loss and its subsequent grief responses. In the mental health field, as in the population as a whole, some people do not take the death of a pet seriously and may trivialize or discount the genuine feelings of loss and grief experienced by the client. It goes without saying that this type of professional would not be an appropriate resource person.

It would be wise to contact these professionals before they are actually needed in order to determine the best possible resources available to you. Evaluating a mental health worker's sensitivity to and familiarity with pet loss issues should be your prime consideration.

2. How do I refer a client to a mental health professional? Traditionally, it may have been viewed as inappropriate for a veterinarian to make this type of referral. However, with the field of veterinary medicine changing in many ways and for many reasons, referring clients to other helping professionals can demonstrate that your concern and caring extends to them as well as to their animals.

One way of referring is to use an analogy like, "If you had a broken leg, you would not try to care for it yourself. You also would not ignore it for days and weeks at a time as you experienced a lot of pain. I can see that you are in a great deal of pain right now and that you are trying to take care of it by yourself. I would like to tell you about someone who can help support you through this painful time." Another way is to offer concrete explanations of why you believe in making referrals to outside professionals. You might say, "If your child or parent was dying, a natural support system would exist for you within the hospital or the medical field. Unfortunately, this does not, as yet, exist within the veterinary medicine field, so it is necessary for us to form them ourselves. Although I myself am not trained to deal with grief issues, I know a professional therapist who is." Only rarely will clients take offense at a gentle suggestion that they seek additional help. Even if the client refuses your offer, you have demonstrated concern, and the client may take you up on it at a later date.

3. How can I best help my staff deal with euthanasias and pet loss issues? Health care professionals need to be aware of each others' feelings and needs. Because the time to perform euthanasias varies from client to client, technician to technician, and veterinarian to veterinarian, potential conflicts and anxieties can occur. For the average health care team [veterinarian(s), animal health technician(s), and receptionist(s)], it is important to communicate and discuss the many issues surrounding loss, grief, and euthanasias. This way, hospital or practice policies and procedures can be somewhat standardized.

Formal and informal meetings that allow free and open expression of problems or "staffings" of tough cases (discussions focusing on one case in particular with treatment strategizing as the goal) help ease the isolation and remorse that all veterinary professionals feel. Debriefing and support group sessions within the veterinary practice itself is healthy and helps manage stress build-up.

In addition, everyone involved in a case should clearly understand that client confusion and angry outbursts are normal responses to loss and common manifestations of the grief process. The most important aspects of dealing with confusion and anger are patience and detachment. Knowing that clients are angry at the situation and not at the veterinary professional helps calm everyone involved. Don't take anger personally as it will only make a difficult situation even harder.

4. What can I say to clients who ask me, "What shall I tell my kids?" Children who are told about death in an honest and open way can resolve losses just as favorably as adults. In order for this to happen, they need to receive prompt and accurate information about what has occurred and be allowed to ask questions and explore their feelings. Two of the best ways to include children in the grief process and to show them that their questions and feelings are welcome are to consistently support them with words ("You're not alone, I'm with you") and touch (hugs, hand-holding, backrubs, a light touch on the arm).

Children often believe that their own thoughts, wishes, and actions have the power to cause a death (*i.e.*, "I wished Pepper was dead so he'd leave me alone and now he is!"). The clear message that must be given to children is, "Pepper's death was not your fault. He died because he had a disease called cancer. There was nothing you could have done to make things different."

Parents sometimes think of a pet's death as a rehearsal for the "real thing." They feel that children will deal with a human loss better once they've experienced pet loss. This belief can tend to diminish the importance of a pet's death in adult eyes. Consequently, it may not be given it's due attention. Parents should understand

that pet loss is not a rehearsal. It is the "real thing" to a child. Whether or not they are better able to deal with the loss of a human loved one later depends, to a large extent, on the quality of care they receive during their first experience with death. Parents should talk openly about the dead pet and about their memories of it. Children need to know that each and every member of the family is important and always will be important. If the pet becomes a taboo subject, dramatic anxieties and behavior problems can occur (*i.e.*, "If you can forget that quickly about Pepper, you won't remember me when I die either!").

5. How can I help clients deal with guilt? Guilt is the critic inside our heads. The voice that judges our thoughts, actions, behaviors, decisions, and feelings comes from childhood experiences, parents, teachers, and societal expectations. Two ways to help clients deal with guilt are to ask them to stop judging themselves and to help them learn something from the experience. When people stop judging their decisions (euthanasia, treatment) or behaviors (crying, confusion), they begin to see that most of life is not right or wrong, black and white, but gray. They understand that they did the best they could at the time and they can't ask for more of themselves than that. Veterinarians can help reinforce this by validating feelings, decisions, behaviors, and thoughts and by gently saying, "I believe that you did everything that you could. What would you have done differently?" Usually, people realize that they would not have done anything differently and will soon get on with the business of grieving.

Many clients also have the ability to learn a positive lesson from an otherwise negative experience. Helping clients learn about themselves through the process of grieving is a skill that everyone dealing with bereavement will find helpful.

Sometimes clients have done or not done something that promotes genuine guilt. Negligent or abusive treatment of animals are two examples of this. Once clients have recognized their errors, however, some of the guilt can be alleviated. It is more beneficial to help them make a decision about what they will do *next* time rather than to help them go over and over the past looking for an answer to what went wrong last time. When clients seem to be firmly stuck on the guilt merry-go-round, a referral to a mental health professional is appropriate.

6. What do I do when a client cries? Crying is a normal and natural response to loss. Many people struggle to control their tears because they anticipate and often get unsupportive reactions from others. The negative reactions from others, though, are more often due to their own feelings of helplessness than to feelings of embarrassment or disgust. In one study, 80% of the women and 74% of the men reported feeling sympathetic when other people cried. Several people also indicated that they wanted to respond in a supportive manner when someone else cried, but they didn't know what to do or say.[14]

Experts in bereavement recommend several supportive ways to respond to a crying client:

Stay quietly nearby
Maintain an open body posture, but do not initiate conversation
Cry along with the client if it feels natural, but refrain from losing control
When the client stops crying, demonstrate a willingness to listen by asking questions like, "How can I help?" This will communicate respect for the client's emotions and reassurance that the tears have not offended or caused any discomfort.

Crying is an effective way to relieve stress and to express emotions. People who are actively encouraged to cry may develop more resiliency when in crisis and may even be more in touch with the healing aspects of the grief process.

REFERENCES

1. Veevers J: The social meaning of pets: Alternative roles for companion animals. Marriage and Family Review 8:3,4, 1985

2. Cain A: Pets as family members. Marriage and Family Review 8:3,4, 1985

3. Voith V: Attachment of people to companion animals. In Quackenbush J, Voith V (eds): Symposium on the Human–Companion Animal Bond. Vet Clin North Am (Small Anim Pract) 15:2, 1985

4. Charles, Charles and Associates Marketing Management Consultants: Studies summary and report on promoting veterinary services. The Veterinary Services Market, Vol. I. Overland Park, Kansas, July, 1983

5. Bernbaum M: The veterinarian's role in grief and bereavement at pet loss. Cornell Feline Health Center News 7:1–7, 1982

6. Kubler–Ross E: On Death and Dying. New York, Macmillan, 1969

7. Worden JW: Bereavement. Semin Oncol 12:472–475, 1985

8. Kahn RL, Wolfe DM, Quinn RP, Snoek JD, Rosenthal RA: Organizational stress: Studies in Role Conflict and Ambiguity. New York, Wiley, 1964

9. French JRP, Caplan RD: Psychosocial factors in coronary heart disease. Ind Med 39:383–397, 1970

10. Kahn RL: Conflict, ambiguity, and overload: Three elements in job stress. Occup Ment Health 3:2–9, 1973

11. Cook A, Oltjenbruns K, Lagoni L: The "ripple effect" of a university sponsored death and dying symposium. Omega 15:2, 1984–1985

12. Wilbur RH: Pets, pet ownership, and animal control: Social and psychological attitudes. In Proceedings of the National Conference on Dog and Cat Control, pp. 21–34. Denver, American Humane Association, 1976

13. Cornish E: Outlook '86—and beyond. The Futurist, Dec, 51–60, 1985

14. Frey WH: Crying: The mystery of tears. Minneapolis, Winston Press, 1985

GUIDELINES FOR HANDLING CYTOTOXIC AGENTS

E. Gregory MacEwen

In the past few years there has been an increasing concern regarding the risk for nurses and physicians handling cytotoxic agents. Although there is no evidence that handling antineoplastic drugs has caused cancer, concern about the potential occupational risk to pharmacists, nurses, and physicians has prompted several studies that have attempted to determine whether mutagenic activity is a reliable assay of occupational exposure. A letter published in the *Lancet* in 1979[1] reported that significant levels of mutagenic activity could be detected in the urine of nurses preparing chemotherapeutic augents, and in that of patients receiving the drugs. Mutagenic activity could not, however, be detected in the urine of exposed control subjects working in the same general environment. More recent studies have evaluated individuals wearing protective clothing who prepare drugs using vertical or horizontal lamina or airflow cabinets.[2,3] These studies have demonstrated that mutagenic activity could not be detected in the urine when vertical-flow laminar safety cabinets were used, but that it could be detected when horizontal-flow laminar airflow cabinets were used. These data suggest that aerosolization of the agents during reconstitution represents a source of exposure. Based on the results of these studies, some recommendations have been developed by the Division of Safety of the National Institutes of Health.[4,4a]

1. Whenever possible, a special area should be set aside for the preparation of injectable agents. Drug reconstitution in a Class II vertical-flow biologic safety cabinet is considered preferable to a horizontal airflow cabinet, but not essential. In the absence of a vertical-flow hood, a mask and safety glasses are recommended

2. A disposable, plastic-backed sheet of absorbent paper should be used to cover the work surface area inside the cabinet to allow complete cleanup of inadvertent spills. The paper should be changed after any overt spills.

3. Latex gloves should be worn and discarded if holes develop. A long-sleeved gown should be worn to protect the skin from drug contact.

4. Drug ampules should be opened away from the face. The ampules should be wrapped with sterile gauze at the anticipated break point to minimize the risk of inhaling powders or aerosols and to protect against broken glass.

5. When a drug is reconstituted, the dilutant should be injected slowly down the side of the vial. The needle should be kept from coming in contact

with the solution, and the air should be allowed back into the syringe to equalize pressure.

6. A sterile alcohol swab should be placed over the needle as it is withdrawn from the vial to prevent aerosolization.

7. The needle should be covered by a sterile alcohol swab, or a sealed waste bottle when air bubbles are injected from a filled syringe to prevent aerosolization.

8. After reconstitution, the old needle should be replaced by a new one. A volume of air that is less than the volume of the drug solution to be withdrawn should be introduced into the vial. When the reconstituted drug is withdrawn, excess solution should be injected into a waste bottle.

9. The external surface of syringes and IV drug bottles should be wiped clean after reconstitution or admixture procedures and properly labeled and dated.

10. When the chemotherapy is mixed with large volumes of fluid for administration it is safer to use plastic fluid bags rather than glass in case the container is dropped.

11. Tablets should not be crushed or broken except in flow hoods due to aerosolization of powder.

12. Contaminated needles and syringes should be disposed of in a leak-proof, puncture-resistant container. Clipping needles is not recommended because the process can generate aerosols.

13. Hands should be washed carefully after gloves have been removed.

The disposal of antineoplastic drugs and contaminated material presents another potential source of drug exposure. Ideally, contaminated materials should be disposed of as hazardous waste.[5] It is advisable to contact the Environmental Protection Agency for specific disposal instructions. It is also very important to label all syringes and IV bottles and fluids containing chemotherapeutic agents with appropriate caution labels and disposal instructions.

In veterinary hospitals it is important to specifically train the people that are going to be preparing and administering these cytotoxic agents. It is advisable to minimize the number of people who come in contact with these substances. Ideally, one or two people should be the ones responsible for the preparation and administration of these drugs. Since some chemotherapeutic agents are administered orally by the owner at home, it is important to also educate the client about the potential risks regarding these agents. Owners should be advised to wear gloves when administering these drugs to their pets.

REFERENCES

1. Falck K, Grohn P, Sorsa M, et al: Mutagenicity in urine of nurses handling cytotoxic drugs. Lancet 1:1250–1251, 1979

2. Staiano N, Gallelli JF, Adamson RH, et al: Letter: Lack of mutagenic activity in urine from hospital pharmacists admixing antitumor drugs. Lancet 1:615–616, 1981

3. Anderson RW, Puciatt WH, Dana WJ, et al: Risk of handling injectable antineoplastic agents. Am J Hosp Pharm 39:881–887, 1982

4. Division of Safety, National Institutes of Health: Recommendations for Safe Handling of Parenteral Antineoplastic Drugs. NIH publ #83-2621, 1982

4a. Hubbard SM, Seipp CA: Administration of cancer treatments: Practical guide for physicians and oncology nurses. In DeVita VT Jr, Hellman S, Rosenberg SA (eds): Cancer: Principles and Practice of Oncology, 2nd ed, pp 2189–2222. Philadelphia, JB Lippincott, 1985

5. Vaccari PL, Tonat K, Dechristoforo R, et al: Disposal of antineoplastic waste at the National Institutes of Health. Am J Hosp Pharm 41:87–93, 1984

B

WORLD HEALTH ORGANIZATION
T N M
CLASSIFICATION OF TUMORS
IN DOMESTIC ANIMALS

Edited By

L. N. Owen

First Edition, Geneva—1980

C O N T E N T S

Introduction   448

The T N M system   449

The anatomical sites   453

Skin (excluding lymphosarcoma and   454
mastocytoma)

Skin—mastocytoma   456

Mammary glands   457

Head and neck   461

Alimentary system, pancreas, liver   466

Urological system   471

Genital system   473

Bones and joints   481

Lymphoid and haemopoietic tissues (including lymphosarcoma of skin)   483

Respiratory system   484

Endocrine glands (thyroid, adrenal)   486

INTRODUCTION

THE PURPOSE OF CLASSIFICATION

The practice of dividing cancer cases into groups according to "stages" has already been established for tumors of man.* The system arose from the fact that survival rates were higher for cases in which the disease was localized than for those in which the disease had extended beyond the organ of origin. These groups were often referred to as "early cases" and "late cases" implying some regular progression with time.

---

*UICC TNM Classification of Malignant Tumours, Ed. M. Harmer, 3rd ed., Geneva, 1978.

The stage of disease at the time of diagnosis may be a reflectiion, not only of the rate of growth and extension of the neoplasm, but also of the type of tumour, the tumour-host relationship and the interval between recognition of the first symptom or sign and the diagnosis or treatment.

The principal purpose of international agreement on classification of cancer cases by extent of disease is to provide a method of conveying one person's clinical observations to others without ambiguity.

The veterinary clinician's task is to make a provisional prognosis and a decision on the most effective course of treatment. These require, among other things, an objective assessment of the anatomical extent of the disease.

The objectives of staging animal tumours are:

1.   to aid the veterinary clinician in planning treatment
2.   to give some indication of prognosis
3.   to assist in evaluation of treatment results
4.   to facilitate the exchange of information between treatment centres
5.   to contribute to the continuing investigation of animal cancer
6.   to contribute information that is of comparative value between man and animal.

To meet these objectives a system of classification is required (1) in which the basic principles are applicable to all sites, regardless of treatment and (2) which may be supplemented later by information that becomes available from histopathology or surgery.

The TNM system meets these requirements. It provides an essential communication and information exchange device and a useful guide for prognosis and therapy.

THE TNM SYSTEM

The TNM system is based on the assessment of:

— the extent of the primary tumour   T
— the condition of the regional lymph nodes   N
— the absence/presence of distant metastases   M

The addition of numbers to these three components (e.g. T1, T2 . . . etc., N0, N1 . . . etc., M0, M1 . . . etc.) indicates the extent of the malignant disease.

For example, a veterinarian familiar with the system might describe a dog with cancer of the mammary gland as "T3b N2 M0". This would indicate that the tumour was of a certain size (more than 3 cm in diameter) with fixation to the underlying fascia or muscle; that either the axillary or inguinal lymph nodes were palpable and fixed; and that there was no clinical evidence of distant metastases.

In other words it is a kind of shorthand notation for the description of a malignant tumour.

General rules

The general rules applicable to all sites are as follows:

1.   In all cases confirmation of malignancy by histological or cytological examination is obligatory. Any cases not so proved must be recorded separately.

At many sites several distinct types of cancer may occur, differing not only in their histological pattern but also in their clinical behaviour. It would clearly be wrong to consider all such types together.

An example is cancer of the mammary gland of the dog. Well differentiated tubular adenocarcinomas have a good prognosis following mastectomy but anaplastic carcinomas have a poor prognosis.

2.   All cases are identified by T, N and M categories, which must be determined and recorded prior to definitive treatment. They remain unchanged although they may be qualified by additional histopathological or surgical information.

The reason for this is clear. The condition of many animals with cancer precludes surgery when they first attend for treatment. Consequently they would be excluded from a universal classification if evidence obtained only at operation were required.

The TNM system in man describes two classifications for each site:

(a) pre-treatment, clinical classification
(b) post-surgical histopathological classification designated pTNM

For most tumours the pTNM categories correspond to the TNM categories but differences have been noted and additions made for thyroid, breast, oesophagus, stomach, bladder, prostate and melanoma. This dual classification has not been attempted at this stage for tumours in domestic animals. It is the pre-treatment clinical TNM classification which is of paramount importance for purposes of reporting and evaluation.

It is recognized, however, especially in the allocation of animals with certain tumours in clinical trials, that detailed histopathological information supplementing the clinical diagnosis is essential, e.g. grading of mastocytomas, invasion or lack of invasion by mammary tubular adenocarcinoma.

3.   In the clinical assessment of an animal tumour numerous investigations may be done. It is important to distinguish obligatory investigations from those which add refinement to the diagnosis of the extent of the malignant disease. For each site minimum criteria for TNM classification are listed. The regional lymph nodes for each site are defined.

4.   After assigning T, N and M categories (with degree of extension) these may be grouped into a number of clinical stages for certain tumours.

It is obvious that tumours of some sites lend themselves more easily and satisfactorily to classification than others. These are the accessible sites where eye and hand can assess by direct vision, palpation and measurement the primary tumour and its regional lymph nodes. The mammary gland, the upper air and food passages, the skin and long bones are examples. The least satisfactory sites for classification of their tumours are the deep-seated viscera, e.g. stomach, colon, kidney and ovary.

It is necessary therefore that, although the rules of the TNM system should be rigidly observed, there must be, for any particular site, some method for the identification and recording of additional information considered essential for that site. The following is an example of such additional information.

Most dogs with mammary cancer of posterior glands have a mastectomy, which usually means the inguinal lymph node is removed and examined histologically. If mobile nodes are palpable clinically before operation the designation N1 is applied to the case. If these nodes are found on histological examination to be tumour-free, the cypher $(-)$ (minus) is added, thus: $N1(-)$. If they contain tumour deposits, the cypher $(+)$ (plus) is added, thus: $N1(+)$.

PRIMARY TUMOUR (T)

T1, T2, T3, T4 indicate increasing degrees of extent of the primary tumour. The number of these T categories may vary according to the particular site but it is recommended that in general there should be four. For each site the ideal situation is when tumours can be accurately defined, accurately assessed on clinical examination and have precise "boundaries", such as a size-limitation or a "yes or no" distinction, e.g. movable or fixed.

1.   The tumours easiest to classify are those which arise in a single organ. In these the tumour can be simply described in terms of its anatomical extent.

In the mammary gland of the dog for instance, the three main qualities which determine the T category are size, involvement of skin and involvement of underlying tissues. There are four degrees of T and any agreed clinical feature can determine the degree of T, as indicated in the following simplified table:

	T1	T2	T3	T4
Size	Less than 3 cm	3–5 cm	More than 5 cm	
Skin	Minor involvement			Major involvement
Fascia, Muscle and Thoracic wall	with or without fascia or muscle fixation			Thoracic or abdominal wall fixation

It is not known if the localization of the tumour within the mammary gland(s) is as important in animals as it is in women. However, although position is not included in the T definitions, there is no difficulty in comparing, for example, a group of T3 outer half cases and a group of T3 inner half cases, provided this information is recorded in the animal's hospital chart.

2.   A second group of tumours occurs in situations which are not so circumscribed and in which the size and extent cannot be so easily ascertained, e.g. tumours of the bladder are assessed on cystoscopy, radiography, manual examination under anaesthesia and the extent of penetration of the bladder wall by the tumour (as indicated by the microscopic examination of tissue removed for biopsy).

3.   A third type cannot be diagnosed at all without taking operative findings into account, e.g. laparotomy in ovarian tumours and surgico-pathological findings in colon and bone tumours.

Multiple tumours have to be considered under several headings:

(a) those occurring simultaneously in paired organs (e.g. chain of mammary glands) should be classified independently.

(b) those occurring simultaneously in the skin should have the actual number recorded. The tumour with the highest T category is selected and the number of tumours indicated in parenthesis, thus T2(5).

(c) those occurring in hollow viscera or cavities, e.g. bladder, vagina, penis, and in which the exact number is immaterial, are denoted by addition of the suffix (m) thus: T3(m). This may also be applied to the histopathological classification, thus: P2(m)— see "Histopathological extent and grading," page 452.

In addition to the degrees of T needed to describe the local extent of a tumour, other T symbols require mention:

T0 means "no evidence of primary tumour". This category is necessary to cover cases where lymphatic or blood-borne metastases occur while the primary neoplasm remains occult.

TX means that it is impossible to assess fully the extent of the primary tumour.

Tis is reserved exclusively for carcinoma in situ (preinvasive carcinoma). This is an essential category in some sites, e.g. cornea and sclera, eyelids and nose.

REGIONAL LYMPH NODES (N)

N1, N2, N3 indicate the characteristics of lymph nodes, which may be assessed by palpation, lymphangiography or other procedures. The number of these categories varies according to site.

Example of N classification: oral cavity.

N0   No palpable regional lymph nodes, i.e. no regional lymph nodes are palpable or they appear to be normal on other diagnostic procedures

N1   Movable regional ipsilateral lymph nodes

N2   Movable contralateral or bilateral lymph nodes

N3   Fixed lymph nodes

Histological information concerning the state of the lymph nodes obtained from a biopsy or following operation may be added to any N category by the use of the cyphers $(-)$ (minus) or $(+)$ (plus), indicating the absence or presence of metastatic involvement. This is also applicable to NX, thus: NX$-$ or NX$+$.

When regional lymph nodes are palpable they must be classified as N1 or N2 but an examining clinician may wish to include his assessment of whether a lymph node contains metastatic tumour or not. Thus for all lymph nodes draining head and neck tumours the definitions are:

N1   Movable regional nodes
   N1a   nodes not considered to contain growth
   N1b   nodes considered to contain growth

N2   Movable ipsilateral or bilateral nodes
   N2a   nodes not considered to contain growth
   N2b   nodes considered to contain growth

DISTANT METASTASES (M)

The absence or presence of metastases is indicated by the letter M.

M0   No metastases are detected clinically

M1   Metastasis other than to regional lymph nodes is present
   If necessary M1 may be subdivided into further categories to indicate the type of metastasis, e.g. to bone, liver, lung, etc.

MX   Impossible to assess the presence of metastases.

Histopathological extent (P) and grading (G)

Information obtained at operation is not generally considered admissible for clinical classification but may be used as an addition. Two aspects of histopathology may be recorded. The symbol P refers to the depth of infiltration of the tumour within the organ or tissue, while the symbol G refers to the pathological grading of the tumour.

For example, for tumours of some hollow organs the histopathological extent is expressed in four degrees of P:

P1   Tumour confined to the mucosa

P2   Tumour involves the mucosa and the submucosa and extends to or into the serosa, but does not penetrate through the serosa

P3   Tumour penetrates through the serosa with or without invasion of contiguous structures

P4   Tumour diffusely involves the entire thickness of the organ wall without obvious boundaries.

Pathological grading is expressed in three degrees:

G1   Low grade malignancy

G2   Medium grade malignancy

G3   High grade malignancy

Additional pathological categories may be used in certain sites, for example, to record invasion of lymphatics or veins in urological sites. These are designated L and V.

Thus for tumours of the bladder the definitions are:

L0   No lymphatic invasion

L1   Superficial lymphatics invaded

L2   Deep lymphatics invaded

For tumours of the kidney the definitions are:

V0   The veins do not contain tumour

V1   Renal vein contains tumour

V2   Vena cava contains tumour

Stage grouping

As stated earlier the "staging" of tumours has been practiced for many years in medicine, and the system can be applied equally well to animal tumours. Classification by T, N and M aims at a more precise recording of the apparent extent of the disease and the cases can then be grouped according to criteria that are statistically predictive. In a tumour with four possible degrees of T, four degrees of N and two degrees of M, the number of groups, extending from T1 N0 M0 at one end of the scale to T4 N3 M1 at the other, is 32. To record individual cases in these groups is simple; to reproduce tables containing that number is impractical except for very large series.

A theoretical example may contain the following stage-grouping:

TNM Groups		Clinical Stage	No of Groups per Stage
T1 N0 M0	T2 N0 M0	I	2
T1 N1 M0	T2 N1 M0	II	2
T1 N2,3 M0 T3 N0,1,2,3 M0	T2 N2,3 M0 T4 N0,1,2,3 M0	III	12
Any TN symbols + M1		IV	16

It will be seen that the 12 TNM groups in Stage III span a range from T1 N2 M0 to T4 N3 M0. The one-year survival of the first group may be about 60% while of the last group only 15%. This shows the limitation of staging where it includes such dissimilar groups and demonstrates at the same time the advantage of TNM categories.

THE ANATOMICAL SITES

The sites now classified cover the greater part of the veterinary field for dogs and cats and most are suitable for other animals. Each site is considered in the same general manner, the following details being set out in short introductory remarks:

1.   Description of the site and regions
2.   Definition of the regional and, where applicable, the juxta-regional lymph nodes for each site
3.   Where necessary, the clinical and surgical methods recommended for establishing the TNM categories.

The sites are grouped under 11 headings:

1.   Skin (excluding lymphosarcoma and mastocytoma)

2.   Skin (mastocytoma)

3.   Mammary glands

4.   Head and neck

5.   Alimentary system, including pancreas, liver

6.   Urological system

7.   Genital system

8.   Bones and joints

9.   Lymphoid and haematopoietic tissues (including lymphosarcoma of skin)

10.   Respiratory system

11.   Endocrine glands (thyroid, adrenal)

Tumours of the eye, CNS, heart and endocrine glands (other than adrenal and thyroid) are not included because it is difficult to classify them clinically at the present time and many of this group are only locally invasive.

1.   SKIN

(excluding lymphosarcoma and mastocytoma)

The classification applies to primary tumours of the skin. There must be histological verification to permit grouping of cases by histological type.

The classification is based on division into six regions.

In defining the lymph nodes for each region, the body is divided vertically at the umbilicus.

The regions and regional nodes are as follows:

Regions	Regional nodes
(a) eyelid, ear and nose	cervical (bilateral)
(b) face (excluding "a"), scalp and neck	cervical (bilateral) submandibular (bilateral) auricular (bilateral)
(c) upper limb	axillary and prescapular (ipsilateral)
(d) trunk anterior to the umbilicus	axillary (bilateral) Prescapular (bilateral)
(e) trunk posterior to the umbilicus	inguinal (bilateral)
(f) lower limb	inguinal and popliteal (ipsilateral)

The extent of the disease is assessed on clinical examination and radiography. The primary tumour is assessed on size, infiltration of subcutis or involvement of other structures such as fascia, muscle, bone or cartilage. The size, to be recorded in cm., may be measured by calliper.

The pathological grade of tumour should be recorded when available but does not modify the classification.

$\overline{T}0$ = no evidence of tumour. Use for rechecks for malignancy after surgical removal of primary tumour.

Multiple tumours

In the case of multiple simultaneous tumours, the tumour with the highest T category should be identified and the number of separate tumours indicated in parenthesis, e.g. T2(5). Successive tumours should be classified independently.

CLINICAL STAGES (TNM) OF CANINE OR FELINE TUMOURS
OF EPIDERMAL OR DERMAL ORIGIN (EXCLUDING LYMPHOSARCOMA AND MASTOCYTOMA)

Case number . . . .   Name of owner . . . .   Date . . . .

Cat/Dog . . . .   Age . . . .   Sex . . . .   Breed . . . .   Body weight . . . . lbs

(1 kg = 2.2 lbs) . . . .   kgs

Circle appropriate category

T: Primary Tumour

Tis   Pre-invasive carcinoma (carcinoma in situ)

T0   No evidence of tumour

T1   Tumour <2 cm. maximum diameter, superficial or exophytic

T2   Tumour 2–5 cm. maximum diameter, or with minimal invasion irrespective of size

T3   Tumour >5 cm. maximum diameter, or with invasion of the subcutis, irrespective of size

T4   Tumour invading other structures such as fascia muscle, bone or cartilage

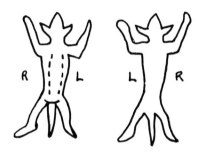

Circle site(s) involved

Tumours occurring simultaneously should have the actual number recorded. The tumour with the highest T category is selected and the number of tumours indicated in parenthesis, e.g. T2(5). Successive tumours should be classified independently.

N: Regional Lymph Nodes (RLN)*

N0   No evidence of RLN involvement

N1   Movable ipsilateral nodes

N1a   Nodes not considered to contain growth**
N1b   Nodes considered to contain growth**

N2   Movable contralateral or bilateral nodes

N2a   Nodes not considered to contain growth**
N2b   Nodes considered to contain growth**

N3   Fixed nodes

---

*For RLN see introduction
**(−) = histologically negative, (+) = histologically positive

M: Distant Metastasis

    M0   No evidence of distant metastasis

    M1   Distant metastasis detected*** — specify site(s) ....

STAGE GROUPING: No stage grouping is at present recommended

Comments: ....
....
....

    ***Including lymph nodes beyond the region in which the primary tumour is situated

2. SKIN

(Mastocytoma)

The extent of disease is assessed on clinical examination and radiography. The primary tumour is assessed on size, infiltration of subcutis or involvement of other structures such as fascia, muscle, bone or cartilage. The size, to be recorded in cm., may be measured by calliper.

In the case of multiple simultaneous tumours, the tumour with the highest T category should be identified and the number of separate tumours indicated in parenthesis, e.g. T2(5). Successive tumours should be classified independently.

The pathological grade of tumour should be recorded when available but does not modify the classification.

Systemic signs include gastric and duodenal ulceration, peritonitis, coagulation defects and glomerulo-nephritis. Because these tumours can be present with or without systemic signs the TNM system is not entirely suitable. The tumours can, however, be clinically staged into four categories.

CLINICAL STAGES OF CANINE MASTOCYTOMA

Case number .... Name of owner .... Date ....

Age .... Sex .... Breed .... Body weight .... lbs

                                                                 (1 kg = 2.2 lbs) .... kgs

---

Circle appropriate category

Clinical Stage

    I One tumour confined to the dermis without regional lymph node involvement

        Ia   without systemic signs

        Ib   with systemic signs

    II One tumour confined to dermis, with regional lymph node involvement

        IIa   without systemic signs

        IIb   with systemic signs

III Multiple dermal tumours or large infiltrating tumour with or without regional lymph node involvement

   IIIa   without systemic signs

   IIIb   with systemic signs

IV Any tumour with distant metastasis or recurrence with metastasis*

Multiple tumours

Tumours occurring simultaneously should have the actual number recorded. The tumour with the highest T category is selected and the number of tumours indicated in parenthesis, e.g. T2(5). Successive tumours should be classified independently.

---

*Including blood and/or bone marrow involvement

3.   MAMMARY GLANDS

The classification applies only to carcinoma.

The extent of disease is assessed on clinical examination and radiography of the thorax. The primary tumour is assessed on size, and involvement of skin and underlying structures. The size, to be recorded in cm., may be measured by calliper.

The position of the tumour in the mammary gland should be recorded but has no bearing on classification.

The pathological grade of tumour should be recorded when available but does not modify the classification.

Multiple tumours should be classified independently.

The regional lymph nodes are the axillary and inguinal nodes.

CLINICAL STAGES (TNM) OF CANINE MAMMARY TUMOURS

Case number . . . . Name of owner . . . . Date . . . .

Age . . . . Sex . . . . Breed . . . . Body weight . . . . lbs

                                       (1 kg = 2.2 lbs) . . . . kgs

---

Number of primary tumours:

Mammary gland location of primary tumours:	Right Chain					Left Chain				
	1	2	3	4	5	1	2	3	4	5

Largest single diameter (cm):

                       R   L

SINGLE   ☐ (Mark √ where applicable)
MULTIPLE ☐

                       Circle all glands involved

The following are the minimum requirements for assessing the T, N and M categories. (If these cannot be met, the symbols TX, NX and MX should be used.)

T categories : Clinical and surgical examination

N categories : Clinical and surgical examination

M categories : Clinical and surgical examination, radiography of thorax

---

Circle appropriate category

T: Primary Tumour

T0   No evidence of tumour

T1   Tumour <3 cm. maximum diameter
     T1a   not fixed   T1c   fixed to muscle
     T1b   fixed to skin

T2   Tumour 3–5 cm. maximum diameter
     T2a   not fixed   T2c   fixed to muscle
     T2b   fixed to skin

T3   Tumour >5 cm. maximum diameter
     T3a   not fixed   T3c   fixed to muscle
     T3b   fixed to skin

T4   Tumour any size, inflammatory carcinoma*

     Multiple tumours should be classified independently.

N: Regional Lymph Nodes (RLN):**

Mark √ where applicable

Circle appropriate category	RLN evaluated		Method of RLN evaluation	
	Inguinal	Axillary	Clinical	Histological***
N0 – no evidence of RLN involvement	☐	☐	☐	☐
N1 – ipsilateral RLN involved				
N1a not fixed	☐	☐	☐	☐
N1b fixed	☐	☐	☐	☐
N2 – bilateral RLN involved				
N2a not fixed	☐	☐	☐	☐
N2b fixed	☐	☐	☐	☐

M: Distant Metastasis

Mark √ where applicable
Method of M Evaluation

Circle appropriate category	Clinical	Radiographic	Histological
M0 – no evidence of distant metastasis	☐	☐	☐

---

*Locally invading skin without infection or trauma as the cause.
**The RLN are the axillary and inguinal nodes
***(−) = histologically negative, (+) = histologically positive

M1 – distant metastasis including
distant nodes ☐ ☐ ☐

Specify site(s) . . . .

STAGE GROUPING:

	T	N	M
I	T1a, b or c	N0(−) or N1a(−) or N2a(−)	M0
II	T0	N1(+)	M0
	T1a, b, or c	N1(+)	
	T2a, b or c	N0(+) or N1a(+)	
III	Any T3	Any N	M0
	Any T	Any Nb	
IV	Any T	Any N	M1

Final Clinical Stage:

	T	N	M	
TNM Evaluation	——	——	——	Stage . . . .

Comments: . . . .
. . . .
. . . .

CLINICAL STAGES (TNM) OF FELINE MAMMARY TUMOURS

Case number . . . . Name of owner . . . . Date . . . .

Age . . . . Sex . . . . Breed . . . . Body weight . . . . lbs
(1 kg = 2.2 lbs) . . . . kgs

Number of primary tumours:

Mammary gland location of primary tumours:

	Right Chain				Left Chain			
	1	2	3	4	1	2	3	4

Largest single diameter (cm): —— —— —— —— —— —— —— ——

SINGLE ☐
MULTIPLE ☐ (Mark √ where applicable)

Circle all glands involved ↗

The following are the minimum requirements for assessing the T, N and M categories. (If these cannot be met, the symbols TX, NX and MX should be used.)

T categories : Clinical and surgical examination

N categories : Clinical and surgical examination

M categories : Clinical and surgical examination, radiography of thorax

---

Circle appropriate category

T: Primary Tumour

  T0   No evidence of tumour

  T1   Tumour <1 cm. maximum diameter

   T1a   not fixed   T1c   fixed to muscle
   T1b   fixed to skin

  T2   Tumour 1–3 cm. maximum diameter

   T2a   not fixed   T2c   fixed to muscle
   T2b   fixed to skin

  T3   Tumour >3 cm. maximum diameter

   T3a   not fixed   T3c   fixed to muscle
   T3b   fixed to skin

  T4   Tumour any size, inflammatory carcinoma*

  Multiple tumours should be classified independently.

N: Regional Lymph Nodes (RLN):**

| | RLN evaluated | | Method of RLN evaluation | |
Circle appropriate category	Inguinal	Axillary	Clinical	Histological***
N0 – no evidence of RLN involvement	☐	☐	☐	☐
N1 – ipsilateral RLN involved				
N1a not fixed	☐	☐	☐	☐
N1b fixed	☐	☐	☐	☐
N2 – bilateral RLN involved				
N2a not fixed	☐	☐	☐	☐
N2b fixed	☐	☐	☐	☐

Mark √ where applicable

M: Distant Metastasis

Mark √ where applicable
Method of M Evaluation

Circle appropriate category	Clinical	Radiographic	Histological
M0 – no evidence of distant metastasis	☐	☐	☐
M1 – distant metastasis including distant nodes	☐	☐	☐

  Specify site(s) ....

---

*Locally invading skin without infection or trauma as the cause.
**The RLN are the axillary and inguinal nodes
***(−) = histologically negative, (+) = histologically positive

STAGE GROUPING:

	T	N	M
I	T1a, b or c	N0(−) or N1a(−) or N2a(−)	M0
II	T0	N1(+)	M0
	T1a, b, or c	N1(+)	
		N0(+) or N1a(+)	
	T2a, b or c		
III	Any T3	Any N	M0
	Any T	Any Nb	
IV	Any T	Any N	M1

Final Clinical Stage:

	T	N	M
TNM Evaluation	——	——	——	Stage . . . .

Comments: . . . .

. . . .

. . . .

4. HEAD AND NECK

(excluding larynx)

The extent of disease is assessed on clinical examination, radiography of the thorax and endoscopy. Radiographic examination is mandatory.

The regional lymph nodes are the cervical, the submandibular and the parotid nodes.

LIPS

1. Lower lip
2. Upper lip
3. Commissures

ORAL CAVITY (BUCCAL CAVITY)

The oral cavity includes the anterior two-thirds of the tongue, floor of mouth, buccal mucosa, the alveoli and the hard palate.

1. Buccal mucosa
2. Lower alveolus and gingiva
3. Upper alveolus and gingiva
4. Hard palate
5. Tongue: (a) dorsal surface and lateral borders (anterior two-thirds); (b) inferior surface
6. Floor of mouth

In the case of multiple tumours, the symbol (m) is added to the appropriate T category.

OROPHARYNX

The oropharynx extends from the junction of the hard and soft palates to the level of the floor of the glossoepiglottic folds.

1. Anterior wall (glossoepiglottic area): (a) tongue (posterior third); (b) glossoepiglottic folds; (c) anterior (lingual) surface of epiglottis
2. Lateral wall and tonsils
3. Posterior oropharyngeal wall
4. Superior wall — inferior surface of soft palate and uvula

The hypopharynx is included with the oropharynx. It extends from the pharyngoepiglottic fold to the upper end of the oesophagus and posterior pharyngeal wall.

In the case of multiple tumours, the symbol (m) is added to the appropriate T category.

CLINICAL STAGES (TNM) OF CANINE / FELINE TUMOURS OF THE LIPS

Case number . . . .   Name of owner . . . .   Date . . . .

Cat/Dog . . . .   Age . . . .   Sex . . . .   Breed . . . .   Body weight . . . . lbs

(1 kg = 2.2 lbs) . . . .   kgs

The following are the minimum requirements for assessing the T, N and M categories. (If these cannot be met, the symbols TX, NX and MX should be used.)

T categories : Clinical and surgical examination

N categories : Clinical and surgical examination

M categories : Clinical and surgical examination, radiography of thorax

Circle appropriate category

T: Primary Tumour

Tis   Preinvasive carcinoma (carcinoma in situ)

T0   No evidence of tumour

T1   Tumour <2 cm. maximum diameter, superficial or exophytic

T2   Tumour <2 cm. maximum diameter, with minimal invasion in depth

T3   Tumour >2 cm. diameter, or with deep invasion irrespective of size

T4   Tumour invading bone

N: Regional Lymph Nodes (RLN)*

N0   No evidence of RLN involvement

N1   Movable ipsilateral nodes

N1a   Nodes not considered to contain growth**
N1b   Nodes considered to contain growth**

   N2   Movable contralateral or bilateral nodes

      N2a   Nodes not considered to contain growth**
      N2b   Nodes considered to contain growth**
   N3   Fixed nodes

M: Distant Metastasis

   M0   No evidence of distant metastasis

   M1   Distant metastasis (including distant nodes) detected — specify site(s) ....

      ....

STAGE GROUPING: No stage grouping is at present recommended

Comments: ....

....

....

      *The RLN are the cervical, submandibular and parotid nodes
   **(−) = histologically negative, (+) = histologically positive

CLINICAL STAGES (TNM) OF CANINE/FELINE TUMOURS OF THE ORAL CAVITY (BUCCAL CAVITY)

Case number .... Name of owner .... Date ....

Cat/Dog .... Age .... Sex .... Breed .... Body weight .... lbs

                                                    (1 kg = 2.2 lbs) .... kgs

This classification applies to the anterior two-thirds of the tongue, floor of mouth, buccal mucosa, the alveoli and the hard palate.

The following are the minimum requirements for assessing the T, N and M categories. (If these cannot be met, the symbols TX, NX and MX should be used.)

   T categories : Clinical and surgical examination

   N categories : Clinical and surgical examination

   M categories : Clinical and surgical examination, radiography of thorax

Circle appropriate category

T: Primary Tumour

   Tis   Preinvasive carcinoma (carcinoma in situ)

   T0   No evidence of tumour

   T1   Tumour <2 cm. maximum diameter

      T1a   without bone invasion   T1b   with bone invasion

T2   Tumour 2–4 cm. maximum diameter

    T2a   without bone invasion   T2b   with bone invasion

T3   Tumour >4 cm. maximum diameter

    T3a   without bone invasion   T3b   with bone invasion

The symbol (m) added to the appropriate T category indicates multiple tumours.

N: Regional Lymph Nodes (RLN)*

N0   No evidence of RLN involvement

N1   Movable ipsilateral nodes

    N1a   Nodes not considered to contain growth**   N1b   Nodes considered to contain growth**

N2   Movable contralateral or bilateral nodes

    N2a   Nodes not considered to contain growth**   N2b   Nodes considered to contain growth**

N3   Fixed nodes

M: Distant Metastasis

M0   No evidence of distant metastasis

M1   Distant metastasis (including distant nodes) detected — specify site(s) ....
....

STAGE GROUPING:

	T	N	M
I	T1	N0, N1a or N2a	M0
II	T2	N0, N1a or N2a	M0
III***	T3 Any T	N0, N1a or N2a N1b	M0
IV	Any T Any T	Any N2b or N3 Any N	M0 M1

Comments: ....
....
....

*The RLN are the cervical, submandibular and parotid nodes
**(−) = histologically negative, (+) = histologically positive
***Any bone involvement

CLINICAL STAGES (TNM) OF CANINE/FELINE/EQUINE TUMOURS OF THE OROPHARYNX*

Case number .... Name of owner .... Date ....

Species .... Age .... Sex .... Breed .... Body weight .... lbs
                                                                  (1 kg = 2.2 lbs) .... kgs

The following classification applies from the junction of the hard and soft palates to the level of the floor of the glossoepiglottic folds.

The following are the minimum requirements for assessing the T, N and M categories. (If these cannot be met, the symbols TX, NX and MX should be used.)

T categories : Clinical, surgical and radiological examination, endoscopy

N categories : Clinical and surgical examination

M categories : Clinical and surgical examination, radiography of thorax

Circle appropriate category

T: Primary Tumour

Tis   Preinvasive carcinoma (carcinoma in situ)

T0   No evidence of primary tumour

T1   Tumour superficial or exophytic

   T1a   without systemic signs   T1b   with systemic signs

T2   Tumour with invasion of tonsil only

   T2a   without systemic signs   T2b   with systemic signs

T3   Tumour with invasion of surrounding tissue

   T3a   without systemic signs   T3b   with systemic signs

The symbol (m) added to the appropriate T category indicates multiple tumours.

N: Regional Lymph Nodes (RLN)**

N0   No evidence of RLN involvement

N1   Movable ipsilateral nodes

   N1a   Nodes not considered to contain growth***
   N1b   Nodes considered to contain growth***

N2   Movable contralateral or bilateral nodes

   N2a   Nodes not considered to contain growth***
   N2b   Nodes considered to contain growth***

N3   Fixed nodes

M: Distant Metastasis

M0   No evidence of distant metastasis

M1   Distant metastasis (including distant nodes) detected — specify site(s) . . . .

STAGE GROUPING: No stage grouping is at present recommended

Comments: . . . .

*Mainly tonsillar carcinoma; **The RLN are the cervical, submandibular and parotid nodes
***(−) = histologically negative, (+) = histologically positive

5. ALIMENTARY SYSTEM*

OESOPHAGUS

Tumours of the oesophagus are rare in animals except in geographic areas where the canine oesophageal parasite Spirocerca lupi exists and where herbivorous animals have a high intake of bracken fern (Pteridium aquilinum).

The extent of disease is assessed by clinical examination, radiography of the thorax and endoscopy.

STOMACH

In single-stomached animals there are two regions and the tumour is assigned to that region in which the bulk of it is situated.

(a) anterior half
(b) posterior half

In herbivores the anatomical site is recorded e.g. rumen, abomasum.

The extent of disease is assessed by clinical examination, radiography of the thorax and endoscopy or laparotomy.

The regional lymph nodes are the gastric and splenic nodes.

PANCREAS

The extent of disease is assessed by laparotomy or laparoscopy, and radiography of the thorax.

The regional lymph nodes are the splenic and hepatic nodes.

LIVER

The extent of disease is assessed by clinical examination, radiography of the thorax, and laparotomy or laparoscopy.

The regional lymph nodes are the hepatic and diaphragmatic nodes.

INTESTINES

The extent of disease is assessed by clinical examination, radiography of the thorax and subsequent laparotomy.

The regional lymph nodes are the mesenteric, caecal, colic and rectal nodes.

---

*With the exception of tumours of the pancreas, in the case of multiple tumours the symbol (m) is added to the appropriate T category.

CLINICAL STAGES (TNM) OF TUMOURS OF THE OESOPHAGUS (ALL SPECIES)

Case number . . . . Name of owner . . . . Date . . . .

Species . . . . Age . . . . Sex . . . . Breed . . . . Body weight . . . . lbs

(1 kg = 2.2 lbs) . . . . kgs

The following are the minimum requirements for assessing the T, N and M categories. (If these cannot be met, the symbols TX, NX and MX should be used.)

T categories : Clinical and surgical examination, endoscopy

N categories : Clinical and surgical examination

M categories : Clinical and surgical examination, radiography of thorax

Circle appropriate category

T: Primary Tumour

T0   No evidence of tumour

T1   Tumour confined to the oesophagus

T2   Tumour invading neighbouring structures

The symbol (m) is added to the appropriate T category indicates multiple tumours.

N: Regional Lymph Nodes (RLN)*

N0   No evidence of RLN involvement

N1   RLN involved

M: Distant Metastasis

M0   No evidence of distant metastasis

M1   Distant metastasis detected — specify site(s) . . . .

STAGE GROUPING: No stage grouping is at present recommended

Comments: . . . .

. . . .

. . . .

*The RLN are:

– for the cervical oesophagus, the cervical and prescapular nodes
– for the thoracic oesophagus, the mediastinal nodes

CLINICAL STAGES (TNM) OF TUMOURS OF THE STOMACH (ALL SPECIES)

Case number . . . . Name of owner . . . . Date . . . .

Species . . . . Age . . . . Sex . . . . Breed . . . . Body weight . . . . lbs

(1 kg = 2.2 lbs) . . . . kgs

The following are the minimum requirements for assessing the T, N and M categories. (If these cannot be met, the symbols TX, NX and MX should be used.)

T categories : Clinical and surgical examination (laparotomy or laparoscopy, endoscopy)

N categories : Surgical examination (laparotomy, laparoscopy)

M categories : Clinical and surgical examination, radiography of thorax

Circle appropriate category

T: Primary Tumour

T0   No evidence of tumour

T1   Tumour not invading serosa

T2   Tumour invading serosa

T3   Tumour invading neighbouring structures

The symbol (m) added to the appropriate T category indicates multiple tumours

N: Regional Lymph Nodes (RLN)*

N0   No evidence of RLN involvement

N1   RLN involved

N2   Distant LN involved

M: Distant Metastasis

M0   No evidence of distant metastasis

M1   Distant metastasis detected — specify site(s) ....

STAGE GROUPING: No stage grouping is at present recommended

Comments: ....
....
....

―――――――――
*The RLN are the gastrosplenic nodes

CLINICAL STAGES (TNM) OF TUMOURS OF THE PANCREAS (ALL SPECIES)

Case number .... Name of owner .... Date ....

Species .... Age .... Sex .... Breed .... Body weight .... lbs
(1 kg = 2.2 lbs) .... kgs

The following are the minimum requirements for assessing the T, N and M categories. (If these cannot be met the symbols TX, NX and MX should be used.)

T categories : Clinical and surgical examination (laparotomy or laparoscopy)

N categories : Surgical examination (laparotomy, laparoscopy)

M categories : Clinical and surgical examination, radiography of thorax

Circle appropriate category

T: Primary Tumour

    T0   No evidence of tumour

    T1   Tumour present — state anatomical site:

N: Regional Lymph Nodes (RLN)*

    N0   No evidence of RLN involvement

    N1   RLN involved

    N2   Distant LN involved

M: Distant Metastasis

    M0   No evidence of distant metastasis

    M1   Distant metastasis detected — specify site(s) . . . .

STAGE GROUPING: No stage grouping is at present recommended.

Comments: . . . .
. . . .
. . . .

_____

    *The RLN are the splenic and hepatic nodes

CLINICAL STAGES (TNM) OF TUMOURS OF THE LIVER (ALL SPECIES)

Case number . . . . Name of owner . . . . Date . . . .

Species . . . . Age . . . . Sex . . . . Breed . . . . Body weight . . . . lbs

                                      (1 kg = 2.2 lbs) . . . . kgs

The following are the minimum requirements for assessing the T, N and M categories. (If these cannot be met, the symbols TX, NX and MX should be used.)

    T categories : Clinical and surgical examination (laparotomy or laparoscopy, endoscopy)

    N categories : Surgical examination (laparotomy, laparoscopy)

    M categories : Clinical and surgical examination, radiography of thorax

Circle appropriate category

T: Primary Tumour

    T0   No evidence of tumour

    T1   Tumour involving one lobe

T2   Tumour involving more than one lobe

T3   Tumour invading neighbouring structures

The symbol (m) added to the appropriate T category indicates multiple tumours

N: Regional Lymph Nodes (RLN)*

N0   No evidence of RLN involvement

N1   RLN involved

N2   Distant LN involved

M: Distant Metastasis

M0   No evidence of distant metastasis

M1   Distant metastasis detected — specify site(s) ....

STAGE GROUPING: No stage grouping is at present recommended

Comments: ....

....

....

---

*The RLN are the hepatic and diaphragmatic nodes

CLINICAL STAGES (TNM) OF TUMOURS OF THE INTESTINES (ALL SPECIES)

Case number .... Name of owner .... Date ....

Species .... Age .... Sex .... Breed .... Body weight .... lbs

(1 kg = 2.2 lbs) .... kgs

The following are the minimum requirements for assessing the T, N and M categories. (If these cannot be met, the symbols TX, NX and MX should be used.)

T categories : Clinical and surgical examination (laparotomy or laparoscopy)

N categories : Surgical examination (laparotomy, laparoscopy)

M categories : Clinical and surgical examination, radiography of thorax

---

Circle appropriate category

T: Primary Tumour

T0   No evidence of tumour

T1   Tumour not invading serosa

T2   Tumour invading serosa

T3   Tumour invading neighbouring structures

The symbol (m) added to the appropriate T category indicates multiple tumours.

N: Regional Lymph Nodes (RLN)*

    N0   No evidence of RLN involvement

    N1   RLN involved

    N2   Distant LN involved

M: Distant Metastasis

    M0   No evidence of distant metastasis

    M1   Distant metastasis detected — specify site(s) ....

STAGE GROUPING: No stage grouping is at present recommended

Comments: ....

....

....

---

*The RLN are the mesenteric, caecal, colic and rectal nodes

6.   UROLOGICAL SYSTEM

KIDNEY AND BLADDER

As well as clinical examination, radiography of the thorax and laparotomy, techniques such as lymphangiography or arteriography may be helpful in the assessment of these tumours. For bladder tumours cystoscopy, urography and cystography are of considerable value. It is recognized that facilities for these techniques are not uniformly available and veterinary clinicians who do not have them cannot classify these tumours according to the system proposed.

In the case of multiple tumours of the bladder, the symbol (m) is added to the appropriate T category.

The regional lymph nodes for the kidney are the lumbar nodes and for the bladder, the external and internal iliac lymph nodes.

CLINICAL STAGES (TNM) OF CANINE TUMOURS OF THE KIDNEY

Case number .... Name of owner .... Date ....

Age .... Sex .... Breed .... Body weight .... lbs

(1 kg = 2.2 lbs) .... kgs

The following are the minimum requirements for assessing the T, N and M categories. (If these cannot be met, the symbols TX, NX and MX should be used.)

    T categories : Clinical and surgical examination (laparotomy or laparoscopy)

    N categories : Surgical examination (laparotomy, laparoscopy)

    M categories : Clinical and surgical examination, radiography of thorax

Circle appropriate category

T: Primary Tumour

T0   No evidence of tumour

T1   Small tumour without deformation of the kidney

T2   Solitary tumour with deformation and/or enlargement of the kidney

T3   Tumour invading perinephric structures (peritoneum) and/or pelvis, ureter and/or renal blood vessels (renal vein)

T4   Tumour invading neighbouring structures

N: Regional Lymph Nodes (RLN)*

N0   No evidence of RLN involvement

N1   Ipsilateral RLN involved

N2   Bilateral RLN involved

N3   Other LN involved (abdominal and pelvic LN)

M: Distant Metastasis

M0   No evidence of distant metastasis

M1   Distant metastasis detected — specify site(s) . . . .
. . . .

M1a   Single metastasis in one organ

M1b   Multiple metastases in one organ

M1c   Multiple metastases in various organs

STAGE GROUPING: No stage grouping is at present recommended

Comments . . . .
. . . .

*The RLN are the lumbar nodes

CLINICAL STAGES (TNM) OF CANINE TUMOURS OF THE URINARY BLADDER

Case number . . . .   Name of owner . . . .   Date . . . .

Age . . . .   Sex . . . .   Breed . . . .   Body weight . . . . lbs

(1 kg = 2.2 lbs) . . . . kgs

The following are the minimum requirements for assessing the T, N and M categories. (If these cannot be met, the symbols TX, NX and MX should be used.)

   T categories : Clinical examination, cystoscopy, urography or cystography, laparotomy

   N categories : Surgical examination (laparotomy or laparoscopy)

   M categories : Clinical and surgical examination, radiography of thorax, laparotomy

Circle appropriate category

T: Primary Tumour

Tis   Carcinoma in situ

T0   No evidence of tumour

T1   Superficial papillary tumour

T2   Tumour invading the bladder wall, with induration

T3   Tumour invading neighbouring organs (prostate, uterus, vagina, anal canal)

The symbol (m) added to the appropriate T category indicates multiple tumours

N: Regional Lymph Nodes (RLN)*

N0   No evidence of RLN involvement

N1   RLN involved

N2   RLN and juxta RLN involved

M: Distant Metastasis

M0   No evidence of distant metastasis

M1   Distant metastasis detected — specify site(s):   . . . .

STAGE GROUPING: No stage grouping is at present recommended

Comments: . . . .

. . . .

. . . .

*The RLN are the internal and external iliac nodes. The juxta RLN are the lumbar nodes

7(a).   FEMALE GENITAL SYSTEM

OVARY

The extent of disease is assessed on clinical examination and the findings at operation, but before definitive treatment is commenced. Radiography of the thorax is mandatory. It is recognized that some cases will remain unclassified.

The regional lymph nodes are the lumbar nodes.

UTERUS

Cervical tumours are very rare in animals and no staging classification is provided. Uterine tumours are infrequent.

There are two areas of the uterus, the body and horns.

The extent of disease is assessed by clinical examination, radiography of the thorax and laparoscopy or laparotomy.

In the case of multiple tumours, the symbol (m) is added to the appropriate T category.

The regional lymph nodes are the internal and external iliac and sub-lumbar and sacral nodes.

VAGINA AND VULVA

Tumours of the vulva are classified as those of skin. Tumours present in the vagina as secondary growths from either genital or extra-genital sites should be excluded.

The extent of disease is assessed on clinical examination and/or following surgical exposure, and radiography of the thorax is required.

In the case of multiple tumours, the symbol (m) is added to the appropriate T category.

The regional lymph nodes are the superficial inguinal, sacral and internal iliac nodes.

CLINICAL STAGES (TNM) OF CANINE TUMOURS OF THE OVARY*

Case number .... Name of owner .... Date ....

Age .... Breed .... Body weight .... lbs

(1 kg = 2.2 lbs) .... kgs

The following are the minimum requirements for assessing the T, N and M categories. (If these cannot be met, the symbols TX, NX and MX should be used.)

T categories : Clinical and surgical examination (laparotomy, laparoscopy)

N categories : Surgical examination (laparotomy, laparoscopy)

M categories : Clinical and surgical examination (laparotomy) and radiography of thorax

Circle appropriate category

T: Primary Tumour

T0   No evidence of tumour

T1   Tumour limited to one ovary

T2   Tumours limited to both ovaries

T3   Tumour invading the ovarian bursa

T4   Tumour invading neighbouring structures

N: Regional Lymph Nodes (RLN)**

N0   No evidence of RLN involvement

N1   RLN involved

M: Distant Metastasis

M0   No evidence of distant metastasis

M1   Evidence of implantation(s) or other metastases:

M1a   in the peritoneal cavity
M1b   beyond the peritoneal cavity — specify site(s): ....
M1c   both peritoneal cavity and beyond

STAGE GROUPING: No stage grouping is at present recommended

Comments: ....

....

....

*General principles apply to all species
**The RLN are the lumbar nodes

CLINICAL STAGES (TNM) OF TUMOURS OF THE UTERUS (ALL SPECIES)

Case number .... Name of owner .... Date ....

Species .... Age .... Breed .... Body weight .... lbs

(1 kg = 2.2 lbs) .... kgs

The following are the minimum requirements for assessing the T, N and M categories. (If these cannot be met, the symbols TX, NX and MX should be used.)

T categories : Clinical and surgical examination (laparotomy or laparoscopy)

N categories : Surgical examination (laparotomy or laparoscopy)

M categories : Clinical and surgical examination, radiography of thorax

Circle appropriate category

T: Primary Tumour

T0   No evidence of tumour

T1   Small non-invasive tumour

T2   Large or invasive tumour

T3   Tumour invading neighbouring structures

The symbol (m) added to the appropriate T category indicates multiple tumours

N: Regional Lymph Nodes (RLN)*

N0   No evidence of RLN involvement

N1   Pelvic RLN involved

N2   Para-aortic RLN involved

M: Distant Metastasis

M0   No evidence of distant metastasis

M1   Evidence of metastasis:

M1a   in the peritoneal cavity
M1b   beyond the peritoneal cavity — specify site(s) ....
M1c   in and beyond the peritoneal cavity

STAGE GROUPING: No stage grouping is at present recommended

Comments: ....

....

....

*The RLN are the pelvic nodes distal to the bifurcation of the common iliac arteries and intra-abdominal para-aortic nodes proximal to the bifurcation of the common iliac arteries.

CLINICAL STAGES (TNM) OF CANINE TUMOURS OF THE VAGINA AND VULVA*

Case number .... Name of owner .... Date ....

Age .... Breed .... Body weight .... lbs

(1 kg = 2.2 lbs) .... kgs

The following are the minimum requirements for assessing the T, N and M categories. (If these cannot be met, the symbols TX, NX and MX should be used.)

T categories : Clinical and surgical examination

N categories : Surgical examination

M categories : Clinical and surgical examination, radiography of thorax

Circle appropriate category

T: Primary Tumour

T0   No evidence of tumour

T1   Tumour <1 cm maximum diameter, superficial

T2   Tumour 1–3 cm maximum diameter, with minimal invasion

T3   Tumour >3 cm or every tumour with deep invasion

T4   Tumour invading neighbouring structures (skin, perineum, urethra, paravaginal wall, anal canal)

The symbol (m) added to the appropriate T category indicates multiple tumours

N: Regional Lymph Nodes (RLN)**

N0   No evidence of RLN involvement

N1   Movable, ipsilateral nodes

N2   Movable, bilateral nodes

N3   Fixed nodes

M: Distant Metastasis

M0   No evidence of distant metastasis

M1   Distant metastasis detected — specify site(s) ....

STAGE GROUPING: No stage grouping is at present recommended

Comments: . . . .

. . . .

---

*Tumours present in the vagina as secondary growths from either genital or extragenital sites should be excluded.

**The RLN are the superficial inguinal, sacral and internal iliac nodes, except that for the cranial part of the vagina they are only the internal iliac nodes.

7(b).   MALE GENITAL SYSTEM

TESTIS

Tumours of the testis may be in the descended testicle (scrotum) or undescended testicle (abdomen or inguinal).

The extent of disease is assessed on clinical examination, radiography of the thorax and (for abdominal testicle) laparotomy.

In the case of multiple tumours, the symbol (m) is added to the appropriate T category.

The regional lymph nodes are the sub-lumbar, inguinal nodes.

PENIS

There are three anatomical regions:

  (a)   preputium or prepuce

  (b)   glans

  (c)   shaft of penis

The extent of disease is assessed on clinical examination and radiography of the thorax.

In the case of multiple tumours, the symbol (m) is added to the appropriate T category.

The regional lymph nodes are the superficial inguinal nodes.

PROSTATE

While hyperplasia of the prostate is common in the dog malignant prostatic tumours in this and other domestic animal species are uncommon.

The extent of disease is assessed on clinical examination, supplemented by (T) urography, endoscopy or laparotomy and biopsy, (N) lymphography and/or urography, laparotomy, (M) pelvic, thoracic and skeletal x-rays.

The regional lymph nodes are the external and internal iliac lymph nodes.

CLINICAL STAGES (TNM) OF CANINE TUMOURS OF THE TESTIS

Case number . . . . Name of owner . . . . Date . . . .

Age . . . . Breed . . . . Body weight . . . . lbs

(1 kg = 2.2 lbs) . . . . kgs

Site: Mark √ where applicable

Right testis   ☐   Scrotal   ☐

Left testis   ☐   Inguinal   ☐

Both testes   ☐   Abdominal   ☐   Feminization present   ☐

The following are the minimum requirements for assessing the T, N and M categories. (If these cannot be met, the symbols TX, NX and MX should be used.)

T categories : Clinical and surgical examination (laparotomy for abdominal testicle only)

N categories : Clinical and surgical examination

M categories : Clinical and surgical examination, radiography of thorax

Circle appropriate category

T: Primary Tumour

T0   No evidence of tumour
T1   Tumour restricted to the testis
T2   Tumour invading the tunica albuginea
T3   Tumour invading the rete testis and/or the epididymis
T4   Tumour invading the spermatic cord and/or the scrotum

The symbol (m) added to the appropriate T category indicates multiple tumours

N: Regional Lymph Nodes (RLN)*

N0   No evidence of RLN involvement
N1   Ipsilateral RLN involved
N2   Contralateral or bilateral RLN involved

M: Distant Metastasis

M0   No evidence of distant metastasis
M1   Distant metastasis detected — specify site(s) . . . .

STAGE GROUPING: No stage grouping is at present recommended

Comments: ....

....

....

_____

*The RLN are the sub-lumbar, inguinal nodes

CLINICAL STAGES (TNM) OF CANINE TUMOURS OF THE THE PENIS (PREPUCE AND GLANS)

Case number .... Name of owner .... Date ....

Age .... Breed .... Body weight .... lbs

(1 kg = 2.2 lbs) .... kgs

The following are the minimum requirements for assessing the T, N and M categories. (If these cannot be met the symbols TX, NX and MX should be used.)

T categories : Clinical and surgical examination, radiography of thorax

N categories : Surgical examination

M categories : Clinical and surgical examination, radiography of thorax

Circle appropriate category

T: Primary Tumour

T0   No evidence of tumour

T1   Tumour <1 cm maximum diameter, strictly superficial

T2   Tumour 1–3 cm maximum diameter with minimal invasion

T3   Tumour >3 cm or every tumour with deep invasion

T4   Tumour invading neighbouring structures

The symbol (m) added to the appropriate T category indicates multiple tumours.

N: Regional Lymph Nodes (RLN)*

N0   No evidence of RLN involvement

N1   Movable ipsilateral nodes

N2   Movable bilateral nodes

N3   Fixed nodes

M: Distant Metastasis

M0   No evidence of distant metastasis

M1   Distant metastasis detected — specify site(s) ....

STAGE GROUPING: No stage grouping is at present recommended

Comments: ....
....
....
_____

*The RLN are the superficial inguinal nodes

CLINICAL STAGES (TNM) OF CANINE TUMOURS OF THE PROSTATE

Case number .... Name of owner .... Date ....

Age .... Breed .... Body weight .... lbs

(1 kg = 2.2 lbs) .... kgs

The following are the minimum requirements for assessing the T, N and M categories. (If these cannot be met, the symbols TX, NX and MX should be used.)

T categories : Clinical and surgical examination, urography, endoscopy and biopsy

N categories : Clinical and surgical examination, lymphography and/or urography

M categories : Clinical and surgical examination, radiography of pelvis, thorax and skeleton

Circle appropriate category

T: Primary Tumour

T0   No evidence of tumour

T1   Intracapsular tumour, surrounded by normal gland

T2   Diffuse intracapsular tumour

T3   Tumour extending beyond the capsule

T4   Tumour fixed, or invading neighbouring structures

N: Regional Lymph Nodes (RLN)*

N0   No evidence of RLN involvement

N1   RLN involved

N2   RLN and juxta RLN involved

M: Distant Metastasis

M0   No evidence of distant metastasis

M1   Distant metastasis detected — specify site(s) ....

STAGE GROUPING: No stage grouping is at present recommended

Comments: ....
....
....
_____

*The RLN are the external and internal iliac nodes. The juxta RLN are the lumbar nodes

8.   BONES AND JOINTS

The extent of disease is assessed on clinical and radiographic examination. Radiographic examination of the affected bone or joint together with the thorax (for metastases) is mandatory.

Multiple tumours should be classified independently.

CLINICAL STAGES (TM) OF CANINE / FELINE TUMOURS OF THE BONE

Case number .... Name of owner .... Date ....

Cat/Dog .... Age .... Sex .... Breed .... Body weight .... lbs

(1 kg = 2.2 lbs) .... kgs

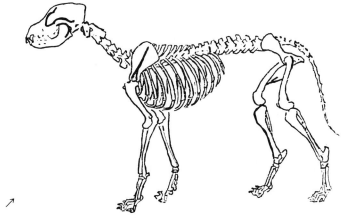

Circle site(s) involved   ↗

The following are the minimum requirements for assessing the T and M categories. (If these cannot be met, the symbols TX and MX should be used.)

T categories : Clinical, surgico-pathological and radiographic examination

M categories : Surgico-pathological examination, radiography of thorax

Circle appropriate category

T: Primary Tumour

T0   No evidence of tumour

T1   Tumour confined within the medulla and cortex

T2   Tumour extends beyond the periosteum

Multiple tumours should be classified independently.

M: Distant Metastasis

M0   No evidence of distant metastasis

M1   Distant metastasis detected — specify site(s) ....

STAGE GROUPING: No stage grouping is at present recommended

Comments: ....

....

CLINICAL STAGES (TNM) OF CANINE AND FELINE TUMOURS OF JOINTS AND ASSOCIATED STRUCTURES (TENDONS, TENDON SHEATHS ETC.)

Case number .... Name of owner .... Date ....

Species .... Age .... Sex .... Breed .... Body weight .... lbs

(1 kg = 2.2 lbs) .... kgs

The following are the minimum requirements for assessing the T, N and M categories. (If these cannot be met, the symbols TX, NX and MX should be used.)

T categories : Clinical, surgico-pathological and radiographic examination

N categories : Clinical and surgico-pathological examination

M categories : Surgico-pathological examination, radiography of thorax

Circle appropriate category

T: Primary Tumour

T0   No evidence of tumour

T1   Tumour well-defined, no invasion of surrounding tissues

T2   Tumour invading soft tissues

T3   Tumour invading joints and/or bones

Multiple tumours should be classified independently

N: Regional Lymph Nodes (RLN)*

N0   No evidence of RLN involvement

N1   RLN involved**

M: Distant Metastasis

M0   No evidence of distant metastasis

M1   Distant metastasis detected — specify site(s) ....

STAGE GROUPING: No stage grouping is at present recommended

Comments: ....

....

....

_____

*The RLN are as described in the introduction to skin (page 12)
**(−) = histologically negative, (+) = histologically positive.

9.   LYMPHOID AND HAEMATOPOIETIC TISSUES

(including lymphosarcoma of skin)

Lymphosarcoma in most domestic mammals falls into distinct anatomic types: generalized lymphade-nopathy, organs and nodes of the alimentary tract, thymus, skin, true lymphatic leukemia and occasionally other sites such as renal tissue or eye only.

The TNM system cannot be used. A histological classification is essential and attempts should be made to type these tumours immunologically as well.

The extent of disease is assessed on clinical, radiographic and haematological examination and is described as with or without systemic signs e.g. dyspnoea, dysentery. The recommended method for biopsy in multicentric lymphosarcoma is to excise an entire node e.g. popliteal, prescapular (superficial cervical).

CLINICAL STAGES OF LYMPHOSARCOMA AND LYMPHOID LEUKAEMIA IN DOMESTIC MAMMALS* (INCLUDING LYMPHOSARCOMA OF SKIN)

Case number . . . . Name of owner . . . . Date . . . .

Species . . . . Age . . . . Sex . . . . Breed . . . . Body weight . . . . lbs

(1 kg = 2.2 lbs) . . . . kgs

The extent of disease is assessed by clinical, radiographic and haematological examination.

Circle appropriate category

1.   ANATOMIC TYPE

A.   Generalized

B.   Alimentary

C.   Thymic

D.   Skin

E.   Leukaemia (True)**

F.   Others (including solitary renal)

2.   STAGE GROUPING (to include anatomic type)

I   Involvement limited to a single node or lymphoid tissue in a single organ***

II   Involvement of many lymph nodes in a regional area (± tonsils)

III   Generalized lymph node involvement

IV   Liver and/or spleen involvement (± Stage III)

V   Manifestation in the blood and involvement of bone marrow and/or other organ systems
     (± Stages I-IV)

   Each stage is subclassified into:

     (a) without systemic signs, or (b) with systemic signs

Comments: . . . .

. . . .

. . . .

---

   *Excluding myeloma
  **Only blood and bone marrow involved
 ***Excluding bone marrow

10. RESPIRATORY SYSTEM

NASAL CHAMBER AND SINUSES

The nasal chamber extends from the external nose anteriorly including the alae to the oropharynx posteriorly. Paranasal sinuses include frontal and maxillary in all species, plus sphenopalatine and ethmoidal sinuses in the horse.

The extent of disease is assessed on clinical and radiographic examination.

In the case of multiple tumours, the symbol (m) is added to the appropriate T category.

The regional lymph nodes are the submandibular, anterior cervical and pharyngeal nodes.

LARYNX, TRACHEA AND LUNGS

Primary tumours of the larynx, trachea and lungs are rare in animals. In some geographical regions there is a high incidence in sheep of jaagsiekte, a horizontally transmissible disease.

The extent of disease is assessed by clinical examination, endoscopy and radiography of the thorax.

Multiple tumours of the lungs should be classified independently.

The regional lymph nodes are the anterior cervical and pharyngeal (larynx and anterior trachea) and intrathoracic nodes (trachea, lungs).

CLINICAL STAGES (TNM) OF CANINE AND FELINE TUMOURS
OF THE NASAL CHAMBER AND SINUSES

Case number . . . . Name of owner . . . . Date . . . .

Species . . . . Age . . . . Sex . . . . Breed . . . . Body weight . . . . lbs

                                                                          (1 kg = 2.2 lbs) . . . . kgs

The following are the minimum requirements for assessing the T, N and M categories. (If these cannot be met, the symbols TX, NX and MX should be used.)

> T categories : Clinical, surgical and radiographic examination
>
> N categories : Clinical examination
>
> M categories : Clinical examination, radiography of thorax

Circle appropriate category

T: Primary Tumour

  T0   No evidence of tumour

  T1   Tumour ipsilateral, minimal or no bone destruction

  T2   Tumour bilateral and/or moderate bone destruction

  T3   Tumour invading neighbouring structures

  The symbol (m) added to the appropriate T category indicates multiple tumours

N: Regional Lymph Nodes (RLN)*

  N0   No evidence of RLN involvement

  N1   Movable ipsilateral nodes

    N1a   Nodes not considered to contain growth**
    N1b   Nodes considered to contain growth**

  N2   Movable contralateral or bilateral nodes

    N2a   Nodes not considered to contain growth**
    N2b   Nodes considered to contain growth**

  N3   Fixed nodes

Circle site(s) involved

M: Distant Metastasis

  M0   No evidence of distant metastasis

  M1   Distant metastasis detected (including distant nodes) — specify site(s) . . . .
        . . . .

STAGE GROUPING: No stage grouping is at present recommended

Comments: . . . .
. . . .

*The regional lymph nodes are the submandibular, anterior cervical and pharyngeal nodes
**(−) = histologically negative, (+) = histologically positive

CLINICAL STAGES (TNM) OF TUMOURS OF THE LARYNX, TRACHEA AND LUNGS (ALL SPECIES)

Case number . . . . Name of owner . . . . Date . . . .

Species . . . . Age . . . . Sex . . . . Breed . . . . Body weight . . . . lbs

(1 kg = 2.2 lbs) . . . . kgs

The following are the minimum requirements for assessing the T, N and M categories. (If these cannot be met, the symbols TX, NX and MX should be used.)

T categories : Clinical and surgical examination, endoscopy, bronchoscopy, radiography

N categories : Clinical and Surgical examination

M categories : Clinical and surgical examination, radiography of thorax

Circle appropriate category

T: Primary Tumour

T0   No evidence of tumour

TX   Tumour proven by presence of malignant cells in bronchopulmonary secretions but not seen by radiography or bronchoscopy

T1   Solitary tumour surrounded by lung or visceral pleura

T2   Multiple tumours of any size

T3   Tumour invading neighbouring tissues

Multiple tumours should be classified independently (applicable to lungs only)

N: Regional Lymph Nodes (RLN)*

N0   No evidence of RLN involvement

N1   Bronchial LN involved

N2   Distant LN involved

M: Distant Metastasis

M0   No evidence of distant metastasis

M1   Distant metastasis detected — specify site(s): . . . .

STAGE GROUPING: No stage grouping is at present recommended

Comments: . . . .
. . . .
. . . .

*The regional lymph nodes for the larynx and anterior trachea are the anterior cervical and pharyngeal nodes; for the trachea and lungs they are the intrathoracic nodes

11.   ENDOCRINE GLANDS

THYROID GLAND

The extent of disease is assessed on clinical examination, radiography of the thorax, endoscopy and radio-isotope scanning. There must be histological verification.

The regional lymph nodes are the cervical nodes.

ADRENAL GLANDS

The extent of disease is assessed on clinical examination, radiography of the thorax, endoscopy and hormonal assays.

The regional lymph nodes are the lumbar nodes.

CLINICAL STAGES (TNM) OF CANINE TUMOURS OF THE THYROID GLAND

Case number .... Name of owner .... Date ....

Age .... Sex .... Breed .... Body weight .... lbs

(1 kg = 2.2 lbs) .... kgs

LOCATION:*	LEFT		RIGHT		BOTH		

The following are the minimum requirements for assessing the T, N and M categories. (If these cannot be met, the symbols TX, NX and MX should be used.)

T categories : Clinical, surgical and radiographic examination, endoscopy, radio-isotope scanning

N categories : Clinical and surgical examination

M categories : Clinical and surgical examination, radiography of thorax, radio-isotope scanning

Circle appropriate category

T: Primary Tumour

T0 No evidence of tumour

T1 Tumour <2 cm maximum diameter : T1a not fixed, T1b fixed

T2 Tumour 2–5 cm maximum diameter : T2a not fixed, T1b fixed

T3 Tumour >5 cm maximum diameter : T3a not fixed, T3b fixed

N: Regional Lymph Nodes (RLN)**

N0 No evidence of RLN involvement

N1 Ipsilateral RLN involved : N1a not fixed***   N1b fixed***

N2 Bilateral RLN involved   : N2a not fixed***   N2b fixed***

Assessment: Clinical ......   Radiographic ....   Histological ....

M: Distant Metastasis

M0 No evidence of distant metastasis

M1 Distant metastasis detected — specify site(s) ....

STAGE GROUPING:

	T	N	M
I	T1a, b	N0(−) or N1a(−) or N2a(−)	M0

II	T0	N1(+)		M0
	T1a, b	N1(+)		
	T2a, b	N0(+) or N1a(+)		
III	Any T3	Any N		M0
	Any T	Any Nb		
IV	Any T	Any N		M1

Comments: ....

....

―――――――――

*When both glands are involved, separate staging forms should be used for each
**The RLN are the cervical nodes
***(−) = histologically negative, (+) = histologically positive

CLINICAL STAGES (TNM) OF CANINE TUMOURS OF THE ADRENAL GLANDS

Case number .... Name of owner .... Date ....

Age .... Sex .... Breed .... Body weight .... lbs

(1 kg = 2.2 lbs) .... kgs

The following are the minimum requirements for assessing the T, N and M categories. (If these cannot be met, the symbols TX, NX and MX should be used.)

T categories : Clinical and surgical examination, radiography of primary site, hormonal assays

N categories : Clinical and surgical examination

M categories : Clinical and surgical examination, radiography of thorax, hormonal assays

―――――――――

Circle appropriate category

T: Primary Tumour

T0   No evidence of tumour

T1   Well-defined tumour

T2   Tumour invading neighbouring structures

T3   Tumour invading blood vessels

N: Regional Lymph Nodes (RLN)*

N0   No evidence of RLN involvement

N1   RLN involved

M: Distant Metastasis

M0   No evidence of distant metastasis

M1   Distant metastasis detected — specify site(s) ....

STAGE GROUPING: No stage grouping is at present recommended

Comments: . . . .
. . . .
. . . .

*The RLN are the lumbar nodes

INDEX

Page numbers followed by *f* indicate figures; numbers followed by *t* indicate tabular material.

abortion, FeLV-induced, 374
acanthomatous epuli, 178t, 181
acidosis, hypercalcemia and, 31
acquired immunodeficiency syndrome, feline retroviruses and, 362. *See also* feline acquired immunodeficiency syndrome; feline immunodeficiency virus; feline leukemia virus
acrylonitrite, in etiology of cancer, 8
ACTH. *See* adrenocorticotropic hormone
actinomycin D, for renal cancer, 315
activated macrophage therapy, 26
acute lymphoblastic leukemia, 380, 381. *See also* lymphoma, lymphoid leukemia and
treatment for, 388, 389t
acute myelogenous leukemia, 397. *See also* myeloproliferative disorders
acute myelomonocytic leukemia, 397. *See also* myeloproliferative disorders
adenocarcinoma. *See also* names of specific adenocarcinomas
anal sac, 209–213
apocrine gland, 210, 212–213, 274
gastric, 193–195, 194f, 195f
intestinal, 200–207
liver, 196–199

mammary, 292–304
nasal, 218–222
orbital, 358–359
pancreatic, 192
papillary, 283–284, 284t
perianal, 209–213, 212f
prostatic, canine, 308
pulmonary, 225–228
renal, 313–315
salivary, 190
sebaceous, 145, 147f
sweat gland, 147–148
thyroid, 253–259
uterine, 287–288
adenoma
hepatocellular, 196–199
interstitial cell tumor and, 210
papillary, 283–284, 284t
parathyroid, 274–275
perianal, 209–210, 210f, 211f
sebaceous, 145, 146f
sweat gland, 147–148
thyroid, 254
hyperthyroidism and, 259
adenoviruses, 9, 10f
adrenal cancer, 264–268, 275–277
adrenocortical tumor, hyperadrenocorticism and, 264–268. *See also* hyperadrenocorticism
adrenocorticotropic hormone
ectopic production of, 34
hyperadrenocorticism and, 265, 266
Adriamycin. *See* doxorubicin
air pollutants, in etiology of cancer, 8

Alkeran. *See* melphalan
alkylating agents, 69, 70t, 72. *See also* chemotherapy; names of specific alkylating agents
ALL. *See* acute lymphoblastic leukemia
alloxan, for insulinoma, 272
alopecia
chemotherapy and, 66
radiation therapy and, 85, 86f, 87t
amines, heterocyclic, 11
AML. *See* acute myelogenous leukemia
AMML. *See* acute myelomonocytic leukemia
amputation, for canine osteosarcoma, 239
amyloid, plasma cell neoplasm and, 405
anal sac adenocarcinoma, 209–213
anatomical sites, TNM classification of, 453–454
alimentary system, 466–471
bones and joints, 481–482
endocrine glands, 486–489
female genital system, 473–477
head and neck, 461–465
lymphoid and haematopoietic tisues, 483–484
male genital system, 477–480
mammary glands, 457–461
respiratory system, 484–486
skin, 454–457
urological system, 471–473

anemia, 35t, 35–36
  FeLV-induced, 373
  in myeloproliferative disorders, 397–398
animal models of cancer, pet animals for, 2
anorectal cancer, 205–206
antibiotics, antitumor, 71t, 73. *See also* doxorubicin; *names of specific antitumor antibiotics*
antibody-dependent cellular cytotoxicity, 94
antibody therapy, 101, 132
antimetabolites, 70t, 72–73. *See also* chemotherapy; *names of specific antimetabolites*
antiretroviral agents, 128–129
antithyroid agents, 260–261
antiviral agents, 373
aortic body tumor, 277–278
apocrine gland adenocarcinoma, 274
APUDoma. *See* pancreatic neoplasms
asbestos, in etiology of cancer, 7
  mesothelioma and, 425, 427
asparaginase (Elspar), 71t, 74, 135
  for canine lymphoma, 386t, 387t
  for insulinoma, 272
  for mycosis fungoides, 389
attachment, pet loss and, 437–438
attitudes, toward cancer in pet animals, 1–2
autologous bone marrow transplantation, for canine lymphoma, 388
azathioprine, for immune-mediated thrombocytopenia, 37
3'-azido-3'-deoxythymidine, 129
AZT. *See* 3'-azido-3'-deoxythymidine

baboon endogenous virus, 364
bacille Calmette-Guerin, 96–98
  for bladder cancer, 320

for malignant melanoma, 182
bacterial agents, 96–99, 98f. *See also* immunotherapy
  for mesothelioma, 427
bacterial infections, 372–373
basal cell tumor, 144, 145f, 146f
basophilic leukemia, 396. *See also* myeloproliferative disorders
  diagnosis of, 398
B cell responses, in cell-mediated immunity, 95
BCG. *See* bacille Calmette-Guerin
BCNU, for brain tumor, 334–335
Bence-Jones proteinuria, 37
benzaldehyde, 134–135
beta cell tumor, 268–272. *See also* pancreatic insulin-secreting neoplasm
bile duct carcinoma, 196–199
biologic agents, 96–102, 373. *See also* immunotherapy
  for canine lymphoma, 388
  for hemangiosarcoma, 416
  for mammary gland tumor, 297, 298
  for transmissible venereal tumor, 424
biopsy, 18
  bone marrow, 384–385
  general considerations for, 53–54, 58
  hepatic, 198
  interpretation of, 56–57
  lymph node, 384
  methods for, 54–56
    excisional, 56
    needle punch, 55f, 55–56, 309, 309f
  nasal, 219–220, 221f
  oral, 179
  prostatic, 309, 309f
  skin and subcutaneous, 140–141
  tracts created by, 59
  wound margins for, 59t, 59–60, 60f
bladder cancer, 315–320
  clinical signs and history of, 317
  diagnosis of, 317, 318f

incidence of, 315, 317
  pathology and natural behavior of, 317
  prognosis for, 320
  risk factors for, 315, 317
  treatment for, 317–320, 319f
blast crisis, in myeloproliferative disorders, 400
Blenoxane. *See* bleomycin
bleomycin (Blenoxane), 71t, 73
bone infarcts, osteosarcoma and, 234–235
bone marrow toxicity, chemotherapy and, 65–66
bone marrow transplantation, 135–136, 388
bone tumor, 234–250. *See also names of specific bone tumors*
  canine, 234–249
    benign, 246–249, 247f–249f
    chondrosarcoma as, 242–243, 243f
    cyst as, 248–249
    fibrosarcoma as, 244
    giant cell tumor as, 245
    hemangiosarcoma as, 243–244, 244f, 412–417
    malignant mesenchymoma as, 245–246
    metastatic, 248
    osteoma as, 246–247, 247f
    osteosarcoma as, 234–241. *See also* osteosarcoma
    synovial cell sarcoma as, 244–245, 246f
  feline, 249–250
  in oral cavity, cryosurgery for, 110, 111
  spinal, 337, 337f
Bouin's solution, 20
bracken fern, in etiology of cancer, 7
brain tumor, 325–336. *See also names of specific brain tumors*
  clinical signs and history of, 326, 329f
  comparative aspects of, 336
  congenital, 325
  diagnosis of, 326, 328, 330f–335f

histologic classification of, 326, 327f
incidence of, 325–326
metastatic, 345t, 345–346
pathology of, 327, 327f, 328f
prognosis for, 336
risk factors for, 325–326
secondary, 325, 326
seizures and, 326, 329f
treatment for, 331–335
 chemotherapy as, 334–335
 immunotherapy as, 335
 radiation as, 333–334, 335f, 336
 surgery as, 332–333, 333f
bromocriptine, for hyperadrenocorticism, 266
busulfan (Myleran), 70t, 400. *See also* alkylating agents

cachexia, 29–31, 30t, 37f
calcitonin, for hypercalcemia, 33
calcium, colon cancer and, 9
canines. *See also names of specific conditions and tumors*
bone tumor in, 234–246. *See also* bone tumor, canine
cardiac tumor in, 174, 412–417
genetic factors in, 5
granulosa cell tumor in, 285
incidence of cancer in, 3, 4f
intracutaneous cornifying epithelioma in, 148–149
lymphoma and lymphoid leukemia in, 380–391. *See also* lymphoma, lymphoid leukemia and
lymphomatoid granulomatosis in, 228–230, 230f
malignant histiocytosis in, 230–231
mammary gland tumor in, 293–294, 294f, 295f
 treatment for, 296–298
metastasis rate in, 23
myeloproliferative disorders in, 394–401. *See also* myeloproliferative disorders
ocular dermoids in, 6

ocular melanoma in, 354–356
oral cancer in, 187–188. *See also* oral cancer
oral eosinophilic granuloma in, 185. *See also* oral cancer
osteosarcoma in, 5, 6, 234–241. *See also* osteosarcoma, canine
ovarian tumor in, 283–285, 284t
prostatic tumor in, 308–309, 309f
radiation response of tumor in, 84–85, 85t
skin and subcutaneous tumors in, 139
soft tissue sarcoma in, 174, 174f
spayed, risks of, 292
testicular tumor in, 305–308, 306f, 306t, 307f
thyroid tumor in, 253–259. *See also* thyroid tumor, canine
transmissible venereal tumor in, 421–424
 clinical signs and history of, 422f, 422–423, 423f
 pathology and natural behavior of, 421–422
 penile, 310
 vulvar and vaginal tumors in, 288–290, 289f
carbohydrates, dietary, 8
carcinogenesis
 inhibitors of, 9
 process of, 3, 5
carcinogens, 3, 5, 7–8
carcinoid, 197
carcinoma. *See also names of specific carcinomas*
anal sac, 209–213
bile duct, 196–199
bladder, 317, 318f, 319f
gastric, 193–195
hepatocellular, 196–199
inflammatory, 294, 294f, 295
intestinal, 200–207
lung/pulmonary, 225–228
mammary, 293t, 293–294, 294f
medullary, 258
nasal, 218–222
pancreatic, 192

prostatic, 308
salivary, 190
thyroid, canine, 253–259, 254f–255f
 hyperthyroidism and, 259
transitional cell, 317, 320
cardiac tumor, canine, 174
cardiovascular disorders
hemangiosarcoma and, 413, 415
hyperthyroidism and, 259–260
castration, 12, 62
for perianal tumor, 211
for prostatic tumor, 308–309
for testicular tumor, 307
CDDP. *See cis*-diaminedichloroplatinum
cell cycle, 63–64
cell-mediated immunity, 92–96
effector cell mechanisms in, 94–96
induced, 92–93, 93f
natural, 93–94
cerebrospinal fluid collection
brain tumor and, 328
spinal cord neoplasia and, 338
ceruminous gland tumor, 145–146, 147f
CFM. *See* chemotactic factor for macrophages
CGL. *See* chronic granulocytic leukemia
chemical carcinogens, 3, 5, 7–8
mammary gland tumor and, 12
chemodectoma, 277–278, 278f
chemotactic factor for macrophages, 93, 93f
chemotherapy, 63–76. *See also names of specific chemotherapeutic agents*
advantages of, 63
for ALL, 388, 389t
alopecia and, 66
biologic basis for, 63–64
for bladder cancer, 320
bone marrow toxicity and, 65–66
for brain tumor, 334–335
for canine lymphoma, 385–388, 386t, 387t
for canine osteosarcoma, 239–240

chemotherapy: (*Continued*)
  as cause of anemia, 36
  as cause of cancer, 8
  for CLL, 388, 389t
  combination, 68
  for cutaneous lymphoma, 389
  drug delivery systems for, 129–132
  drug resistance and, 66–68
  drugs used in, 69–74, 70t–71t
    alkylating agents as, 69, 70t, 72
    antibiotics as, 71t, 73
    antimetabolites as, 70t, 72–73
    conversion table for, 69, 72t
    hormones as, 71t, 73–74
    miscellaneous, 71t, 74
    plant alkaloids as, 71t, 73
  for feline lymphoma, 370–371, 371t
  FeLV and, 370–371, 371t
  guidelines for, 68–69, 446–447
  for hemangiosarcoma, 151, 415–416
  hyperthermia and, 114, 114t, 119–121
  for lung cancer, 228–230, 230f
  for mammary gland tumor, 297, 298
  for mast cell tumor, 161–162, 162f
  for mesothelioma, 427
  for metastasis, 26
  in multimodality therapy, 74–76
  for myeloid diseases, 373
  pharmacologic factors in, 64–65
  for plasma cell neoplasm, 407–408, 408f, 409f, 410
  for renal cancer, 315
  for schwannoma, 345
  for skin and subcutaneous tumors, 141
  for soft tissue sarcoma, 171, 172–173
  surgical oncology and, 61
  systemic cancer and, 346
  for testicular tumor, 307
  for thymoma, 420
  toxicity of, 65–66
  for transmissible venereal tumor, 424
children, pet loss and, 444. *See also* pet loss
chlorambucil (Leukeran), 70t, 72. *See also* alkylating agents
  for CLL, 389
  for multiple myeloma, 407–408, 408f, 409f, 410
chondroma rodens, 246–247
chondrosarcoma, osseous, 242–243, 243f
chromaffin cell tumor, 275–277, 276f
chromosome aberrations, in transmissible venereal tumor, 421
chronic granulocytic leukemia, 396. *See also* myeloproliferative disorders
  diagnosis of, 398
  therapy for, 399–400
chronic lymphocytic leukemia, 380, 381. *See also* lymphoid leukemia
  macroglobulinemia in, 405
  treatment for, 388–389
ciliary body epithelial tumor, 356–357
cimetidine (Tagamet), 99
  for mast cell tumor, 162f, 163
cis-diaminedichloroplatinum (Platinol), 74, 71t
cisplatin, for canine osteosarcoma, 239–241
  for squamous cell carcinoma, 144–145
  for bladder cancer, 320
classification systems
  generic, 18, 19t
  importance of, 17–18
  surgical pathology and, 20–21
clinical trials, 429–434
  cooperative, 434
  evaluation criteria for, 433
  follow-up procedures for, 433–434
  general considerations for, 430t, 430–432, 434
  sample size for, 432f, 432–433, 433t
  standardization in, 432
  statistical considerations for, 434
  types of, 429–430, 430t
CLL. *See* chronic lymphocytic leukemia
coagulogram, 296
Codman's triangle, 235, 236f
colon cancer, 11–12. *See also* intestinal tract tumor
  calcium and, 9
colony-stimulating factors, 394f, 394–395
colorectal cancer, 207. *See also* intestinal tract tumor
conjuctival tumor, 353–354
cooperative clinical trials, 434. *See also* clinical trials
corticoids, urinary, hyperadrenocorticism and, 265–266
corticosteroids
  for brain tumor, 331–332
  for CLL, 389
  for lymphoma, 380–402
  for plasma cell tumors, 402–411
  for mast cell tumor, 162
corticotrophin-releasing hormone stimulation testing, for hyperadrenocorticism, 266
cortisol, excessive. *See* hyperadrenocorticism
Corynebacterium parvum therapy, 96, 97f, 182, 183f
cryoglobulinemia, macroglobulinemia in, 405
cryosurgery, 106–111
  advantages of, 111
  cell death from, 107
  contraindications for, 111
  definition of, 106
  disadvantages of, 110–111
  equipment for, 106–107, 107t, 110–111
  for eyelid tumor, 109
  for mast cell tumor, 161
  for oral cancer, 110, 180
  for perianal region, 109–110
  for skin and subcutaneous tumors, 110, 141
  techniques for, 107–108
  tissue response to, 108–109
CSF. *See* colony-stimulating factors
cycasin, in etiology of cancer, 7
cyclophosphamide (Cytoxan), 70t. *See also* chemotherapy

for anemia, 36

for canine lymphoma, 386t, 387t

as cause of bladder cancer, 8, 66, 69, 70t, 72, 317

for CLL, 389

for fibrosarcoma, 173

for multiple myeloma, 407–408, 408f, 409f, 410

for myeloid diseases, 373

pharmacology of, 64

toxicity of, 8, 66, 69, 70t, 72, 317

cyproheptadine

for hyperadrenocorticism, 266

for mast cell tumor, 163

cystadenocarcinoma, renal, 313f, 313–315

cystadenoma, 283–284, 284t

cystectomy, 318, 319f

cystitis

bladder cancer and, 317

cyclophosphamide-induced, 69, 70t, 72

hyperadrenocorticism and, 265

cytochemical stains, for cell type determination, 389f, 399

cytokines, 92–93, 93f

for immunotherapy, 100–101

cytologic diagnosis, 41–51

advantages of, 41–42

limitations of, 42

malignancy criteria in, 49–51, 49f–51f, 50t

microscopic examination for, 48

slide preparation for, 44–47, 45f, 46t, 47f, 48f

specimens for, 42–44

collection of, 43–44, 44f. See also biopsy

types of, 42

cytoreductive surgery, 61

Cytosar-U. See cytosine arabinoside

cytosine arabinoside (Cytosar-U), 70t. See also antimetabolites

for canine lymphoma, 388

for myeloid diseases, 373

for myeloproliferative disorders, 400, 401

cytotoxic agents. See also chemotherapy

guidelines for handling of, 446–447

Cytoxan. See cyclophosphamide

dacarbazine, 70t, 72. See also alkylating agents

for canine lymphoma, 388

death of pet, 436–445. See also pet loss

incidence of cancer as cause of, 1

debulking surgery, 61

dental procedures, prior radiotherapy and, 87–88

dental tumor, 178t, 179. See also oral cancer

dermatofibrosis renal carcinoma, 313f

dermoid cyst, 141

dexamethasone, for brain tumor, 331–332

dexamethasone suppression test, for hyperadrenocorticism, 266

DFMO. See D,L-alpha-Difluoro-methylornithine

DHE. See dihematoporphyrin ether

diabetes

hyperadrenocorticism and, 265

pituitary tumor and, 273

dialkylhydrazines, in etiology of cancer, 7

diazoxide

for hypoglycemia, 272

for insulinoma, 34

DIC. See disseminated intravascular coagulation

diet

for canines or cats with cancer, 31

in etiology of cancer, 5, 8–9, 11–12

diethylstilbestrol, 71t. See also hormone therapy

Diff-Quik stain, 44–47, 47f, 51f

dihematoporphyrin ether, 124–127

disseminated intravascular coagulation, 36–37

in hemangiosarcoma, 414

distant metastases, TNM classification of, 452–453

D,L-alpha-Difluoromethylornithine, 133

DNA, viral, 9, 10f

doxorubicin (Adriamycin), 71t, 73

for fibrosarcoma, 173

for hemangiopericytoma, 173

for hypergammaglobulinemia, 38

for lymphoma, 386, 386t, 387, 387t

for multiple myeloma, 38

for myeloproliferative disorders, 400, 401

for osteosarcoma, 239

resistance to, 67

for thyroid tumor, 257

for transmissible venereal tumor, 424

drug delivery, targeted, 129–132, 130f

drug resistance, 66–68

DTIC. See dacarbazine

dysgerminoma, 284, 284t

ear

ceruminous gland, 145–146, 147f

ectopic hormone production, 31–34, 32t

Efudex cream, 70t. See also 5-fluorouracil

electromyography, for peripheral nerve tumor, 344

electron probe microanalysis, 21

ELISA. See enzyme-linked immunosorbent assay

Elspar. See asparaginase

EMG. See electromyography

endocrine tumor, 253–278

canine thyroid tumor as, 253–259. See also thyroid tumor, canine

chemodectoma as, 277–278, 278f

feline hyperthyroidism and, 259–264. See also hyperthyroidism, feline

hyperadrenocorticism and, 264–268. See also hyperadrenocorticism

endocrine tumor: (*Continued*)
  MEN as, 277
  pancreatic insulin-secreting
    neoplasm as, 268–272. *See
    also* pancreatic insulin-se-
    creting neoplasm
  parathyroid tumor as, 274–275
  pheochromocytoma as, 275–
    277, 276f
  pituitary tumor as, 273
  Zollinger-Ellison syndrome
    and, 275
endometrial cancer, human, 288
environmental contaminants, in
    etiology of cancer, 5, 8
enzyme-linked immunosorbent
    assay
  for FeLV, 368
  for FIV, 365
eosinophilic granuloma, oral
  canine, 185
  feline, 186–187f
eosinophilic leukemia, 396. *See
    also* myeloproliferative
    disorders
  diagnosis of, 398
epidemiology, 3–15
epidermoid cyst, 141, 142f. *See
    also* skin and subcuta-
    neous tumors
epithelial tumor, 19t, 141–149.
    See also adenocarcinoma
  basal cell tumor as, 144, 145f,
    146f
  ciliary body, 356–357
  hair matrix tumor as, 149
  intracutaneous cornifying epi-
    thelioma as, 148f, 148–149
  ovarian tumor as, 283–284,
    284t, 285
  papilloma as, 141–143, 142f
  sebaceous gland tumor as,
    144–146, 146f, 147f
  squamous cell carcinoma as,
    143f, 143–144, 144f
  sweat gland tumor as, 146–148
epulides, oral, 179, 185, 186f.
    See also oral cancer
erythroid diseases, FeLV and,
    373
erythropoietin, 394f, 394–395
  ectopic production of, 34
esophageal cancer, 9, 11, 190–
    191

esophagoscopy, 191
estrogen, in etiology of cancer,
    5–6, 25
estrogen therapy, for perianal tu-
    mor, 211
etiology, of cancer, 3, 4f, 5–9
euthanasia, pet loss and, 439,
    443–444
excisional biopsy, 56. *See also* bi-
    opsy
exocrine pancreas, 192–193
eye. *See* ocular, 351–360
eyelid tumor, 351–353, 352f

FAIDS. *See* feline acquired im-
    munodeficiency syndrome
family
  pet loss and, 436–445. *See also*
    pet loss
  pet's role in, 436
feline acquired immunodeficiency
    syndrome
  FeLV and, 364, 369, 371t,
    371–373. *See also* feline
    leukemia virus
  FIV and, 362, 363t, 374–376,
    375t
feline immunodeficiency virus,
    362, 363t, 374–376, 375t.
    See also retrovirus(es), fe-
    line
feline leukemia virus, 362–374
  antibiotics and, 372–373
  chemotherapy and, 370–371,
    371t
  classification of, 362–363, 363t
  diseases associated with, 369–
    374, 370t
    abortions as, 374
    erythroid diseases as, 373
    FAIDS as, 364, 369, 371t,
      371–373
    glomerulonephritis as, 374
    immunosuppression and,
      372–373
    lymphoid atrophy as, 372
    lymphoma as, 363, 369–371,
      371t
    myeloid diseases as, 373–374
    neurologic syndromes as,
      374
    resorption syndromes as, 374

  thymic atrophy as, 371t,
    371–372
  endogenous sequences of, 364–
    367
    exposure and, 367, 367t
    FeLV genome in, 364, 365f
    FeLV replication in, 364,
      366f
    infection in, 364–365, 372–
      373
  epidemiology of, 367–368
    effects and, 363t
    occurrence and, 363, 367
    testing methods and, 367t
    transmission and, 363t
  FIV compared to, 375, 375t
  human AIDS and, 372
  immune response for, 368,
    371t, 372–373
  latent, 365–366
  prevention of spread of, 368–
    369
  spinal cord neoplasia and, 337
  subgroups of, 363t, 364
  thymic lymphoma and, 419
  vaccines for, 369
  virology of, 363t, 363–364
feline oncornavirus-associated cell
    membrane antigen anti-
    body, 366, 368, 370
felines. *See also* names of specific
    conditions and tumors
  fibrosarcoma in, 374
  granulosa cell tumor in, 285–
    286
  hyperthyroidism in, 259–264.
    See also hyperthyroidism,
    feline
  mammary gland tumor in,
    294–295
    incidence of, 292–293
    prevalence of, 292
    treatment for, 298
  metastasis rate in, 23
  oral eosinophilic granuloma in,
    186–187f
  ovarian tumor in, 285–286
  pituitary tumor in, 273–274
  skin and subcutaneous tumors
    in, 139. *See also* skin and
    subcutaneous tumors
  soft tissue sarcoma in, 173–174
  testicular tumor in, 308
  thyroid tumor in, 258, 258t

vulvar and vaginal tumors in, 289f, 290f, 290–291
feline sarcoma virus, 362, 363t, 374
FeLV. *See* feline leukemia virus
FeLV-neutralizing antibody, 368
ferrous sulfate, 36
FeSV. *See* feline sarcoma virus
fever, cancer-associated, 38
fiber, dietary, 8
fibroameloblastoma, inductive, 185–186, 186f
fibroblastoma, perineural, 342
fibroepithelial hyperplasia, of feline mammary glands, 294–295
fibroma, 168, 168t
    fibrosarcoma and, 149, 150f
    treatment of, 172–173
fibronectin therapy, 102, 102f
fibrosarcoma, 149, 168, 168t
    feline, 374
    oral, 177, 178t, 180f, 183. *See also* oral cancer
    osseous, 244
    prognosis for, 173
    treatment of, 172–173
fine-needle aspiration, 24–25, 42–43. *See also* cytologic diagnosis
    for cutaneous tumor, 140
    for histiocytoma, 153
    for mast cell tumor, 160, 160f
    for thymoma, 418–419, 419f
    for transmissible venereal tumor, 423, 424f
FIV. *See* feline immunodeficiency virus
5-fluorouracil (Efudex cream), 70t. *See also* antimetabolites
FOCMA. *See* feline oncornavirus-associated cell membrane antigen antibody
follicular cyst, 141
food additives, in etiology of cancer, 7–8
fracture, management of, 407
Franzen syringe holder, 43–44, 55f
fungal infections, 372–373
    treatment for, 389
furosemide, for hypercalcemia, 33

gammopathies, in plasma cell neoplasm, 402–405
gastric cancer, 193–195, 194f, 195f
gastroduodenostomy, 194
gastrointestinal tract tumor, 177–213
    chemotherapy and, 65
    esophageal cancer as, 9, 11, 190–191
    gastric cancer as, 193–195, 194f, 195f
    hepatic tumor as, 196–199, 198f, 270, 271
    intestinal tract tumor as, 200–207. *See also* intestinal tract tumor
    oral cancer as, 177–188. *See also* oral cancer
    pancreatic cancer as, 192–193
    perianal tumor as, 209–213. *See also* perianal tumor
    salivary gland cancer as, 190
gastroscopy, 194
genetic factors, in etiology of cancer, 5
genetic probes, 21
germ cell tumor, 283–284, 284t, 285
giant cell tumor
    extraskeletal, 151–152
    osseous, 245
glioma, 325–326. *See also* brain tumor
glomerulonephritis, FeLV-induced, 374
glucagon tolerance test, for hyperadrenocorticism, 266
glucocorticoid therapy, for mast cell tumor, 161–163
glucose-insulin ratio, insulinoma and, 270
glucose tolerance testing, 270
glutaraldehyde, 20
Gompertzian growth, 26, 64
granular cell myoblastoma, 184–185, 185f
granulomatous histiocytic dermatosis, 389
granulosa cell tumor, 284t, 284–286
grief, pet loss and, 438–439, 442–445. *See also* pet loss

hair loss. *See* alopecia
hair matrix tumor, 149
H_2 antagonists, 99, 163
heart tumors, 174. *See also* chemodectoma, 277–278, *and* hemangiosarcoma, 412–417
hemangioendothelioma, malignant, 412–417. *See also* hemangiosarcoma
hemangioma, 168t, 169
    conjunctival, 353–354
    hemangiosarcoma and, 150–151
hemangiopericytoma, 149–150, 151f, 168t, 168–169
    prognosis for, 173
    treatment of, 173
hemangiosarcoma, 168t, 169, 412–417
    clinical signs and history of, 413–414
    clinical staging for, 416t
    comparative aspects of, 417
    conjunctival, 353–354
    cutaneous, 150–151
    diagnosis of, 414, 415f, 415t
    hemangioma and, 168t, 169, 353–354
    incidence of, 412
    osseous, 243–244, 244f
    pathology and natural behavior of, 413
    prognosis for, 416–417
    risk factors for, 412
    therapy for, 414–416
hematologic-hemostatic abnormalities, 35t, 35–38
hematopoeitic dysplasia, 395
hematopoiesis
    in myeloproliferative disorders, 395
    normal, 394f, 394–395
hematopoietic tumor, 362–410
    canine lymphoma and lymphoid leukemia as, 380–391. *See also* lymphoma, lymphoid leukemia and
    canine myeloproliferative disorders and, 394–401. *See also* myeloproliferative disorders
    feline retroviruses as, 362–376. *See also* retroviruses, feline

hematopoietic tumor: (Continued)
plasma cell neoplasm as, 402–
410. See also plasma cell
neoplasm
hemorrhage
hemangiosarcoma and, 414
transmissible venereal tumor
and, 422
hepatic tumor, 196–199, 198f
metastasis and, 270, 271
hepatocellular tumor, 196–199,
198f
hepatosplenomegaly, canine lymphoma and, 381
herpes viruses, 10f. See also
DNA, viral
histiocytoma, cutaneous, 151–
153, 153f
histiocytosis, malignant, 230–231
hormone-dependent tumor, 292–
303. See also mammary
gland tumor
hormones, in etiology of cancer,
5–6
hormone therapy, 71t, 73–74.
See also chemotherapy;
names of specific hor-
monal agents
for mammary gland tumor,
297–298
Horner's syndrome, 343
H₂ receptor blockers, 99, 163
human immunodeficiency viruses, 362, 363t. See also
retrovirus(es)
hydrazines, 7
Hydrea. See hydroxyurea
hydroxyurea (Hydrea), 34, 71t.
See also chemotherapy
for myeloproliferative disorders, 399–400
hyperadrenocorticism, 264–268
brain tumor and, 326
clinical signs and history of,
264–265
comparative aspects of, 264–
268
diagnosis of, 265–266
incidence of, 264
pathology and natural behavior
of, 264
prognosis for, 268
risk factors for, 264

therapy for, 266–268
hypercalcemia, 31–33, 32t, 256–
257
canine lymphoma and, 275,
381, 390
hyperparathyroidism and, 274–
275
lymphoma and, 275
metastasis and, 25
parathyroid tumor and, 274
plasma cell neoplasm and,
403–404, 407
therapy for, 407
thymic lymphoma and, 419
hyperestrogenism, as evidence of
metastasis, 25
hypergammaglobulinemia, 37–38
hyperparathyroidism, hypercalcemia secondary to, 274–
275
hyperplasia
of feline mammary glands,
294–295
sebaceous, nodular, 145
hypertension
intraoperative, 277
pheochromocytoma and, 276
propranolol and, 277
hyperthermia, 113–121
biologic effects of, 113–115,
114f
chemotherapy and, 114,
114t, 119–121
radiotherapy and, 113–114,
115f, 117–118, 118t, 119f
thermal isoeffect dose for,
114–115
clinical results of, 117–118,
118t, 119f
for mast cell tumor, 161
for oral cancer, 181
physical methods of, 115–117,
116f
whole-body, 116–117, 118–121
hyperthyroidism
canine, 254–255
clinical signs and history of, 259
comparative aspects of, 263–
264
diagnosis of, 259–260
feline, 259–264
cardiovascular disorders and,
259–260

incidence of, 259
pathology and natural behavior of, 259
therapy for, 260–263, 261f,
263f
hypertrophic osteopathy, 34–35,
35f
hyperviscosity syndrome, in
plasma cell neoplasm, 405
hypocalcemia, 256–257
hypoglycemia, 33–34
diazoxide for, 272
glucose test strips for, 270
hepatic tumor and, 198
insulinoma and, 269–272
metastasis and, 25
prednisone for, 271–272
hypoparathyroidism, 256
postoperative, 262
hypothyroidism, canine, 255, 257

ICT. See interstitial cell tumor
IFA. See immunofluorescent antibody
IFN. See interferon therapy
Il-1. See interleukin-1
Il-2. See interleukin-2
Il-3. See interleukin-3
immune identification, 21
immune response, in cell-mediated immunity, 93f, 95–
96. See also cell-mediated
immunity
immune response cascade, 93f,
96
immune suppression, chemotherapy and, 65–66
immunofluorescent antibody, for
FeLV, 367t, 367–368
immunology, 9
immunosurveillance, 95
immunotherapy, 96–102
bacterial products for, 96–99,
98f
for brain tumor, 335
general considerations for,
102–103
for mesothelioma, 427
for metastasis, 26
passive, 101–102
vaccines for, 99–101

incidence of cancer, site of origin and, 3, 4f
incisional biopsy, 56, 56f. *See also* biopsy
indolent ulcer, 186, 187f
inductive fibroameloblastoma, 185–186, 186f
infections, CNS, 356
insulin-glucose ratio, insulinoma and, 270
insulinoma, 268–272. *See also* pancreatic insulin-secreting neoplasm
  glucose tolerance testing for, 270
  hypoglycemia and, 269–272
  surgery for, 33
interferon therapy, 93, 93f, 94, 100–101
interleukin-1, 93, 93f
interleukin-2, 93, 93f, 94
interleukin-3, 93, 93f
interleukins, for immunotherapy, 100–101
interstitial cell tumor
  adenoma and, 210
  testicular, 305–308, 306f, 306t, 307f
intestinal tract tumor, 200–207
  clinical signs and history of, 202
  comparative aspects of, 207
  diagnosis of, 202–203, 203f, 204f
  incidence of, 200–201
  pathology and natural behavior of, 201–202, 202f, 203f
  prognosis for, 206–207
  risk factors for, 200–201
  therapy for, 65, 203–206, 205f, 206f
intracranial neoplasia, 325–336. *See also* brain tumor
intracutaneous cornifying epithelioma, 148f, 148–149
iodine therapy, 261, 262–263
ionizing radiation, in etiology of cancer, 6
iron, 9
islet cell tumor, 268–272. *See also* pancreatic insulin-secreting neoplasm
isoflurane, intraoperative, 277

juxtacortical osteosarcoma, 241–242

keratoacanthoma, 148f, 148–149
ketoconazole, for hyperadrenocorticism, 267
kidney. *See* renal, 312–315
killer cells, 93f, 93–94
Kubler-Ross, Elizabeth, 438, 441

LAP. *See* leukocyte alkaline phosphatase
laparotomy, hepatic tumor and, 198
large bowel cancer, 11–12. *See also* intestinal tract tumor
laryngeal tumor, 222–225
laser therapy, 125, 126t, 127
leiomyoma
  uterine, 287–288
  vulvar and vaginal, 289–291
leiomyosarcoma
  intestinal, 200, 202, 202f, 203f. *See also* intestinal tract tumor
  uterine, 287–288
lemnocytoma, 342. *See also* peripheral nerve tumor
lentiviruses, 362–363, 363t. *See also* retrovirus(es)
leukemia. *See also* feline leukemia virus; myeloproliferative disorders, canine; *names of specific leukemias*
Leukeran. *See* chlorambucil
leukocyte alkaline phosphatase, 399
leukocytosis, 36
levamisole therapy, 99
lid tumor, 351–353, 352f
limb sparing, 239–241, 241t
lipids, dietary, 8
lipoma, 168t, 169, 289
  liposarcoma and, 151, 152f
  treatment of, 172
liposarcoma, 151, 168t, 169
  lipoma and, 151, 152f
  prognosis for, 173

  treatment of, 172
liposomes, for targeted drug delivery, 129–131, 130f
liquid nitrogen vs. nitrous oxide, 106–107, 107t
liver. *See* hepatic, 196–199
lobular hyperplasia, of feline mammary gland, 294
Lonidamine, 134
lumpectomy, for canines, 296
lung cancer, 225–231
  canine lymphomatoid granulomatosis as, 228–230, 230f
  metastatic, 227
  primary, 225–231
    clinical signs and history of, 226
    comparative aspects of, 227–228
    diagnosis of, 226f, 226–227
    incidence of, 225, 227
    pathology and natural behavior of, 225
    prognosis for, 227, 229f
    risk factors for, 225
    therapy for, 227, 228f, 229f
luteoma, 285
lymphadenopathy, 60
lymphangioma, 168t, 169
  cutaneous, 153
lymphangiosarcoma, 169, 169t
lymph nodes
  immunologic response of, 24–25
  removal of, 25, 60–61
lymphoblastic leukemia, feline, 371, 371t
lymphoid atrophy, FeLV and, 371t, 371–372
lymphoid leukemia, canine lymphoma and, 380–391. *See also* lymphoma, lymphoid leukemia and
lymphokines, 92–93, 93f
  for immunotherapy, 100–101
lymphoma
  cutaneous, 384
    treatment for, 389–390
  drug resistance and, 68
  feline, 363, 369–371
    chemotherapy for, 370–371, 371t

lymphoma: (Continued)
 FeLV and, 363, 369–371
  FOCMA and, 368, 370
 hypercalcemia and, 32, 275
 intestinal, 200–201, 203f
 intracranial, 326
 lymphoid leukemia and, 380–391
  clinical signs and history of, 383–384
  comparative aspects of, 390–391
  cutaneous, 384, 389–390
  diagnosis of, 384–385, 385t
  differential diagnosis of, 383
  histologic classification of, 382t, 382–383, 384, 390
  incidence of, 380
  paraneoplastic syndromes and, 383
  pathology and natural behavior of, 381
  prognosis for, 390
  risk factors for, 380–381
  therapy for, 385–390, 386t, 387t
 neuronal, 342, 342f, 344, 345. See also peripheral nerve tumor
 renal, 313–315, 371, 371t
 spinal, 337, 338–339
 thymic, 419
lymphomatoid granulomatosis, canine, 228–230, 230f
lymphoscintigraphy, for metastasis, 25
lymphotoxins, 93, 93f
Lysodren. See o,p'-DDD

MAb. See monoclonal antibodies
macroglobulinemia, 381, 402–410. See also plasma cell neoplasm
macrophage activating factor, 93, 93f, 101
 muramyl dipeptide and, 98
macrophages, 93, 93f, 94
 activated, 26
MAF. See macrophage activating factor

magnetic microspheres, for targeted drug delivery, 131
mammary gland tumor, 292–303
 canine, 293–294, 294f, 295f
  treatment for, 296–298
 clinical signs and history of, 295
 comparative aspects of, 301–303
 cutaneous involvement in, 295, 295f
 diagnosis of, 296
 feline, 294–295
  prevalence and incidence of, 292–293
  treatment for, 298
 hormonal factors in, 5–6
 incidence of, 12
 lymph node involvement in, 297, 299–300
 natural behavior of, 293–294
 pathology of, 293t, 293–294
 prevention of, 12
 prognosis for, 298–301, 299t, 299f–302f
 receptor-positive, 301, 302
 risk factors for, 12, 292–293
mammectomy, for canines, 296
mandibulectomy, 179–180, 181t, 183–184
mast cell tumor, 156–165
 clinical signs and history of, 159
 clinical staging system for, 161
 comparative aspects of, 165
 diagnosis of, 160f, 160–161
 histologic classification of, 157t, 157–158, 158t
 incidence of, 156
 intestinal, 201
 pathology and natural behavior of, 157–159
 prognosis for, 164, 164t
 risk factors for, 156–157
 treatment of, 161–164, 162f
mastectomy
 for canines, 296–297, 298
 palliative, 61
mastocytemia, 160
maxillectomy, 179–180, 182t, 183–184
MBV. See mixed bacterial vaccine

M-component disorders, 37–38
MDP. See muramyl dipeptide
medullary carcinoma, 258
melanoma, 153–154
 bacille Calmette-Guerin and, 182
 genetic factors and, 5
 ocular, 355–356
  canine, 354–356
  feline, 356, 357f
 oral, 177, 178t, 183
melphalan (Alkeran), 70t, 72. See also alkylating agents
 for hypergammaglobulinemia, 38
 for multiple myeloma, 38, 407–408, 408f, 409f, 410
membrana nictitans tumor, 353f, 353–354
membrane transport inhibitors, 133–135
MEN. See multiple endocrine neoplasia
meningioma, 325–326. See also brain tumor
 orbital, 358–359
 spinal, 336–337
MER. See methanol-extractable residue of BCG
6-mercaptopurine (Purinethol), 70t. See also antimetabolites
Merkel cell tumor, 188
mesenchymoma, osseous, 245–246
mesothelioma, 425–427
 clinical signs and history of, 425–426, 426f
 comparative aspects of, 427
 diagnosis of, 426–427
 incidence of, 425
 pathology and natural behavior of, 425
 prognosis for, 427
 sclerosing, 426, 426f
 therapy for, 427
metabolic encephalopathy, systemic cancer and, 346
metastasis, 23–27
 canine osteosarcoma and, 237
 "cure" for, 25–26
 diagnosis of, 25
 hepatic tumor and, 270, 271

neurologic, 345t, 345–346
   pathogenesis of, 23–24
   regional lymph nodes in, 24–25
   therapy for, 26–27
methanol-extractable residue of
      BCG, 97
methimazole, for feline hyperthy-
      roidism, 260–261
methotrexate, 70t. *See also* anti-
      metabolites
   for canine lymphoma, 386t,
      387t
   resistance to, 67
methylene blue stain, 44–47
Michele trephine, 246
microscopic examination, 48–49,
      49f–51f
microspheres, for targeted drug
      delivery, 131
MIF. *See* migration inhibition
      factor
migration inhibition factor, 92,
      93f
minerals and vitamins, 8–9
mithramycin, for hypercalcemia,
      33
mitotane. *See* o,p'-DDD, Lysod-
      rin, 264–268, 273–274
mixed bacterial vaccine, 98
moist desquamation, radiation
      therapy and, 85–87, 86f,
      87t
monoclonal antibodies, 101, 132
monoclonal gammopathies, 37–38
morphological interpretation
   biopsy for, 18
   problems in, 20
   tissue fixation for, 18, 20
MPD. *See* myeloproliferative dis-
      orders
MTP. *See* muramyl tripeptide
mucositis, radiation-induced, 86,
      87t
multiple endocrine neoplasia, 277
multiple myeloma, 406–410. *See
      also* plasma cell neoplasm
   chemotherapy for, 407–408,
      408f, 409f, 410
   clinical stages of, 406, 406f
   diagnosis of, 406
muramyl dipeptide, 97–98, 98f
muramyl tripeptide, 97, 98
Mustragen. *See* nitrogen mustard

myasthenia gravis, thymoma and,
      418, 420
mycosis fungoides, treatment for,
      389
myeloblastopenia, FeLV-in-
      duced, 373–374
myelodysplastic syndrome, 400
myelofibrosis. *See also* myelopro-
      liferative disorders
   diagnosis of, 398
   FeLV and, 373–374
   primary, 396–397
myelography, for spinal cord
      neoplasia, 338, 340f, 341f
myeloma. *See also* multiple mye-
      loma
   plasma cell, 406
   plasmacytoma, 153
myeloma kidney, 404
myeloproliferative disorders
   canine, 394–401
      acute, 395, 397, 400, 401t
      chronic, 395–397
      classification of, 395
      clincial signs and history of,
         397–398
      comparative aspects of, 400–
         401
      diagnosis of, 398–399
      incidence of, 394
      pathology and natural behav-
         ior of, 394–397
      prognosis for, 400
      risk factors for, 394
      therapy for, 399–400, 401t
   FeLV and, 373–374
Myleran. *See* busulfan
myoblastoma, granular cell, 184–
      185, 185f
myxosarcoma, 168t

nasal planum, cancer of, 215–
      218, 216f, 218f
nasal tumor, 218–222, 220f–223f
   differential diagnosis for, 219t
nasopharyngeal polyp, feline,
      186, 187f. *See also* oral
      cancer
National Cancer Institute, Veter-
      inary Medical Data Pro-
      gram of, 23

needle punch biopsy, 55f, 55–56,
      309, 309f. *See also* biopsy
neoplasia, features of, 16, 17t
nephrectomy, for renal cancer,
      315
nephroblastoma, 313–315, 316f
nervous system neoplasia, 325–
      346
   intracranial neoplasia as, 325–
      336. *See also* brain tumor
   metastatic, 345t, 345–346
   peripheral nerve tumor as,
      341–345. *See also* periph-
      eral nerve tumor
   spinal cord neoplasia as, 336–
      341. *See also* spinal cord
      neoplasia
neural crest tumor, 19t
neural sheath tumor, 341–345
neurilemmoma, 342
neurinoma, 342
neuroendocrine cell tumor, 188
neuroepithelioma, spinal, 336–
      337. *See also* spinal cord
      neoplasia
neurofibroma, 168t, 169, 342
neurofibromatosis, 341, 342
neurofibrosarcoma, 168t, 169,
      342
neurolemmoma, 342. *See also*
      peripheral nerve tumor
neurologic disorders
   cancer-associated, 345t, 345–
      346
   FeLV-induced, 374
neuronal tumor, 341–345. *See
      also* peripheral nerve tu-
      mor
neurosurgery, 332–333, 333f
neutropenia
   FeLV-induced, 374
   systemic cancer and, 346
nitrate, in etiology of cancer, 7
nitrite, in etiology of cancer, 7
nitrogen mustard, 70t, 72. *See
      also* alkylating agents
   for mycosis fungoides, 389
nitrous oxide vs. liquid nitrogen,
      106–107, 107t
NK cells, 93f, 94
nodal excision, 25
nodular sebaceous hyperplasia,
      145

502   INDEX

nodulectomy, for canines, 296
non-islet cell tumor, hypoglycemia and, 33–34
nosectomy, for squamous cell
carcinoma, 217–218, 218f

ocular tumor, 351–360
comparative aspects of, 359–
360
conjunctiva tumor as, 353–354
dermoid as, 66
eyelid tumor, 351–353, 352f
membrana nictitans tumor as,
353f, 353–354
orbital tumor as, 358–359, 359f
primary, 354–358
canine ocular melanoma as,
354–356
ciliary body epithelial tumor
as, 356, 357f
feline ocular melanoma as,
356–357f
feline post-traumatic sarcoma
as, 357–358
oncocytoma, laryngeal, 222–225
oncogenes, genetic factors and, 5
Oncovin. See vincristine
oncoviruses, 362–363, 363t. See
also retrovirus(es) 43
oophorectomy, 61–62
o,p'-DDD (Lysodren), 71t, 74
for hyperadrenocorticism, 266–
268
optic nerve tumor, 358–359, 359f
oral cancer, 177–188
clinical signs and history of,
179
common, 178t, 184–188, 185f–
187f
comparative aspects of, 188
diagnosis of, 179, 180f
eosinophilic granuloma as, 185,
186–187, 187f
epulides as, 185, 186f
incidence of, 177
inductive fibroameloblastoma
as, 185–186, 186f
nasopharyngeal polyp as, 186,
186f
neuroendocrine, 188
papillary, 187–188

pathology and natural behavior
of, 177, 179
prevention of, 9, 11
prognosis for, 182–184
risk factors for, 9, 11, 177
therapy for, 179–182
tongue cancer as, 184–185,
185f
tonsillar, 184
undifferentiated, in young canines, 187
viral, 185
orbital tumors. See ocular, 351–
360
osteochondromatosis, 248, 248f
feline, 250
osteolysis, plasma cell neoplasm
and, 403–405, 404f. See
also plasma cell neoplasm
osteoma, 246–247, 247f. See also
bone tumor
osteoporosis, plasma cell neoplasm and, 404–405. See
also plasma cell neoplasm
osteosarcoma. See also bone tumor
canine, 234–241
clinical signs and history of,
235
comparative aspects of, 241
diagnosis of, 235, 236f, 237,
238f, 239
genetic factors and, 5
incidence of, 234–235
lung metastasis from, 237
pathology and natural behavior of, 235
prognosis for, 239–241, 240f,
241f
risk factors for, 234–235
therapy for, 239–241, 241f
trauma and, 6
feline, 249–250
juxtacortical, 241–242
orbital, 358–359
parosteal, 241–242
spinal, 337, 337f
surface, 241–242
trauma and, 6
ovarian tumor, 283–287
canine, 283–285, 284t
clinical signs and history of,
285–286

comparative aspects of, 286–
287
cyst as, 285
diagnosis of, 286
feline, 285–286
incidence of, 283
metastasis and, 285
pathology of, 283–285
prognosis for, 286
therapy for, 286
ovariohysterectomy
fibroepithelial hyperplasia and,
295
mammary cancer and, 12
ovarian cancer and, 286, 287
uterine cancer and, 290, 291

PAH. See polycyclic aromatic hydrocarbons
palliative sugery, 61
pancreatectomy, 271
pancreatic exocrine carcinoma,
192–193
pancreatic insulin-secreting neoplasm, 268–272
clinical signs and history of,
269–270
comparative aspects of, 273
diagnosis of, 270–271
incidence of, 268–269
natural behavior of, 269
pathology of, 269, 269f
prognosis for, 272–273
risk factors for, 268–269
therapy for, 271–272
pancreatitis, postoperative, 271
Papanicolaou stain, 45–47, 46t,
47f, 51f
papillary adenocarcinoma, 283–
284, 284t
papillary squamous cell carcinoma, in young canines,
187–188
papilloma, 141–143, 142f
eyelid, 351–353, 352f
in older canines, 142–143
oral, 185
viral, 142
papillomatosis, viral, 142, 185
papovaviruses, 10f. See also
DNA, viral

paraganglioma, 277–278, 278f
paraneoplastic syndromes, 29–38,
    30t, 226–227
  cancer cachexia in, 29–31, 37f
  ectopic hormone production
      and, 31–34, 32t
  fever in, 38
  hematologic-hemostatic abnor-
      malities in, 35t, 35–38
  neurologic abnormalities in, 38
  systemic cancer and, 346
paraovarian cyst, 285. See also
    ovarian tumor
parasites, in etiology of cancer,
    5–6
parathyroid tumor, 274–275
parosteal osteosarcoma, 241–242
  feline, 249–250
pathology, discipline of, 16–17
PCB. See polychlorobiphenyls, in
    etiology of cancer
PDH. See pituitary-dependent
    hyperadrenocorticism
PEG-asparaginase, for mycosis
    fungoides, 389–390
  for lymphoma, 135
penile tumor, 310
perianal tumor, 209–213
  clinical signs of, 210, 211f, 212f
  comparative aspects of, 213
  diagnosis of, 210–211, 212f
  hormonal factors in, 6
  pathology and natural behavior
      of, 210
  prognosis for, 213
  risk factors for, 209t, 209–210
  therapy for, 211–213
peripheral nerve tumor, 341–345
  clinical signs and history of,
      343–344
  comparative aspects of, 345
  diagnosis of, 344
  incidence of, 341–342
  lymphoma as, 342, 342f, 344,
      345
  metastatic, 345t, 345–346
  natural behavior of, 342–343
  pathology of, 342–343, 343f
  prognosis for, 345
  risk factors for, 341–342
  treatment for, 344–345
pesticides, in etiology of can-
    cer, 8

pet loss, 436–445
  attachment and, 437–438
  euthanasia and, 439, 443–444
  grief and, 438–439, 442–445
  pet's role in family and, 436
  veterinarian's role in, 439–445
    common questions and an-
        swers for, 443–445
    educator's role in, 441
    facilitation in, 441–442
    grief management in, 442–
        445
    guidelines for, 437
    guilt and, 444–445
    support in, 441
phenobarbital, for seizures, 332
phenoxybenzamine, preopera-
    tive, 277
phenytoin, for insulinoma, 272
pheochromocytoma, 275–277,
    276f
phlebotomy, 34
photodynamic therapy, 124–127,
    125t, 126t
Photofrin II, 124–127
photoradiation therapy, 124–125
pilomatrixoma, 149
pituitary-dependent hyperadren-
    ocorticism, 264–268
pituitary tumor, 273, 273–274
  non-ACTH-producing, 273
plamacytoma, in plasma cell neo-
    plasm, 403–404
plant alkaloids, 71t, 73. See also
    names of specific plant al-
    kaloids
plasma cell neoplasm, 402–410.
    See also multiple mye-
    loma; Waldenstrom's mac-
    roglobulinemia
  clinical signs and history of, 405
  comparative features of, 410
  incidence of, 403
  pathology and natural behavior
      of, 403–405, 404f
  prognosis for, 408, 408f, 409f,
      410
  risk factors for, 403
  therapy for, 406–408
plasma cells, 95
plasmacytoma, 406. See also
    plasma cell neoplasm
  cutaneous, 153

plasmaphoresis, for hypergam-
    maglobulinemia, 38
Platinol. See cisplatin
pleiotropic drug resistance, 67
pleural effusions, lung cancer
    and, 227
polyamine biosynthesis, inhibi-
    tors of, 133
polychlorobiphenyls, in etiology
    of cancer, 8
polycyclic aromatic hydrocarbons,
    8
polycythemia, 34
  in transmissible venereal tu-
      mor, 422
polycythemia vera, 395. See also
    myeloproliferative disor-
    ders
  diagnosis of, 398
  therapy for, 399–400
polyethylene glycol-asparaginase,
    135, 389–390. See also
    PEG-asparaginase
polyneuropathy, insulinoma and,
    270–271
polyp
  nasopharyngeal, feline, 186,
      187f
  rectal, 205, 205f, 206f
polyuria, in plasma cell neo-
    plasm, 405
polyvinylchloride, 8
post-traumatic sarcoma, 357–358
poxviruses, 10f. See also DNA,
    viral
prednisolone, 71t
  for brain tumor, 331–332
prednisone
  for anemia, 36
  for brain tumor, 331–332
  for canine lymphoma, 386t,
      387t
  for cyclic neutropenia, 374
  for hypercalcemia, 33
  for hypergammaglobulinemia,
      38
  for hypertrophic osteopathy, 35
  for hypoglycemia, 271–272
  for immune-mediated throm-
      bocytopenia, 37
  for insulinoma, 34
  for mast cell tumor, 161, 162f,
      163

prednisone: (*Continued*)
    for multiple myeloma, 407–
        408, 408f, 409f, 410
    for myeloid diseases, 373
    for oral cancer, 186–187
    pharmacology of, 64
primary tumor, TNM classifica-
    tion of, 450–451
progestins, mammary gland tu-
    mor and, 292–293
propranolol
    hypertension and, 277
    for hypertrophic cardiomyopa-
        thy, 261
    for insulinoma, 34, 272
propylthiouracil, for feline hyper-
    thyroidism, 260
prostatic tumor, 12, 308–310,
    309f
    canine, 308–309
    feline, 309–310
    hormonal factors in, 6
protein A therapy, 98–99
proto-oncogenes, 3
PRT. *See* photoradiation therapy
pseudohypoparathyroidism, 32
P-TS. *See* post-traumatic sarcoma
pulmonary. *See* lung, 225–228
Purinethol. *See* 6-mercaptopurine
PVC. *see* polyvinylchloride
pyrrolizidine alkaloids, 7

radiation, in etiology of cancer,
    6–7
radiation therapy, 79–90
    alopecia and, 85, 86f, 87t
    for anorectal cancers, 205–206
    for brain tumor, 333–334, 335f,
        336
    for canine osteosarcoma, 240
    complications of, 85–88, 86f,
        87t
    dose guidelines for, 80, 82, 88–
        90, 90f
        intraoperative, 82
    for esophageal cancer, 191
    failure of, 88–90, 89f
    for gastric cancer, 195
    for hyperadrenocorticism, 267
    hyperthermia and, 113–114,
        115f, 117–118, 118t, 119f

intraoperative, for bladder can-
    cer, 318, 320
for mammary gland tumor, 297
for mast cell tumor, 162f, 164
for nasal tumor, 220
neurologic complications from,
    346
for oral cancer, 181–182
patient evaluation for, 80–81
rationale for, 79–80, 80f
for skin and subcutaneous tu-
    mors, 141
for soft tissue sarcoma, 171
sources of, 82–83
surgery and, 61, 81–82
technical factors in, 82–84, 83f
for testicular tumor, 307
tissue heterogeneity and, 82,
    83f
for transmissible venereal tu-
    mor, 423–424
tumor response to, 84–85, 85t
radioactive cobalt, 84. *See also*
    radiation therapy
radiographic findings
    in bladder cancer, 317, 318f,
        319f
    in brain tumor, 328, 330f–335f,
        331
    in canine osteosarcoma, 235,
        236f, 237, 239
    in feline hyperthyroidism, 260
    in mast cell tumor, 160–161
    in metastasis, 25
    in nasal tumor, 221
    in peripheral nerve tumor, 344
    in primary lung cancer, 226f,
        226–227
    in spinal cord neoplasia, 338,
        339f, 341f
    in thyroid tumor, 255–256
radioimmunoassay, of serum thy-
    roid hormones, 260
radioiodine therapy, 262–263
radon gas, 6
ranitidine therapy, 99, 163
RD-114 virus, 363t, 364
rectal cancer, 200, 204–205, 205f.
    See also intestinal tract tu-
    mor
regional lymph nodes, TNM clas-
    sification of, 451–452
renal cancer, 312–315, 314f, 315f,
    316f

lymphoma as, 313–315, 371,
    371t
renal disorders, plasma cell neo-
    plasm and, 404–405
renal function, hypercalcemia
    and, 32
reproductive tract tumor, 283–
    291, 305–311
    feline prostatic tumor as, 309–
        310
    male, 305–310
        of penis and external geni-
            talia, 310
        prostatic tumor as, 308–310,
            309f
        testicular tumor as, 305–308,
            306f, 306t, 307f
    ovarian tumor as, 283–287. *See
        also* ovarian tumor
    penile tumor as, 310. *See also*
        transmissible venereal tu-
        mor
    uterine tumor as, 287–288
    vaginal and vulvar tumors as,
        288–291, 290f
        canine, 288–290, 289f
        feline, 290–291
resorption syndromes, FeLV-in-
    duced, 374
respiratory tract tumor, 215–231
    cancer of nasal planum as,
        215–218, 216f, 218f
    lung cancer as, 222–231. *See
        also* lung cancer
    nasal tumor as, 218–222, 220f–
        223f
    tracheal tumor as, 222–225,
        224f, 225f
reticulosis, intracranial, 326,
    328f. *See also* brain tumor
retinoids, 132–133
retrovirus(es), 11f. *See also* DNA,
    viral; RNA, viral
    feline, 362–376
        classification of, 362–363t
        definition of, 362
        FeLV as, 362–374. *See also*
            feline leukemia virus
        FeSV as, 362, 363t, 374
        FIV as, 362, 363t, 374–376,
            375t
        transmission and effects of,
            363t
    leukemia and, 380

lymphoma and, 380
reverse transcriptase, 362
  canine lymphoma and, 380
rhabdomyosarcoma, 168t, 169
RNA, viral, 9, 11f
Rosenthal needle, 43f
round cell tumor, cutaneous,
    152–153, 153f

salivary gland cancer, 190
salt intake, in etiology of cancer,
    11
Sano trichrome stain, 45–47
sarcoma, 19t. *See also names of
    specific sarcomas*
  mammary, 293t, 294, 299
  post-traumatic, feline, 357–358
  soft tissue, 167–175
  synovial cell, 244–245, 246f
SCC. *See* squamous cell carci-
    noma
schwannoma, 341–345, 343f
sclerosing mesothelioma, 426,
    426f. *See also* mesothe-
    lioma
SCT. *See* Sertoli cell tumor, tes-
    ticular
sebaceous gland tumor, 144–146,
    146f, 147f
  eyelid, 352
seizures
  brain tumor and, 326, 329f
  therapy for, 332
selenium, cancer and, 9
SEM. *See* seminoma, testicular
seminoma, testicular, 305–308,
    306f, 306t, 307f
Sertoli cell tumor, testicular,
    305–308, 306f, 306t, 307f
Sertoli-Leydig cell tumor, 284t,
    284–285. *See also* ovarian
    tumor
serum factors, for immunother-
    apy, 101–102
sex-cord stromal tumor, 284t,
    284–285. *See also* ovarian
    tumor
  canine, 285
sex steroids, for mast cell tumor,
    163
skeletal system tumor, 234–250.
    See also bone tumor

skin and subcutaneous tumors,
    139–154
  benign, 140
  clinical signs and history of,
    140
  cryosurgery for, 110, 141. *See
    also* cryosurgery
  dermoid cysts as, 141
  diagnosis of, 140–141
  epidermoid cysts as, 141, 142f
  epithelial tumor as, 141–149
  etiology of, 139–140
  follicular cysts as, 141
  incidence of, 139
  melanocytic tumor as, 153–
    154, 154f
  mesenchymal tumor as, 149–
    152
  natural history of, 140
  pathologic classification of, 140
  prevention of, 13
  risk factors for, 12–13, 139–140
  round cell tumor as, 149–152
  treatment for, 141
  tumorlike lesions as, 141
sodium chromoglycolate, for mast
    cell tumor, 163–164, 165
soft tissue sarcoma, 167–175
  canine, 174, 174f
  common sites for, 175
  comparative aspects of, 174–
    175
  diagnosis of, 170–171
  feline, 173–174
  incidence of, 167
  pathology and natural behavior
    of, 167–170, 168t
  prognosis for, 168t, 173, 173f,
    175
  risk factors for, 167
  treatment of, 171–173, 172f,
    173f, 175
spaying, risks of, 292
spinal cord neoplasia, 336–341
  clinical signs and history of,
    337–338
  comparative aspects of, 339–
    341
  diagnosis of, 338, 339f–341f
  FeLV and, 337
  incidence of, 336–337
  metastatic, 345t, 345–346
  pathology of, 337, 337f
  prognosis for, 339

risk factors for, 336–337
  treatment for, 338–339
Spirocerca lupi
  esophageal cancer and, 190–
    191
  in etiology of cancer, 5–6
splenectomy
  canine lymphoma and, 388
  mast cell tumor and, 161–163f
splenomegaly
  differential diagnosis of, 414
  in lymphoid leukemia, 383–384
  therapy for, 388
spumaviruses, 362–363, 363t. *See
    also* retrovirus(es)
squamous cell carcinoma, 143f,
    143–144, 144f
  conjunctival and membrana
    nictitans, 353f, 353–354
  cytologic features of, 49f
  esophageal, 191
  eyelid, 351–353, 352f
  feline, 5
  laryngeal, 225
  of nasal planum, 215–218,
    216f, 218f
  oral, 178t, 179, 183, 188
  papillary, in young canines,
    187–188
  perianal, 213
  radiation therapy for, 81
  tongue tumor as, 184–185, 185f
  tonsillar, 184
  UV light and, 6, 140
  in young canines, 187–188
squash method, of slide prepara-
    tion, 44, 45f
stains, for cytologic diagnosis,
    44–47, 46t, 47f, 51f
standard blade excision, for skin
    and subcutaneous tumors,
    141
Staphylococcus aureus therapy,
    98–99
stomach. *See* gastric cancer, 193–
    195
stratification, 432
streptozotocin, for insulinoma,
    272
stromal tumor, sex-cord, 284t,
    284–285. *See also* ovarian
    tumor
strontium-90, in etiology of can-
    cer, 6

subcutaneous tumor, 139–154. *See also* skin and subcutaneous tumors
sunlight, in etiology of cancer, 6, 13, 140
suramin, 128–129
surgical oncology, 58–62
 biopsy tracts and, 59
 chemotherapy and, 61
 debulking, 61
 for diagnosis, 58. *See also* biopsy
 general considerations for, 58–59, 62
 indications for, 58–59
 lymph node removal and, 60–61
 miscellaneous, 62
 palliative, 61
 prophylactic, 61–62
 radiation and, 61
 vascular ligation and, 59
 wound margins and, 59t, 59–60, 60f
surgical pathology, 16–17
 tumor staging and, 20–21
sweat gland tumor, 146–148
syndrome of inappropriate secretion of antidiuretic hormone, 34
synovial cell sarcoma, osseous, 244–245, 246f. *See also* bone tumor

TAA. *See* tumor-associated antigens
Tagamet. *See* cimetidine
tamoxifin, 302
T cell activation, 92–93, 93f
teratocarcinoma, 283–284, 284t
teratoma, 283–286, 284t. *See also* ovarian tumor
 canine, 285
 feline, 286
testicular tumor, 305–308
 canine, 305–308, 306f, 306t, 307f
 feline, 308
testosterone, perianal adenoma and, 210
TF. *See* transfer factor

thecoma, 284t, 284–285
6-thioguanine, for myeloproliferative disorders, 400, 401
Thio-Tepa, for mesothelioma, 427
thoracotomy, 227
thrombocythemia, primary, 396. *See also* myeloproliferative disorders
thrombocytopenia, 36–37
 in plasma cell neoplasm, 405
 systemic cancer and, 346
thymic atrophy, FeLV and, 371t, 371–372
thymoma, 418–420
 clinical signs and history of, 418
 comparative aspects of, 420
 diagnosis of, 418–420, 419f
 incidence of, 418
 prognosis for, 420
 risk factors for, 418
 therapy for, 420
thymosin therapy, 101
thyroidectomy, 256, 261–262, 262f
thyroid storm, TSH administration and, 256
thyroid tumor, canine, 253–259
 clinical signs and history of, 254–255, 255f, 256f
 comparative aspects of, 258–259
 diagnosis of, 255–256
 differential diagnosis of, 255
 feline thyroid tumor vs., 258, 258t
 incidence of, 253
 natural behavior of, 254
 pathology of, 254, 254f
 prognosis for, 257–258
 risk factors for, 253
 therapy for, 256–257, 257f, 258f
thyrotropin, 255, 256
tissue fixation, for morphological interpretation, 18, 20
tissue heterogeneity, radiation therapy and, 82, 83f
TLS. *See* tumor lysis syndrome
TNF. *See* tumor necrosis factor
TNM system, of classification of domestic animal tumors, 449–489

tongue tumor, 184–185, 185f. *See also* oral cancer
tonsillar squamous cell carcinoma, 184
total body irradiation, bone marrow transplantation and, 135–136
Toxoplasma gondii, 375
tracheal tumor, 222–225, 224f, 225f
transfer factor, 93, 93f
transitional cell carcinoma, 317, 320
transmissible venereal tumor, 421–424
 clinical signs and history of, 422f, 422–423, 423f
 in etiology of cancer, 7
 pathology and natural behavior of, 421–422
 penile, 310
transplantation, in etiology of cancer, 7
trauma, in etiology of osteosarcoma, 6
triamcinolone, for mast cell tumor, 161, 162f, 163
trichoepithelioma, 149
Tru-cut biopsy needle, 43, 43f
TSH. *See* thyrotropin
tube feeding, for canines or cats with cancer, 31
tuftsin therapy, 101
tumor-associated antigens, 92, 93f
tumor debulking, 102
tumor heterogeneity, 26
tumor lysis syndrome, 388
tumor necrosis factor, 94, 101
tumor staging. *See* classification systems
TVT. *See* transmissible venereal tumor

ultraviolet radiation, in etiology of cancer, 6, 12–13, 140
upper alimentary tract cancer
 prevention of, 11
 risk factors for, 9, 11
ureter, cancer of, 315
ureterostomy, 318

urethral tumor, 320–322
urinary tract infection, hyperadrenocorticism and, 265
urinary tract tumor, 312–322
    bladder cancer as, 315–320. *See also* bladder cancer
    renal cancer as, 312–315, 313f, 314f, 371, 371t
    urethral involvement in, 315, 320–322, 321f
urogram, 314, 314f
    intravenous, 319f
uterine tumor, 287–288
UV radiation. *See* ultraviolet radiation, in etiology of cancer

vaccines
    for canine lymphoma, 388
    for FeLV, 369
    tumor cell, 99–101
vaginal fibroids, 290
vaginal tumor, 288–291, 290f
    canine, 288–290, 289f
    feline, 290–291
vascular ligation, 59
Velban. *See* vinblastine
venereal tumor
    penile, 310
    transmissible, 421–424
        clinical signs and history of, 422f, 422–423, 423f

in etiology of cancer, 7
    pathology and natural behavior of, 421–422
    penile, 310
venography, caudal vena caval, 276
vinblastine (Velban), 71t, 73
    for canine lymphoma, 387
vincristine (Oncovin), 71t, 73. *See also* plant alkaloids
    for canine lymphoma, 386t, 387t
    for multiple myeloma, 407–408, 408f, 409f, 410
    for myeloid diseases, 373
    for transmissible venereal tumor, 424
viral papillomatosis. *See also* oral cancer
virus(es). *See also names of specific viruses;* retrovirus(es), feline
    DNA, 9, 10f
    in etiology of canine osteosarcoma, 234
    in etiology of mast cell tumor, 157
    in etiology of skin and subcutaneous tumors, 139–140
    in etiology of soft tissue sarcoma, 167
    oncogenic, 9, 362–363, 363t
    RNA, 9, 11f

vitamin A, 8, 132–133
vitamin C, 8
vitamin D, 257
vitamin E, 8
vitamins and minerals, 8–9
vulvar tumor, 289–291, 290f
    canine, 288–290, 289f
    feline, 290–291

Waldenstrom's macroglobulinemia, 402–410. *See also* plasma cell neoplasm
weight loss. *See* cachexia
Whipple's triad, 270
WHO Clinical Staging, for lymphosarcoma and lymphoid leukemia, 385, 385t
Wilm's tumor, 313–315, 316f
World Health Organization staging system
World Health Organization TNM classification of tumors in domestic animals, 448–489
Wright stain, 44–47, 47f, 51f

zinc, 9
Zollinger-Ellison syndrome, 269, 275

ISBN 0-397-50784-4

90000

9 780397 507849